FITZGERALD'S
Clinical Neuroanatomy
and Neuroscience

FITZGERALD'S
Clinical Neuroanatomy
and Neuroscience

8TH EDITION

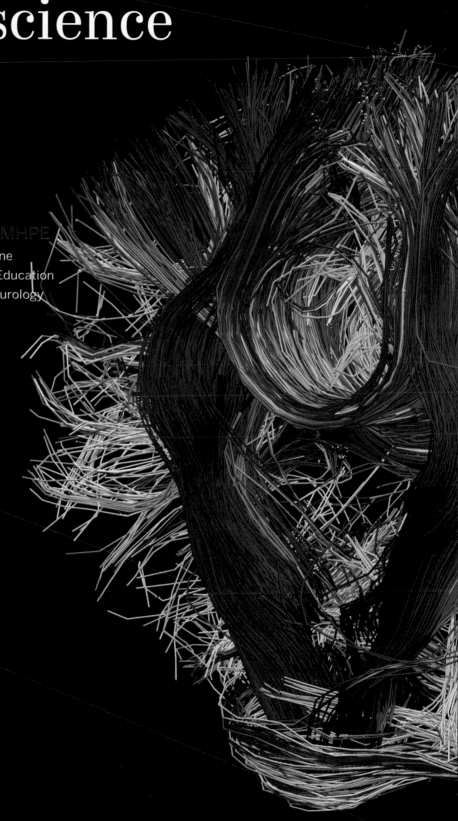

Estomih Mtui, MD
Professor of Anatomy in Radiology
Chief, Division of Anatomy
Weill Cornell Medical College
New York, New York

Gregory Gruener, MD, MBA, MHPE
Vice Dean for Education, Stritch School of Medicine
Ralph P. Leischner Jr., MD, Professor of Medical Education
Professor and Associate Chair, Department of Neurology
Loyola University Chicago
Maywood, Illinois

Peter Dockery, BSc, PhD
Professor of Anatomy
School of Medicine
College of Medicine, Nursing & Health Sciences
National University of Ireland, Galway
Galway, Ireland

ELSEVIER

Notice

Practitioners and researchers must always rely on their own experience and knowledge in evaluating and using any information, methods, compounds, or experiments described herein. Because of rapid advances in the medical sciences, in particular, independent verification of diagnoses and drug dosages should be made. To the fullest extent of the law, no responsibility is assumed by Elsevier, authors, editors, or contributors for any injury and/or damage to persons or property as a matter of products liability, negligence or otherwise, or from any use or operation of any methods, products, instructions, or ideas contained in the material herein.

ISBN: 978-0-702-07909-2

Content Strategist: Marybeth Thiel
Content Development Manager: Meghan B. Andress
Content Development Specialist: Deborah Poulson
Publishing Services Manager: Shereen Jameel
Project Manager: Manikandan Chandrasekaran
Cover Design and Design Direction: Amy L. Buxton

Printed in China
Last digit is the print number: 9 8 7 6 5 4 3

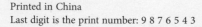

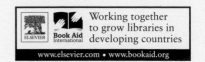

To my wife, Elizabeth, and our children and grandchildren, who have supported me; my professional colleagues and role models; and students. This edition is dedicated to you.

Estomih Mtui

To my wife, Catherine, our children, Ethan, Michael, and Margaret and our grandchildren, Henry, Madeline, and Oliver. Thanks for your love and support. This book is dedicated to you.

Gregory Gruener

To my wife, Angela, and our children, Lucy and Clyde, who make my life worthwhile. To my brother Robert who gifted me a lifelong love of learning.
Thanks to Elsevier and my co-authors for retaining the connection with Galway.

Peter Dockery

Professor M.J. Turlough FitzGerald (1929—2014) was highly distinguished for both his teaching and research in anatomy. After an outstanding undergraduate career, he qualified in Medicine from University College Dublin in 1952. Following a short period in clinical work, he became a Statutory (Senior) Lecturer in Anatomy at University College Cork in 1954, where he remained for 9 years. During this time, he spent a sabbatical year and several shorter research study periods in UK Anatomy Departments. From 1964 to 1968, he worked in the United States, in St. Louis and Seattle. He returned to Ireland to the Chair at University College Galway, now National University of Ireland, Galway. He remained there for the rest of his professional career, consistently developing and enhancing the department as a centre of high excellence in anatomical teaching.

Turlough FitzGerald was especially distinguished as a teacher and educator. The range and depth of his knowledge extended across the spectrum of anatomical disciplines, encompassing topographical anatomy, embryology, histology, and neuroanatomy. His teaching was enhanced throughout by the background of his clinical training. His lectures were typified by a unique and memorable lucidity. Inevitably, his enthusiasm for teaching led to publications, including a book of anatomy multiple choice questions, a book on embryology with his wife Maeve as co-author (1994), and most notably, his Clinical Neuroanatomy (1985). Its standing was enhanced with each new edition, incorporating contemporary developments from the rapidly changing world of structural and functional neuroscience. It has become one of the leading neuroanatomy texts worldwide; the fourth edition won first prize in the BMA Medical Book competition. In the seventh edition, the title was changed, involving the ultimate accolade: it became eponymic. That it will henceforth be called *FitzGerald's Clinical Neuroanatomy and Neuroscience* confirms its status, quality, and value in this crowded field of publications.

Turlough FitzGerald was also distinguished in research and published widely over a wide range of topics. His main area of contribution was to the light microscopy of the peripheral nervous system, and in particular cutaneous sensory innervation. His principal studies dealt with the morphology, development, and maturation of peripheral nerve endings. Other publications in the field of neuroanatomy concerned topics as diverse as the connections of lingual proprioceptors, the ganglia within the tongue, transmedian innervation, the nerve supply to skin grafts, and the fibre composition of peripheral nerves.

Maurice John Turlough FitzGerald held the PhD, MD, and DSc degrees of the National University of Ireland. He was a Member of the Royal Irish Academy.

John Fraher MB, FRCSEdin, PhD, DSc, FAS(hon), MRIA
Professor Emeritus of Anatomy
University College Cork

When I first arrived in Galway in 2005, Professor FitzGerald sat outside of my office, I believe to ensure that his cherished department was in safe hands.

He recalled to me that during his first term in action in Galway, a student asked was 'cerebellum' a misspelling of 'cerebrum'. This may well have set the seed for the first edition of this book.

During his tenure, he transformed the teaching of anatomy in Galway and, while retaining the importance of safe anatomical knowledge, he introduced some very modern methods of delivery.

I hope that his endorsement of my appointment was justified and that I have maintained his strong belief that modern anatomy places function in a structural and clinically relevant context.

Peter Dockery BSc(hon), PhD
Established Professor of Anatomy
School of Medicine
National University of Ireland Galway

Professor FitzGerald began the preface of the sixth edition by stating it was "...designed as a vade mecum ('go with me') for medical students." Knowing that neuroscience is first introduced within the classroom, he believed his textbook would also support students as they transition into the hospital and clinic. For students to understand the clinical manifestations of nervous system disorders first requires familiarity with normal structure and function at a gross and microscopic level. In order to foster that appreciation, clinical examples were interwoven throughout the text. While he did not intend to write a clinical textbook, it would be impossible to appreciate (or perhaps remember) the functional neuroanatomy without the consequences of its breakdown. Perhaps he summarised his beliefs best as, "Sequential fusion of descriptive structure, function, and malfunction is known as vertical integration and is highly recommended owing to its manifest logic."

CHAPTERS AND PAGES

Each chapter of this edition was revised or updated with the hope of increasing readability, as well as relevance. Following a brief account of nervous system development in Chapter 1, the topography of the brain and spinal cord and their meningeal surrounds occupies Chapters 2, 3, and 5. Chapter 4 discusses the clinically very important blood supply. Microscopic and ultramicroscopic anatomy of neurons (nerve cells) and neuroglia (their surrounding "nerve glue") come to the fore in Chapter 6, along with the consequences of expanding neuroglial tumours.

Chapter 7 changes the context by describing electrical events underlying the impulses that are triggered at the point of origin of axons and travel along those axons and their branches to their final termination where they liberate excitatory or inhibitory molecules onto target neurons. These molecules, pillars of the science of neuropharmacology, are examined in Chapter 8. Chapters 9–11 explore the structure and distribution of the peripheral nerves attached to the spinal cord, innervating the muscles and skin of the trunk and limbs. Electrical activity returns in Chapter 12 in the form of electromyography, a technique widely used in the detection of disorders of the peripheral nervous system.

The autonomic nervous system is the subject of Chapter 13 and controls the smooth musculature of the vascular system and of the alimentary, urinary, and reproductive tracts. The spinal nerves (Chapter 14), attached to the whole length of the spinal cord, are "mixed" (both motor and sensory) and innervate all the voluntary muscles and skin in the trunk and limbs. Description of the contents of the spinal cord itself occupies Chapters 15 and 16.

The brainstem (medulla oblongata, pons, and midbrain) connects the spinal cord to the cerebral hemispheres, as described by means of transverse sections in Chapter 17. The cranial nerves attached to it (nerves III to XII) are described in Chapters 18–23. Chapter 24 is devoted to the reticular formation of the brainstem which, inter alia, links cranial nerves to one another and the neuromodulatory system that facilitates the different states of arousal, attention, sleep, and wakefulness.

The thalamus and epithalamus (Chapter 25) have numerous vital connections between subcortical structures and the cerebral cortex and play a role in sensorimotor integration, emotion, memory, and consciousness.

The basal ganglia (Chapter 26) are a group of nuclei within the base of the brain primarily involved in the execution of learned motor programs, motor learning, appropriate sequencing of serial motor actions, and giving a physical expression to the current emotional state The most frequent failure of control takes the form of Parkinson disease. The cerebellum, Chapter 27, occupies the posterior cranial fossa and with the basal ganglia plays a prominent role in motor control by indirectly affecting motor activity and matching the intended action to what occurs in real time, but also plays an integrative role in cognition, behaviour, speech, affect, and executive functioning.

Chapter 28 examines the histological structure of the cerebral cortex and provides a summary of the function of the different cortical areas. Electrical activities are examined by means of electroencephalography (Chapter 29) and evoked potentials (Chapter 30).

The visual pathways chapter (Chapter 31) lays out the largest of all horizontal pathways, stretching from the very front end of the brain (the retina) to the very back (the occipital cortex). Its clinical significance is obvious. Functional inequalities between the left and right sides of the brain are the subject of Chapter 32, hemispherical asymmetries.

The final anatomic structures, analysed in Chapter 33, are the olfactory system and the limbic system, the latter being involved in memory as well as emotional expression. The pituitary and hypothalamus (Chapter 34) can be traced in nature to reptiles. It still operates basic survival controls, including food and fluid intake, temperature control, and sleep.

Chapter 35 is about cerebrovascular disease. The main purpose of this chapter is to highlight the functional defects that follow cerebral haemorrhage or thrombosis, but it also serves to highlight that stroke remains a major worldwide cause of morbidity and mortality. The global lifetime risk of stroke from the age of 25 years and onwards is about 25%.

CHAPTER TITLE PAGES FEATURE:

- **Study Guidelines.** A running commentary on the subject matter stressing features of clinical importance.
- **Tables.** Concise summaries of facts and relevant information.
- **Clinical** and **Basic Science Panel Boxes.** Clinical disorders related to the section as well as emerging basic science discoveries that expand on relevant concepts.

- **Core Information.** A summary of and list of the items to be dealt with in the chapter.
- **Suggested References.** Relevant and timely references that expand on chapter topics.

WEBSITE FEATURES — LEARNING RESOURCES

- **Case studies.** Case studies demonstrating the clinical consequences of physical or other injury to the nervous system.
- **Tutorials.** A "Web tutorial" is available for each chapter, and clicking that link will deliver a session on the relevant topic and in many cases a self-assessment quiz.

- **MCQs.** Multiple-choice questions are available for each chapter, with over 200 questions in USMLE format. Half contain an illustration; half are text only.

FACULTY RESOURCES

An image bank is available to help you prepare lectures via our Evolve website. Contact your local sales representative for more information, or go directly to the Evolve website to request access: http://evolve.elsevier.com/Mtui/clinicalneuro/

EM

GG

PD

2020

ACKNOWLEDGMENTS

The authors wish to first express their sincere appreciation and gratitude to the family of M.J. Turlough FitzGerald for entrusting *FitzGerald's Clinical Neuroanatomy and Neuroscience* to our care. With this new eighth edition, the authors want to acknowledge, with appreciation, the strong tradition on which this text is built and repeat our pledge to further develop and refine this book and its online resources so that it remains relevant and formative for its readers for years to come.

Our work on this, the eighth edition, has been facilitated and made possible by Marybeth Thiel, Denise Roslonski, Meghan Andress, Deborah Poulson, and Manikandan Chandrasekaran at Elsevier. While there were revisions made to the illustrations, they remain superb enhancements as they exquisitely capture the meaning of the text. Finally, a special thanks to Elsevier's Amy Buxton, who as the designer was responsible for a format that is crisp and appealing to the eye.

It is a pleasure for us to acknowledge the support of our Panel of Consultants and the input of our students, whose comments and participation we will further develop in future editions.

CLINICAL AND BASIC SCIENCE PERSPECTIVES

Chapters	Perspectives
1 Embryology	Prosencephalon. Telencephalon. Diencephalon. Mesencephalon. Rhombencephalon. Metencephalon. Myelencephalon. Choroid capillary plexus. Ventricular system.
2 Cerebral topography	Paresis. Space-occupying lesions. Magnetic Resonance Imaging. Diffusion Tensor Imaging.
3 Midbrain, hindbrain, spinal cord	Basilar region. Tegmentum. Tectum. Decussation. Ipsilateral. Contralateral. Cauda equina.
4 Blood supply of the brain	Blood—brain barrier pathology.
5 Meninges	Extradural hematoma. Subdural hematoma. Hydrocephalus. Meningitis. Spinal tap. Epidural analgesia. Caudal analgesia.
6 Neurons and neuroglia: overview	Brain tumours. Multiple sclerosis. Neuronal transport disorders.
7 Electrical events	Local anaesthetics — how they work. The node, paranode, and juxtaparanode.
8 Transmitters and receptors	Stiff person spectrum disorder. Botulinum toxin administration for movement disorders. Neuromyelitis optica spectrum disorder.
9 Peripheral nerves	Degeneration and regeneration.
10 Innervation of muscles and joints	Myofascial pain syndrome. (Explanatory layout)
11 Innervation of skin	Neurogenic inflammation. Leprosy.
12 Electrodiagnostic examination	Entrapment neuropathies. Peripheral neuropathies. Abnormal motor unit action potentials (MUAPs). Myasthenia gravis and myasthenic syndromes.
13 Autonomic nervous system	Horner syndrome. Raynaud syndrome. Stellate block. Lumbar sympathectomy. Irritable bowel syndrome. Visceral pain. Drug actions on the sympathetic and parasympathetic systems.
14 Nerve roots	Spina bifida. Cervical spondylosis. Prolapsed intervertebral disc.
15 Spinal cord: ascending pathways	Syringomyelia.
16 Spinal cord: descending pathways	Upper motor neuron disease. Lower motor neuron disease. Spinal cord injury.
17 Brainstem	Cranial nerve cell columns. Pyramidal decussation. Head-righting reflexes. Respiratory reticular nuclei.
18 The lowest four cranial nerves	Supranuclear, nuclear, infranuclear lesions.
19 Vestibular nerve	Vestibular disorders. Lateral medullary syndrome.
20 Cochlear nerve	Conduction deafness. Sensorineural deafness.
21 Trigeminal nerve	Trigeminal neuralgia. Referred pain in diseases of the head and neck.
22 Facial nerve	Lesions of the facial nerve. Acoustic neuroma.
23 Ocular motor nerves	Ocular palsies.
24 Reticular formation and the neuromodulatory system	Congenital central hypoventilation syndrome ('Ondine's curse'). Higher-level urinary bladder control. Locomotor pattern generator.
25 Thalamus, epithalamus	Thalamic territory strokes. Fatal familial insomnia (FFI).
26 Basal ganglia	Hypokinetic-rigid syndromes. Other movement disorders. Deep brain stimulation for Parkinson disease.
27 Cerebellum	Clinical disorders of the cerebellum and higher brain functions. Posturography. Paraneoplastic syndrome: cerebellar degeneration.
28 Cerebral cortex	Stiff person syndrome. (Explanatory layout)
29 Electroencephalography	Narcolepsy. Seizures.
30 Evoked potentials	Motor training. Acupuncture.
31 Visual pathways	Lesions of the visual pathway.
32 Hemispheric asymmetries	Bedside evaluation of aphasia. Frontal lobe dysfunction. Parietal lobe dysfunction.
33 Olfactory and limbic systems	Anosmia. Alzheimer disease. Complex partial seizure. Schizophrenia. Drug addiction.
34 Pituitary and hypothalamus	Hypothalamic disorders. Major depression.
35 Cerebrovascular disease	Anterior choroidal artery occlusion. Anterior cerebral artery syndrome. Middle cerebral artery syndrome. Lacunar syndromes. Internal carotid artery occlusion. Posterior circulation syndromes. Posterior cerebral artery syndromes. Subarachnoid haemorrhage. Motor recovery after stroke.

PANEL OF CONSULTANTS

Ritwik Baidya, MD
Assistant Professor of Anatomy in Radiology
Division of Anatomy, Department of Radiology
Weill Cornell Medical College
New York, New York

Michael F. Dauzvardis, PhD
Assistant Professor, Department of Medical Education
Loyola University Chicago Stritch School of Medicine
Maywood, Illinois

Robert J. Frysztak, PhD
Associate Professor, Department of Medical Education
Loyola University Chicago Stritch School of Medicine
Maywood, Illinois

Martin D. Hamburg, PhD
Associate Professor of Anatomy in Radiology
Division of Anatomy, Department of Radiology
Weill Cornell Medical College
New York, New York

Janet Kelly, PhD
Assistant Professor, Department of Medical Education
Loyola University Chicago Stritch School of Medicine
Maywood, Illinois

Sushil Kumar, MBBS, MD
Assistant Professor of Anatomy in Radiology
Division of Anatomy, Department of Radiology
Weill Cornell Medical College
New York, New York

Mange Manyama, MD, MSc, PhD
Assistant Professor of Anatomy in Radiology, Department of
    Radiology
Weill Cornell Medical College in Qatar
Doha, Qatar

Santosh Sangari, MD
Associate Professor of Anatomy in Radiology
Division of Anatomy, Department of Radiology
Weill Cornell Medical College
New York, New York

STUDENT CONSULTANTS

Daniel Burkett
Loyola University Chicago Stritch School of Medicine
Maywood, Illinois
Year of graduation: 2017

Elizabeth Carroll
Loyola University Chicago Stritch School of Medicine
Maywood, Illinois
Year of graduation: 2017

Lucy Dockery
National University of Ireland Galway
Galway, Ireland
Year of graduation: 2019

William Ford
Weill Cornell Medical College
New York, New York
Year of graduation: 2022

Jared M. Miller
Loyola University Chicago Stritch School of Medicine
Maywood, Illinois
Year of graduation: 2017

Brendan Moran
National University of Ireland, Galway
Galway, Ireland
Year of graduation: 2018

Anjana Rajan
Weill Cornell Medical College
New York, New York
Year of graduation: 2022

David Rosenthal
Weill Cornell Medical College
New York, New York
Year of graduation: 2022

Noreen Tagney
National University of Ireland, Galway
Galway, Ireland
Year of graduation: 2018

Amanda Williams
Loyola University Chicago Stritch School of Medicine
Maywood, Illinois
Year of graduation: 2017

CONTENTS

Embryology

CHAPTER SUMMARY

STUDY GUIDELINES

This chapter aims to give you sufficient insight into the embryologic development of the brain and spinal cord to account for the arrangement of structures in the mature nervous system. If not already familiar with adult brain anatomy, we suggest you read this chapter again following your study of Chapters 2 and 3.

For descriptive purposes, the embryo is in the prone (face-down) position, whereby the terms *ventral* and *dorsal* correspond to the adult *anterior* and *posterior*, and *rostral* and *caudal* correspond to *superior* and *inferior*.

SPINAL CORD

Neurulation

The entire nervous system originates from the **neural plate**, which arises from an ectodermal thickening of the floor of the amniotic sac (Fig. 1.1). During the third week after fertilisation, the neural plate forms paired **neural folds**, which unite to create the **neural tube** and **neural canal**. Union of the folds commences in the future neck region of the embryo and proceeds rostrally and caudally. The open cranial and caudal ends of the neural tube, the **neuropores**, are closed off before the end of the fourth week. The process of formation of the neural tube from the ectoderm is known as *neurulation*.

Cells at the edge of each neural fold escape from the line of union and form the **neural crest** alongside the tube. Cell types derived from the neural crest include spinal and autonomic ganglion cells, melanocytes, and the Schwann cells of peripheral nerves.

Spinal Nerves

The dorsal part of the neural tube is called the **alar plate** and the ventral part is called the **basal plate** (Fig. 1.2). Neurons developing from the alar plate are predominantly sensory in function and receive *dorsal nerve roots* arising from the spinal ganglia, and those in the basal plate are predominantly motor neurons and give rise to *ventral nerve roots*. At appropriate levels of the spinal cord, the ventral roots also contain axons from developing autonomic neurons. The dorsal and ventral roots unite to form the *spinal nerves*, which emerge from the vertebral canal through the intervertebral foramina lying in between the neural arches.

The cells of the spinal (dorsal root) ganglia are initially bipolar. They become unipolar by the coalescence of their two processes on one side of the parent cells.

BRAIN

Brain Parts

Late in the fourth week of embryonic development, the rostral part of the neural tube undergoes flexion at the level of the future midbrain (Fig. 1.3A). This region is known as the **mesencephalon**. A slight constriction marks its junction with the **prosencephalon** (future forebrain) and **rhombencephalon** (future hindbrain).

The alar plate of the prosencephalon expands on each side (Fig. 1.3A) to form the **telencephalon** (cerebral hemispheres). The basal plate remains in place as the **diencephalon**. Finally, an **optic outgrowth** from the diencephalon is the forerunner of the retina and optic nerve.

The diencephalon, mesencephalon, and rhombencephalon constitute the embryonic brainstem.

The brainstem buckles as development proceeds. As a result, the mesencephalon is carried to the summit of the brain. The rhombencephalon folds on itself, causing the alar plates to flare and creating the rhomboid (diamond-shaped) fourth ventricle of the brain. The rostral part of the rhombencephalon gives rise to the pons and cerebellum. The caudal part gives rise to the medulla oblongata (Fig. 1.4).

Ventricular System and Choroid Plexuses

The neural canal dilates within the cerebral hemispheres, forming the lateral ventricles; these communicate with the third ventricle contained within the diencephalon. The two lateral ventricles communicate with the third ventricle through the **foramen of Monro** (*interventricular foramen*). The third and fourth ventricles communicate through the **cerebral aqueduct** (or *aqueduct of Sylvius*) in the midbrain (Fig. 1.5).

The thin roofs of the forebrain and hindbrain are invaginated by tufts of capillaries, which form the choroid plexuses of

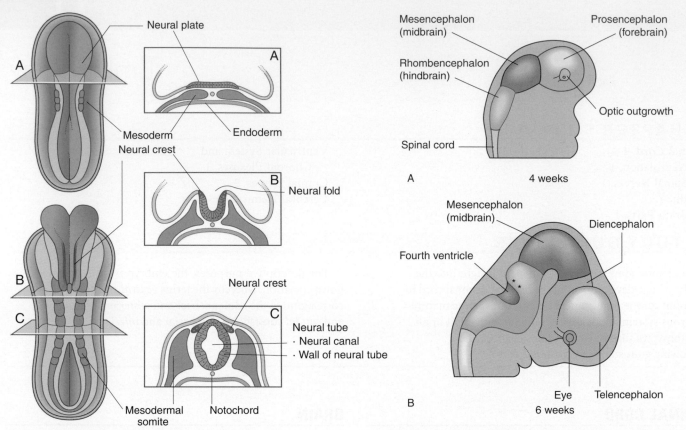

Fig. 1.1 (A) Cross-sections from a three-somite (20-day) embryo. (B and C) Cross-sections from an eight-somite (22-day) embryo.

Fig. 1.3 (A) Early development of the three primary brain vesicles. (B) *Asterisks* indicate the site of initial development of the cerebellum.

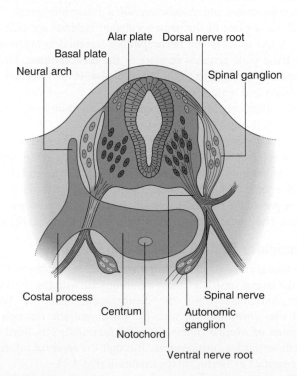

Fig. 1.2 Neural tube, spinal nerve, and mesenchymal vertebra of an embryo at 6 weeks.

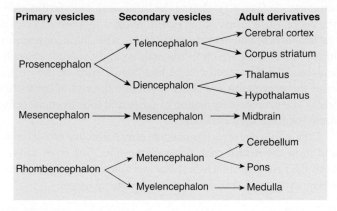

Fig. 1.4 Some derivatives of the brain vesicles.

the lateral, third, and fourth ventricles. The choroid plexuses secrete cerebrospinal fluid (CSF), which flows through the ventricular system. CSF exits the fourth ventricle through three apertures in its roof known as foramen Magendie (in the midline) and the right and left foramen Luschka (Fig. 1.6).

Cranial Nerves

Fig. 1.7 illustrates the state of development of the cranial nerves during the sixth week after fertilization.

- The olfactory nerve (I) arises from bipolar neurons developing in the epithelium lining the olfactory pit.
- The optic nerve (II) grows centrally from the retina.

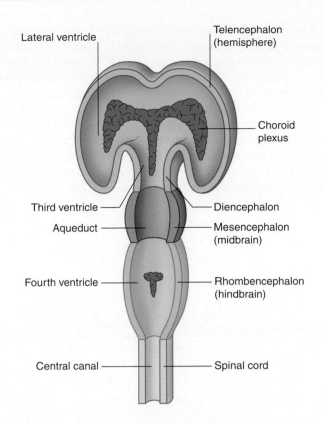

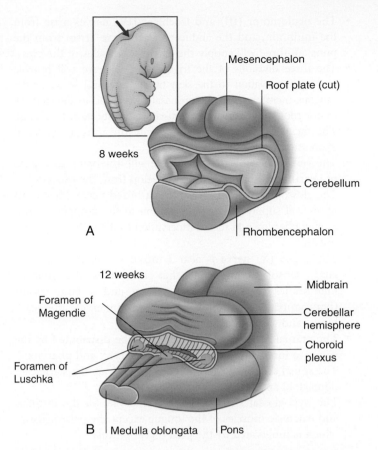

Fig. 1.5 The developing ventricular system. Choroid plexuses are shown in red.

Fig. 1.6 Dorsal views of the developing hindbrain *(see arrow in inset)*. (A) At 8 weeks, the cerebellum is emerging from the fourth ventricle. (B) At 12 weeks, the ventricle is becoming hidden by the cerebellum, and three apertures have appeared in the roof plate.

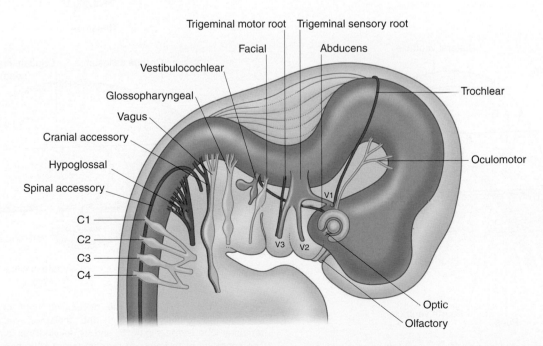

Fig. 1.7 Cranial nerves of a 6-week-old embryo. (Reproduced from Bossy et al. 1990, with permission from Springer-Verlag.)

- The oculomotor (III) and trochlear (IV) nerves arise from the midbrain, and the abducens (VI) nerve arises from the pons; all three will supply the extrinsic muscles of the eye.
- The three divisions of the trigeminal (V) nerve will provide sensory innervation to the skin of the face and scalp, to the mucous membranes of the oronasal cavity, and to the teeth. A motor root will innervate the muscles of mastication (chewing).
- The facial (VII) nerve will innervate the muscles of facial expression.
- The vestibulocochlear (VIII) nerve will innervate the organs of hearing and balance, which develop from the otocyst.
- The glossopharyngeal (IX) nerve is a mixed nerve. Most of its fibres will supply sensory innervation to the oropharynx and laryngopharynx and motor innervation to the stylopharyngeus muscle.
- The vagus (X) nerve is also a mixed nerve. It contains a large sensory component that innervates the mucous membranes of the digestive system and a large motor (parasympathetic) component that will innervate the heart, lungs, and gastrointestinal tract.
- The cranial accessory (XIc) nerve will be distributed by the vagus to innervate the muscles of the larynx and pharynx.
- The spinal accessory (XIs) nerve will innervate the sternocleidomastoid and trapezius muscles.
- The hypoglossal (XII) nerve will innervate all the intrinsic and extrinsic muscles of the tongue except the palatoglossus, which is innervated by the pharyngeal plexus.

Cerebral Hemispheres

In the telencephalon, mitotic activity takes place in the **ventricular zone** just outside the lateral ventricle. Daughter cells migrate to the outer surface of the expanding hemisphere and form the cerebral cortex.

Expansion of the cerebral hemispheres is not uniform. A region on the lateral surface, the **insula** (L. 'island'), is relatively quiescent and forms a pivot around which the expanding hemisphere rotates. Frontal, parietal, occipital, and temporal lobes can be identified at 14 weeks' gestational age (Fig. 1.8).

On the medial surface of the hemisphere, a part of the cerebral cortex, the **hippocampus**, forms a fifth lobe, the **limbic lobe** of the brain. The hippocampus is drawn into the temporal lobe, leaving in its wake a strand of fibres known as the **fornix**. Within the concavity of this arc lies the **choroid fissure**, through which the choroid plexus invaginates into the lateral ventricle (Fig. 1.9).

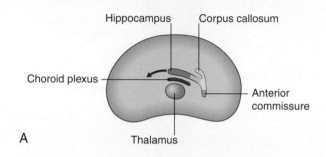

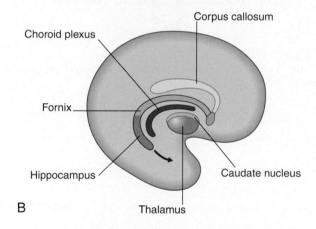

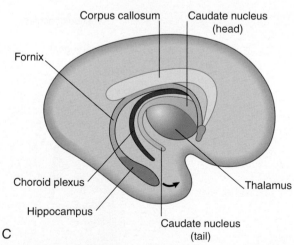

Fig. 1.9 Medial aspect of the developing right hemisphere. The hippocampus, initially dorsal to the thalamus, migrates into the temporal lobe (*arrows* in A, B, and C), leaving the fornix in its wake. The concavity of the arch so formed contains the choroid fissure (the line of insertion of the choroid plexus into the ventricle) and the tail of the caudate nucleus.

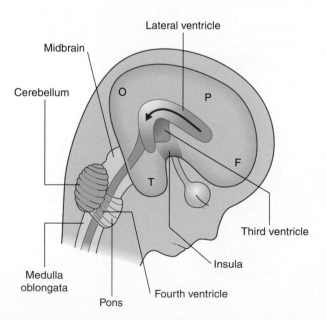

Fig. 1.8 Fetal brain at 14 weeks. The *arrow* indicates the C-shaped growth of the hemisphere around the insula. *F*, Frontal lobe, *O*, occipital lobe; *P*, parietal lobe; *T*, temporal lobe.

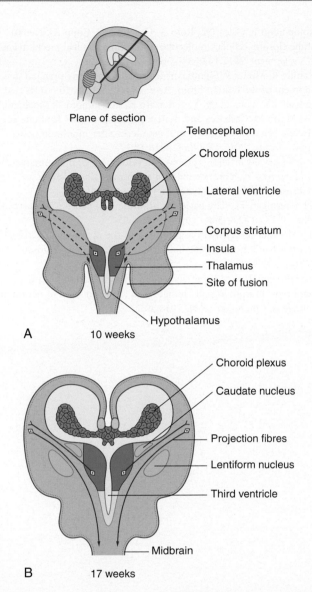

Plane of section

A   10 weeks

- Telencephalon
- Choroid plexus
- Lateral ventricle
- Corpus striatum
- Insula
- Thalamus
- Site of fusion
- Hypothalamus

B   17 weeks

- Choroid plexus
- Caudate nucleus
- Projection fibres
- Lentiform nucleus
- Third ventricle
- Midbrain

Fig. 1.10 Coronal sections of the developing cerebrum. (A) At 10 weeks, the corpus striatum is traversed by axons projecting from thalamus to cerebral cortex and from cerebral cortex to spinal cord. (B) At 17 weeks, the corpus striatum has been divided to form the caudate and lentiform nuclei (fusion persists at the anterior end, not shown here).

The **anterior commissure** develops as a connection linking olfactory (smell) regions of the left and right sides. Above this, a much larger commissure, the *corpus callosum*, links matching areas of the cerebral cortex of the two sides. It extends backward above the fornix.

Coronal sections of the telencephalon reveal a mass of grey matter at the base of each hemisphere, which is the forerunner of the *corpus striatum*. The diencephalon develops into the thalamus and hypothalamus, as well as forming the walls of the third ventricle (Fig. 1.10).

The expanding cerebral hemispheres come into contact with the diencephalon and they fuse with it (see 'site of fusion' in Fig. 1.10A). One consequence is that the term 'brainstem' is

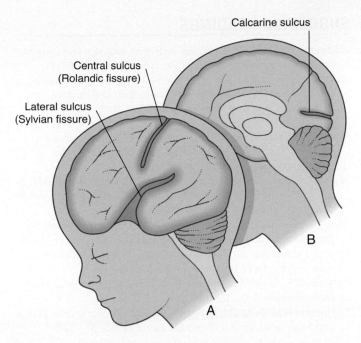

- Calcarine sulcus
- Central sulcus (Rolandic fissure)
- Lateral sulcus (Sylvian fissure)

A

B

Fig. 1.11 Three major cortical sulci in a 28-week fetus. (A) Lateral surface and (B) medial surface of the left cerebral hemisphere.

restricted thereafter to the remaining, free parts: midbrain, pons, and medulla oblongata. A second consequence is that the cerebral cortex is able to project axons directly down to the brainstem. Together with axons projecting from thalamus to the cortex, they split the corpus striatum into *caudate* and *lentiform nuclei* (Fig. 1.10B).

By the 28th week of development, several sulci (fissures) appear on the surface of the brain, notably the *lateral, central,* and *calcarine sulci* (Fig. 1.11).

✳ Core Information

The nervous system takes the initial form of a cellular neural tube derived from the ectoderm and enclosing a neural canal. A ribbon of cells escapes along each side of the tube to form the neural crest. The more caudal part of the neural tube forms the spinal cord. The neural crest forms spinal ganglion cells that send dorsal nerve roots into the sensory part (alar plate) of the spinal cord. The basal plate of the spinal cord contains motor neurons that emit ventral roots to complete the spinal nerves by joining the dorsal roots.

The more rostral part of the neural tube forms three brain vesicles. Of these, the prosencephalon (forebrain) gives rise to the cerebral hemispheres (telencephalon) dorsally and the diencephalon ventrally. The mesencephalon develops into the midbrain, and the rhombencephalon becomes the hindbrain (pons, medulla oblongata, and cerebellum).

The neural tube expands rostrally to create the ventricular system of the brain. CSF is secreted by a choroid capillary plexus that invaginates the roof plates of the ventricles.

The cerebral hemispheres develop frontal, parietal, temporal, occipital, and limbic lobes. The hemispheres are cross-linked by the corpus callosum and posterior and anterior commissures. The grey matter in the base of each hemisphere is the forerunner of the corpus striatum. The hemispheres fuse with the side walls of the diencephalon, whereupon the mesencephalon and rhombencephalon are all that remain of the embryonic brainstem.

SUGGESTED READINGS

Adameyko I, Fried K. The nervous system orchestrates and integrates craniofacial development: a review. *Front Physiol.* 2016;7:49.

Azais M, Agius E, Blanco S, et al. Timing the spinal cord development with neural progenitor cells losing their proliferative capacity: a theoretical analysis. *Neural Dev.* 2019; 14(7):1—19.

Bossy J, O'Rahilly R, Müller F. Ontogenèse du système nerveux. In: Bossy J, ed. *Anatomie Clinique: Neuroanatomie.* Paris: Springer-Verlag; 1990:357—388.

Dubois J, Benders M. Borradori-Tolsa, et al. Primary cortical folding in the human newborn: an early marker of later functional development. *Brain.* 2008;131:2028—2041.

Kang KH, Reichert H. Control of neural stem cell self-renewal and differentiation in Drosophila. *Cell Tissue Res.* 2015;359(1):33—45.

Kiecker C, Lumsden A. The role of organizers in patterning the nervous system. *Annu Rev Neurosci.* 2012;35:347—367.

Lehtinen MK, Walsh CA. Neurogenesis at the brain-cerebrospinal fluid interface. *Annu Rev Cell Dev Biol.* 2011;27:653—679.

Le Douarin NM, Brito JM, Creuzet S. Role of the neural crest in face and brain development. *Brain Res Dev.* 2007;55:237—224.

Nikolopoulou E, Galea GL, Rolo A, Greene ND, Copp AJ. Neural tube closure: cellular, molecular and biomechanical mechanisms. *Development.* 2017;144:552—566.

O'Rahilly R, Muller F. Significant features in the early prenatal development of the human brain. *Ann Anat.* 2008;104:105—118.

Shinotsuka N, Yamaguchi Y, Nakazato K, Matsumoto Y, Mochizuki A, Miura M. Caspases and matrix metalloproteases facilitate collective behavior of non-neural ectoderm after hindbrain neuropore closure. *BMC Dev Biol.* 2018;18:17.

Shiota K. Review article — prenatal development of the human central nervous system, normal and abnormal. *Donald Sch J Ultrasound Obstetrics Gynecology.* 2015;9(1):61—66.

Stiles J, Jernigan TL. The basics of brain development. *Neuropsychol Rev.* 2010;20:327—348.

Sun T, Hevner RF. Growth and folding of the mammalian cerebral cortex: from molecules to malformations. *Nat Rev Neurosci.* 2014;15:217—232.

Yang HJ, Lee DH, Lee YJ, et al. Secondary neurulation of human embryos: morphological changes and the expression of neuronal antigens. *Childs Nerv Syst.* 2014;30:73—82.

STUDY GUIDELINES

1. The most important objective is that you become able to recite **all** the central nervous system items identified in the magnetic resonance images without looking at the labels.
2. Try to get the nomenclature of the component parts of the basal ganglia into long-term memory. Not easily done!

3. Because of its clinical importance, you **must** be able to pop up a mental image of the position and named parts of the internal capsule and to appreciate the continuity of the corona radiata, internal capsule, and crus cerebri (cerebral peduncle).

SURFACE FEATURES

Lobes

The surfaces of the two cerebral hemispheres are furrowed by *sulci*, and the intervening ridges are called *gyri*. Most of the cerebral cortex forms the walls of sulci and, from the lateral surface of the hemispheres, is concealed from view. Although the patterns of the various sulci vary from brain to brain, some are sufficiently constant to serve as descriptive landmarks. The deepest sulci are the *lateral sulcus (Sylvian fissure)* and the *central sulcus (Rolandic fissure)* (Fig. 2.1A). These two serve to divide the hemisphere (lateral view) into four **lobes** with the aid of two imaginary lines, one extending back from the lateral sulcus, the other reaching from the upper end of the *parietooccipital sulcus* (Fig. 2.1B) to a blunt *preoccipital notch* at the lower border of the hemisphere (the sulcus and notch are labelled in Fig. 2.2). The lobes are called *frontal*, *parietal*, *occipital*, and *temporal*.

The blunt tips of the frontal, occipital, and temporal lobes are the respective poles of the hemispheres.

The *opercula* (lips) of the lateral sulcus can be pulled apart to expose the *insula* (Fig. 2.3). The insula was mentioned in Chapter 1 as being relatively quiescent during prenatal expansion of the telencephalon.

The medial surface of the hemisphere is exposed by sectioning the *corpus callosum*, a massive band of white matter connecting matching/homotopic areas of the cortex of the two hemispheres. The corpus callosum consists of a rostrum, genu, body and splenium from anterior to posterior. The anterior commissure lies below the rostrum (Fig. 2.2B). The frontal lobe lies anterior to a line drawn from the upper end of the central sulcus to the trunk or body of the corpus callosum (Fig. 2.2B).

The parietal lobe lies behind this line and is separated from the occipital lobe by the parietooccipital sulcus. The temporal lobe lies in front of a line drawn from the preoccipital notch to the splenium of the corpus callosum. Figs. 2.2 and 2.4 to 2.6 should be consulted along with the following description of surface features of the lobes of the brain.

Frontal Lobe. The lateral surface of the *frontal lobe* contains the *precentral gyrus* bounded in front by the *precentral sulcus*. Further forward, *superior*, *middle*, and *inferior frontal gyri* are separated by *superior* and *inferior frontal sulci*. On the medial surface, the superior frontal gyrus is separated from the *cingulate gyrus* by the *cingulate sulcus*. The inferior or orbital surface is marked by several *orbital gyri*. In contact with this surface are the *olfactory bulb* and *olfactory tract*.

Parietal Lobe. The anterior part of the parietal lobe contains the *postcentral gyrus* bounded behind by the *postcentral sulcus*. The posterior parietal lobe is divided into superior and inferior parietal lobules by an *intraparietal sulcus*. The inferior parietal lobule shows a *supramarginal gyrus* capping the upturned end of the lateral sulcus, and an *angular gyrus* capping the superior temporal sulcus.

The medial surface contains the posterior part of the *paracentral lobule* and, behind this, the *precuneus*. The paracentral lobule (partly contained in the frontal lobe) is so called because of its relationship to the central sulcus.

Occipital Lobe. The lateral surface of the occipital lobe is marked by several *lateral occipital gyri*. The medial surface contains the *cuneus* ('wedge') between the *parietooccipital*

7

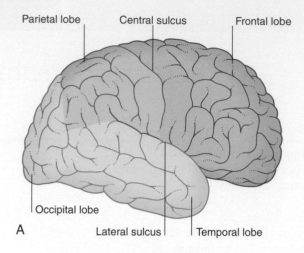

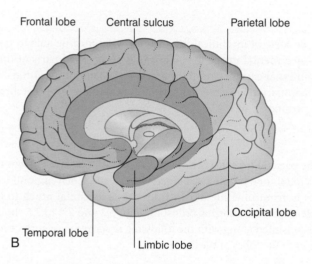

Fig. 2.1 The five lobes of the brain. (A) Lateral surface and (B) medial surface of the right cerebral hemisphere.

sulcus and the important *calcarine sulcus*. The *lingual gyrus* lies between the collateral sulcus and the anterior end of the calcarine sulcus. The inferior surface shows three gyri and three sulci. The *lateral and medial occipitotemporal gyri* are separated by the *occipitotemporal sulcus*.

Temporal Lobe. The lateral surface of the temporal lobe displays *superior*, *middle*, and *inferior temporal gyri* separated by *superior* and *inferior temporal sulci*. The inferior surface shows the anterior parts of the *occipitotemporal gyri*. The *lingual gyrus* continues forward as the *parahippocampal gyrus*, which ends in a blunt medial projection, the *uncus*. As will be seen later in views of the sectioned brain, the parahippocampal gyrus underlies a rolled-in part of the cortex, the *hippocampus*.

Limbic Lobe. A fifth *limbic lobe* of the brain surrounds the medial margin of the hemisphere. Surface contributors to the limbic lobe include the cingulate and parahippocampal gyri. It is more usual to speak of the *limbic system*, which includes the hippocampus, fornix, amygdala, and other elements

connected to or related in function to the limbic lobe (see Chapter 33).

Diencephalon

The largest components of the diencephalon are the *thalamus* and the *hypothalamus* (Figs. 2.6 and 2.7). These nuclear groups form the side walls of the third ventricle. Between them is a shallow *hypothalamic sulcus*, which represents the rostral limit of the embryonic sulcus limitans.

Midline Sagittal View of the Brain

Fig. 2.8 is taken from a midline sagittal section of the head of a cadaver, displaying the brain in relation to its surroundings.

INTERNAL ANATOMY OF THE CEREBRUM

The arrangement of the following structures will now be described: thalamus, caudate and lentiform nuclei, internal capsule; hippocampus and fornix; association and commissural fibres; lateral and third ventricles.

Thalamus, Caudate, and Lentiform Nuclei, Internal Capsule

The two thalami face one another across the slot-like third ventricle. More often than not, they are interconnected across the third ventricle, creating an *interthalamic adhesion/massa intermedia* (Fig. 2.9). In Fig. 2.10, the thalamus and related structures are assembled in a mediolateral sequence. In contact with the upper surface of the thalamus are the *head* and *body* of the *caudate nucleus*. The *tail* of the caudate nucleus passes forward below the thalamus but is not in contact with it.

The thalamus is separated from the lentiform nucleus by the posterior limb of the *internal capsule*, which is a common site for a *stroke* resulting from local arterial embolism (blockage) or haemorrhage. The internal capsule contains fibres running from thalamus to cortex and from cortex to thalamus, brainstem, and spinal cord. In the interval between cortex and internal capsule, these ascending and descending fibres form the *corona radiata*. Below the internal capsule, the *crus* of the midbrain (cerebral peduncle) receives descending fibres continuing down to the brainstem.

The lens-shaped *lentiform nucleus* is composed of two parts: the *putamen* and *globus pallidus*. While not part of the lentiform nucleus, the caudate is of similar structure to the putamen and their anterior ends are fused. In addition, they are linked by strands of grey matter (cellular bridges) that traverse the anterior limb of the internal capsule, hence the term *corpus striatum* (or, simply, *striatum*) used to include the putamen and caudate nucleus. The term *pallidum* refers to the *globus pallidus*.

The caudate and lentiform nuclei belong to the *basal ganglia*, a term originally applied to half a dozen masses of grey matter located near the base of the hemisphere. In current usage, the term designates five nuclei known to be involved in motor control: the caudate, putamen, globus pallidus, and

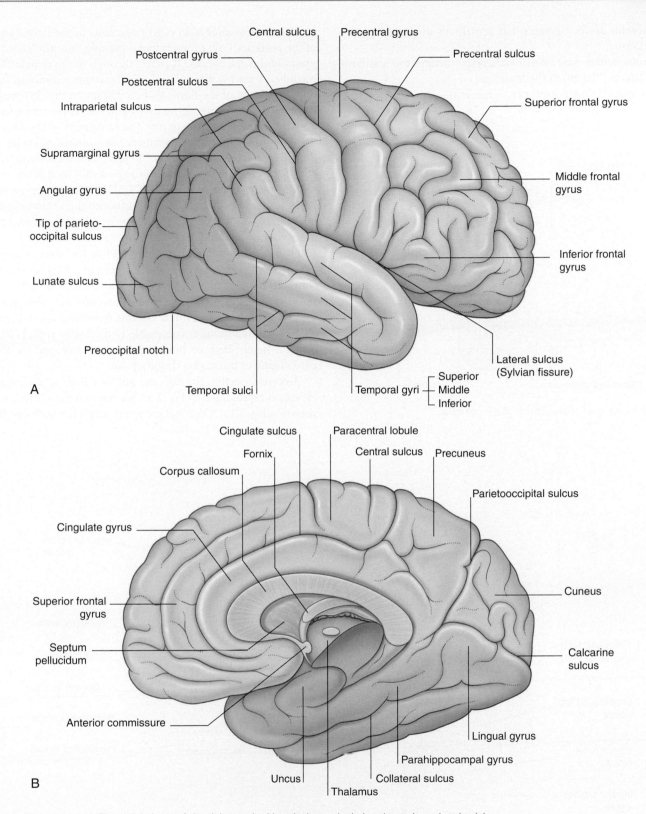

Fig. 2.2 (A) Lateral and (B) medial views of the right cerebral hemisphere, depicting the main gyri and sulci.

subthalamic nucleus in the diencephalon, and the *substantia nigra* in the midbrain (Fig. 2.11).

In horizontal section, the internal capsule has a dog-leg shape (see photograph of a fixed-brain section in Fig. 2.12, and in vivo magnetic resonance image [MRI] in Fig. 2.13).

The internal capsule has five named parts in horizontal sections:

1. ***anterior limb***, between the lentiform nucleus and the head of the caudate nucleus;

2. ***genu***;

3. ***posterior limb***, between the lentiform nucleus and the thalamus;
4. ***retrolenticular part*** (visual radiations), behind the lentiform nucleus and lateral to the thalamus;
5. ***sublenticular part*** (auditory radiations).

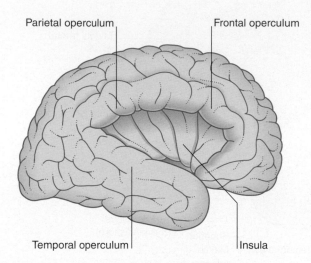

Fig. 2.3 Insula, seen on retraction of the opercula.

The ***corticospinal tract*** (CST) descends in the lateral aspect of the posterior limb of the internal capsule. It is also called the ***pyramidal tract***, because it passes through the pyramids of the medulla. A *tract* is a bundle of fibres serving a common function. Over 50% of the fibres that contribute to the CST mainly originate from the precentral gyrus and the cortex immediately anterior to the precentral gyrus. The remainder of the fibres in the CST originate from the primary somatosensory cortex and the parietal association cortex. The CST descends through the corona radiata, the lateral part of the posterior limb of the internal capsule, and the intermediate 3/5th of the crus of the midbrain (cerebral peduncle) and continues to the spinomedullary junction before crossing to the opposite side of the spinal cord in the motor (pyramidal) decussation.

From a clinical standpoint, *the CST is the most important pathway in the entire central nervous system (CNS)* for two reasons. First, it mediates voluntary movement of all kinds. Interruption of the CST leads to motor weakness (called *paresis*) or motor paralysis. Second, it extends the entire vertical length of the CNS, rendering it vulnerable to disease or trauma in the cerebral hemisphere or brainstem on one side and to spinal cord disease or trauma on the other side.

A coronal section through the anterior limb of the internal capsule is represented in Fig. 2.14; a corresponding MRI view is shown in Fig. 2.15. A coronal section through the posterior limb

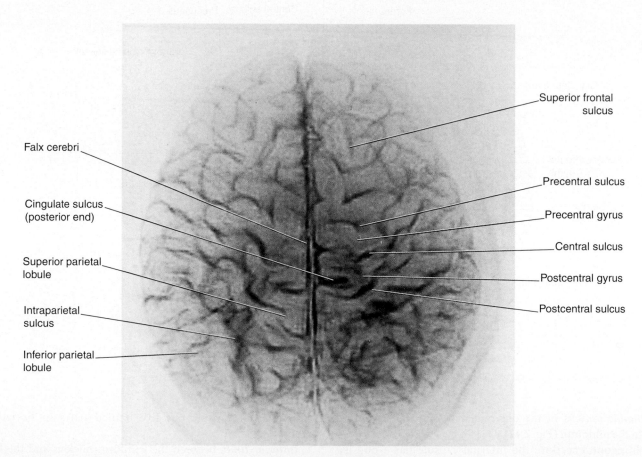

Fig. 2.4 'Thick slice' surface anatomy brain Magnetic Resonance Imaging scan from a healthy volunteer. (From Katada K. MR imaging of brain surface structures: surface anatomy scanning (SAS). *Neuroradiology*. 1990;3(5):439–448.)

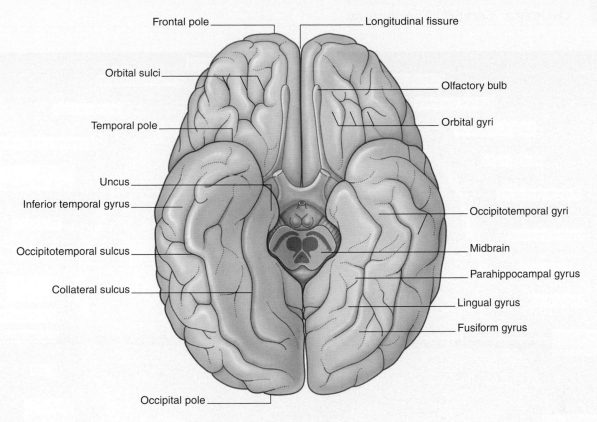

Fig. 2.5 Cerebrum viewed from inferior aspect, depicting the main gyri and sulci.

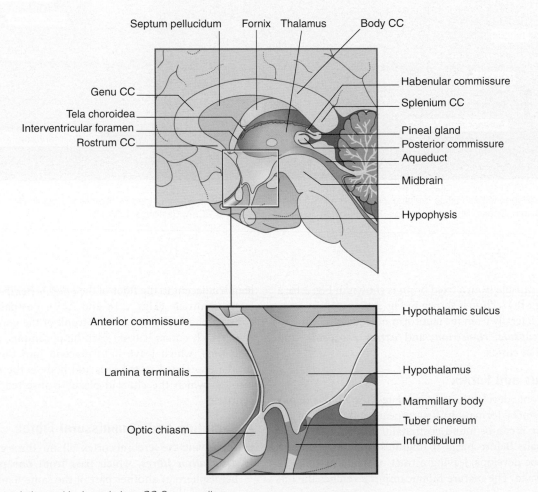

Fig. 2.6 The diencephalon and its boundaries. *CC,* Corpus callosum.

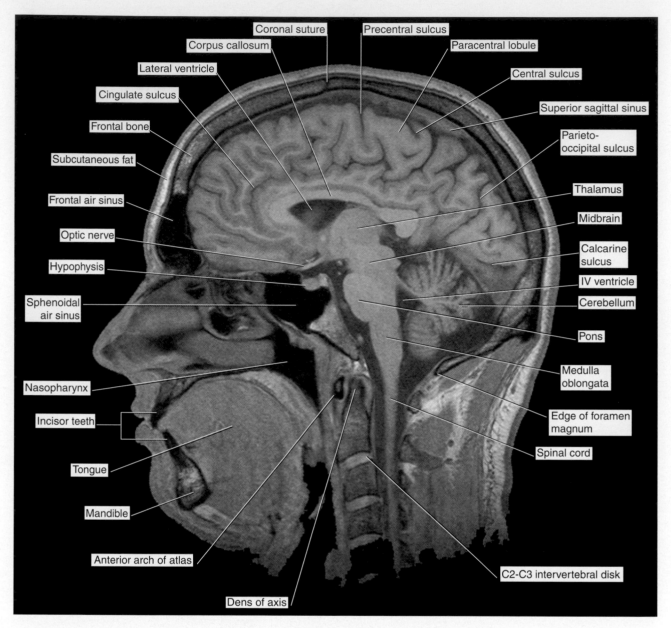

Fig. 2.7 Sagittal Magnetic Resonance Imaging 'slice' of the living brain. (From a series kindly provided by Professor J. Paul Finn, Director, Magnetic Resonance Research, Department of Radiology, David Geffen School of Medicine at UCLA, California, USA.)

of the internal capsule from a fixed brain is shown in Fig. 2.16; a corresponding MRI section is shown in Fig. 2.17.

Proceeding laterally from the lentiform nucleus can be found the *external capsule*, *claustrum*, and *extreme capsule*, and finally the insular cortex.

Hippocampus and Fornix

During embryonic development in primates, the *hippocampus* (crucial for memory formation) first appears above the corpus callosum where it can be found postnatally in phylogenetically earlier mammals. Before birth, it migrates into the temporal lobe as this lobe develops, leaving a tract of white matter, the *fornix*, in its wake. The mature hippocampus stretches the full length adjacent to the floor of the *inferior (temporal) horn* of the lateral ventricle (Figs. 2.18 and 2.19). Postnatally, the fornix consists of a *body* beneath the trunk of the corpus callosum, a *crus*, which enters it from each hippocampus, and two *pillars (columns)*, which leave it to descend into the diencephalon. Intimately related to the crus and body is the *choroid fissure*, through which the choroid plexus is inserted into the lateral ventricle.

Association and Commissural Fibres

Fibres leaving the cerebral cortex fall into three groups:

1. *association fibres*, which pass from one part of a single hemisphere to another part of the same hemisphere;

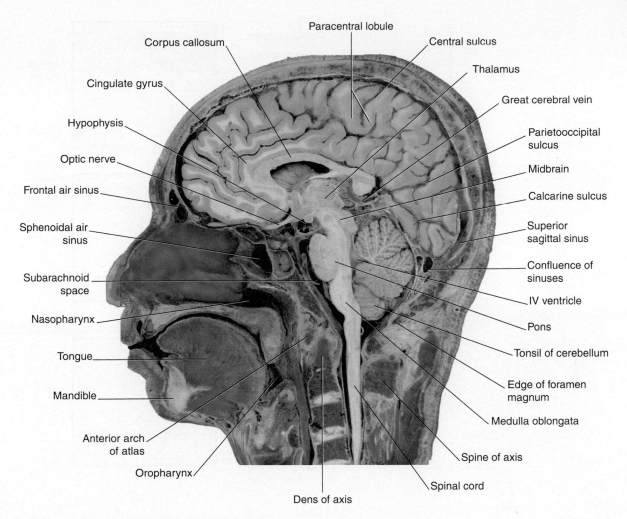

Fig. 2.8 Sagittal section of fixed cadaver brain. (From Liu S, et al., eds. *Atlas of Human Sectional Anatomy*. Jinan: Shantung Press of Science and Technology; 2003, with permission from Shantung Press of Science and Technology.)

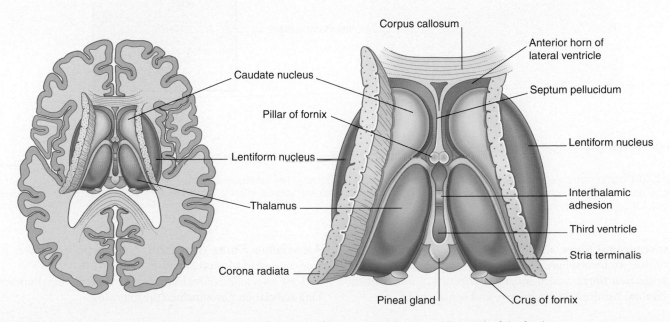

Fig. 2.9 Thalamus and corpus striatum, seen on removal of the body of the corpus callosum and the trunk of the fornix.

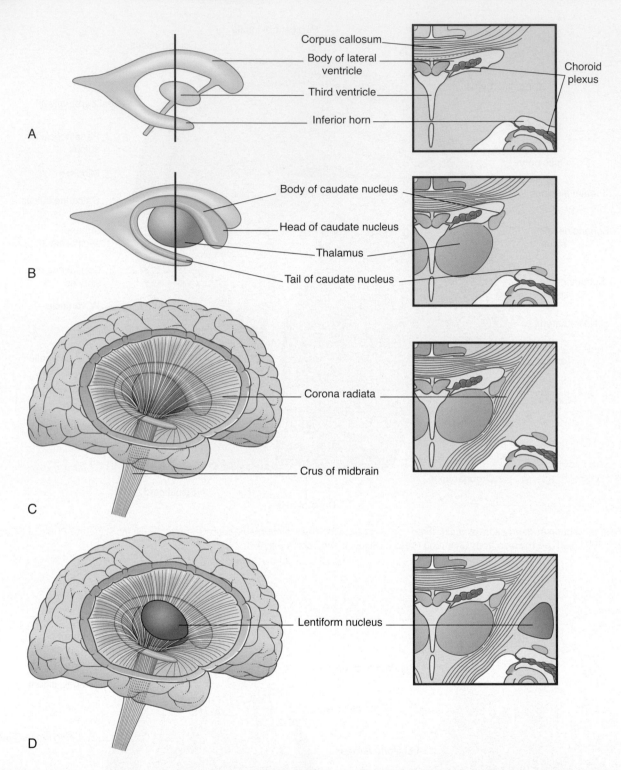

Fig. 2.10 Diagrammatic reconstruction of corpus striatum and related structures. The *vertical lines* on the left in A and B indicate the level of the coronal sections on the right. (A) Ventricular system. (B) Thalamus and caudate nucleus in place. (C) Addition of projections to and from cerebral cortex. (D) Lentiform nucleus in place.

2. ***commissural fibres***, which link matching/homotopic areas of the two hemispheres; and
3. ***projection fibres***, which innervate subcortical nuclei in the cerebral hemisphere, brainstem, and spinal cord.

Association Fibres (Fig. 2.20). *Short association fibres* pass from one gyrus to another within a lobe.

Long association fibres link one lobe with another. Bundles of long association fibres include the following:

- the *superior longitudinal fasciculus*, linking the frontal and occipital lobes;
- the *inferior longitudinal fasciculus*, linking the occipital and temporal lobes;
- the *arcuate fasciculus*, linking the frontal lobe with the occipitotemporal cortex;

- the *uncinate fasciculus*, linking the frontal and anterior temporal lobes;
- the *cingulum*, underlying the cortex of the cingulate gyrus.

Cerebral Commissures. *Corpus callosum.* The *corpus callosum* is the largest of the commissures linking matching areas of the left and right cerebral cortex (Fig. 2.21). From the body, some fibres pass laterally and upward, intersecting the corona radiata. Other fibres pass laterally and then bend ventrally as the *tapetum* (a thin band of fibres) to reach the inferior parts of the temporal and occipital lobes. Fibres travelling to the medial wall of the occipital lobe emerge from the *splenium* on each side and form the *occipital (major) forceps*. The *frontal (minor) forceps* emerges from each side of the genu to reach the medial wall of the frontal lobe.

Minor commissures. The *anterior commissure* interconnects the anterior parts of the temporal lobes with the two olfactory tracts.

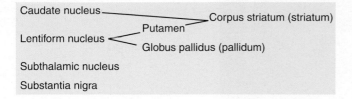

Caudate nucleus — Corpus striatum (striatum)
— Putamen
Lentiform nucleus — Globus pallidus (pallidum)
Subthalamic nucleus
Substantia nigra

Fig. 2.11 Nomenclature of basal ganglia.

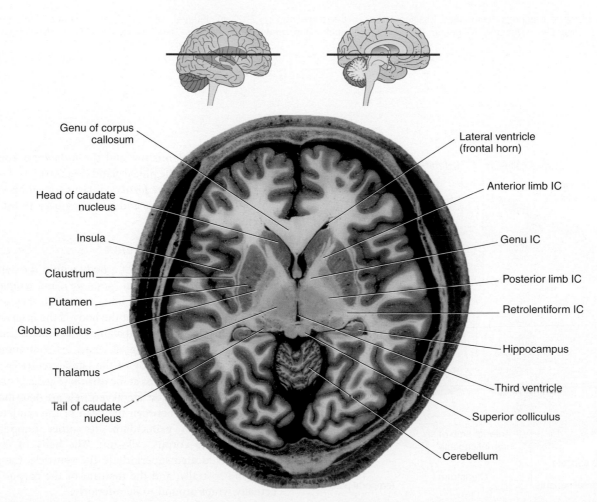

Fig. 2.12 Horizontal section of fixed cadaver brain at the level indicated at top. *IC*, internal capsule. (From Liu S, et al., eds. *Atlas of Human Sectional Anatomy*. Jinan: Shantung Press of Science and Technology; 2003, with permission from Shantung Press of Science and Technology.)

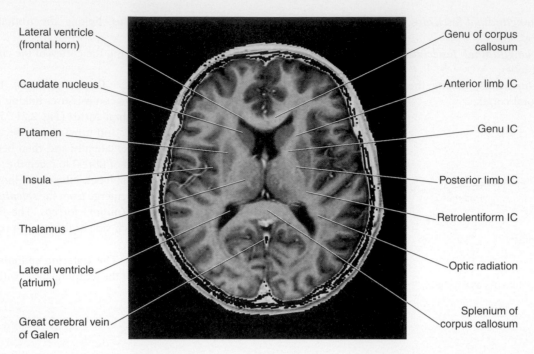

Fig. 2.13 Horizontal Magnetic Resonance Imaging 'slice' in the plane of Fig. 2.12. *IC*, internal capsule. (From a series kindly provided by Professor J. Paul Finn, Director, Magnetic Resonance Research, Department of Radiology, David Geffen School of Medicine at UCLA, California, USA.)

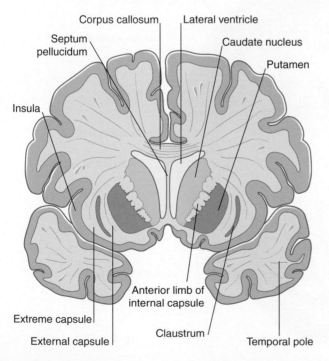

Fig. 2.14 Drawing of a coronal section through the anterior limb of the internal capsule.

The *posterior commissure* and the *habenular commissure* lie directly in front of the pineal gland (Fig. 2.6).

The *commissure of the fornix* contains some fibres originating from one hippocampus and travelling back to the other by way of the two crura.

Lateral and Third Ventricles

The *lateral ventricle* consists of a *body* within the parietal lobe and *frontal (anterior)*, *occipital (posterior)*, and *temporal (inferior) horns* extending into the lobes for which they are named (Fig. 2.22). The anterior limit of the body is the *interventricular foramen*, located between the thalamus and anterior pillar of the fornix, through which the lateral ventricles communicate with the third ventricle. The body of the lateral ventricles joins the occipital and temporal horns at the *atrium* (Figs. 2.23 and 2.24).

The relationships of the lateral ventricle are described here:

- *Frontal horn*: Lies between the head of the caudate nucleus and the septum pellucidum. Its other boundaries are formed by the corpus callosum. The body of the corpus callosum is located superiorly to the ventricle, the genu can be found rostrally, and the rostrum of the corpus callosum actually wraps around to lie inferiorly.
- *Body*: Lies inferior to the body of the corpus callosum and superior to the thalamus and anterior part of the body of

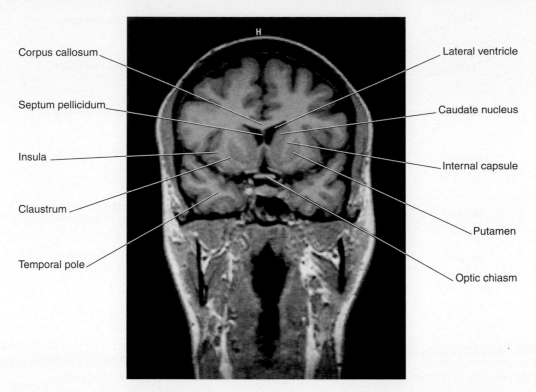

Fig. 2.15 Coronal Magnetic Resonance Imaging 'slice' at the level of Fig. 2.14. (From a series kindly provided by Professor J. Paul Finn, Director, Magnetic Resonance Research, Department of Radiology, David Geffen School of Medicine at UCLA, California, USA.)

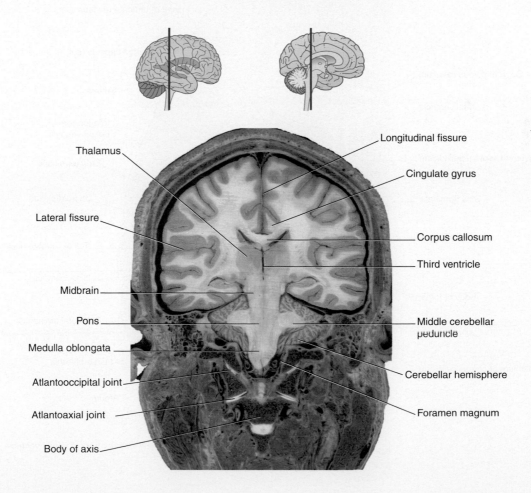

Fig. 2.16 Coronal section of fixed cadaver brain at the level indicated at top of image. (From Liu S, et al., eds. *Atlas of Human Sectional Anatomy*. Jinan: Shantung Press of Science and Technology; 2003, with permission of Shantung Press of Science and Technology.)

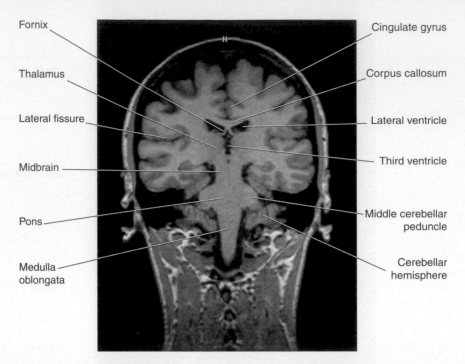

Fig. 2.17 Coronal Magnetic Resonance Imaging 'slice' at the level of Fig. 2.16. (From a series kindly provided by Professor J. Paul Finn, Director, Magnetic Resonance Research, Department of Radiology, David Geffen School of Medicine at UCLA, California, USA.)

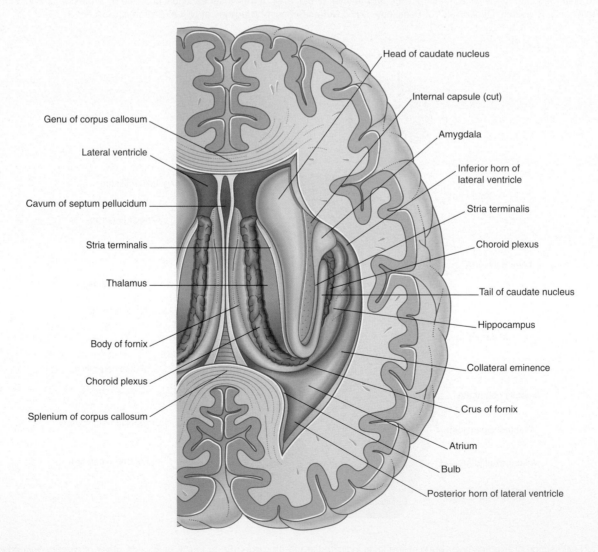

Fig. 2.18 Tilted view of the ventricular system, showing the continuity of structures in the body and inferior horn of the lateral ventricle. *Note:* The amygdala, stria terminalis, and tail of caudate nucleus occupy the roof of the inferior horn; the hippocampus occupies the floor. (The choroid plexus is 'reduced' in order to show related structures.)

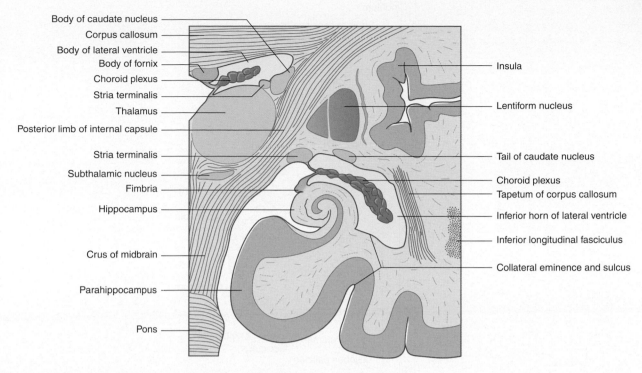

Body of caudate nucleus
Corpus callosum
Body of lateral ventricle
Body of fornix
Choroid plexus
Stria terminalis
Thalamus
Posterior limb of internal capsule
Stria terminalis
Subthalamic nucleus
Fimbria
Hippocampus
Crus of midbrain
Parahippocampus
Pons

Insula
Lentiform nucleus
Tail of caudate nucleus
Choroid plexus
Tapetum of corpus callosum
Inferior horn of lateral ventricle
Inferior longitudinal fasciculus
Collateral eminence and sulcus

Fig. 2.19 Coronal section through the body and inferior horn of the lateral ventricle.

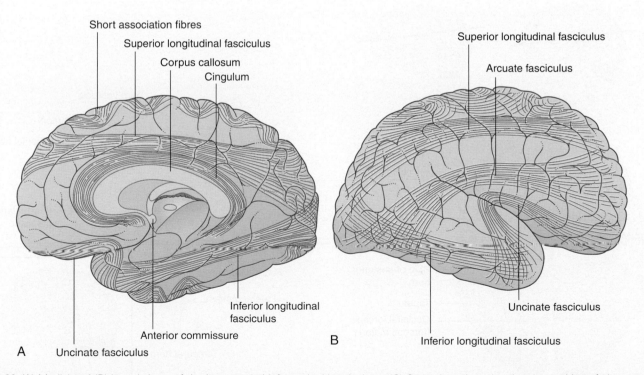

Short association fibres
Superior longitudinal fasciculus
Corpus callosum
Cingulum

Superior longitudinal fasciculus
Arcuate fasciculus

Inferior longitudinal fasciculus

Uncinate fasciculus

Inferior longitudinal fasciculus

A Uncinate fasciculus
Anterior commissure

B

Fig. 2.20 (A) Medial and (B) lateral views of the 'transparent' left cerebral hemisphere. (C) Coronal section, showing the position of short and long association fibre bundles.

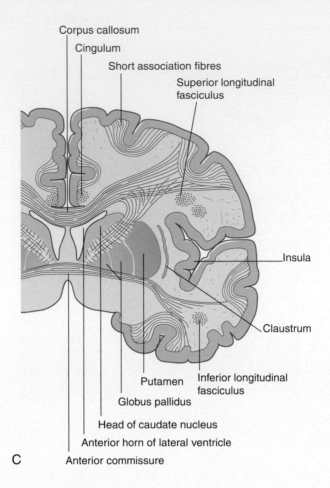

C

Fig. 2.20 (Continued).

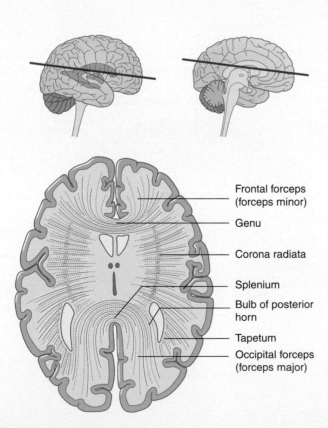

Fig. 2.21 Horizontal section through the genu and splenium of the corpus callosum. Fibres passing laterally from the body of the corpus callosum intersect the corona radiata.

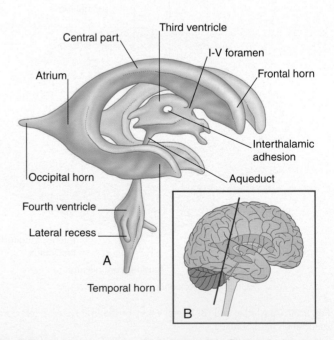

Fig. 2.22 Ventricular system. (A) Isolated cast. (B) Ventricular system in situ.

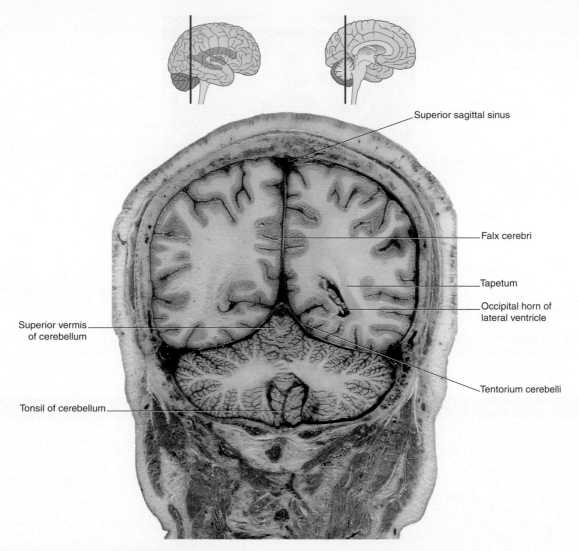

Superior sagittal sinus

Falx cerebri

Tapetum

Occipital horn of
lateral ventricle

Tentorium cerebelli

Superior vermis
of cerebellum

Tonsil of cerebellum

Fig. 2.23 Coronal section of fixed cadaver brain at the level indicated at top of image. (From Liu S, et al., eds. *Atlas of Human Sectional Anatomy*. Jinan: Shantung Press of Science and Technology; 2003, with permission of Shantung Press of Science and Technology.)

the fornix. Medially is the septum pellucidum, which tapers away posteriorly where the fornix rises to meet the corpus callosum. The **septum pellucidum** is formed by the fusion of the thinned-out walls of the two cerebral hemispheres. Its bilateral origin explains the occasional presence of a central cavity known as the *cavum*.

- **Occipital horn**. Lies inferior to the splenium and medial to the tapetum of the corpus callosum. On its medial side, the forceps major forms the *bulb* of the posterior horn.
- **Temporal horn**. Lies below the tail of the caudate nucleus and, at its anterior end, can be found the **amygdala** (*Gr.* 'almond') (Fig. 2.18), a nucleus belonging to the limbic system. The hippocampus and its associated structures occupy the full length of the floor of the inferior horn.
- Laterally can be found the **collateral eminence**, an indentation into the temporal horn created by the collateral sulcus (Fig. 2.18).

The **third ventricle** is the cavity of the diencephalon. Its boundaries are shown in Fig. 2.6. A **choroid plexus** hangs from its roof, which is formed from a double layer of pia mater fused with the ependyma/capillary complex of the ventricles, called the **tela choroidea**. Superior to this can be found the fornix of both sides and the corpus callosum. On either side of the third ventricle can be found the thalamus and hypothalamus. The anterior wall is formed by the anterior commissure, the **lamina terminalis**, and the **optic chiasm**. On the floor can be found the **infundibulum**, the **tuber cinereum**, the **mammillary bodies** and the rostral portion of the midbrain. The **pineal gland** and adjacent commissures form the posterior wall. The pineal gland is often calcified, and the **habenular commissure** is sometimes calcified as early as the second decade of life, thereby becoming detectable even on plain radiographs of the skull. The pineal gland is sometimes displaced to one side by a tumour, hematoma, or other masses (space-occupying lesions) within the cranial cavity.

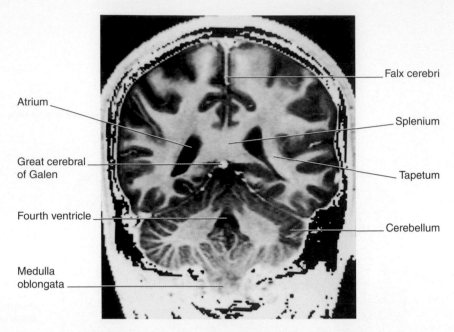

Falx cerebri

Atrium

Splenium

Great cerebral of Galen

Tapetum

Fourth ventricle

Cerebellum

Medulla oblongata

Fig. 2.24 Coronal Magnetic Resonance Imaging 'slice' at the level of Fig. 2.22B. (From a series kindly provided by Professor J. Paul Finn, Director, Magnetic Resonance Research, Department of Radiology, David Geffen School of Medicine at UCLA, California, USA.)

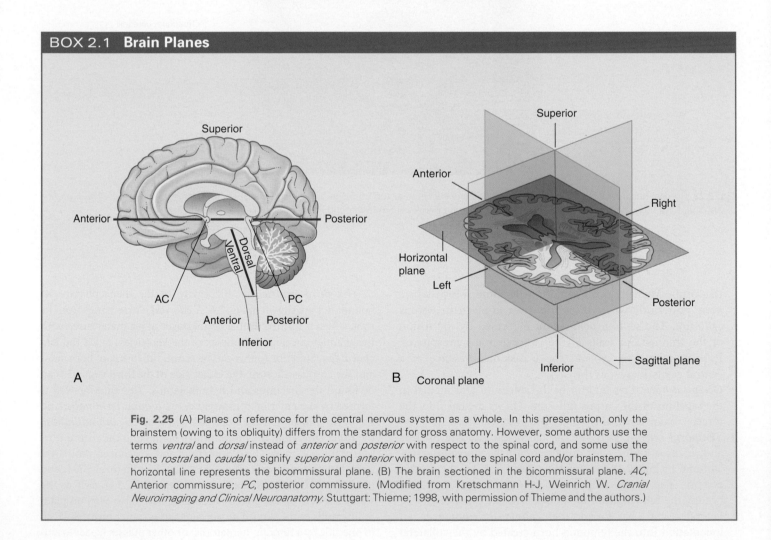

BOX 2.1 Brain Planes

Fig. 2.25 (A) Planes of reference for the central nervous system as a whole. In this presentation, only the brainstem (owing to its obliquity) differs from the standard for gross anatomy. However, some authors use the terms *ventral* and *dorsal* instead of *anterior* and *posterior* with respect to the spinal cord, and some use the terms *rostral* and *caudal* to signify *superior* and *anterior* with respect to the spinal cord and/or brainstem. The horizontal line represents the bicommissural plane. (B) The brain sectioned in the bicommissural plane. *AC*, Anterior commissure; *PC*, posterior commissure. (Modified from Kretschmann H-J, Weinrich W. *Cranial Neuroimaging and Clinical Neuroanatomy*. Stuttgart: Thieme; 1998, with permission of Thieme and the authors.)

BOX 2.2 **Magnetic Resonance Imaging**

Magnetic resonance imaging of the CNS is immensely useful for the detection of tumours and other space-occupying lesions (masses). When properly used, it is quite safe, even for young children and pregnant women. As will be shown later on, it can be adapted to the study of normal brain physiology in healthy volunteers.

The original name for the technique is *nuclear MRI*, because it is based on the behaviour of atomic nuclei in applied magnetic fields. The simplest atomic nucleus is that of the element hydrogen, consisting of a single proton, and this is prevalent in many substances (e.g., water) throughout the body.

Nuclei possess a property known as *spin* (Fig. 2.26), and it may be helpful to visualise this as akin to a spinning gyroscope. Normally, the direction of the spin (the axis of the gyroscope in our analogy) for any given nucleus is random. Spin produces a magnetic moment (vector) that makes it behave like a tiny dipole (north and south) magnet. In the absence of any external magnetic field, the dipoles are randomly arranged.

In the presence of a magnetic field, however, the dipoles will orient themselves along the direction of the magnetic field z (vertical) line.

The cylindric external magnet of an MRI machine (Fig. 2.27) is immensely powerful, capable of lifting the weight of several cars at one time. When the magnet is switched on, individual nuclear magnetic moments undergo a process called *precession*, analogous to the wobbling of a gyroscope, whereby they adopt a cone-shaped spin around the z axis of the external magnetic field.

Excitatory pulses are transmitted from radiofrequency coils set at right angles to the z axis of the external magnetic field. The effect is to tilt the net nuclear magnetic moment into the x—y axis, with all the nuclei precessing 'in phase'. When the radiofrequency coils are switched off, the nuclei '*dephase*' while still in the x—y axis and then *relax* back to vertical alignment. The time constant involved is called *T2*. The external magnet then restores the conical precession around the z axis; the time constant here is much slower and is called *T1*.

Because of the spinning, precessing nuclei behave like little magnets; if they are surrounded by a coil of wire, they will induce a current in that coil that can then be measured. The radio transmitter coil is able to receive and measure this current and is hence termed *transceiver* in the diagram.

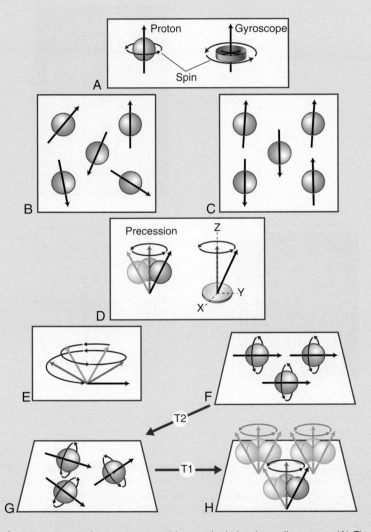

Fig. 2.26 Basis of nuclear magnetic resonance and its manipulation by radio waves. (A) The proton of the hydrogen nucleus is in a constant state of spin, analogous to that of a gyroscope. (B) At rest, the orientation of the axes of the spinning protons is random. (C) When the external magnet is switched on, all the axes become oriented along its longitudinal, z axis. The great majority are parallel with a small minority antiparallel, as indicated. (D) At the same time, the magnetic moments immediately precess around the axis like a wobbling gyroscope, being oriented in an intermediate state between the z axis of the magnetic field and the x—y axis at right angles to it. (E) An excitatory radiofrequency pulse at right angles to the axis of the external magnetic field tips the net magnetic moment along a 'snail shell' spiral into the x—y plane. (F) While the radiofrequency transceiver pulse is 'on', the nuclei are precessing in phase. (G) Switching off the radio frequency allows the nuclei to dephase immediately, with a brief T2 time constant. (H) Conical precession is resumed under the influence of the external magnet with a longer T1 time constant. (The assistance of Professor Hugh Garavan, Department of Psychology, Trinity College, Dublin, is gratefully appreciated.)

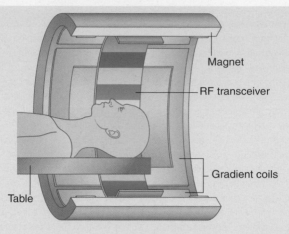

Fig. 2.27 The Magnetic Resonance Imaging machine. Outermost is the magnet. Innermost is the radiofrequency transceiver. In-between are the gradient coils. *RF*, Radiofrequency.

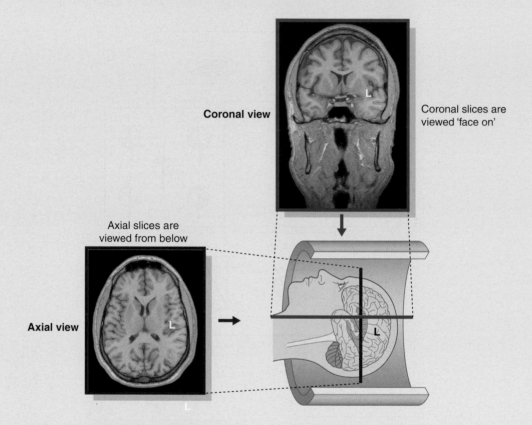

Fig. 2.28 Standard orientation of magnetic resonance images. Coronal sections are viewed from the front. Axial sections are viewed from below.

This is the basic principle of nuclear magnetic resonance. However, to be able to construct an actual image, it is required to *spatially* resolve the detected signal. This can be achieved by introducing *gradient coils*. Superimposition of a second magnetic field, set at right angles to that of the main magnet, causes the resonant frequency to be disturbed along the axis of the new field, with the proton spin being highest at one end and lowest at the other. The magnetic resonance machine in fact contains three gradient coils, one set in each of the three planes of space. The three coils are activated sequentially, allowing three-dimensional localisation of tissue signals. In this way, it is possible to 'slice' through the patient, detecting the signals emitted from different components in each selected plane of the patient and building up an image piece by piece.

The varying densities within the magnetic resonance images reflect the varying rates of dephasing and of relaxation of protons in different locations. The protons of the cerebrospinal fluid (CSF), for example, are free to resonate at maximum frequency, whereas in the white matter they are largely bound to lipid molecules. The grey matter has intermediate values, with some protons being protein bound. The radiofrequency pulses can be varied to exploit these differences. Almost all the images shown in textbooks (including this one) are T1-weighted, favouring the very weak signal provided by free protons during the relaxation period. This accounts for the different densities of CSF, grey matter, and white matter, the last being strongest. The reverse is true for T2-weighted images. T2-weighted images are especially useful for the detection of lesions in the white matter. For example, they can indicate an increase in free protons resulting from patchy loss of myelin sheath lipid in multiple sclerosis (see Chapter 6), or local oedema of brain tissue resulting from a vascular stroke.

The standard orientation of coronal and axial slices is shown in Fig. 2.28.

BOX 2.3 Diffusion Tensor Imaging

Terms

- *Diffusion tensor imaging* is a technique developed in the mid-1990s that uses MRI to measure diffusion constants of water molecules along many (more than 6) directions and that characterises diffusion anisotropy.
- An *isotropic* liquid has uniform diffusion properties on all sides (e.g., a drop of milk, which diffuses uniformly all around when released in water). *Isotropy* is uniformity in all directions and can be represented by a sphere.
- An *anisotropic* (*Gr.* 'not isotropic') liquid diffuses along a preferred axis and can be represented graphically as an ellipsoid.
- A *tensor* describes the shape of the ellipsoid. Diffusion tensors are second-order tensors (special cases of tensors are scalar [zero order or single digits] and vectors [first order or {1 × n} matrices]). A tensor can be reduced to its component axes (eigenvalues), termed lambda 1, 2, and 3, that describe the relative rate of diffusion along the length, breadth, and width of the ellipsoid (eigenvectors).

Fractional anisotropy (FA) describes the relationship between lambda 1, 2, and 3 as a fraction. The value of FA therefore ranges from 0 to 1. In the nervous system, diffusion of intracellular water in the white matter is restricted by the cell membranes. Extracellular water circulating in the ventricles and subarachnoid space, and water in grey matter, diffuses in a more isotropic manner. The interstitial fluid among myelinated fibre bundles preferentially diffuses parallel to the long axis of the fibres. The higher the FA, the more compact and uniform the bundles of fibres. This is particularly useful when comparing the relative integrity of matching myelinated pathways on each side of the brain or spinal white matter. One can reconstruct the three-dimensional trajectories of white matter tracts using tractography together with colour encoding to denote direction. The reconstruction algorithm is based on fibre orientation information obtained from diffusion tensor imaging. A more advanced method that addresses the limitations of the tensor model (i.e., that summarises information to one principal direction as the basis of tractography) and results in more accurate reconstruction is constrained spherical deconvolution (CSD). CSD uses information in multiple directions for each voxel and has begun to address the problems for tractography that occur in regions where fibre bundles cross.

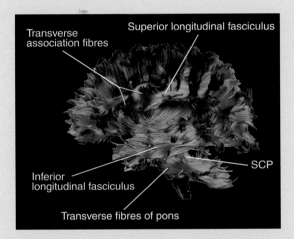

Fig. 2.29 Deterministic tractography across the entire brain performed using *ExploreDTI software. This image uses the common convention in diffusion tensor and tractography images where tracts in the anterior–posterior orientation are represented in green, superior–inferior in blue, and right–left in red. *SCP*, Superior cerebellar peduncle.

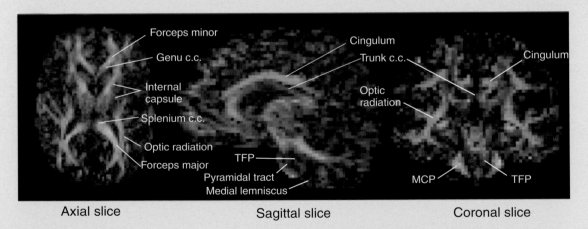

Axial slice   Sagittal slice   Coronal slice

Fig. 2.30 Fractional anisotropy is shown in three planes of space, with the same colour coding as in Fig. 2.29. *c.c.*, corpus callosum; *MCP*, middle cerebellar peduncle; *TFP*, transverse fibres of pons.

*ExploreDTI.com provided by Dr Alexander Leemans, Image Sciences Institute, University Medical Center, Utrecht. (The assistance of Dr Dara M. Cannon, Co-Director, Clinical Neuroimaging Laboratory, Department of Psychiatry, National University of Ireland, Galway is gratefully acknowledged.)

✳ Core Information

On the lateral surface of the cerebrum, four lobes are defined by the lateral and central sulci and an imaginary T-shaped line. The frontal lobe has six named gyri, the parietal lobe seven, the occipital lobe five, and the temporal lobe four. The insula is in the floor of the lateral sulcus.

On its medial surface, the corpus callosum can be divided into a splenium, body, genu, and rostrum. The septum pellucidum stretches from the corpus callosum to the body of the fornix. Separating the fornix from the thalamus is the choroidal fissure, through which the choroid plexus is inserted into the lateral ventricle. The third ventricle has the fornix as its roof; the thalamus and hypothalamus in its side walls; and the infundibulum, tuber cinereum, and mammillary bodies as its floor. Caudally can be found the pineal gland, which is often calcified.

The basal ganglia consist of the corpus striatum (caudate and lentiform nuclei), subthalamic nucleus, and substantia nigra. The lentiform nucleus comprises the putamen and globus pallidus. The striatum is made up of the caudate nucleus and putamen, and the pallidum refers to the globus pallidus alone.

The internal capsule is the white matter separating the lentiform nucleus from the thalamus and head of the caudate nucleus. The CST descends through the corona radiata and the posterior limb of the internal capsule to reach the brainstem.

Association fibres (e.g., the longitudinal, arcuate, uncinate fasciculi) link different areas within each hemisphere. Commissural fibres (e.g., the corpus callosum, anterior and posterior commissures) link matching/homotopic areas across the midline. Projection fibres (e.g., corticothalamic, corticobulbar, corticopontine, corticospinal) descend to the thalamus and brainstem. The lateral ventricles consist of a body, frontal, occipital, and temporal horns. Structures determining ventricular shape include corpus callosum, caudate nucleus, thalamus, amygdala, and hippocampus.

SUGGESTED READINGS

Clarke C, Howard R. Nervous system structure and function. In: Clarke C, Howard R, Rossor M, Shorvon S, eds. *Neurology: A Queen Square Textbook*. London: Wiley-Blackwell; 2009:13−74.

England MA, Wakely J. *A Colour Atlas of the Brain and Spinal Cord*. St. Louis: Mosby; 2005.

Garcia KB, Fernandez CI. Review − What we know about the brain structure−function relationship. *Behav Sci*. 2018;8(4):39.

Katada K. MR imaging of brain surface structures: surface anatomy scanning (SAS). *Neuroradiology*. 1990;3(5):439−448.

Kretschmann H-J, Weinrich W. *Cranial Neuroimaging and Clinical Neuroanatomy*. Stuttgart: Thieme; 1998.

Liu S, et al., eds. *Atlas of Human Sectional Anatomy*. Jinan: Shantung Press of Science and Technology; 2003.

Messé A, Rudrauf D, Benali H, Marrelec G. Relating structure and function in the human brain: relative contributions of anatomy, stationary dynamics, and non-stationarities. *PLoS Computat Biol*. 2014;10(3):1−9.

Pukenas B. Normal brain anatomy on magnetic resonance imaging. *Magn Reson Imaging Clin N Am*. 2011;19(3):429−437, vii.

van der Kolk AG, Hendrikse J, Zwanenburg JJM, Visser F, Luijten PR. Clinical applications of 7 T MRI in the brain. *Eur J Radiol*. 2013;82(5):708−718.

Midbrain, Hindbrain, Spinal Cord

CHAPTER SUMMARY

STUDY GUIDELINES

1. Be able to recognise and label the locations of the ascending and descending pathways in the horizontal sections of the brainstem and spinal cord.
2. Be able to describe or trace the four decussations that occur as part of a simple motor action. (Box 3.1 deserves special attention because it indicates why certain pathways cross the midline and others do not. The brainstem crossings are formally addressed in Chapters 15 and 16.)
3. Identify the major 'constituents' of the midbrain, pons, and medulla (prominent structures) and the location of the dorsal column—medial lemniscal pathways and corticospinal tracts and their decussations, as well as the superior cerebellar peduncles.
4. List the spinal cord segments and describe the anatomic reason for the prominent enlargements.
5. Describe the relationships of the three cerebellar peduncles to the fourth ventricle as seen in cross-sections.

The midbrain connects the diencephalon to the hindbrain. As explained in Chapter 1, the hindbrain is made up of the pons, medulla oblongata, and cerebellum. The medulla oblongata joins the spinal cord at the spinomedullary junction within the foramen magnum of the skull.

In this chapter, the cerebellum (part of the hindbrain) is considered *after* the spinal cord for the sake of continuity of motor and sensory pathway descriptions.

BRAINSTEM

Ventral View (Figs. 3.1 and 3.2A)

Midbrain. The ventral surface of the midbrain shows two *cerebral peduncles* bordering the *interpeduncular fossa*. The *optic tracts* wind around the midbrain at its junction with the diencephalon. Lateral to the midbrain is the uncus of the temporal lobe. The *oculomotor nerve* (CN III) exits the brainstem on the medial surface of the cerebral peduncle, whereas the *trochlear nerve* (CN IV) exits the brainstem from the lateral surface of the cerebral peduncle.

Pons. The bulk of the pons is composed of **transverse fibres** (the *pontocerebellar tract*) that raise numerous surface ridges. On each side, the pons is marked off from the middle cerebellar peduncle by the attachment of the *trigeminal nerve* (V). The *middle cerebellar peduncle* enters into the hemisphere of the cerebellum.

At the lower border of the pons are the attachments of the *abducens* (VI), *facial* (VII), and *vestibulocochlear* (VIII) *nerves* (Table 3.1).

Medulla Oblongata. The pyramids are on either side of the anterior median fissure. Just above the spinomedullary junction, this fissure is traversed by the *decussation of the corticospinal tracts*, where the majority of the corticospinal fibres from the two pyramids decussate in the midline. Lateral to the pyramids are the *olives* while posterior to the olives lies the inferior cerebellar peduncle. Attached between the pyramid and the olive in the preolivary sulcus are the rootlets of the *hypoglossal nerve* (CN XII). Attached between the olive and inferior cerebellar peduncle in the postolivary sulcus are the *glossopharyngeal* (CN IX), *vagus* (CN X), and *cranial accessory* (CN XIc) *nerves*. The *spinal accessory nerve* (CN XIs) arises from the upper five spinal segments of the spinal cord and enters the foramen magnum to join the cranial accessory nerve.

Dorsal View (Fig. 3.2B)

The roof or *tectum* of the midbrain is composed of four *colliculi* (*corpora quadrigemina*). The *superior colliculi* process visual information, and the *inferior colliculi* process auditory information. The *trochlear nerve* (CN IV) emerges below the inferior colliculus on each side.

The diamond-shaped *fourth ventricle* lies dorsal to the pons and upper medulla oblongata, under cover of the cerebellum. The upper half of the diamond is bounded by the *superior cerebellar peduncles*, which are attached to the midbrain. The lower half is bounded by the *inferior cerebellar peduncles*, which are attached to the medulla oblongata. The *middle cerebellar peduncles* enter from the pons and overlap the other two.

Close to the midline in the midregion of the floor of the fourth ventricle is the *facial colliculus*, which is created by the axons of the facial nerve curving around the nucleus of the abducens nerve. The *vestibular area* and the *vagal* and *hypoglossal trigones* overlie the corresponding cranial nerve nuclei. The *obex* is located in the inferior angle of the floor of the fourth ventricle.

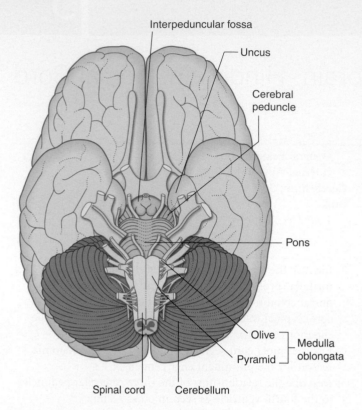

Interpeduncular fossa

Uncus

Cerebral
peduncle

Pons

Olive
Pyramid ⎤ Medulla
        ⎦ oblongata

Spinal cord   Cerebellum

Fig. 3.1 Ventral view of the brainstem in situ.

Below the fourth ventricle, the medulla oblongata has a pair of *gracile tubercles* flanked by a pair of *cuneate tubercles*.

Sectional Views

In the midbrain, the lumen of the embryonic neural tube is represented by the *cerebral/Sylvian aqueduct*. Behind the pons and upper medulla oblongata (Fig. 3.3), it is represented by the fourth ventricle, which is tent-shaped in this view. The central canal forms at mid-medullary level and it is continuous with the central canal of the spinal cord. The flow of the cerebrospinal fluid within the central canal of the spinal cord is negligible.

The intermediate region of the brainstem is called the *tegmentum*, which in the midbrain contains the paired *red nuclei*. Ventral to the tegmentum in the pons is the *basilar region*. Ventral to the tegmentum in the medulla oblongata are the pyramids.

The tegmentum of the entire brainstem is permeated by an important network of neurons, the *reticular formation*. The tegmentum also contains *ascending sensory pathways* carrying general sensory information from the trunk and limbs. Illustrated in Figs. 3.4 to 3.6 are the *dorsal column–medial lemniscal (DCML) pathways*, which inform the brain about the position of the limbs in space. At spinal cord level, the label **DCML** is used because these pathways occupy the *dorsal columns* of white matter in the spinal cord. In the brainstem, the label DCML is used because they continue upward as the **medial lemnisci**.

The most important *motor pathways* from a clinical standpoint are the *corticospinal tracts* (CSTs), the pathways for execution of voluntary movements. The CSTs are placed ventrally, occupying the cerebral crura of the midbrain, the basilar pons, and the pyramids of the medulla oblongata.

Note that, in the medulla oblongata, the DCML pathways and CSTs *decussate*: one of each of the paired tracts intersects with the other to cross over to the contralateral (opposite) side of the neuraxis (brainstem–spinal cord). The four most important decussations are illustrated in Box 3.1.

In the following account of seven horizontal sections of the brainstem, the positions of the cranial nerve nuclei are not included.

Midbrain (Fig. 3.4). The main landmarks have already been identified. On each side, the medial lemniscal component of the DCML pathway occupies the lateral part of the tegmentum *(upper section)*, on its way to the ventroposterolateral (VPL) nucleus of the thalamus immediately above this level. The CST has arisen in the cerebral cortex, and it is descending in the midregion of the cerebral crus on the same (ipsilateral) side.

The *decussation of the superior cerebellar peduncles* straddles the midline at the level of the inferior colliculi *(lower section)*.

Pons (Fig. 3.5). In the *upper section*, the cavity of the fourth ventricle is bordered laterally by the superior cerebellar peduncles, which are ascending *(arrows)* to decussate in the lower midbrain. In the floor of the ventricle is the central grey matter. The medial lemniscus occupies the ventral part of the tegmentum on each side. The basilar region contains millions of *transverse fibres*, some of which separate the CST into individual fascicles. The transverse fibres enter the cerebellum via the middle cerebellar peduncles and *appear* to form a bridge (hence, *pons*) connecting the cerebellar hemispheres. But the *individual* transverse fibres arise on one side of the pons and cross the midline to enter the contralateral cerebellar hemisphere. The transverse fibres belong to the giant *corticopontocerebellar pathway*, which travels from the cerebral cortex of one side to the contralateral cerebellar hemisphere, as depicted in Box 3.1.

The *lower section* contains the inferior cerebellar peduncle, about to enter into the cerebellum (Fig. 3.6). Follow the CST from above down. It descends through sections A and B as the *pyramid*. In C, it intersects with its opposite number in the *motor decussation*, prior to entering the contralateral side of the spinal cord.

Follow the **DCML** pathway from below upward. In section C, it takes the form of the *gracile* and *cuneate fasciculi*, known in the spinal cord as the *dorsal columns* of white matter. In section B, the dorsal columns terminate in the *gracile* and *cuneate nuclei*. From these nuclei, the second-order neurons swing around the central grey matter and decussate with their opposite numbers in the *sensory decussation*. Having crossed the midline, the fibres turn upward. In section A, they form the medial lemniscal component of the DCML pathway.

On the left side of the medulla is shown the *dorsal spinocerebellar tract*. Its function (nonconscious) is to inform the cerebellum of the state of activity of the ipsilateral (same side) skeletal muscles in the trunk and limbs.

The upper half of the medulla shows the wrinkled *inferior olivary nucleus*, which creates the olive in the ventral midmedullary region lying lateral to the pyramids.

Sections of brainstem in situ are shown in Figs. 3.8 to 3.12.

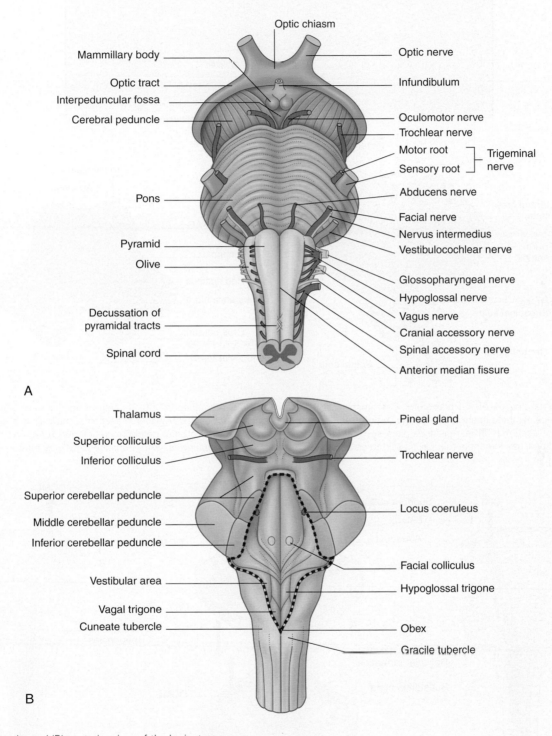

Optic chiasm

Mammillary body

Optic nerve

Optic tract

Infundibulum

Interpeduncular fossa

Cerebral peduncle

Oculomotor nerve

Trochlear nerve

Motor root ⎫ Trigeminal
           ⎬ nerve
Sensory root ⎭

Pons

Abducens nerve

Facial nerve

Nervus intermedius

Pyramid

Vestibulocochlear nerve

Olive

Glossopharyngeal nerve

Hypoglossal nerve

Vagus nerve

Decussation of
pyramidal tracts

Cranial accessory nerve

Spinal accessory nerve

Spinal cord

Anterior median fissure

A

Thalamus

Pineal gland

Superior colliculus

Inferior colliculus

Trochlear nerve

Superior cerebellar peduncle

Middle cerebellar peduncle

Locus coeruleus

Inferior cerebellar peduncle

Vestibular area

Facial colliculus

Hypoglossal trigone

Vagal trigone

Cuneate tubercle

Obex

Gracile tubercle

B

Fig. 3.2 (A) Anterior and (B) posterior view of the brainstem.

TABLE 3.1	**The Cranial Nerves.**
Number	**Name**
I	Olfactory, enters the olfactory bulb from the nose
II	Optic
III	Oculomotor
IV	Trochlear
V	Trigeminal
VI	Abducens
VII	Facial
VIII	Vestibulocochlear
IX	Glossopharyngeal
X	Vagus
XI	Accessory
XII	Hypoglossal

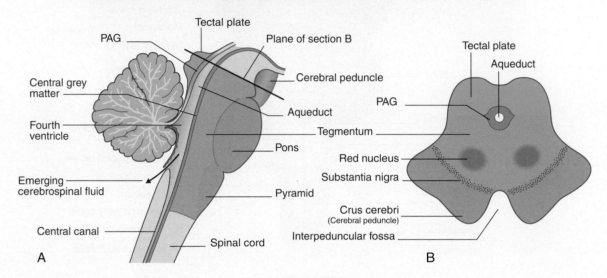

Fig. 3.3 (A) Sagittal section of the brainstem. Cerebrospinal fluid descends along the aqueduct into the fourth ventricle and emerges into the subarachnoid space via three apertures, including the median aperture of Magendie *(arrow)*. (B) Transverse section of midbrain at the level indicated in (A) as 'plane of section B'. The substantia nigra separates the tegmentum from the two crura cerebri (cerebral peduncle). The interpeduncular fossa is so called because the entire midbrain is said to be made up of a pair of cerebral peduncles. *PAG*, Periaqueductal grey matter.

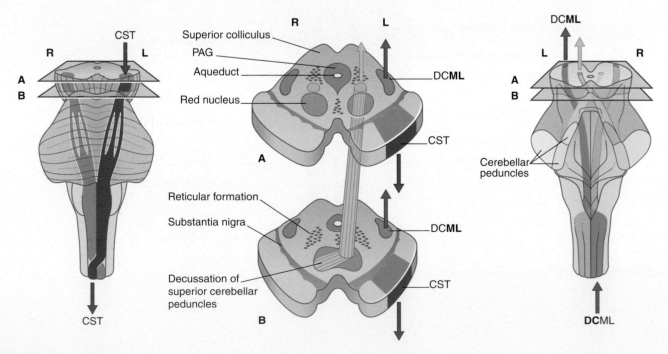

Fig. 3.4 Transverse sections of midbrain. (A) At the level of superior colliculi. (B) At the level of inferior colliculi. In this and following diagrams, the corticospinal tract *(CST)* and dorsal column–medial lemniscal *(DCML)* pathway connected to the *left* cerebral hemisphere are highlighted. *PAG*, Periaqueductal grey matter.

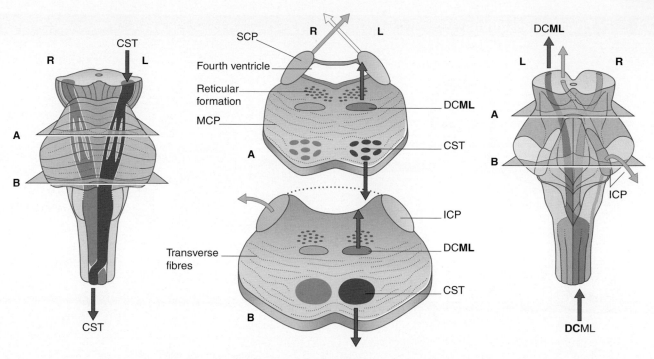

Fig. 3.5 Transverse sections of pons. (A) Upper pons. (B) Lower pons. *CST*, Corticospinal tract; *DCML*, dorsal column—medial lemniscal pathway; *ICP*, inferior cerebellar peduncle; *MCP*, middle cerebellar peduncle; *SCP*, superior cerebellar peduncle.

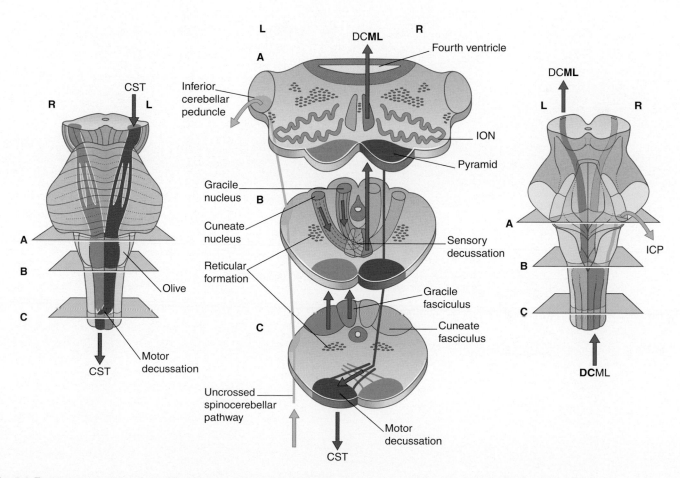

Fig. 3.6 Transverse sections of medulla oblongata. (A) Level of inferior olivary nucleus *(ION)*. (B) Level of sensory decussation. (C) Level of motor decussation. *CST*, Corticospinal tract; *DCML*, dorsal column—medial lemniscal pathway; *ICP*, inferior cerebellar peduncle.

BOX 3.1   Four Decussations

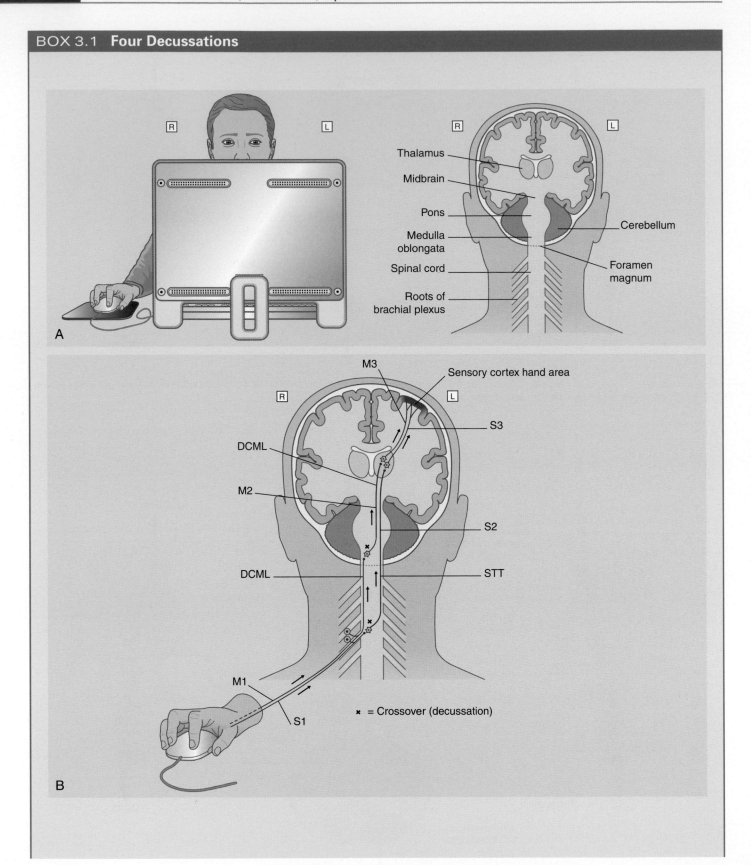

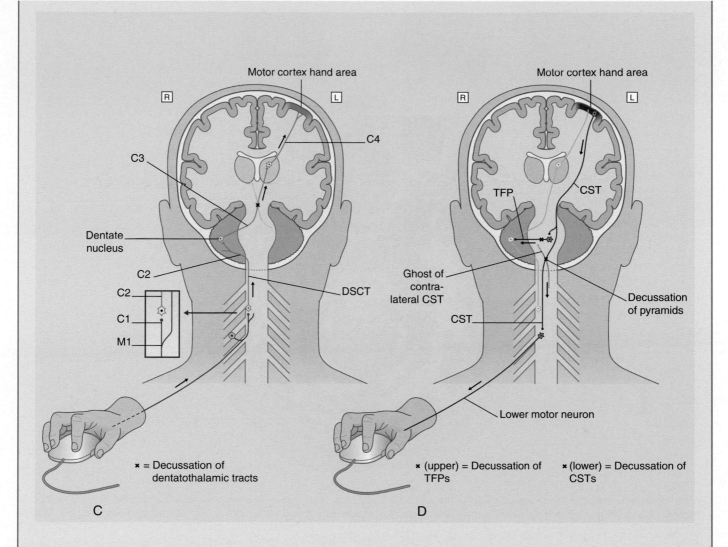

Fig. 3.7 (A) The stage is set. The subject's right hand is about to click a mouse while the eyes are directed elsewhere. The coronal section identifies key structures. (B) Afferents. The left parietal lobe constructs a map of the right hand in relation to the mouse, based on the information sent to the left somatic sensory cortex (postcentral gyrus) from the skin and deep tissues. The information is relayed by three successive sets of neurons from the skin and by another set of three from the deep tissues. The first set in each case is composed of *first-order* or *primary afferent neurons*. These neurons are called *pseudo-unipolar*, because each axon emerges from a single point (or pole) of the cell body and divides in a T-shaped manner to provide continuity of impulse conduction from tissue to central nervous system. The primary afferent neurons terminate by forming contacts known as *synapses* on the *multipolar* (more or less star-shaped) cells of the *second-order (secondary)* set. The axons of the second-order neurons project across the midline before turning up to terminate on *third-order (tertiary)* multipolar neurons projecting to the postcentral gyrus. Primary afferents activated by contacts with the skin of the hand (S1) terminate in the posterior horn of the grey matter of the spinal cord. Second-order cutaneous afferents (S2) cross the midline in the anterior white commissure and ascend to the thalamus within the *spinothalamic tract* (STT), to be relayed by third-order neurons to the hand area of the sensory cortex.

The most significant deep tissue sensory organs are *neuromuscular spindles* (muscle spindles) contained within skeletal muscles. The primary afferents supplying the muscle spindles of the intrinsic muscles of the hand belong to large unipolar neurons whose axons (labelled M1) ascend ipsilaterally (on the same side of the spinal cord) within the dorsal funiculus, as already seen in Fig. 3.5. They synapse in the nucleus cuneatus in the medulla oblongata. The multipolar second-order neurons send their axons across the midline in the sensory decussation (seen in Fig. 3.6). The axons ascend (M2) through pons and midbrain before synapsing on third-order neurons (M3) projecting from VPL nucleus of the thalamus to sensory cortex.

(C) Cerebellar control. Before the brain sends an instruction to click the mouse, it requires information on the current state of contraction of the muscles. This information is constantly being sent from the muscles to the cerebellar hemisphere on the same side. As indicated in the diagram, M1 neurons are dual-purpose sensory neurons. At their point of entry to the dorsal funiculus, they give off a branch, here labelled C1, to a *spinocerebellar* neuron that projects (C2) to the ipsilateral cerebellum. From here, a *cerebellothalamic* neuron (C3) is shown projecting across the midbrain to the contralateral thalamus, where a further neuron (C4) relays information to the hand area of the *motor* cortex in the precentral gyrus. (D) Motor output. Multipolar neurons in the left motor cortex now fire impulses along the upper motor neurons that constitute the corticospinal tract (CST), which crosses to the opposite side in the motor decussation, as already described in Fig. 3.6. The CST synapses on *lower motor neurons* projecting from the anterior horn of the spinal grey matter to activate flexor muscles of the index finger and local stabilising muscles. Note that a copy of the outgoing message is sent to the right cerebellar hemisphere by way of *transverse fibres of the pons* (TFP) originating in multipolar neurons located on the left side of the pons.
DCML, Dorsal column—medial lemniscal pathway.

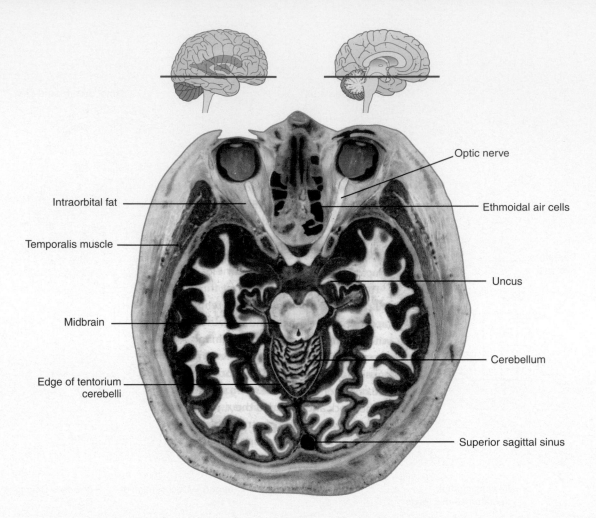

Optic nerve

Intraorbital fat

Ethmoidal air cells

Temporalis muscle

Uncus

Midbrain

Cerebellum

Edge of tentorium
cerebelli

Superior sagittal sinus

Fig. 3.8 Horizontal section of fixed cadaver, taken at the level of the midbrain. The cerebellum is seen through the tentorial notch. (From Liu S, et al., eds. *Atlas of Human Sectional Anatomy*. Jinan: Shantung Press of Science and Technology; 2003, with permission from Shantung Press of Science and Technology.)

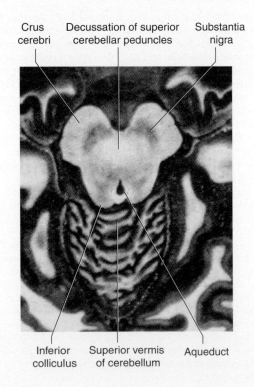

Crus
cerebri

Decussation of superior
cerebellar peduncles

Substantia
nigra

Inferior
colliculus

Superior vermis
of cerebellum

Aqueduct

Fig. 3.9 Enlargement of Fig. 3.8.

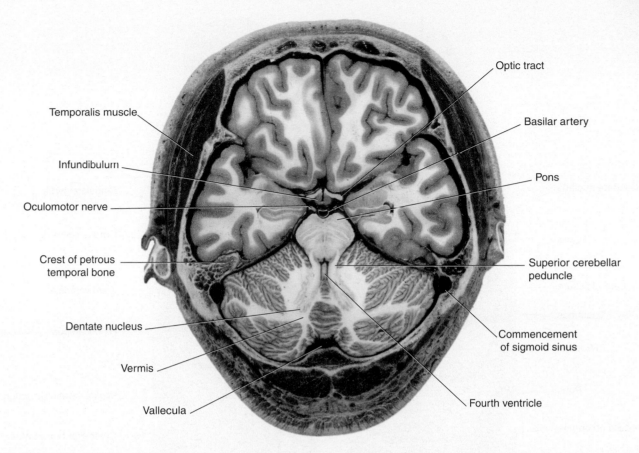

Temporalis muscle

Infundibulum

Oculomotor nerve

Crest of petrous
temporal bone

Dentate nucleus

Vermis

Vallecula

Optic tract

Basilar artery

Pons

Superior cerebellar
peduncle

Commencement
of sigmoid sinus

Fourth ventricle

Fig. 3.10 Horizontal section taken at the level of the upper pons. The fourth ventricle is slot-like at this level; on each side is a superior cerebellar peduncle travelling upward and medially from the dentate nucleus towards the contralateral thalamus. (From Liu S, et al., eds. *Atlas of Human Sectional Anatomy*. Jinan: Shantung Press of Science and Technology; 2003, with permission from Shantung Press of Science and Technology.)

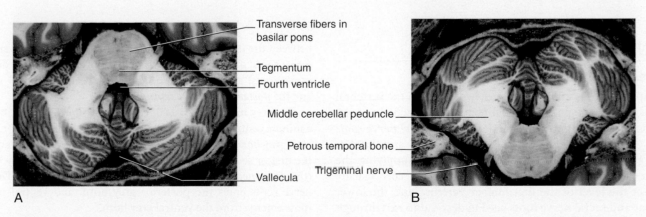

Transverse fibers in
basilar pons

Tegmentum
Fourth ventricle

Middle cerebellar peduncle

Petrous temporal bone

Trigeminal nerve

Vallecula

A   B

Fig. 3.11 Horizontal section taken through the middle of the pons. (A) In axial brain scans, the pons would be in the position shown, i.e., in the roof of the fourth ventricle. (B) In standard anatomic descriptions including histologic sections (see Chapter 17), the pons occupies the floor of the fourth ventricle, as shown here. Note the massive size of the middle cerebellar peduncles. (From Liu S, et al., eds. *Atlas of Human Sectional Anatomy*. Jinan: Shantung Press of Science and Technology; 2003, with permission from Shantung Press of Science and Technology.)

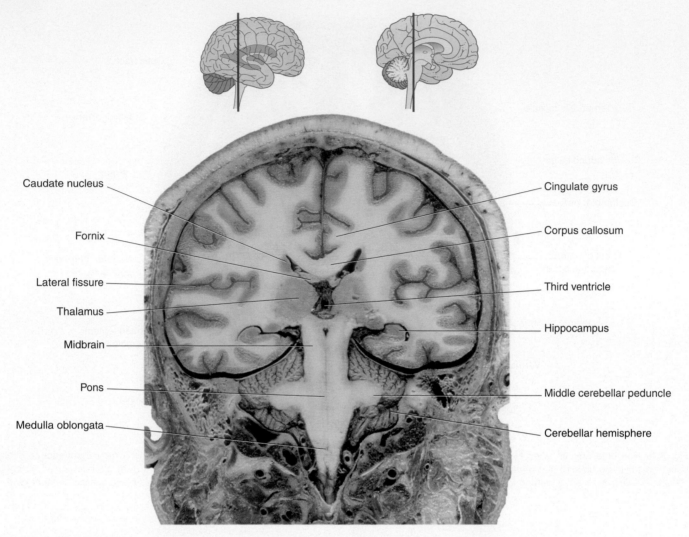

Fig. 3.12 Coronal section of brainstem and cerebellum at the level shown at top. Note that the section passes through the tegmentum of the midbrain. The spinal and trigeminal lemnisci are entering the ventral posteromedial nucleus of the thalamus. The periaqueductal grey matter is sectioned longitudinally; the aqueduct itself is seen below the third ventricle.

SPINAL CORD

General Features

The spinal cord occupies the upper two-thirds of the vertebral canal. Thirty-one pairs of spinal nerves are attached to it by means of *ventral (anterior)* and *dorsal (posterior) nerve roots* (Fig. 3.13A). The spinal cord shows *cervical* and *lumbar enlargements* that accommodate nerve cells supplying the upper and lower limbs. In the adult the spinal cord usually ends at the level of the first lumbar vertebra and the lower lumbar and sacral nerve roots need to descend to exit through their appropriate intervertebral foramina. This collection of nerve roots is referred to as the *cauda equina* (Figs. 3.14 and 3.15).

Internal Anatomy

In transverse sections the cord shows butterfly-shaped grey matter surrounded by three columns or *funiculi* of white matter on each side (Fig. 3.13B): a *ventral funiculus* in the interval between the *anterior median fissure* and the emerging *ventral nerve roots*; a *lateral funiculus* between the ventral and dorsal nerve roots; and a *dorsal funiculus* between the dorsal roots and the *posterior median septum*.

The grey matter consists of *central grey matter* surrounding a minute central canal, and *ventral (anterior)* and *dorsal (posterior) grey horns* on each side. At the levels of the first thoracic to the first or second lumbar spinal segments, a *lateral grey horn* (the *intermediolateral cell column*) is also present. Dorsal nerve roots enter the posterior grey horn, and ventral nerve roots emerge from the ventral grey horn.

Axons pass from one side of the spinal cord to the other in the *anterior white* and *grey commissures* deep to the anterior median fissure.

The LCST descends the spinal cord within the lateral funiculus. Its principal targets are neurons in the anterior grey horn concerned with activation of skeletal muscles. *Special note:* In Chapter 16, it will be seen that a small, *ventral CST* separates from the main bundle and descends within the ventral

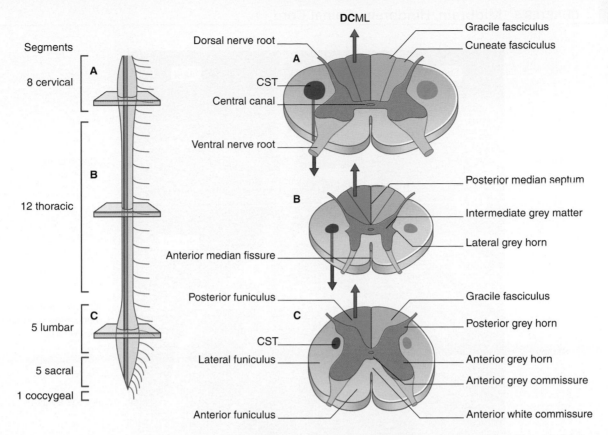

Fig. 3.13 Spinal cord. On the *left* is an anterior view of the cord with nerve attachments enumerated. On the *right* are (A) cervical enlargement level, (B) thoracic level, and (C) lumbar enlargement level, showing the arrangement of the largest motor and sensory pathways in the white matter, namely the corticospinal tract *(CST)* and the dorsal column–medial lemniscal pathway *(DCML)* comprising the gracile and cuneatus fasciculus.

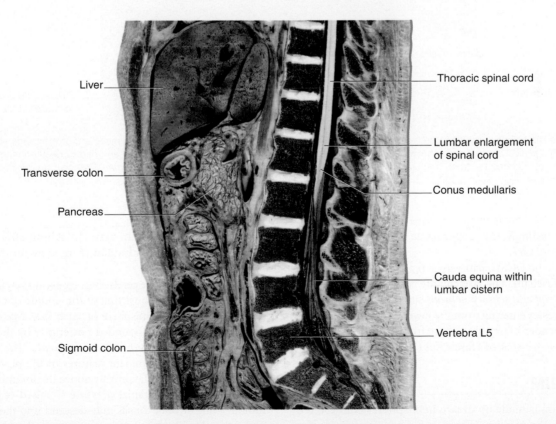

Fig. 3.14 Midline sagittal section of fixed cadaver, displaying the spinal cord and cauda equina in situ. It should be borne in mind that the cauda equina contains not only the motor and sensory nerve roots of the lumbosacral plexus supplying the lower limbs, but also the autonomic motor nerves supplying smooth muscle of the hindgut (sigmoid colon and rectum), bladder, uterus, and erectile tissues. (From Liu S, et al., eds. *Atlas of Human Sectional Anatomy*. Jinan: Shantung Press of Science and Technology; 2003, with permission from Shantung Press of Science and Technology.)

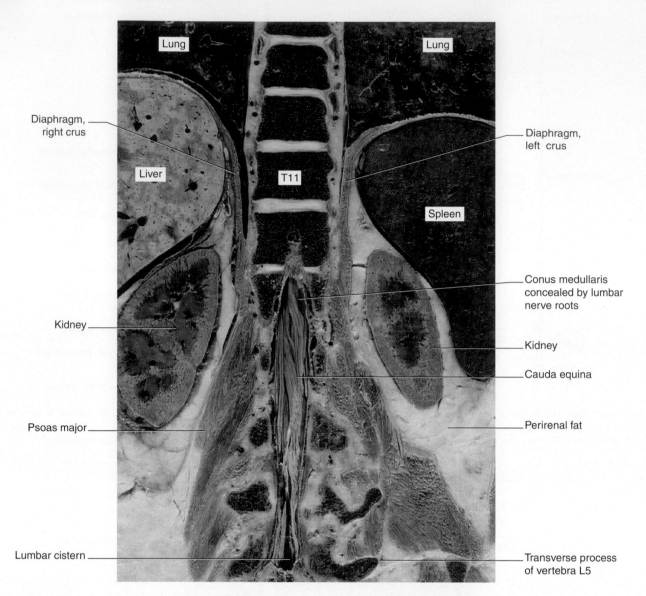

Fig. 3.15 Remarkable photograph of a coronal section of fixed cadaver, confirming the high level of commencement of the cauda equina as viewed from in front. In a clinical context, this photograph is a reminder of the hazard to somatic (notably sciatic) and parasympathetic (notably to bladder and rectum) nerves incurred by crush fractures of lumbar vertebrae. (From Liu S, et al., eds. *Atlas of Human Sectional Anatomy*. Jinan: Shantung Press of Science and Technology; 2003, with permission from Shantung Press of Science and Technology.)

funiculus. Accordingly, the proper name of the bundle depicted here is the *lateral CST*.

In the cord, the DCML pathway is represented by the **gracile** and **cuneate fasciculi**. The fasciculi are composed of the *central processes of peripheral sensory neurons* supplying muscles, joints, and skin. Processes entering from the lower part of the body form the gracile ('slender') fasciculus; those from the upper part form the cuneate ('wedge-shaped') fasciculus (Fig. 3.13).

CEREBELLUM

The cerebellum is made up of two hemispheres connected by the **vermis** in the midline (Fig. 3.16). The vermis is distinct only on the undersurface, where it occupies the floor of a deep groove, the **vallecula**. The hemispheres show numerous deep **fissures**, with **folia** in between. About 80% of the cortex (surface grey matter) is hidden from view on the surfaces of the folia.

The oldest part of the cerebellum (present even in fishes) is the **flocculonodular lobe** consisting of the **nodule** of the vermis and the **flocculus** in the hemisphere on each side. More recent is the **anterior lobe**, which is bounded posteriorly by the **primary fissure** and contains the **pyramis** and the **uvula**. The most recent is the **posterior lobe**. Prominent features of the posterior lobe are the **tonsils**. The tonsils lie directly above the foramen magnum of the skull; if the intracranial pressure is raised (e.g., by a brain tumour), one or both tonsils may descend into the foramen and pose a threat to life by compressing the medulla oblongata.

The white matter contains several deep nuclei. The largest of these is the **dentate nucleus** (Fig. 3.17).

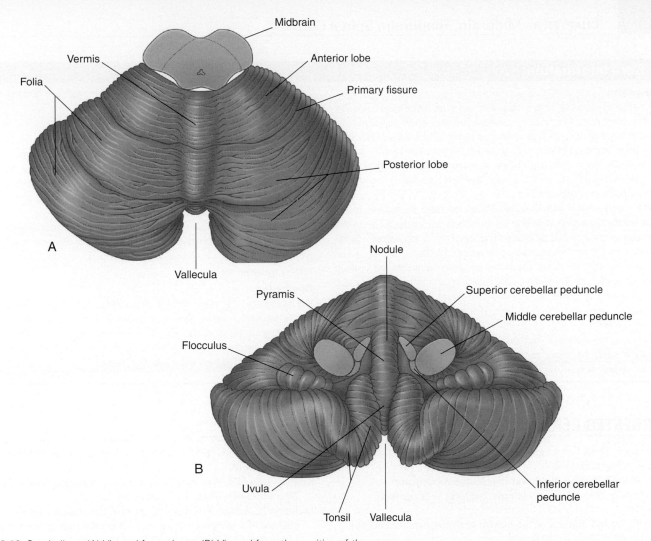

Fig. 3.16 Cerebellum. (A) Viewed from above. (B) Viewed from the position of the pons.

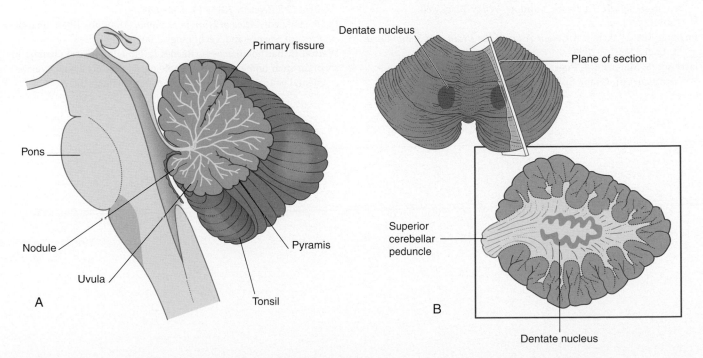

Fig. 3.17 (A) Sagittal section of hindbrain. (B) Oblique section of cerebellum.

✳ Core Information

Brainstem

The midbrain comprises the tectum, tegmentum, and a crus cerebri on each side. The cerebral aqueduct is surrounded by periaqueductal grey matter. The tegmentum contains the red nucleus at the level of the upper part of the midbrain and elements of the reticular formation at all levels of the brainstem. The largest component of the pons is the basilar region containing millions of transverse fibres belonging to the corticopontocerebellar pathways. The most prominent structure in the medulla oblongata is the inferior olivary nucleus.

The CST descends in the intermediate 3/5th of the crus of the midbrain, basilar pons, and medullary pyramid. Its principal component, the lateral CST, enters the pyramidal decussation and descends the spinal cord in the opposite lateral funiculus. Most of its fibres terminate in the anterior grey horn.

The dorsal columns of the spinal cord comprise the gracile and cuneate fasciculi, which terminate in the lower medulla by synapsing upon neurons of the corresponding nuclei. A second set of fibres traverses the sensory decussation before ascending, as the medial lemniscus, to the contralateral sensory thalamus.

The dorsal spinocerebellar tract carries information about ipsilateral muscular activity. It enters the inferior cerebellar peduncle. The cerebellum responds by sending signals through the superior cerebellar peduncle of that side to the contralateral motor thalamus via the superior cerebellar peduncle decussation in the lower midbrain.

Spinal Cord

The spinal cord occupies the upper two-thirds of the vertebral canal, the sacral nerve roots being attached to it at the level of the first lumbar vertebra. In all, 31 pairs of roots are attached. The grey matter is most abundant at the levels of attachment of the brachial and lumbosacral plexuses. Anterior and posterior horns are present at all levels, and lateral horns at the levels of the first thoracic to second or third lumbar vertebrae. The white matter comprises ventral, lateral, and dorsal funiculi. Axons cross the midline in the grey commissures and in the white commissure. In general, propriospinal pathways are innermost, motor pathways are intermediate, and sensory pathways are outermost.

Cerebellum

The hemispheres are deeply fissured and are linked by the vermis. The oldest part is the flocculonodular lobe; more recent is the anterior lobe; and the most recent is the posterior lobe, which includes the tonsils. The white matter contains several nuclei, including the dentate nucleus, the interposed nuclei, emboliform/globose and the fastigial nucleus.

SUGGESTED READINGS

Anderson C, Stern CD. Organizers in development. *Curr Top Dev Biol.* 2016;117:435−454.

Barker RA, Cicchetti F, Robinson ESJ. *Neuroanatomy and Neuroscience at a Glance.* Newark, NJ: John Wiley & Sons; 2017.

Bazier JS. Unique features of the human brainstem and cerebellum. *Front Hum Neurosci.* 2014;8:202.

Clarke C, Howard R. Nervous system structure and function. In: Clarke C, Howard R, Rossor M, Shorvon S, eds. *Neurology: A Queen Square Textbook.* London: Wiley-Blackwell; 2009:13−74.

England MA, Wakely J. *A Colour Atlas of the Brain and Spinal Cord.* St. Louis: Mosby; 2005.

Jacobson S, Marcus EM, Pugsley S. *Neuroanatomy for the Neuroscientist.* Cham: Springer; 2017.

Kiernan J, Rajakumar R. *Barr's The Human Nervous System: An Anatomical Viewpoint.* Philadelphia, PA: Lippincott Williams & Wilkins; 2013.

Kretschmann H-J, Weinrich W. *Cranial Neuroimaging and Clinical Neuroanatomy.* Stuttgart: Thieme; 2004.

Lachman N, Acland RD, Rosse C. Anatomical evidence for the absence of a morphologically distinct cranial root of the accessory nerve in man. *Clin Anat.* 2002;15:4−10.

Lippmann ES, Williams CE, Ruhl DA, et al. Deterministic HOX patterning in human pluripotent stem cell-derived neuroectoderm. *Stem Cell Reports.* 2015;4(4):632−644.

Liu S, et al., eds. *Atlas of Human Sectional Anatomy.* Jinan: Shantung Press of Science and Technology; 2003.

Watson C, Bartholomaeus C, Puelles L. Time for radical changes in brain stem nomenclature − applying the lessons from developmental gene patterns. *Front Neuroanat.* 2019;13:1−12.

Blood Supply of the Brain

STUDY GUIDELINES

1. On simple outline drawings of the lateral, medial, and inferior surfaces of a cerebral hemisphere, learn to shade in the territories of the three cerebral arteries.
2. Identify the main sources of arterial supply to the internal capsule.
3. Become familiar with carotid and vertebral angiograms.
4. Be able to list the territories supplied by the vertebral and basilar arteries.

5. Identify the two blood—brain barriers. Be able to understand why shallow breathing following abdominal surgery in a critical patient may induce coma.

Because interpretation of the symptoms caused by cerebro-vascular accidents requires prior understanding of brain function, Clinical Panels on this subject are placed in the final chapter.

A Clinical Panel on blood—brain barrier pathology is placed in the present chapter because the symptoms are of a general nature.

The brain is absolutely dependent on a continuous supply of oxygenated blood. It controls the delivery of blood by sensing the momentary pressure changes in its main arteries of supply, the internal carotid and vertebral arteries. The arterial oxygen tension is controlled by a medullary chemosensitive area that monitors respiratory gas levels in the internal carotid artery and in the cerebrospinal fluid. The control systems used by the brain are exquisitely sophisticated, but they can be fatally affected due to poor perfusion as a result of a raptured arterial aneurysm or a thromboembolic phenomenon.

ARTERIAL SUPPLY OF THE FOREBRAIN

The blood supply to the forebrain is derived from the two *internal carotid arteries* and from the *basilar artery* (Fig. 4.1).

Each internal carotid artery enters the subarachnoid space by piercing the roof of the cavernous sinus. In the subarachnoid space, it gives off *ophthalmic*, *posterior communicating*, and *anterior choroidal arteries* before dividing into the *anterior* and *middle cerebral arteries*.

The basilar artery divides at the upper border of the pons into the two *posterior cerebral arteries*. The *cerebral arterial circle (circle of Willis)* is completed by the union of the posterior communicating artery with the posterior cerebral artery on each side, and by the union of the two anterior cerebral arteries by the *anterior communicating artery*.

The choroid plexus of the lateral ventricle is supplied from the *anterior choroidal branch* of the internal carotid artery and by the *posterior choroidal branch* from the posterior cerebral artery.

Dozens of fine *central (perforating) branches* are given off by the constituent arteries of the circle of Willis. They enter the brain through the *anterior perforated substance* next to the optic chiasm and through the *posterior perforated substance* lying behind the mammillary bodies. (These designations refer to both the location on the ventral surface of the brain and the small perforations that appear when the numerous small penetrating arteries that supply these areas are pulled away from their points of entry.) These small perforating arteries have been classified in various ways but can be conveniently grouped into short and long branches. *Short central branches* arise from all the constituent arteries and from the two choroidal arteries. They supply the optic nerve, chiasm, and tract, and the hypothalamus. *Long central branches* arise from the three cerebral arteries. They supply the thalamus, corpus striatum, and internal capsule. They include the *striate (lenticulostriate) branches* of the anterior and middle cerebral arteries.

Anterior Cerebral Artery (Fig. 4.2)

The anterior cerebral artery passes above the optic chiasm to gain the medial surface of the cerebral hemisphere. It forms an arch around the genu of the corpus callosum, making it easy to

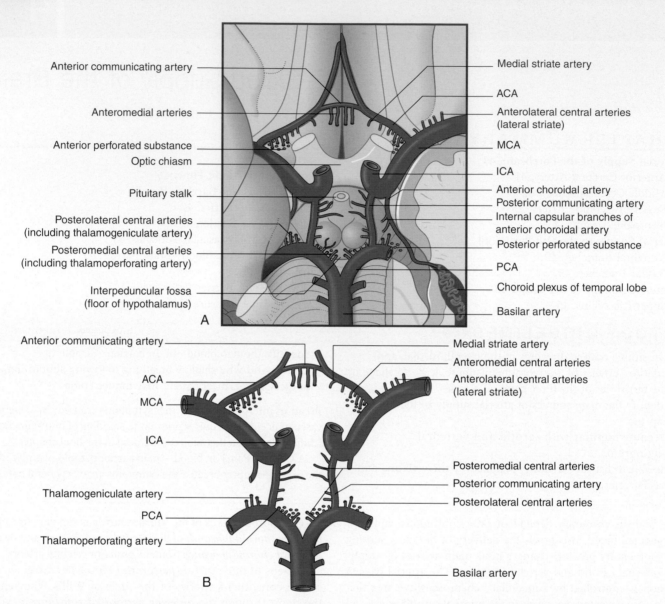

Fig. 4.1 (A) Brain viewed from below, showing background structures related to the circle of Willis. Part of the left temporal lobe (to the right of the picture) has been removed to show the choroid plexus in the inferior horn of the lateral ventricle. (B) The arteries comprising the circle of Willis. The four groups of central branches are shown; the thalamoperforating artery belongs to the posteromedial group, and the thalamogeniculate artery belongs to the posterolateral group. *ACA,* Anterior cerebral artery; *ICA,* internal carotid artery; *MCA,* middle cerebral artery; *PCA,* posterior cerebral artery.

identify in a carotid angiogram (see later). Close to the anterior communicating artery, it gives off the ***medial striate artery***, also known as the *recurrent artery of Heubner* (*pronounced* 'Hoibner'), which contributes to the arterial blood supply of the internal capsule and the head of the caudate nucleus. Cortical branches of the anterior cerebral artery supply the medial surface of the hemisphere as far back as the parietooccipital sulcus (Table 4.1). The branches overlap onto the orbital and lateral surfaces of the hemisphere.

Middle Cerebral Artery (Fig. 4.3)

The middle cerebral artery is the main continuation of the internal carotid, receiving 60% to 80% of the carotid blood flow. It

immediately gives off important central branches and then passes along the depth of the lateral fissure to reach the surface of the insula. There it usually divides into upper and lower divisions. The upper division supplies the frontal and parietal lobes; the lower division supplies the parietal and temporal lobes and the mid-region of the optic radiation. Named branches and their territories are listed in Table 4.2. Overall, the middle cerebral supplies two thirds of the lateral surface of the brain.

The ***central branches*** of the middle cerebral include the ***lateral striate arteries*** (Fig. 4.4). These arteries supply the corpus striatum, internal capsule, and thalamus. Occlusion or rapture of a lateral striate artery causes a classic stroke syndrome (contralateral pure motor hemiplegia — paralysis of the arm, leg,

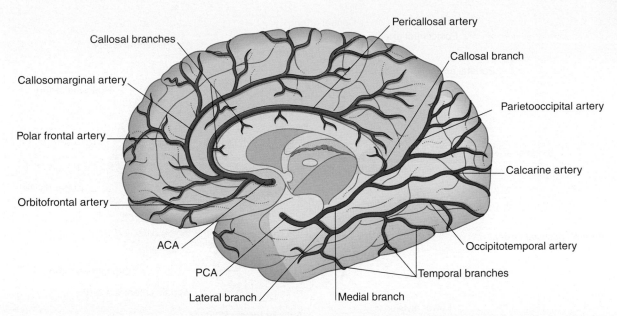

Fig. 4.2 Medial view of the right hemisphere, showing the cortical branches and territories of the three cerebral arteries. *ACA*, Anterior cerebral artery; *PCA*, posterior cerebral artery.

TABLE 4.1 Named Cortical[a] Branches of the Anterior Cerebral Artery.	
Branch	**Territory**
Orbitofrontal	Orbital surface of frontal lobe
Polar frontal	Frontal pole
Callosomarginal	Cingulate and superior frontal gyri; paracentral lobule
Pericallosal	Corpus callosum

[a]The term cortical is conventional. Terminal is better, because these arteries also supply the underlying white matter.

and lower part of the face) due to loss of perfusion in the corticospinal tract in the posterior limb of the internal capsule.

Note: Additional information on the blood supply of the internal capsule is provided in Chapter 35.

Posterior Cerebral Artery (Figs. 4.2 and 4.5)

The two posterior cerebral arteries are the terminal branches of the basilar artery. However, in embryonic life they arise from the internal carotid, and in about 25% of individuals the internal carotid persists as the primary source of blood on one or both sides by way of a large *posterior communicating artery*.

Close to its origin, each posterior cerebral artery gives branches to the midbrain and a *posterior choroidal artery* to the choroid plexus of the lateral ventricle. Additionally, **central branches** pass through the posterior perforated substance (Fig. 4.1). The main artery winds around the midbrain in company with the optic tract. It supplies the splenium of the corpus callosum and the cortex of the occipital and temporal lobes. Named cortical branches and their territories are shown in Table 4.3.

The central branches, called ***thalamoperforating*** and ***thalamogeniculate***, supply the thalamus, subthalamic nucleus, and optic radiation.

Note: Additional information on the central branches is provided in Chapter 35.

Neuroangiography

The cerebral arteries and veins can be displayed under general anaesthesia by rapid injection of a radiopaque dye into the internal carotid or vertebral artery, followed by serial radiography every 2 seconds. The dye completes its course through the arteries, brain capillaries, and veins in about 10 seconds. The *arterial phase* yields either a *carotid angiogram* or a *vertebrobasilar angiogram*. Improved vascular definition in radiographs of the arterial phase or of the *venous phase* can be procured by a process of *subtraction*, whereby positive and negative images of the overlying skull are superimposed on one another, thereby virtually deleting the skull image.

A relatively recent technique, *three-dimensional angiography*, is based on simultaneous angiography from two slightly separate perspectives. In addition, with the use of *magnetic resonance angiography (MRA)* similar imagery of the intracranial and extracranial vessels can be obtained. The noninvasiveness of this method has resulted in its increasing use to substitute for conventional angiographic techniques.

Arterial phases of carotid angiograms are shown in Figs. 4.6 to 4.8.

Fig. 4.9 was taken at the *parenchymal phase*, when the dye is filling a web of minute terminal branches of the anterior and middle cerebral arteries, some of these anastomosing on the brain surface but most occupying the parenchyma (the cortex and subjacent white matter).

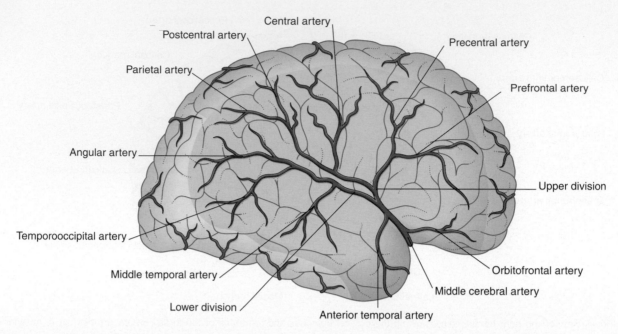

Fig. 4.3 Lateral view of the right cerebral hemisphere, showing the cortical branches and territories of the three cerebral arteries.

TABLE 4.2 **Cortical Branches of the Middle Cerebral Artery.**		
Origin	**Branch(es)**	**Territory**
Stem	Frontobasal	Orbital surface of frontal lobe
	Anterior temporal	Anterior temporal cortex
Upper division	Prefrontal	Prefrontal cortex
	Precentral	Premotor areas
	Central	Pre- and postcentral gyri
	Postcentral	Postcentral and anterior parietal cortex
	Parietal	Posterior parietal cortex
Lower division	Middle temporal	Midtemporal cortex
	Temporooccipital	Temporal and occipital cortex
	Angular	Angular and neighbouring gyri

ARTERIAL SUPPLY TO THE HINDBRAIN

The brainstem and cerebellum are supplied by the vertebral and basilar arteries and their branches (Fig. 4.10).

The two *vertebral arteries* arise from the subclavian arteries and ascend in the neck through the *transverse foramina* of the upper six cervical vertebrae. They enter the skull through the foramen magnum and unite at the lower border of the pons to form the *basilar artery*. The basilar artery ascends on the basilar surface of the pons and at its rostral end divides into two posterior cerebral arteries (Figs. 4.11 and 4.12).

All primary branches of the vertebral and basilar arteries give branches to the brainstem and cerebellum.

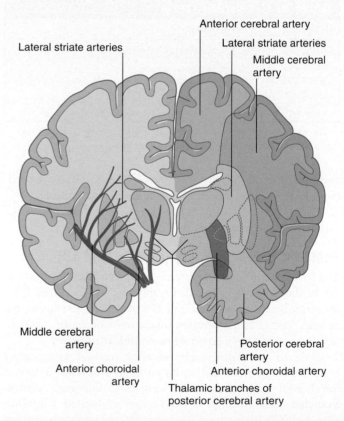

Fig. 4.4 Distribution of perforating branches of the middle cerebral, anterior choroidal, and posterior cerebral arteries (schematic). The anterior choroidal artery arises from the internal carotid.

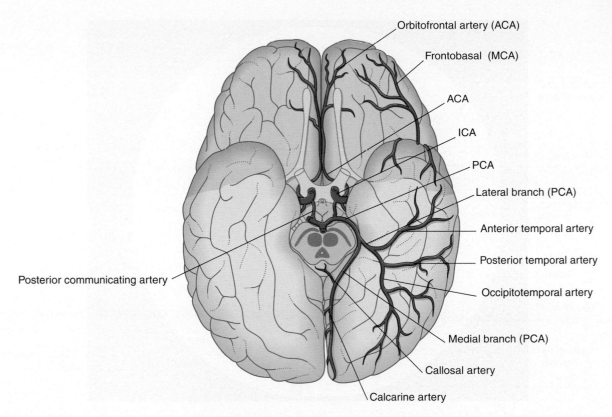

Fig. 4.5 View from below the cerebral hemispheres, showing the cortical branches and territories of the three cerebral arteries. *ACA*, Anterior cerebral artery; *ICA*, internal carotid artery; *MCA*, middle cerebral artery; *PCA*, posterior cerebral artery.

TABLE 4.3 Named Cortical Branches of the Posterior Cerebral Artery.

Branch	Artery	Territory
Lateral	Anterior temporal	Anterior temporal cortex
	Posterior temporal	Posterior temporal cortex
	Occipitotemporal	Posterior temporal and occipital cortex
Medial	Calcarine	Calcarine cortex
	Parietooccipital	Cuneus and precuneus
	Callosal	Splenium of corpus callosum

Vertebral Branches

The *posterior inferior cerebellar artery* supplies the side of the medulla before giving branches to the cerebellum. *Anterior* and *posterior spinal arteries* supply the ventral and dorsal medulla, respectively, before descending through the foramen magnum.

Basilar Branches

The *anterior inferior cerebellar* and *superior cerebellar arteries* supply the side of the pons before giving branches to the cerebellum. The anterior inferior cerebellar and usually the labyrinthine to the inner ear arises directly from the basilar artery.

About a dozen *pontine arteries* supply the full thickness of the medial part of the pons.

The midbrain is supplied by the *posterior cerebral artery* and by the *posterior communicating artery* that links the posterior cerebral artery to the internal carotid artery.

VENOUS DRAINAGE OF THE BRAIN

Venous drainage of the brain is of great importance in relation to neurosurgical procedures. It is also important to the neurologist, because a variety of clinical syndromes that may be produced by venous obstruction, venous thrombosis, and congenital arteriovenous communications. In medical practice, however, complications (other than subdural hematomas, Chapter 5) due to diseases involving cerebral veins are rare in comparison with those affecting cerebral arteries. The cerebral hemispheres are drained by superficial and deep cerebral veins, which, like the intracranial venous sinuses, are devoid of valves.

Superficial Veins

The *superficial cerebral veins* lie in the subarachnoid space overlying the hemispheres. They drain the cerebral cortex and underlying white matter, and empty into intracranial venous sinuses (Figs. 4.13A, 4.14, and 4.15).

The upper part of each hemisphere drains into the *superior sagittal sinus*. The middle part drains into the *cavernous sinus* (as a rule) by way of the *superficial middle cerebral vein*. The lower part drains into the transverse sinus.

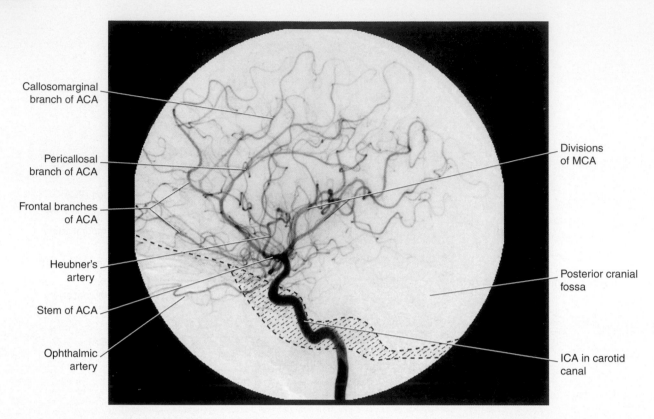

Fig. 4.6 Digital subtracted angiogram (DSA)—Arterial phase of a carotid angiogram, lateral view. Contrast medium injected into the left internal carotid artery is passing through the ACA and MCA. The base of the skull is shown in hatched outline. *ACA*, Anterior cerebral artery; *ICA*, internal carotid artery; *MCA*, middle cerebral artery. (From an original series kindly provided by Dr Michael Modic, Department of Radiology, The Cleveland Clinic Foundation, Cleveland, Ohio, USA.)

Deep Veins (Fig. 4.13B)

The deep cerebral veins drain the corpus striatum, thalamus, and choroid plexuses.

A ***thalamostriate vein*** drains the thalamus and caudate nucleus. Together with a ***choroidal vein***, it forms the ***internal cerebral vein***. The two internal cerebral veins unite beneath the corpus callosum to form the ***great cerebral vein (of Galen)***.

A ***basal vein*** is formed beneath the anterior perforated substance by the union of ***anterior*** and ***deep middle cerebral veins***. The basal vein runs around the crus cerebri and empties into the great cerebral vein.

Finally, the great cerebral vein enters the midpoint of the tentorium cerebelli. As it does so, it unites with the ***inferior sagittal sinus*** to form the ***straight sinus***. The straight sinus empties in turn into the left (or occasionally, right, as we shall see) ***transverse sinus***.

REGULATION OF BLOOD FLOW

Under normal conditions, cerebral blood flow (perfusion) amounts to 700 to 850 mL per minute (approximately 55 mL of blood for every 100 g of brain tissue per minute), accounting for 20% of the total cardiac output. The blood flow is primarily controlled by *autoregulation*, which is defined as the capacity of a tissue to regulate its own blood supply.

The most rapid source of autoregulation is the *intraluminal pressure* within the arterioles. Any increase in pressure elicits a direct *myogenic* response. When other factors are controlled (in animal experiments), the myogenic response is sufficient to maintain steady-state perfusion of the brain within a systemic blood pressure range of 80 to 180 mm Hg (11–24 kPa).

A second powerful source of autoregulation in the central nervous system (CNS) is the H^+ *ion concentration* in the extracellular fluid (ECF) surrounding the arterioles within the brain parenchyma. Generalised relaxation of arteriolar smooth muscle tone is produced by hypercapnia (excess plasma PCO_2). On the other hand, hypocapnia leads to arteriolar constriction.

Local blood flow increases within cortical areas and deep nuclei involved in particular motor, sensory, or cognitive tasks. Local arteriolar relaxation can be accounted for by a rise in K^+ levels caused by propagation of action potentials and by a rise in H^+ caused by increased cell metabolism.

THE BLOOD–BRAIN BARRIER

The nervous system is isolated from the blood by a barrier system that provides a stable and chemically optimal environment for neuronal function. The neurons and neuroglia are

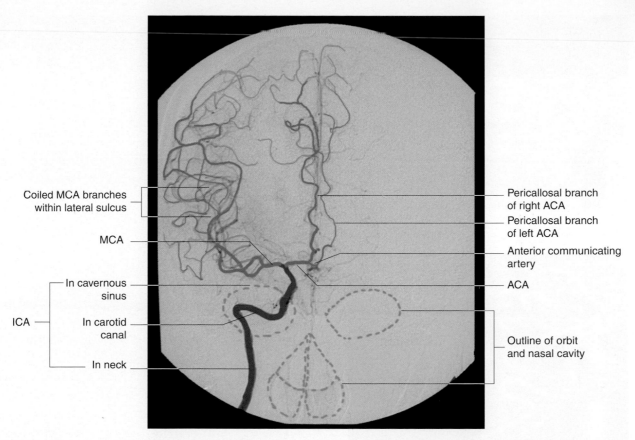

Coiled MCA branches within lateral sulcus

MCA

ICA
- In cavernous sinus
- In carotid canal
- In neck

Pericallosal branch of right ACA

Pericallosal branch of left ACA

Anterior communicating artery

ACA

Outline of orbit and nasal cavity

Fig. 4.7 Digital subtracted angiogram (DSA)—Arterial phase of the right carotid angiogram, anteroposterior view. Note some perfusion of left anterior cerebral artery (ACA) territory (via the anterior communicating artery). *ICA*, internal carotid artery; *MCA*, middle cerebral artery. (Angiogram kindly provided by Dr Pearse Morris, Director, Interventional Neuroradiology, Wake Forest University School of Medicine, Winston-Salem, North Carolina, USA.)

bathed in *brain ECF*, which accounts for 15% of total brain volume.

The extracellular compartments of the CNS are shown diagrammatically in Fig. 4.16. As described elsewhere (Chapter 5), the CSF secreted by the choroid plexuses circulates through the ventricular system and the subarachnoid space before passing through the arachnoid villi into the dural venous sinuses. In addition, the CSF diffuses passively through the ependyma—glial membrane lining the ventricles and enters the brain extracellular spaces. It adds to the ECF produced by the capillary bed and by cell metabolism, and it diffuses through the pia—glial membrane into the subarachnoid space. This 'sink' movement of fluid compensates for the absence of lymphatics in the CNS.

Metabolic water is the only component of the CSF that does not pass through the blood—brain barrier. It carries with it any neurotransmitter substances that have not been recaptured following liberation by neurons, and it accounts for the presence in the subarachnoid space of transmitters and transmitter metabolites that could not penetrate the blood—brain barrier.

Relative contributions to the CSF obtained from a spinal tap are approximately as follows:
- choroid plexuses, 60%
- capillary bed, 30%
- metabolic water, 10%

The blood—brain barrier has two components. One is at the level of the choroid plexus, and the other resides in the CNS capillary bed.

Blood—CSF Barrier (Fig. 4.17)

The blood—CSF barrier resides in the specialised ependymal lining of the choroid plexuses. This choroidal epithelium differs from the general ependymal epithelium in three ways.
1. Cilia are almost completely replaced by microvilli.
2. The cells are connected by tight junctions. These pericellular belts of membrane fusion are the actual site of the blood—CSF barrier.
3. The epithelium contains numerous enzymes specifically involved in the transport of ions and metabolites.

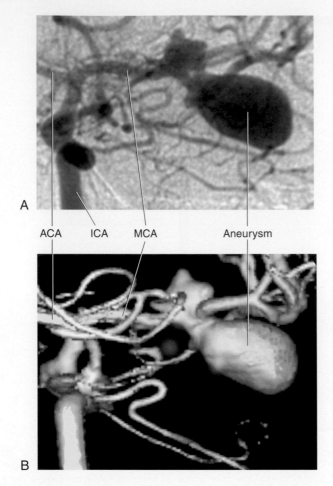

Fig. 4.8 (A) Excerpt from a conventional carotid angiogram, antero-posterior view, showing an aneurysm attached to the middle cerebral artery. (B) Excerpt from a three-dimensional image of the same area. *ACA*, Anterior cerebral artery; *ICA*, internal carotid artery; *MCA*, middle cerebral artery. (Originals kindly provided by Dr Pearse Morris, Director, Interventional Neuroradiology, Wake Forest University School of Medicine, Winston-Salem, North Carolina, USA.)

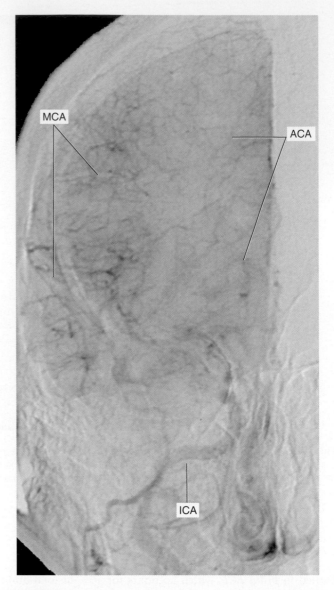

Fig. 4.9 Digital subtracted angiogram (DSA) — Parenchymal phase of a carotid angiogram, anteroposterior view. *ACA*, Anterior cerebral artery; *ICA*, internal carotid artery; *MCA*, middle cerebral artery. (Angiogram kindly provided by Dr Pearse Morris, Director, Interventional Neuroradiology, Wake Forest University School of Medicine, Winston-Salem, North Carolina, USA.)

Blood—ECF Barrier (Fig. 4.18)

The blood—ECF barrier resides in the CNS capillary bed, which differs from that of other capillary beds in three ways:
1. The endothelial cells are connected by tight junctions.
2. Pinocytotic vesicles are rare, and fenestrations are absent.
3. The cells contain the same transport systems as those of the choroidal epithelium.

Roles of Microvascular Pericytes

Pericytes are in cytoplasmic continuity with the endothelial cells by way of gap junctions. Tissue culture studies have provided strong evidence for their primary roles in capillary angiogenesis during development and in the production and maintenance of tight junctions.

Pericytes express receptors for vasoactive mediators, including norepinephrine (noradrenaline), vasopressin, and angiotensin II, all indicative of a role in cerebrovascular autoregulation. In the presence of chronic hypertension, they strengthen the capillary bed by undergoing hypertrophy, hyperplasia, and internal production of cytoplasmic contractile protein filaments.

Pericytes are equipped for a haemostatic function, having an appropriate membrane surface for assembly of the prothrombin complex.

Pericytes are also phagocytic and possess immunoregulatory cytokines.

The surface area of the brain capillary bed is about the size of a tennis court! This huge area accounts for the brain's

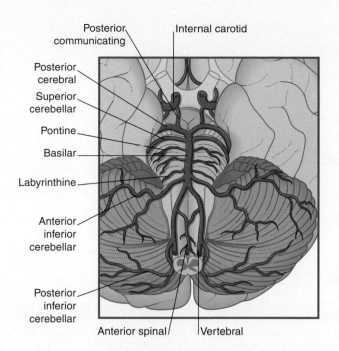

Posterior communicating
Internal carotid
Posterior cerebral
Superior cerebellar
Pontine
Basilar
Labyrinthine
Anterior inferior cerebellar
Posterior inferior cerebellar
Anterior spinal
Vertebral

Fig. 4.10 Arterial supply of hindbrain.

consumption of 20% of basal oxygen intake by the lungs. The density of the cortical capillary bed is demonstrated in the latex cast shown in Fig. 4.19.

Functions of the Blood—Brain Barrier

• Modulation of the entry of metabolic substrates. Glucose, in particular, is a fundamental source of energy for neurons. The level of glucose in the brain ECF is more stable than that in the blood, because the specific carrier becomes saturated when blood glucose rises and becomes hyperactive when it falls.
• Control of ion movements. Na^+-K^+ ATPase in the barrier cells pumps sodium into the CSF and pumps potassium out of the CSF into the blood.
• Prevention of access to the CNS by toxins and by peripheral neurotransmitters escaping into the bloodstream from autonomic nerve endings.

For some clinical notes concerning the blood—brain barrier, see Clinical Panel 4.1. Clinical Panel 4.2 describes the effects of raised intracranial pressure (ICP).

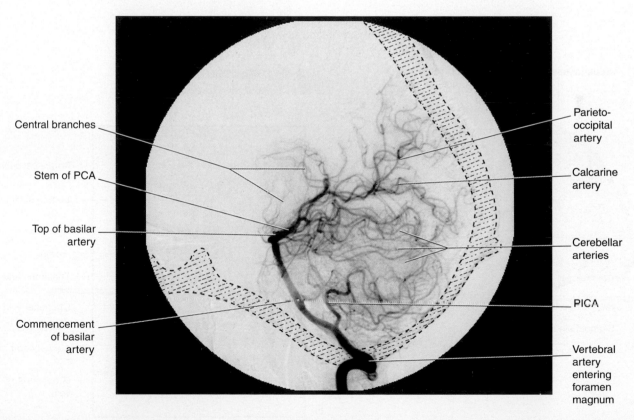

Central branches
Stem of PCA
Top of basilar artery
Commencement of basilar artery
Parieto-occipital artery
Calcarine artery
Cerebellar arteries
PICA
Vertebral artery entering foramen magnum

Fig. 4.11 Digital subtracted angiogram (DSA) — Vertebrobasilar angiogram, lateral view. Contrast medium was injected into the left vertebral artery. Basilar supply to the upper half of the cerebellum is somewhat obscured by overlying posterior parietal branches of the posterior cerebral artery. *PCA*, Posterior cerebral artery; *PICA*, posterior-inferior cerebellar artery. (From an original series kindly provided by Dr Michael Modic, Department of Radiology, The Cleveland Clinic Foundation, Cleveland, Ohio, USA.)

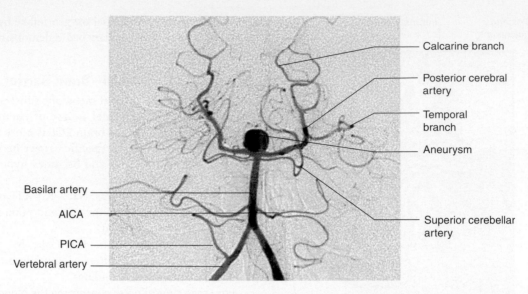

Fig. 4.12 Digital subtracted angiogram (DSA)—Vertebrobasilar angiogram, Towne view (from above and in front), showing the vertebrobasilar arterial system. Note the large aneurysm arising from the bifurcation point of the basilar artery and accounting for the patient's persistent headache. *AICA*, Anterior-inferior cerebellar artery; *PICA*, posterior-inferior cerebellar artery. (Angiogram kindly provided by Dr Pearse Morris, Director, Interventional Neuroradiology, Wake Forest University School of Medicine, Winston-Salem, North Carolina, USA.)

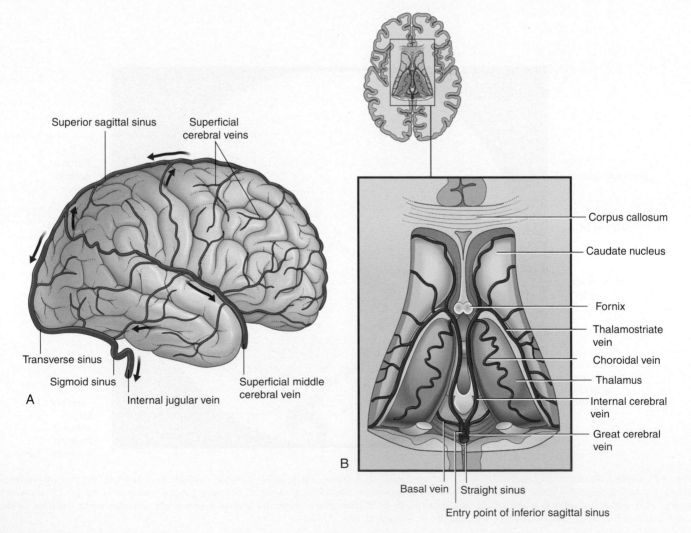

Fig. 4.13 Cerebral veins. (A) Superficial veins viewed from the right side; *arrows* indicate the direction of blood flow. (B) Deep veins viewed from above.

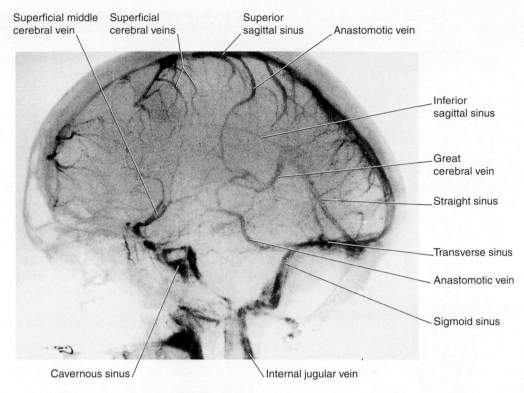

Superficial middle cerebral vein

Superficial cerebral veins

Superior sagittal sinus

Anastomotic vein

Inferior sagittal sinus

Great cerebral vein

Straight sinus

Transverse sinus

Anastomotic vein

Sigmoid sinus

Cavernous sinus

Internal jugular vein

Fig. 4.14 Internal carotid angiogram, venous phase, and lateral view. The dye is draining into the dural venous sinuses. (Photograph kindly provided by Dr James Toland, Department of Radiology, Beaumont Hospital, Dublin, Ireland.)

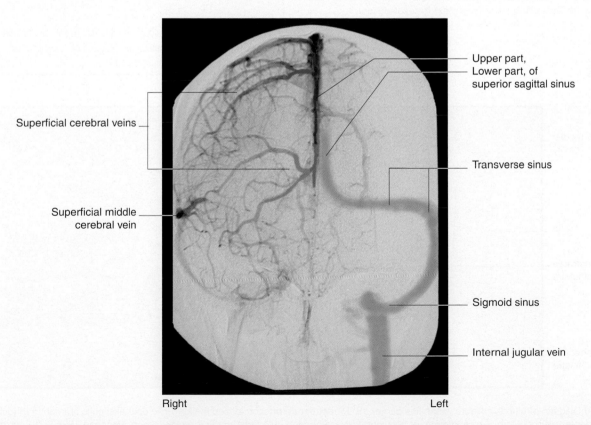

Superficial cerebral veins

Superficial middle cerebral vein

Upper part,
Lower part, of superior sagittal sinus

Transverse sinus

Sigmoid sinus

Internal jugular vein

Right   Left

Fig. 4.15 Internal carotid angiogram, venous phase, and anteroposterior view. Same patient as in Fig. 4.6; this picture taken about 8 seconds later. The vascular pattern is unusual, in that the left rather than the right transverse sinus is dominant. (Angiogram kindly provided by Dr Pearse Morris, Director, Interventional Neuroradiology, Wake Forest University School of Medicine, Winston-Salem, North Carolina, USA.)

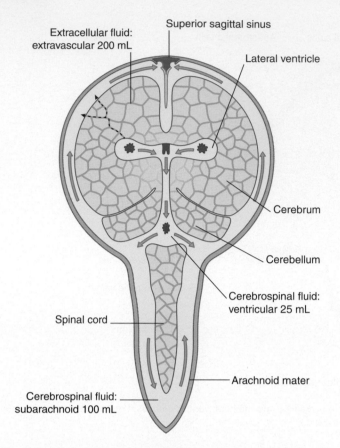

Extracellular fluid: extravascular 200 mL

Superior sagittal sinus

Lateral ventricle

Cerebrum

Cerebellum

Cerebrospinal fluid: ventricular 25 mL

Spinal cord

Arachnoid mater

Cerebrospinal fluid: subarachnoid 100 mL

Fig. 4.16 Extracellular compartments of the brain. Green arrows indicate circulation of the cerebrospinal fluid. Flow of extracellular fluid is shown by the dashed black lines (see text for explanation).

✳ Core Information

Arteries

The circle of Willis comprises the anterior communicating artery and two anterior cerebral arteries, the internal carotids, two posterior communicating arteries, and the two posterior cerebral arteries.

The anterior cerebral artery gives off the medial striate artery (recurrent artery of Heubner) to the anteroinferior internal capsule, then arches around the corpus callosum and supplies the medial surface of the hemisphere as far back as the parietooccipital sulcus, with overlap onto the lateral surface.

The middle cerebral artery enters the lateral sulcus and supplies two thirds of the lateral surface of the hemisphere. Its central branches include the lateral striate supplying the upper part of the internal capsule.

The posterior cerebral artery arises from the basilar artery; it supplies the splenium of the corpus callosum and the occipital and temporal cortex.

The vertebral arteries enter the foramen magnum. They supply the spinal cord, posterior-inferior cerebellum, and medulla oblongata before uniting to form the basilar artery. The basilar artery supplies the anterior-inferior and superior cerebellum, the pons, and inner ear before dividing into posterior cerebral arteries.

Veins

Superficial cerebral veins drain the cerebral cortex and empty into dural venous sinuses. The internal cerebral veins drain the thalami and unite as the great cerebral vein. The great veins drain the corpus striatum via the basal vein before entering the straight sinus.

Autoregulation

Hypercapnia causes arteriolar dilatation; hypocapnia causes constriction. A rise in intraluminal pressure produces a direct myogenic response by arteriolar walls.

Blood–Brain Barrier

A blood–CSF barrier resides in the choroidal epithelium (modified ependyma) of the ventricles. A blood–ECF barrier resides in the endothelium of the brain capillary bed.

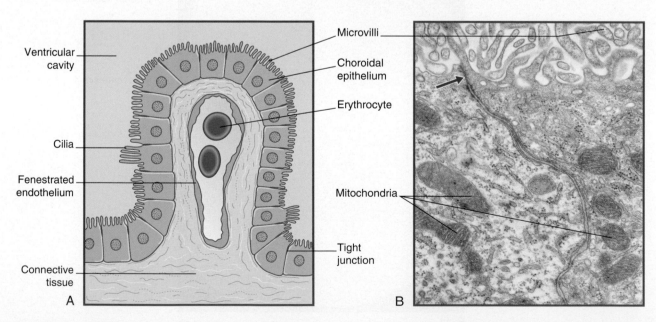

Ventricular cavity

Microvilli

Choroidal epithelium

Erythrocyte

Cilia

Fenestrated endothelium

Mitochondria

Tight junction

Connective tissue

A

B

Fig. 4.17 (A) Diagram of blood–cerebrospinal fluid barrier. (B) Ultrastructure of choroidal epithelium. The epithelial cells are rich in mitochondria and granular endoplasmic reticulum. Apical regions of adjacent cells are bonded by a tight junction *(arrow)*. (From Pannese 1994, with permission from Thieme.)

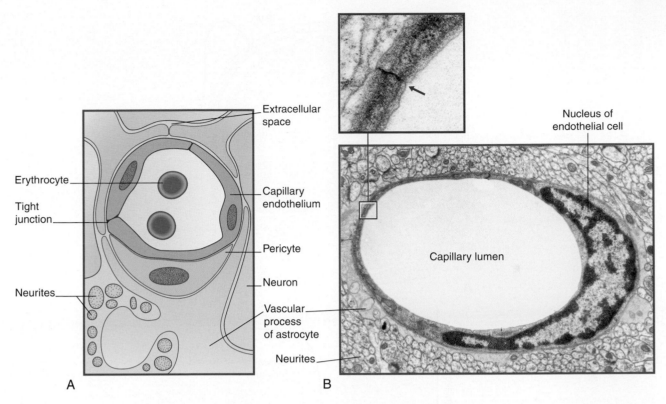

Labels in figure A:
- Extracellular space
- Erythrocyte
- Tight junction
- Neurites
- Capillary endothelium
- Pericyte
- Neuron
- Vascular process of astrocyte
- Neurites

A

Labels in figure B:
- Nucleus of endothelial cell
- Capillary lumen
- Neurites

B

Fig. 4.18 (A) Diagram of the blood–extracellular fluid barrier. (Astrocytes are described in Chapter 6.) (B) Central nervous system capillary. In this transverse section, a single endothelial cell completely surrounds the lumen, its edges being sealed by a tight junction *(inset)*. Outside its basement membrane, the capillary is invested with an astrocytic sheath. (From Pannese 1994, with permission from Thieme.)

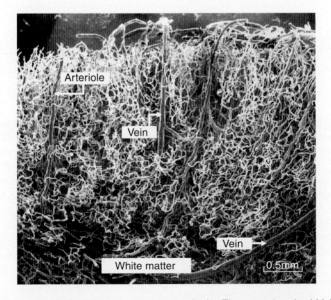

Labels in figure:
- Arteriole
- Vein
- Vein
- White matter
- 0.5mm

Fig. 4.19 Latex injection cast of the blood vessels in a human postmortem brain. The convoluted whitish threads represent cortical capillaries. (From Duvernoy et al. 1981, with permission from Thieme.)

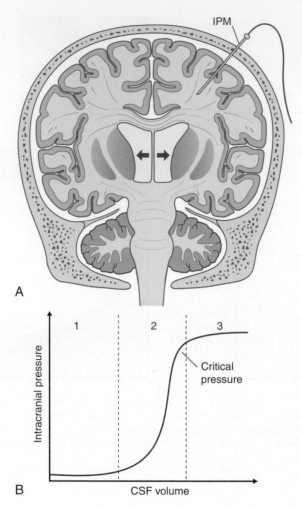

A

B

Intracranial pressure

CSF volume

1   2   3

Critical pressure

Fig. 4.20 (A) Adult hydrocephalus. *Arrows* indicate compression of the cerebral parenchyma by expanding lateral ventricles. (B) Intracranial pressure—CSF volume curve. *CSF,* Cerebrospinal fluid; *IPM,* intraparenchymal pressure monitor. (Based on Steiner and Andrews 2006.)

CLINICAL PANEL 4.1   Blood—Brain Barrier Pathology

The following five conditions are associated with breakdown of the blood—brain barrier:

1. Patients suffering from hypertension are liable to attacks of *hypertensive encephalopathy* should the blood pressure exceed the power of the arterioles to control it. The pressure may then open the tight junctions of the brain capillary endothelium. Rapid exudation of plasma causes *cerebral oedema* with severe headache and vomiting, sometimes progressing to convulsions and coma.

2. In patients with severe *hypercapnia* brought about by reduced ventilation of the lungs (as in pulmonary or heart disease, or after surgery), relaxation of arteriolar muscle may be sufficient to induce cerebral oedema even if the blood pressure is normal. In this case, the oedema may be expressed by mental confusion and drowsiness progressing to coma.

3. *Brain injury,* whether from trauma or spontaneous haemorrhage, leads to oedema owing to the osmotic effects of tissue damage (and other factors).

4. *Infections* of the brain or meninges are accompanied by breakdown of the blood—brain barrier, perhaps because of the large-scale emigration of leukocytes through the brain capillary bed. The breakdown can be exploited because the porous capillary walls will permit the passage of non-lipid-soluble antibiotics.

The capillary bed of *brain tumours* is fenestrated. As a result, radioactive tracers too large to penetrate healthy brain capillaries can be detected within tumours.

CLINICAL PANEL 4.2 Intracranial Pressure Curve

Fig. 4.20 represents progressive ventricular expansion in an adult case of hydrocephalus. As noted in Clinical Panel 5.3, hydrocephalus can result from obstruction of the fourth ventricular outlets by leptomeningeal webs caused by meningitis. The same effect can be induced by accumulated blood around the base of the brain following spontaneous arterial haemorrhage into the subarachnoid space.

The lateral ventricles are expanding progressively *(arrows)*. The rising intracranial pressure is being monitored by an intraparenchymal pressure monitor. The vascular perfusion pressure rises in parallel.

(1) The pressure—volume curve commences with a relatively flat part: interstitial fluid is displaced into the subarachnoid space; subarachnoid cerebrospinal fluid (CSF) is shifted into the spinal dural sac; and venous blood is squeezed through the intracranial sinuses into the internal jugular vein. (2) Intracranial pressure rises with increasing speed during the steep part. (3) A critical pressure point is reached where *decompensation* takes place: the vascular circulation is completely blocked, the vital centres run out of oxygen, and the patient loses consciousness and will die unless the CSF is urgently drained through a burr (drill) hole.

SUGGESTED READINGS

Abbott NJ, Pizzo ME, Preston JE, Janigro D, Thorne RG. The role of brain barriers in fluid movement in the CNS: is there a 'glymphatic' system? *Acta Neuropathol.* 2018;135:387—407.

Balabanonov B, Dore-Duffy P. Role of the microvascular pericyte in the blood—brain barrier. *J Neurosci Res.* 1998;53:637—644.

Bartanusz V, Jezova D, Alajajian B, Digicaylioglu M. The blood—spinal cord barrier: morphology and clinical implications. *Ann Neurol.* 2011;70:194—206.

Benarroch EE. Blood—brain barrier: recent developments and clinical correlations. *Neurology.* 2012;78:1268—1276.

Dalkara T, Gursoy-Ozdemir Y, Yemisci M. Brain microvascular pericytes in health and disease. *Acta Neuropathol.* 2011;122:1—9.

Horng S, Therattil A, Moyon S, et al. Astrocytic tight junctions control inflammatory CNS lesion pathogenesis. *J Clin Invest.* 2017;127:3136—3151.

Kaur C, Rathnasamy G, Ling E-A. The choroid plexus in healthy and diseased brain. *J Neuropathol Exp Neurol.* 2016;75:198—213.

Mastorakos P, McGavern D. The anatomy and immunology of vasculature in the central nervous system. *Sci Immunol.* 2019;4:1—14.

Morita S, Furube E, Mannari T, et al. Heterogeneous vascular permeability and alternative diffusion barrier in sensory circum-ventricular organs of adult mouse brain. *Cell Tissue Res.* 2016;363:497—511.

Pannese E. *Neurocytology: Fine Structure of Neurons, Nerve Processes, and Neuroglial Cells.* New York: Thieme; 1994.

Popescu BO, Toescu EC, Popescu LM, et al. Blood—brain barrier alterations in ageing and dementia. *J Neurol Sci.* 2009;283:99—106.

Scremin IU. Cerebral vascular system. In: Paxinos G, Mai JK, eds. *The Human Nervous System.* 2nd ed. Amsterdam: Elsevier; 2004.

Steiner LA, Andrews PJD. Monitoring the injured brain: ICP and CBF. *Br J Anaesth.* 2006;1:26—38.

Meninges

STUDY GUIDELINES

1. Be able to contrast the structure of the dura mater with that of the pia—arachnoid.
2. Be able to follow a drop of venous blood from the superior sagittal sinus to the internal jugular vein and from an ophthalmic vein to the sigmoid sinus.
3. Name the nerves supplying (a) the supratentorial dura and (b) the infratentorial dura.
4. Identify the different vessels responsible for extradural, subdural, and subarachnoid bleeding.
5. Explain the mechanism of papilloedema and why spinal tap (lumbar puncture) should not be undertaken in its presence.
6. Trace a drop of the cerebrospinal fluid from a lateral ventricle to (a) its point of entry into the bloodstream, and (b) an in situ lumbar puncture needle.
7. Know about a major cause of hydrocephalus (a) in infancy, (b) in adults, and why both are examples of 'outlet obstruction'.

The meninges surround the central nervous system (CNS) and suspend it in the protective jacket provided by the cerebrospinal fluid (CSF). The meninges comprise the tough *dura mater* or *pachymeninx* (*Gr.* 'thick membrane') and the *leptomeninges* (*Gr.* 'slender membranes') consisting of the *arachnoid mater* and *pia mater*. Between the arachnoid and the pia is the *sub-arachnoid space* filled with the CSF.

CRANIAL MENINGES

Dura Mater

The terminology used to describe the cranial dura mater varies among different authors. It seems best to regard it as a single, tough layer of fibrous tissue that is fused with the endosteum (inner periosteum) of the skull, except where it is reflected into the interior of the vault or is stretched across the skull base. Wherever it separates from the periosteum, the intervening space contains dural venous sinuses (Fig. 5.1).

Two great dural folds extend into the cranial cavity and help to stabilise the brain. These are the *falx cerebri* and the *tentorium cerebelli*.

The falx cerebri occupies the longitudinal fissure between the cerebral hemispheres. Its attached border extends from the *crista galli* of the ethmoid bone to the upper surface of the tentorium cerebelli. Along the vault of the skull, it encloses the *superior sagittal sinus*. Its free border contains the *inferior sagittal sinus* that unites with the *great cerebral vein of Galen* to form the *straight sinus*. The straight sinus travels along the line of attachment of the falx cerebri to tentorium cerebelli and meets the superior sagittal sinus at the *confluence of the sinuses*.

The crescentic *tentorium cerebelli* arches like a tent above the posterior cranial fossa, being lifted up by the falx cerebri in the midline. The attached margin of the tentorium encloses the *transverse sinuses* on the inner surface of the occipital bone and the *superior petrosal sinuses* along the upper border of the petrous temporal bone. The attached margin reaches to the posterior clinoid processes of the sphenoid bone. Most of the blood from the superior sagittal sinus usually empties into the right transverse sinus (Fig. 5.2).

The free margin of the tentorium is U-shaped. The tips of the U are attached to the anterior clinoid processes. Just behind this, the two limbs of the U are linked by a sheet of dura, the *diaphragma sellae*, which is pierced by the pituitary stalk. Laterally, the dura falls away into the middle cranial fossae from the limbs of the U, creating the *cavernous sinus* on each side (Fig. 5.3). Behind the sphenoid bone, the concavity of the U encloses the midbrain.

The cavernous sinus receives blood from the orbit via the ophthalmic veins. The superior petrosal sinus joins the transverse sinus at its junction with the *sigmoid sinus*. The sigmoid sinus descends along the occipital bone and drains into the bulb of the internal jugular vein. The bulb also receives the *inferior*

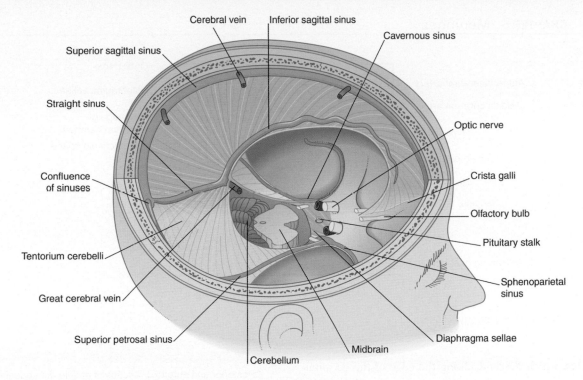

Fig. 5.1 Dural reflections and venous sinuses. The midbrain occupies the tentorial notch.

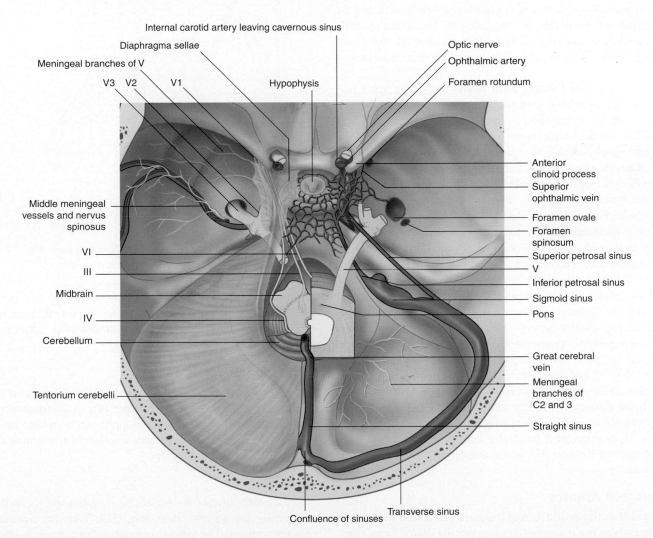

Fig. 5.2 Venous sinuses on the base of the skull. The dura mater has been removed on the right side. The inset indicates where grooves for sinuses are seen on the dry skull. On the left, the midbrain is seen at the level of the tentorial notch. On the right, a lower level section shows the trigeminal nerve attached to the pons.

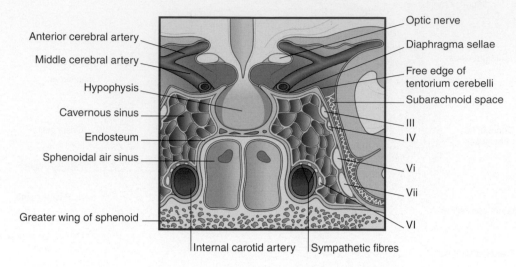

Anterior cerebral artery

Middle cerebral artery

Hypophysis

Cavernous sinus

Endosteum

Sphenoidal air sinus

Greater wing of sphenoid

Optic nerve

Diaphragma sellae

Free edge of tentorium cerebelli

Subarachnoid space

III

IV

Vi

Vii

VI

Internal carotid artery | Sympathetic fibres

Fig. 5.3 Coronal section of the cavernous sinus.

petrosal sinus, which descends along the edge of the occipital bone.

The tentorium cerebelli divides the cranial cavity into a **supratentorial compartment** containing the forebrain, and an **infratentorial compartment** containing the hindbrain. A small **falx cerebelli** is attached to the undersurface of the tentorium cerebelli and to the internal occipital crest of the occipital bone.

Innervation of the Cranial Dura Mater. The dura mater lining the supratentorial compartment of the cranial cavity receives sensory innervation from the trigeminal nerve: the lining of the anterior cranial fossa, anterior part of the falx cerebri, and tentorium cerebelli is supplied by the nerve's ophthalmic branch, and the lining of the middle cranial fossa and midregion of the vault is mainly supplied by the recurrent meningeal nerve **(nervus spinosus)** (Fig. 5.2). The trigeminal nerve leaves the mandibular branch outside the foramen ovale to return via the foramen spinosum and accompany the **middle meningeal artery** and its branches. Stretching or inflammation of the supratentorial dura gives rise to frontal or parietal headache.

The dura mater lining the infratentorial compartment is supplied by branches of the upper three cervical spinal nerves entering the foramen magnum (and also distributed by the vagus or hypoglossal nerves) (Fig. 5.2). All meningeal nerves have an autonomic component (postganglionic sympathetic). Occipital and posterior neck pains accompany the disturbance of the infratentorial dura. Acute meningitis involving posterior cranial fossa meninges is associated with **neck rigidity** and often with **head retraction** brought about by reflex contraction of the posterior nuchal muscles, which are supplied by cervical nerves. Violent occipital headache follows **subarachnoid haemorrhage** (see Chapter 35), where free blood swirls around the hindbrain.

Meningeal Arteries

Embedded in the endosteum of the skull are several **meningeal arteries** whose main function is to supply the **diploë** (bone marrow). The largest is the **middle meningeal artery**, which

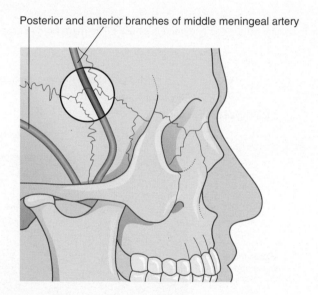

Posterior and anterior branches of middle meningeal artery

Fig. 5.4 Side view of skull. The circle encloses the pterion.

ramifies over the inner surface of the temporal and parietal bones. Tearing of this artery, with its accompanying vein, is the usual source of an **extradural hematoma** (Fig. 5.4, Clinical Panel 5.1).

Arachnoid Mater

The arachnoid (*Gr.* 'spidery') mater is a thin, fibrocellular layer in direct contact with the dura mater (Fig. 5.5). Its outermost cells are bonded to one another by tight junctions that seal the **subarachnoid space**. Innumerable **arachnoid trabeculae** cross the space to reach the pia mater.

Pia Mater

The pia mater invests the brain closely, following its contours and lining the various sulci (Fig. 5.5). Like the arachnoid, it is fibrocellular. The cellular component of the pia is external and permeable to the CSF. The fibrous component occupies a

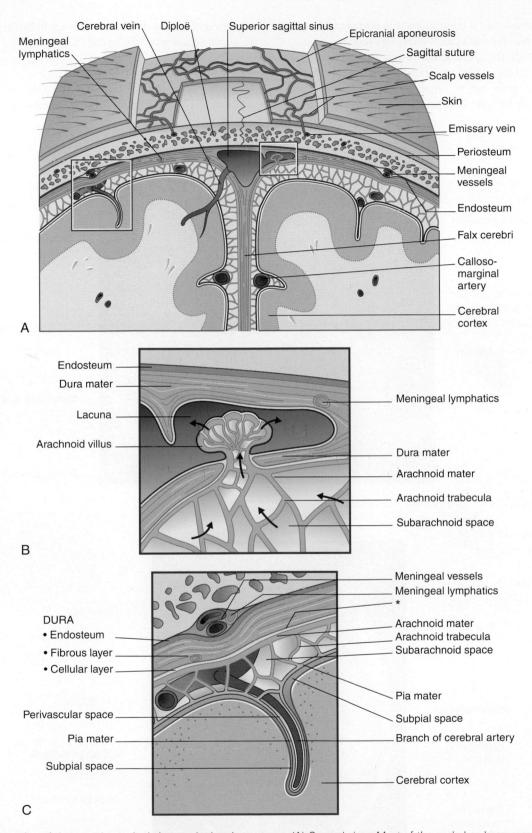

Fig. 5.5 Coronal section of the superior sagittal sinus and related structures. (A) General view. Most of the scalp has been removed to show two emissary veins transferring blood from the diploë into scalp veins on the surface of the epicranial aponeurosis. On the right, the diploë is being fed and drained by meningeal vessels. Also seen is a cerebral vein draining into the superior sagittal sinus. (B) Enlargement from (A), showing an arachnoid granulation transferring cerebrospinal fluid from the subarachnoid space to a lacuna connected to the superior sagittal sinus. *Arrows* indicate direction of flow. (C) Enlargement from (A), showing an artery sequentially surrounded by a perivascular space, pia, and a subpial space. The *asterisk* marks the potential space between dura and arachnoid for spread of subdural blood from a torn cerebral vein. Note the extradural position of the meningeal vessels.

narrow **subpial space** that is continuous with **perivascular spaces** around cerebral blood vessels penetrating the brain surface.

Note: Although the subarachnoid and subpial spaces are proven, there is no sign of any 'subdural space' in properly fixed material. Such a space can be created, however, by leakage of blood into the cellular layer of the dura mater following a tear of

a cerebral vein at its point of anchorage to the fibrous layer. (See *Subdural hematomas* in Clinical Panel 5.1.)

Subarachnoid Cisterns

Along the base of the brain and the sides of the brainstem, pools of CSF occupy subarachnoid cisterns (Figs. 5.6 and 5.7).

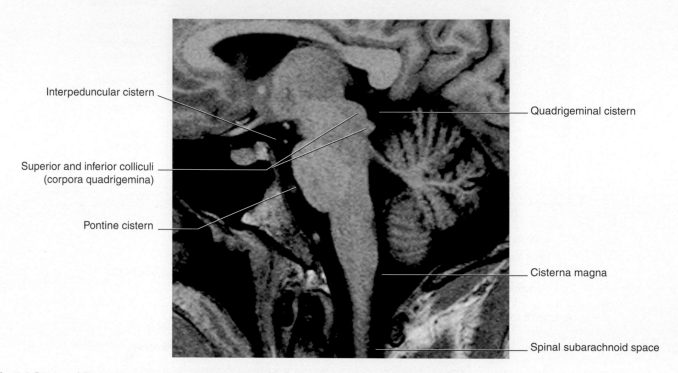

Fig. 5.6 Portion of Fig. 2.7 showing subarachnoid cisterns.

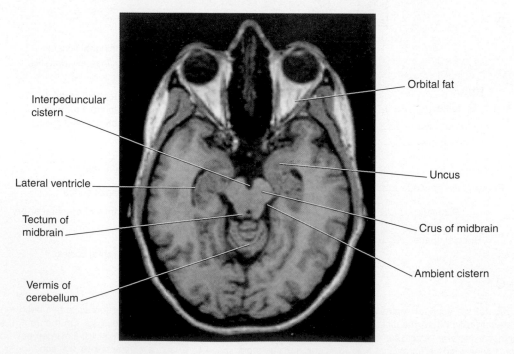

Fig. 5.7 Horizontal MRI. Note the proximity of the uncus to the crus of the midbrain (cf. *uncal herniation,* Clinical Panel 6.2). (From a series kindly provided by Professor J. Paul Finn, Director, Magnetic Resonance Research, Department of Radiology, David Geffen School of Medicine at UCLA, California, USA.)

TABLE 5.1 Subarachnoid Cisterns.

Cistern	Location
Ambient (cisterna ambiens)	On each side of the midbrain
Chiasmatic	Behind and above the optic chiasm
Cistern of lateral cerebral fossa	Along the lateral sulcus (Sylvian fissure)
Cisterna magna	Between the cerebellum and the dorsal surface of medulla oblongata
Interpeduncular	Interpeduncular fossa
Lateral cerebellomedullary	Along each side of the medulla
Lumbar cistern	In the spinal canal and below the spinal cord proper
Pontine cistern	Ventral to pons
Quadrigeminal	Surrounding the great cerebral vein dorsal to the midbrain colliculi (quadrigeminal bodies)

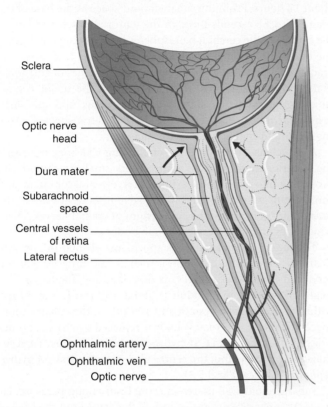

Fig. 5.8 Horizontal section of the left orbit. The subarachnoid space extends forward to the level of fusion of dura mater with the scleral coat of the eyeball (arrows).

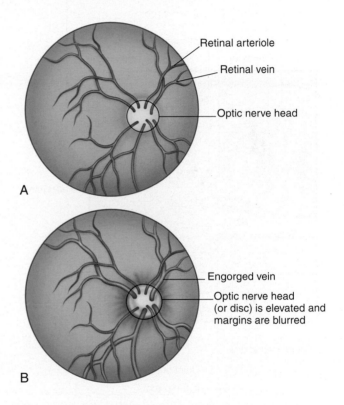

Fig. 5.9 Fundus oculi as seen with an ophthalmoscope. (A) Normal. (B) Papilloedema resulting from raised intracranial pressure.

The largest of these is the **cisterna magna**, in the interval between the cerebellum and medulla oblongata. More rostrally are the **cisterna pontis** ventral to the pons, the **interpeduncular cistern** between the cerebral peduncles, and the **cisterna ambiens** at the side of the midbrain. The complete list of cisterns is in Table 5.1.

Sheath of the Optic Nerve

The optic nerve is composed of CNS white matter, and it has a complete meningeal investment. The dura mater fuses with the **scleral shell** of the eyeball; the subarachnoid space is a tubular **cul de sac** (dead end). The central vessels of the retina pierce the meninges to enter it (Fig. 5.8). Any sustained elevation of intracranial pressure will be transmitted to the subarachnoid sleeve surrounding the nerve. The **central vein** will be compressed, resulting in swelling of the retinal tributaries of the vein and oedema of the **optic nerve head** (or **optic disc**), where the optic nerve begins. The condition is known as **papilloedema** (Fig. 5.9). It can be recognised on inspection of the retina with an ophthalmoscope.

SPINAL MENINGES (FIG. 5.10)

The spinal dural sac is like a test tube, attached to the rim of the foramen magnum and reaching down to the level of the second sacral vertebra. The outer surface of the tube is adherent to the posterior longitudinal ligament of the vertebrae in the midline; elsewhere, it is surrounded by fat containing the

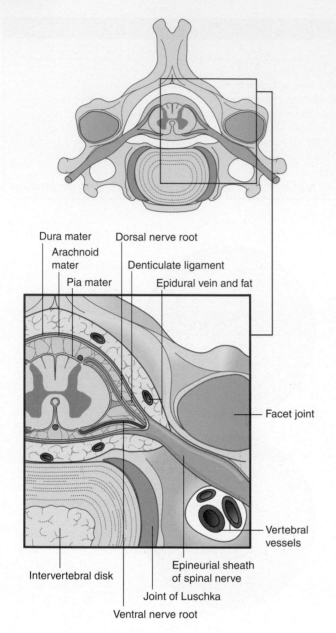

Dura mater

Arachnoid mater

Pia mater

Dorsal nerve root

Denticulate ligament

Epidural vein and fat

Facet joint

Vertebral vessels

Intervertebral disk

Epineurial sheath of spinal nerve

Joint of Luschka

Ventral nerve root

Fig. 5.10 Contents of cervical vertebral canal. The dura mater blends with the epineurium of the spinal nerve trunk.

epidural, ***internal vertebral venous plexus of Batson*** (see Chapter 14).

The internal surface of the dura is lined with arachnoid mater. The pia mater lines the surface of the spinal cord and is attached to the dura mater at regular intervals by the serrated ***denticulate*** (toothed) ***ligament***.

Because the spinal cord reaches only to the level of the first or second lumbar vertebra, a large ***lumbar cistern*** is created, containing the free-floating motor and sensory roots of the sacral and lower lumbar spinal nerves (see Chapter 14). The lumbar cistern may be tapped to procure samples of CSF for analysis (Fig. 5.12, Clinical Panel 5.2) or to deliver a spinal anaesthetic (see Chapter 14).

The spinal dura mater (with its arachnoid lining) is sometimes referred to as the ***thecal sac*** (*Gr.* 'enclosing capsule').

CIRCULATION OF THE CEREBROSPINAL FLUID (FIG. 5.11)

The source of the CSF is from the secretion of the ***choroid plexuses*** into the ventricles of the brain. From the lateral ventricles, the CSF enters the third ventricle via the ***interventricular foramen (of Monro)***. It descends to the fourth ventricle through the aqueduct and squirts into the subarachnoid space through the ***median aperture (foramen of Magendie)*** and ***lateral aperture***. (Flow within the central canal of the spinal cord is negligible.)

Within the subarachnoid space, some of the CSF descends through the foramen magnum, reaching the lumbar cistern in about 12 hours. From the subarachnoid space at the base of the brain, the CSF ascends through the tentorial notch and bathes the surface of the cerebral hemispheres before being returned to the blood through the ***arachnoid granulations*** (Fig. 5.5). The arachnoid granulations are pinhead-sized pouches of arachnoid mater projecting through the dural wall of the major venous sinuses, especially the superior sagittal sinus and the small ***venous lacunae*** that open into it. The CSF is transported across the arachnoid epithelium in giant vacuoles.

As much as a quarter of the circulating CSF may not reach the superior sagittal sinus. Some enters small arachnoid villi projecting into spinal veins exiting intervertebral foramina, and some drains into lymphatics in the adventitia of arteries at the base of the brain and in the epineurium of cranial nerves. These lymphatics drain into cervical lymph nodes.

The rate of CSF formation is approximately 500 mL per day (300 mL secreted by the choroid plexus and another 200 mL produced from other sources, as described in Chapter 4). The total CSF volume in an adult is about 150 mL (25 to 50 mL within the ventricular system and 100 mL in the subarachnoid space); therefore, this total volume is replaced two to three times a day. A disturbance in CSF hydrodynamics will cause an accumulation of CSF within the ventricular system: a state of ***hydrocephalus*** (Clinical Panel 5.3).

Subarachnoid CSF passes into the brain along paravascular spaces that encircle arterioles and, at this level or at the level of the capillary endothelium, can pass into the closely opposed ***astroglial end-feet***, which contribute to the formation of the ***blood–brain barrier***. This paravascular system or glymphatic system provides a functional waste clearance pathway for the central nervous system. This is an active process that occurs via water channels or pores within the plasma membrane of the astrocyte end-feet and involves the integral membrane protein aquaporin-5 (AQP5). The water is released from the astrocytes and distributed into the extracellular space where it combines with water produced by metabolic processes of brain cells. This interstitial fluid 'flows' through the brain and can leave via the pial or ependymal surfaces to enter the CSF and eventually be transported out of the brain into the blood circulation.

The presence of a meningeal lymphatic system has been around in the literature for almost 200 years but largely ignored. However, a recent discovery shows that the dural sinuses and meningeal arteries are in fact lined with conventional lymphatic

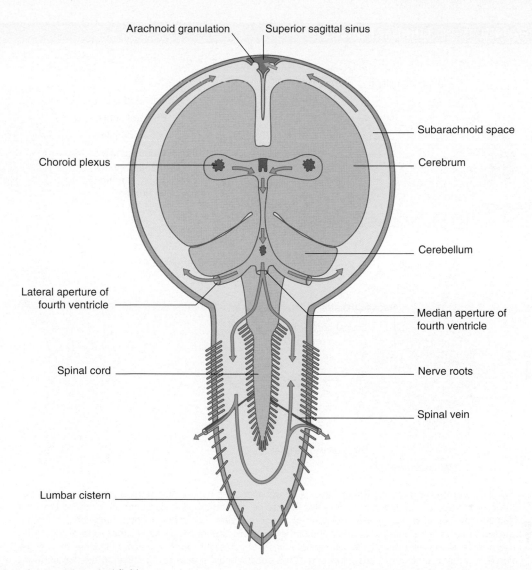

Arachnoid granulation   Superior sagittal sinus

Subarachnoid space

Choroid plexus

Cerebrum

Cerebellum

Lateral aperture of
fourth ventricle

Median aperture of
fourth ventricle

Spinal cord

Nerve roots

Spinal vein

Lumbar cistern

Fig. 5.11 Circulation of the cerebrospinal fluid.

vessels, and that this long-elusive vasculature forms a connecting pathway to the glymphatic system.

Understanding the nature of fluid dynamics within the brain is essential to the understanding of pathologies such as Alzheimer disease and the aging process. The activity of meningeal lymphatics could also affect levels of immune neuromodulators such as cytokines in the brain parenchyma; this may in turn affect their influence on brain function.

CLINICAL PANEL 5.1 Extradural and Subdural Hematomas

An *extradural (epidural) hematoma* is typically caused by a blow to the side of the head severe enough to cause a fracture with associated tearing of the anterior or posterior branch of the middle meningeal artery. Most cases remain unconscious unless treated. Occasionally, following the initial *concussion* of the brain, with loss of consciousness, there may be a *lucid interval* of several hours. Onset of increasing headache and drowsiness signals *cerebral compression* produced by expansion of the hematoma. Coma and death will supervene unless the hematoma is drained. The favoured site of access is the H-shaped suture complex known as the *pterion*, which overlies the anterior branch of the middle meningeal artery (Fig. 5.4).

Subdural hematomas are caused by rupture of superficial cerebral veins in transit from the brain to an intracranial venous sinus. An *acute subdural* *hematoma* most often follows severe head injury in children. It must always be suspected where a child remains unconscious after a head injury. Child-battering is a possible explanation if this situation arises in the home. A *subacute subdural hematoma* may follow head injury at any age. Symptoms and signs of raised intracranial pressure (described in Chapter 6) develop up to 3 weeks after the injury.

Chronic subdural hematomas occur in older people, where the transit veins have become brittle and made taut by shrinkage of the aging brain. Head injury may be mild or even absent. A significant number of these patients have a coagulopathy (e.g. from anticoagulant therapy or excess alcohol intake). Presenting symptoms are variable and include personality changes, headaches, and epileptic seizures.

CLINICAL PANEL 5.2   Lumbar Puncture

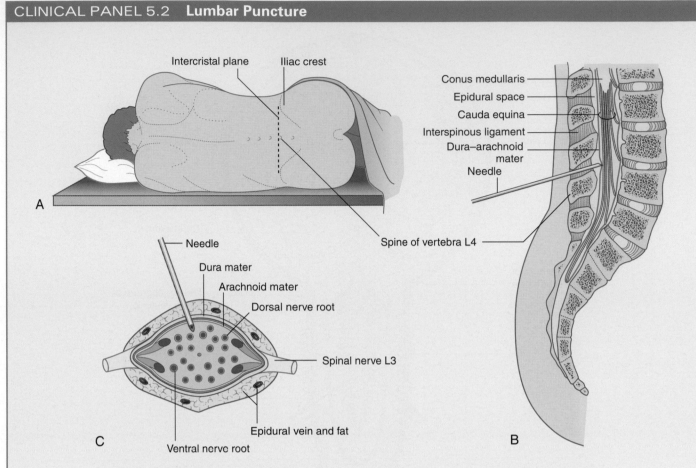

Fig. 5.12 Lumbar Puncture (Spinal Tap). (A) The patient lies on one side, curled forward to open the interspinous spaces of the lumbar region. The spine of vertebra L4 is identified in the intercristal (supracristal) plane at the level of the tops of the iliac crests. (B) Under aseptic conditions, a lumbar puncture needle is introduced obliquely above the spine of vertebra L4, parallel to the plane of the spine. The needle is passed through the interspinous ligament. A slight 'give' is perceived when the needle pierces the dura–arachnoid mater and enters the subarachnoid space. (C) Transverse section showing the cauda equina floating in the subarachnoid space. The ventral and dorsal roots of spinal nerve L3 are coming together as they leave the lumbar cistern.

CLINICAL PANEL 5.3   Hydrocephalus

Hydrocephalus (*Gr.* 'water in the head') denotes accumulation of the cerebrospinal fluid (CSF) in the ventricular system. With the exception of overproduction of the CSF by a rare papilloma of the choroid plexus, hydrocephalus is a pathologic state that results in an excessive accumulation of the CSF within the ventricles (and their consequent dilatation) or within the subarachnoid space. (The term hydrocephalus is not used to describe the 'accumulation' of fluid in the ventricles and subarachnoid space in association with senile atrophy of the brain, but the term **hydrocephalus ex vacuo** is occasionally used.) There are several different pathophysiologic processes that can lead to hydrocephalus (e.g. inflammation, neoplasms, trauma, and changes in CSF osmolality), suggesting that our currently preferred explanation that it only reflects 'blockage' of CSF pathways may be too simplistic and perhaps incorrect.

One developmental syndrome where hydrocephalus is encountered in infancy is the *Arnold–Chiari malformation*, where the cerebellum is partly extruded into the vertebral canal during foetal life because the posterior cranial fossa is underdeveloped. In untreated cases, the child's head may become as large as a football and the cerebral hemispheres paper-thin. The condition is nearly always associated with spina bifida (see Chapter 14). Early treatment is essential to prevent severe brain damage. Attempts to treat the hydrocephalus involve the use of a shunt or a catheter with one end inserted into a lateral ventricle and the other inserted into the internal jugular vein.

An abrupt or subacute form of hydrocephalus can occur if CSF flow is disrupted by the displacement of the cerebellum into the foramen magnum or to obstruct the fourth ventricle, caused by a space-occupying lesion (mass) such as a tumour or hematoma (see Chapter 6).

Meningitis can cause hydrocephalus at any age. One component of the mechanism(s) that may be responsible for its development is leptomeningeal adhesions that compromise CSF circulation at the level of the ventricular outlets, the tentorial notch, and/or the arachnoid granulations.

Core Information

Meninges

The meninges comprise dura, arachnoid, and pia mater. The subarachnoid space contains the cerebrospinal fluid (CSF).

The cranial dura mater shows two large folds: the falx cerebri and tentorium cerebelli. The attached edge of the falx encloses the superior sagittal sinus, which usually enters the right transverse sinus. The free edge of the falx encloses the inferior sagittal sinus, which joins the great cerebral vein of Galen, forming the straight sinus that enters the confluence of the superior sagittal and transverse sinuses. The attached edge of the tentorium encloses the transverse sinus, which descends and continues as the sigmoid sinus to join the internal jugular vein. The midbrain is partly surrounded by the free edge of the tentorium, which is attached to the anterior clinoid processes of the sphenoid bone and provides a U-shaped gap for passage of the midbrain. Dura drapes from each side of the U into the middle cranial fossa, creating the cavernous sinus. This sinus receives blood from the ophthalmic veins and drains via petrosal sinuses into each end of the sigmoid sinus.

The supratentorial dura mater is innervated by the trigeminal nerve, the infratentorial dura by upper cervical nerves. The meningeal vessels run extradurally to supply the diploë; if torn by skull fracture, they may form an extradural hematoma and compress the brain. A subdural hematoma may be caused by leakage from a cerebral vein in transit to the superior sagittal sinus.

Cerebrospinal Fluid

Pools of CSF at the base of the brain include the cisterna magna, cisterna pontis, interpeduncular cistern, and cisterna ambiens. The CSF also extends along the meningeal sheath of the optic nerve, and raised intracranial pressure may compress the central vein of the retina, causing papilloedema. The spinal dural sac extends down to the level of the second sacral vertebra. The lumbar cistern contains spinal nerve roots and is accessible for lumbar puncture (spinal tap). The CSF secreted by the choroid plexuses escapes into the subarachnoid space through the three apertures of the fourth ventricle. Some descends to the lumbar cistern. The CSF ascends through the tentorial notch and the cerebral subarachnoid space to reach the superior sagittal sinus and its lacunae via the arachnoid granulations. A disturbance in CSF hydrodynamics can lead to hydrocephalus.

SUGGESTED READINGS

Adeeb N, Deep A, Griessenauer CJ, et al. The intracranial arachnoid mater: a comprehensive review of its history, anatomy, imaging, and pathology. *Child Nerv Syst*. 2013;29:17−33.

Adeeb N, Mortazavi MM, Tubbs RS, et al. The cranial dura mater: a review of its history, embryology, and anatomy. *Child Nerv Syst*. 2012;28:827−837.

Begley DJ. Brain superhighways. *Sci Transl Med*. 2012;4(147):147fs29.

Charbonneau F, Williams M, Lafitte F, et al. No more fear of the cavernous sinuses! *Diagn Interv Imaging*. 2013;95:1003−1016.

Da Mesquita S, Fu Z, Kipnis J. The meningeal lymphatic system: a new player in neurophysiology. *Neuron*. 2018;100(2):375−388.

Iliff JJ, Lee H, Yu M, et al. Brain-wide pathway for waste clearance captured by contrast-enhanced MRI. *J Clin Invest*. 2013;123: 1299−1309.

Kemp WJ, Tubbs RS, Cohen-Gadol AA. The innervation of the cranial dura mater: neurosurgical case correlates and a review of the literature. *World Neurosurg*. 2012;78:505−510.

Strittmatter WJ. Bathing the brain. *J Clin Invest*. 2013;123: 1013−1015.

Neurons and Neuroglia

STUDY GUIDELINES

1. Give an account of neuronal structure.
2. Give an account of synaptic structure and function and outline the lock and key analogy used in pharmacology.
3. Explain how a demyelinating disorder can compromise conduction.
4. Draw up a structure–function list for neuroglial cells.
5. Gliomas interfere with brain function in the region they grow. Explain how they may exert effects at a 'distance'.

Nerve cells, or **neurons**, are the structural and functional units of the nervous system. They generate and conduct electrical changes in the form of nerve impulses. They communicate chemically with other neurons at points of contact called **synapses**. **Neuroglia** (literally, 'nerve glue') is the connective tissue of the nervous system. Neuroglial cells are as numerous as neurons in the brain. They have important nutritive and supportive functions.

NEURONS

Neurons are highly polarised cells, with a long process known as the axon and shorter ones known as the dendrites. In the central nervous system (CNS), almost all neurons are multipolar, their cell bodies or somas having multiple poles or angular points. At every pole but one, a dendrite emerges and divides repeatedly (Fig. 6.1). On some neurons the shafts of the dendrites are smooth; on others the shafts show numerous short spines (Fig. 6.2). The dendrites receive synaptic contacts from other neurons, some on the spines and others on the shafts.

The remaining pole of the soma gives rise to the **axon**, which conducts nerve impulses. This electrical excitability stems from the fact that the cell membrane is rich in voltage-gated ion channels and ion pumps. Axons vary greatly in length. Some are short and end by synapsing with neurons in the neighbourhood of the cell body.

Others may be as long as several tens of centimetres. Terminal branches synapse on target neurons. Most synaptic contacts between neurons are either axodendritic or axosomatic. Axodendritic synapses are usually excitatory in their effect on target neurons, whereas most axosomatic synapses have an inhibitory effect. The dendrites receive synaptic

contacts from other neurons, some on the spines and others on the shafts.

The remaining pole of the soma gives rise to the **axon**, which conducts nerve impulses. Most axons give off *collateral* branches (Fig. 6.3). *Terminal* branches synapse on target neurons.

Internal Structure of Neurons

The growth and maintenance of the neuron and axon is enabled by bidirectional axonal transport which is composed of molecular motors and an elaborate cytoskeleton. All parts of neurons are permeated by **microtubules** and **neurofilaments** (Fig. 6.4). At the core of the typical neuron is the cell body or soma. The soma contains the nucleus and the cytoplasm or **perikaryon** (*Gr.* 'around the nucleus'). The perikaryon contains clumps of granular endoplasmic reticulum known as *Nissl bodies* (Fig. 6.5), as well as Golgi complexes, free ribosomes, mitochondria, and smooth endoplasmic reticulum (SER) (Fig. 6.4).

Intracellular Transport. Turnover of membranous and skeletal materials takes place in all cells. In neurons, fresh components are continuously synthesised in the soma and moved into the axon and dendrites by a process of **anterograde transport**. At the same time, worn-out materials are returned to the soma by **retrograde transport** for degradation in lysosomes (see also *target recognition*, later).

Anterograde transport is of two kinds: *rapid* and *slow*. Included in rapid transport (at a speed of 300–400 mm/day) are free elements such as synaptic vesicles, transmitter substances (or their precursor molecules), and mitochondria. Also included are lipid and protein molecules (including receptor

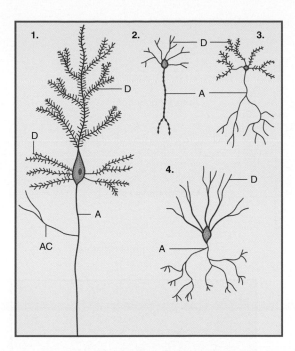

Fig. 6.1 Profiles of neurons from the brain. *(1)* Pyramidal cell, cerebral cortex. *(2)* Neuroendocrine cell, hypothalamus. *(3)* Spiny neuron, corpus striatum. *(4)* Basket cell, cerebellum. Neurons 1 and 3 show dendritic spines. *A*, Axon; *AC*, axon collateral; *D*, dendrites.

proteins) for insertion into the plasma membrane. Included in slow transport (at 5—10 mm/day) are the skeletal elements and soluble proteins, including some of those involved in transmitter release at nerve endings. Microtubules seem to be largely constructed within the axon. They are exported from the soma in preassembled short sheaves that propel one another along the initial segment of the axon; further progress is mainly by a process of elongation (up to 1 mm apiece) performed by the addition of tubulin polymers at their distal ends, with some disassembly at their proximal ends. The bulk movement of neurofilaments slows down to almost zero distally; there, the filaments are refreshed by the insertion of filament polymers moving from the soma by slow transport.

Retrograde transport of worn-out mitochondria, SER, and plasma membrane (including receptors therein) is fairly rapid (150—200 mm/day). In addition to its function in waste disposal, retrograde transport is involved in *target cell recognition*. At synaptic contacts, axons constantly 'nibble' the plasma membrane of target neurons by means of endocytotic uptake of protein-containing *signalling endosomes*. These proteins are known as *neurotrophins* ('neuron foods'). They are brought to the soma and incorporated into Golgi complexes there. In addition, the uptake of target cell 'marker' molecules is important

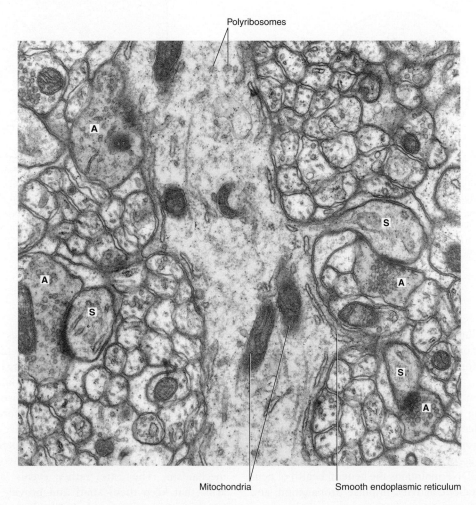

Fig. 6.2 Dendritic spines. This section is taken from the cerebellum, where the dendrites of the giant cells of Purkinje are studded with spines. In this field three spines *(S)* are in receipt of synaptic contacts by axonal boutons *(A)*. A fourth axon *(top left)* is synapsing on the shaft of the dendrite. (From Pannese 1994, with permission of Thieme.)

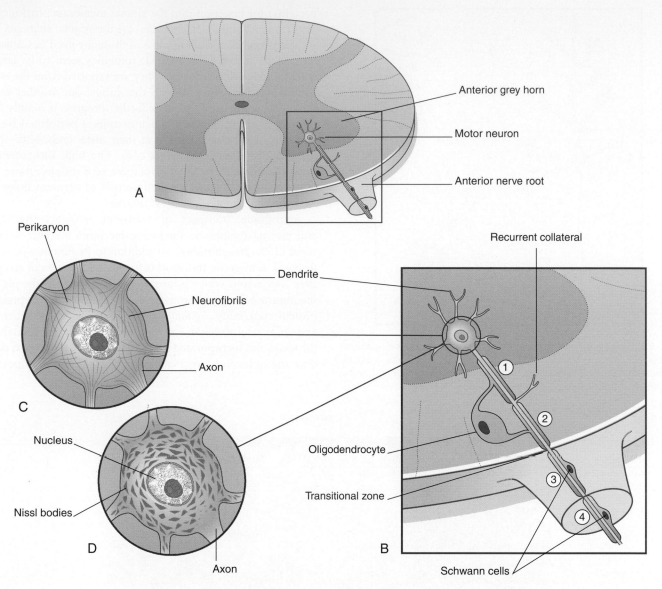

Fig. 6.3 (A) Motor neuron in the anterior grey horn of the spinal cord. (B) Enlargement from (A). Myelin segments *1* and *2* occupy central nervous system white matter and have been laid down by an oligodendrocyte; a recurrent collateral branch of the axon originated from the node. Myelin segments *3* and *4* occupy peripheral nervous system and have been laid down by Schwann cells; the node at the transitional zone is bounded by an oligodendrocyte and a Schwann cell. (C) Neurofibrils (matted neurofilaments) are seen after staining with silver salts. (D) Nissl bodies (clumps of granular endoplasmic reticulum) are seen after staining with a cationic dye such as thionin.

for cell recognition during development. It may also be necessary for viability later on because adult neurons shrink and may even die if their axons are severed proximal to their first branches.

The longest-known neurotrophin is *nerve growth factor*, on which the developing peripheral sensory and autonomic systems are especially dependent. Adult brain neurons synthesise *brain-derived neurotrophic factor (BDNF)* in the soma and send it to their nerve endings by anterograde transport. Animal studies have shown that BDNF maintains the general health of neurons in terms of metabolic activity, impulse propagation, and synaptic transmission.

Transport Mechanisms. Microtubules are the supporting structures for neuronal transport. Microtubule-binding proteins, in the form of ATPases, propel organelles and molecules along the outer surface of the microtubules. Distinct ATPases are used for anterograde and retrograde work. Retrograde transport of signalling endosomes is performed by the *dynein ATPase*. Failure of dynein performance has been found in motor neuron disease, described in Chapter 16.

Neurofilaments do not seem to be involved in the transport mechanism. They are rather evenly spaced, having side arms that keep them apart and provide skeletal stability by attachment to proteins beneath the axolemmal membrane.

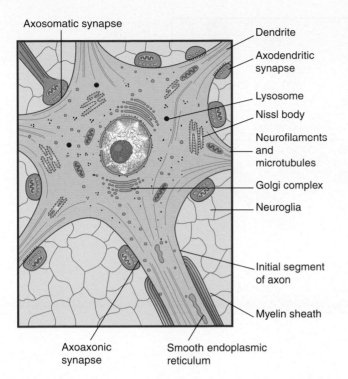

Fig. 6.4 Ultrastructure of a motor neuron. Stems of five dendrites are included, as well as three excitatory synapses *(red)* and six inhibitory synapses (including the axosomatic one).

Neurofilament numbers are in direct proportion to axonal diameter and may in truth *determine* axonal diameter.

Some points of clinical relevance are highlighted in Clinical Panel 6.1.

SYNAPSES

Synapses are the points of contact between neurons. A neural network function is founded on the patterns and types of connections made between neurons. Neuronal synapses are specialised junctions for communication and come in two types, chemical and electrical.

Electrical Synapses

Electrical synapses are scarce in the mammalian nervous system. They consist of *gap junctions (nexuses)* between dendrites or somas of contiguous neurons, where there is cytoplasmic continuity through 1.5-nm channels. No transmitter is involved, and there is no synaptic delay. They permit electrotonic changes to pass from one neuron to another. Being tightly coupled, modulation is not possible. Their function is to ensure synchronous activity of neurons having a common action. An example is the inspiratory centre in the medulla oblongata, where all the cells exhibit synchronous discharge during inspiration. A second example is among neuronal circuits

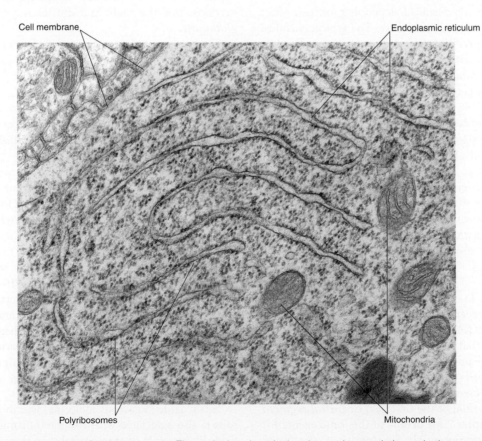

Fig. 6.5 Nissl substance in the soma of a motor neuron. The endoplasmic reticulum has a characteristic stacked arrangement. Polyribosomes are studded along the outer surface of the cisternae; many others lie free in the cytoplasm. (*Note:* Faint colour tones have been added here and later for ease of identification.) (From Pannese 1994, with permission of Thieme.)

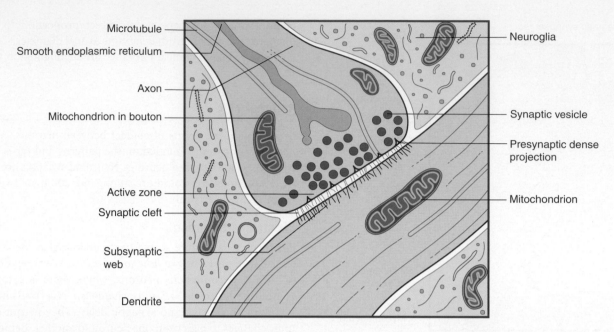

Labels (clockwise from upper left): Microtubule; Smooth endoplasmic reticulum; Axon; Mitochondrion in bouton; Active zone; Synaptic cleft; Subsynaptic web; Dendrite; Neuroglia; Synaptic vesicle; Presynaptic dense projection; Mitochondrion

Fig. 6.6 Ultrastructure of an axodendritic synapse.

controlling *saccades*, where the gaze darts from one object of interest to another.

Chemical Synapses

Conventional synapses are *chemical*, depending for their effect on the release of a *transmitter substance*. The typical chemical synapse comprises a **presynaptic membrane**, a **synaptic cleft**, and a **postsynaptic membrane** (Fig. 6.6). The presynaptic membrane belongs to the terminal bouton, the postsynaptic membrane to the target neuron. Transmitter substance is released from the bouton by exocytosis, traverses the narrow synaptic cleft, and activates receptors in the postsynaptic membrane. Underlying the postsynaptic membrane is a **subsynaptic web**, in which numerous biochemical changes are initiated by receptor activation.

The bouton contains **synaptic vesicles** loaded with transmitter substance, together with numerous mitochondria and sacs of SER (Fig. 6.7). Following conventional methods of fixation, *presynaptic dense projections* are visible, and microtubules seem to guide the synaptic vesicles to active zones in the intervals between the projections.

Receptor Activation. Transmitter molecules cross the synaptic cleft and activate receptor proteins that straddle the postsynaptic membrane (Fig. 6.8). The activated receptors initiate ionic events that either depolarise the postsynaptic membrane (*excitatory postsynaptic effect*) or hyperpolarise it (*inhibitory postsynaptic effect*). The voltage change passes over the soma in a decremental wave called *electrotonus*, and alters the resting potential of the first part or **initial segment** of the axon. (See Chapter 7 for details of the ionic events.) If excitatory postsynaptic potentials are dominant, the initial segment will be depolarised to threshold and generate action potentials.

In the CNS the most common excitatory transmitter is *glutamate*; the most common inhibitory one is γ-*aminobutyric acid* (GABA). In the peripheral nervous system the transmitter for motor neurons supplying striated muscle is *acetylcholine*; the main transmitter for sensory neurons is *glutamate*.

The sequence of events involved in *glutamatergic* synaptic transmission is shown in Fig. 6.8A. In the case of peptide *cotransmission* with glutamate, release of (one or more) peptides is *nonsynaptic*, as shown in Fig. 6.8B.

Many sensory neurons liberate one or more peptides in addition to glutamate; the peptides may be liberated from any part of the neuron, but their usual role is to *modulate* (raise or lower) the effectiveness of the transmitter.

A further kind of transmission is known as *volume transmission*. This kind is typical of *monoamine (biogenic amine) neurons*, which fall into two categories. One category synthesises a *catecholamine*, namely *norepinephrine (noradrenaline)* or *dopamine*, both synthesised from the amino acid tyrosine. The other synthesises *serotonin*, derived from tryptophan. As illustrated in Fig. 6.9, for dopamine, the transmitter is liberated from *varicosities* (where the transmitters are also synthesised) as well as from synaptic contacts. The transmitter enters the extracellular fluid of the CNS and activates specific receptors up to 100 μm away before being degraded. The monoamine neurons have enormous territorial distribution, and deviation from normal function is implicated in a variety of ailments, including Parkinson disease, schizophrenia, and major depression.

Nitric oxide (a gaseous molecule) within glutamatergic neurons is also associated with volume transmission. Excess nitric oxide liberation is *cytotoxic*, notably in areas rendered avascular by cerebral arterial thrombosis. Glutamate itself is also potentially cytotoxic.

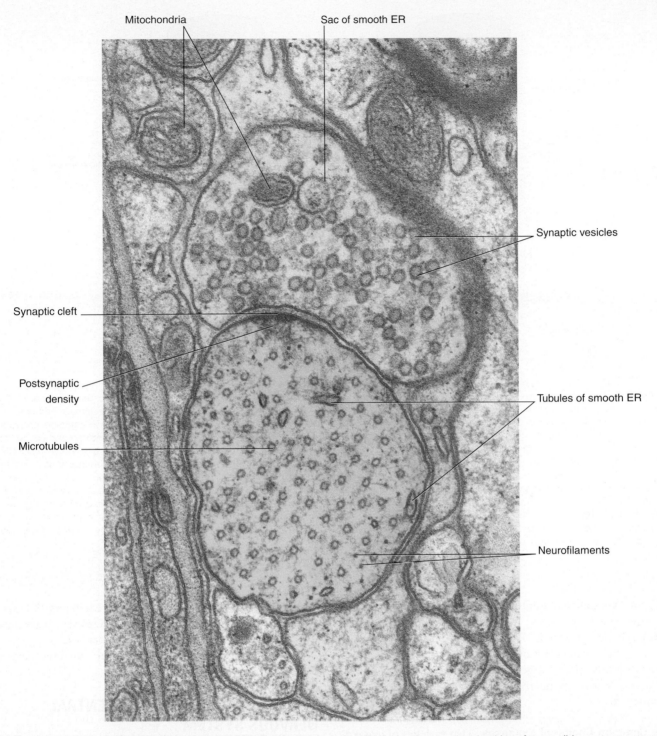

Mitochondria · Sac of smooth ER · Synaptic vesicles · Synaptic cleft · Postsynaptic density · Microtubules · Tubules of smooth ER · Neurofilaments

Fig. 6.7 Axodendritic synapse. Section of spinal cord showing an axon terminal synapsing on the dendrite of a possible motor neuron. The spherical synaptic vesicles together with the asymmetric morphology (strong postsynaptic density) indicate an excitatory synapse. The dendrite is cut transversely, as are the numerous microtubules; some of the neurofilaments can also be seen. The synapse is invested by a protoplasmic astrocyte. *ER*, Endoplasmic reticulum. (From Pannese 1994, with permission of Thieme.)

In the context of volume transmission, the conventional kind is called 'wiring' to indicate its relatively fixed nature.

Lock and Key Analogy for Drug Therapy. The receptor may be likened to a lock, the transmitter being the key that operates it. The transmitter output of certain neurons may falter as a consequence of age or disease, and a duplicate key can often be provided in the form of a drug that mimics the action of the transmitter. Such a drug is called an *agonist*. On the other hand, excessive production of a transmitter may be countered by a *receptor blocker*—the equivalent of a dummy key that will occupy the lock without activating it.

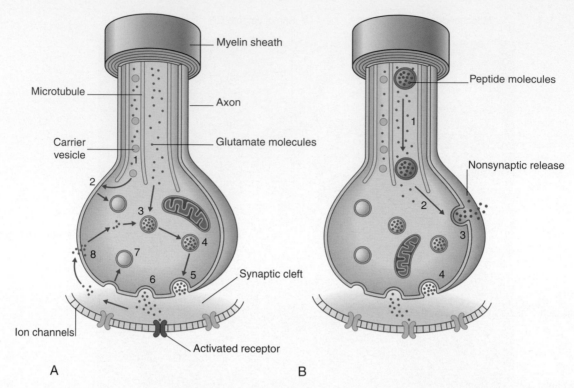

Fig. 6.8 Dynamic events at two types of nerve terminals. (A) Small molecule transmitter, exemplified by a glutamatergic nerve ending. *(1)* Carrier vesicles containing synaptic vesicle membrane proteins are rapidly transported along microtubules and stored in the plasma membrane of the terminal bouton. At the same time, enzymes and glutamate molecules are conveyed by slow transport. *(2)* Vesicle membrane proteins are retrieved from the plasma membrane and form synaptic vesicles. *(3)* Glutamate is taken into the vesicles, where it is stored and concentrated. *(4)* Loaded vesicles approach the presynaptic membrane. *(5)* Following depolarisation, the 'docked' vesicles undergo exocytosis. *(6)* Released transmitter diffuses across the synaptic cleft and activates specific receptors in the postsynaptic membrane. *(7)* Vesicular membranes are retrieved by means of endocytosis. *(8)* Some glutamate is actively transported back into the bouton for recycling. (B) Neuropeptide cotransmission. The example here is peptide *substance P* cotransmission with glutamate, a combination found at the central end of unipolar neurons serving pain sensation. *(1)* The vesicles and peptide precursors (propeptides) are synthesised in Golgi complexes in the perikaryon and taken to the terminal bouton by rapid transport. *(2)* As they enter the bouton, peptide formation is being completed, whereupon the vesicle approaches the plasma membrane. *(3)* Following membrane depolarisation, the vesicular contents are sent into the intercellular space by means of exocytosis. *(4)* Glutamate is simultaneously released into the synaptic cleft.

Inhibition Versus Disinhibition. Spontaneously active neurons are often held in check by inhibitory neurons (usually GABAergic), as shown in Fig. 6.10A. The inhibitory neurons may be silenced by others of the same kind, leading to *disinhibition* of the target cell (Fig. 6.10B). Disinhibition is a major feature of neuronal activity in the basal ganglia (Chapter 26).

Less Common Chemical Synapses. Two varieties of *axoaxonic* synapses are recognised. In both cases the boutons belong to inhibitory neurons. One variety occurs on the initial segment of the axon, where it exercises a powerful veto on impulse generation (Fig. 6.11). In the second kind the boutons are applied to excitatory boutons of other neurons, and they inhibit transmitter release. The effect is called *presynaptic inhibition*, conventional contact being *postsynaptic* in this context (Fig. 6.12).

Dendrodendritic (D-D) synapses occur between dendritic spines of contiguous spiny neurons and alter the electrotonus of the target neuron rather than generating nerve impulses. In *one-way* D-D synapses, one of the two spines contains synaptic

vesicles. In *reciprocal* synapses, both do. Excitatory D-D synapses are shown in Fig. 6.13. Inhibitory D-D synapses are numerous in relay nuclei of the thalamus (Chapter 26).

Somatodendritic and *somatosomatic* synapses have also been identified, but they are scarce.

NEUROGLIAL CELLS OF THE CENTRAL NERVOUS SYSTEM

Four different types of neuroglial cells are found in the CNS: astrocytes, oligodendrocytes, microglia, and ependymal cells.

Astrocytes

Astrocytes are often regarded as the support cells of the CNS. Astrocytes are the most abundant cell type in the CNS and provide an elaborate cellular tapestry throughout the CNS. Astrocytes are bushy cells with dozens of fine radiating processes. The cytoplasm contains abundant intermediate filaments; this confers a degree of rigidity on these cells, which helps to support the brain as a whole. Glycogen granules, which are also abundant,

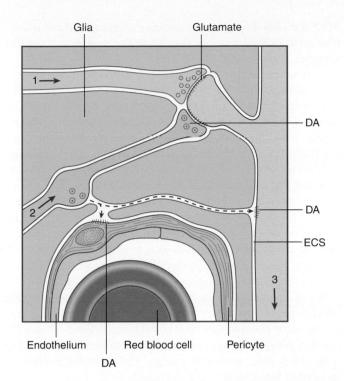

Fig. 6.9 Volume transmission in the brain. The axons of a glutamatergic neuron *(1)* and of a dopaminergic neuron *(2)* are making conventional synaptic contacts on the spine of a spiny stellate cell *(3)* in the striatum. Dopamine *(DA)* is also escaping from a varicosity and diffusing through the extracellular space *(ECS)* to activate dopamine receptors on the dendritic shaft and on the wall of a capillary pericyte (Chapter 4).

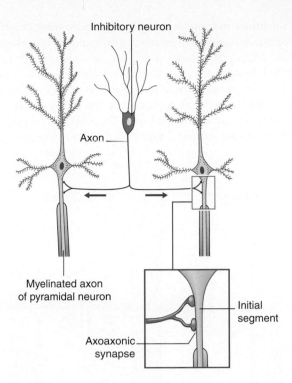

Fig. 6.11 Axoaxonic synapses in the cerebral cortex. *Arrows* indicate direction of impulse conduction.

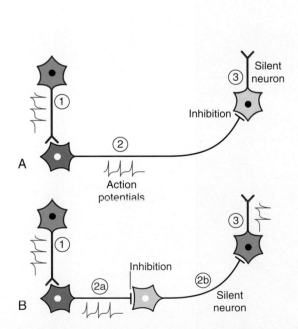

Fig. 6.10 Disinhibition. (A) Excitatory neuron *1* is activating inhibitory neuron *2* with consequent silencing of neuron *3* by neuron *2*. (B) Interpolation of a second inhibitory neuron *(2b)* has the opposite effect on neuron *3*, because *2b* is silenced. Neuron *3* (spontaneously active unless inhibited) is released.

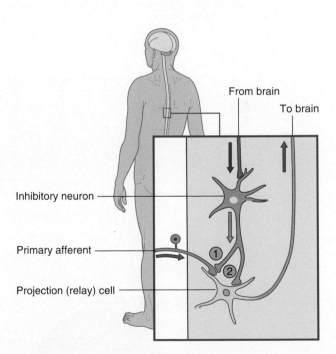

Fig. 6.12 *(1)* Presynaptic and *(2)* postsynaptic inhibition of a spinal neuron projecting to the brain. *Arrows* indicate directions of impulse conduction (relay cell may be silenced by inhibitory cell activity).

provide an immediate source of glucose for the neurons. Some astrocyte processes form glial-limiting membranes on the inner (ventricular) and outer (pial) surfaces of the brain. Other processes invest synaptic contacts between neurons. In addition, vascular processes invest brain capillaries (Fig. 6.14).

Two broad morphologies have classically been described: protoplasmic astrocytes having long unbranched processes and fibrous astrocytes whose processes are short and highly branched. Protoplasmic astrocytes are mainly found in the grey matter, while fibrous astrocytes are mainly found in the white matter. Functionally, protoplasmic astrocytes associate with both synapses and endothelial cells, thus directly participating in the 'neurovascular unit.' Fibrous astrocytes may participate in CNS myelination. There is evidence of functional and molecular heterogeneity possibly suggesting the existence of distinct subtypes of astrocytes.

Astrocytes perform many essential functions in the healthy CNS. Astrocytes use specific channels (Chapter 8) to mop up K^+ ion accumulation in the extracellular space during periods of intense neuronal activity. They participate in recycling certain neurotransmitter substances following release, notably the chief excitatory CNS transmitter, glutamate, and the chief inhibitory transmitter, GABA. Astrocytes also have a role in the formation, function, and elimination of synapses within the brain.

Astrocytes can multiply at any time. As part of the healing process following CNS injury, proliferation of astrocytes and their processes results in dense glial scar tissue (astrogliosis). More importantly, spontaneous local proliferation of astrocytes may give rise to a brain tumour (Figs. 6.15 and 6.16, Clinical Panel 6.2). Reactive astrogliosis is not a simple response but a series of changes that occur in context-dependent manners which are regulated by key signalling events. The molecular repertoire of the reactive astrocytes is still being defined. These cells can potentially serve as novel therapeutic targets. It is critical to understand how astrocytes execute their diverse supportive tasks while maintaining neuronal health.

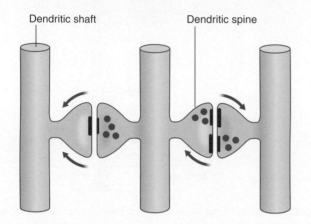

Fig. 6.13 Dendrodendritic excitation. The dendrites belong to three separate neurons. On the right is a reciprocal synapse. *Arrows* indicate direction of electrotonic waves.

Oligodendrocytes

Oligodendrocytes are responsible for wrapping myelin sheaths around axons in the white matter, where they help to maintain

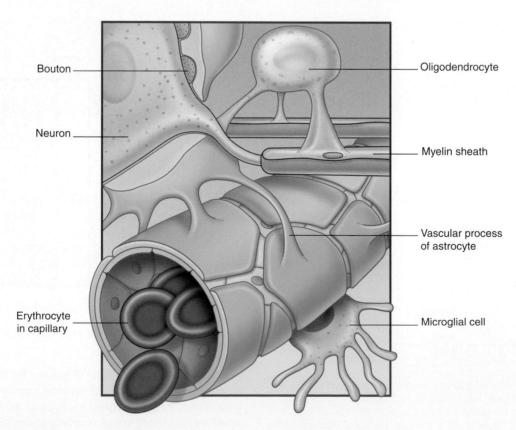

Fig. 6.14 The cellular relationships of three neuroglial cell types: oligodendrocyte, astrocyte and microglia.

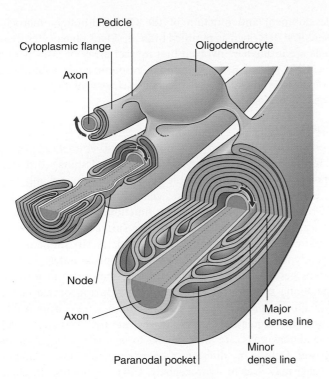

Fig. 6.15 Myelination in the central nervous system. *Arrows* indicate movement of the growing edge of the cytoplasmic flange of oligodendrocytes.

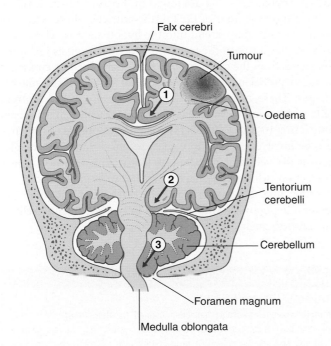

Fig. 6.16 Brain herniations. For numbers see text in Clinical Panel 6.2.

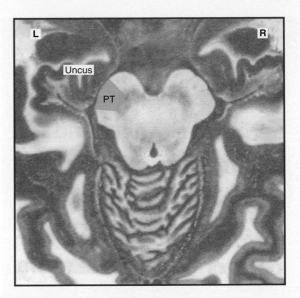

Fig. 6.17 Enlargement from Fig. 3.8 emphasising the proximity of the uncus to the pyramidal tract *(PT)*. (From Liu S, et al., eds. *Atlas of Human Sectional Anatomy*. Jinan: Shantung Press of Science and Technology; 2003, with permission from Shantung Press of Science and Technology.)

axon structure and function. In the grey matter they form satellite cells that seem to participate in ion exchange with neurons.

Myelination. Myelinated nerve fibres have evolved to enable fast and efficient transduction of electrical signals in the nervous system. Myelination commences during the middle period of gestation and continues well into the second decade. The myelin sheath is a greatly extended and modified glial plasma membrane wrapped around an axon segment in a spiral fashion. The myelin-forming cell is the Schwann cell in the peripheral nervous system (PNS) and the oligodendrocyte in the CNS.

The myelin sheath acts as an electric insulator. The subsequent withdrawal of cytoplasm and compaction of the membranes results in the characteristic periodicity. The inner and outer faces of the plasma membrane form the alternating major and minor dense lines seen in transverse sections of the myelin sheath (Fig. 6.15). In the PNS a Schwann cell myelinates a single segment of only one axon. In the CNS, each oligodendrocyte myelinates several (commonly 50 or so) segments of different axons. The part of the oligodendrocyte responsible for myelinating a single axon segment is called a **glial unit**. Thus, each oligodendrocyte includes several glial units.

The short gaps between the glial wrappings are known as the nodes of Ranvier. The myelinated intervals between the nodes are called internodes.

The myelin sheath is more than an inert insulating structure. The neuroglial cells are functionally connected to the subjacent axon via regions of cytoplasmic continuity (myelinic channels and Schmidt–Lanterman incisures (in PNS)). Myelination greatly increases the speed of impulse conduction because the depolarisation process jumps from node to node. This is known as saltatory conduction (Chapter 9). During myelination, K^+ ion channels are deleted from the underlying axolemma. For this reason, demyelinating diseases such as multiple sclerosis (Fig. 6.18, Clinical Panel 6.3) are accompanied by progressive failure of impulse conduction. Unmyelinated axons abound in the grey matter. They are fine (0.2 μm or less in diameter) and not individually ensheathed.

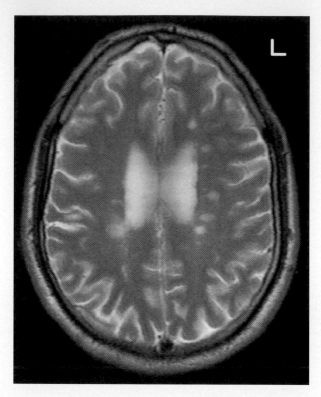

Fig. 6.18 An axial T$_2$-weighted magnetic resonance image of a 28-year-old man with multifocal demyelination secondary to multiple sclerosis showing multiple high signal intensity lesions in the white matter. On the left side of the brain, at least five of these plaques are periventricular. (Kindly provided by Dr Joe Walsh, Department of Radiology, University College Hospital, Galway, Ireland.)

Microglia

Microglia (Fig. 6.14) are of mesodermal origin, seem to have the same parentage as ependymal cells, and are capable of self-renewal. *Resting* microglial cells are minute (hence the name), but when *activated* by inflammation or by myelin sheath breakdown, they enlarge and become motile phagocytes. Microglia are dynamic and versatile cells with the capacity to morphologically and functionally adapt and respond to changes in their local environment. The microglia constantly scan the CNS and act as key sentinels monitoring the internal microenvironment of the CNS. Microglia seem to be essential for normal development and function of the CNS. Although microglia were first described as ramified brain-resident phagocytes these cells are intimately involved in a myriad array of tasks within the CNS related to both immune response and maintaining homeostasis including synaptogenesis. Dysregulation can give rise to neurological disease.

Ependyma

Ependymal cells form a simple ciliated epithelium which lines the ventricular system of the brain and spinal cord. The ependymal cells possess motile cilia, micro villi, and adherens junctions and may mediate cellular infiltration into the CNS to indicate that it may be functioning as an immunological barrier. The cilia on their free surface help the flow of cerebrospinal fluid through the ventricles. In humans, the ependymal lining is complete by approximately 26–28 weeks gestation. They provide trophic support and possibly metabolic support for progenitor cells during development. Aquaporins present in the cell membranes have been implicated in regulating water fluxes at the ventricle wall. Ependymal cells are susceptible to a variety of common viruses. Defects in adhesion of ependymal cells and formation of cilia may lead to hydrocephaly. Cilia dysfunction in ependymal cells may also be associated with microcephaly induced by Zika virus.

Other Ependymal-Associated Cell Types. Tanycytes are special ependymal cells that are found in the third ventricle of the brain and on the floor of the fourth ventricle. These cells have basal processes that extend into the hypothalamus. These cells seem to play a role in the transfer of chemical signals including hormones from the cerebrospinal fluid to the median eminence of the hypothalamus. **Supraependymal or epiplexus macrophages**: These macrophage-like cells are also called **Kolmer cells** which are found on the ventricular surface. Their main function is to act as intraventricular macrophages. They may also be involved in immunological responses and iron regulation in the ventricular system or the brain as a whole. Their interactions with ependymal cells are not well understood.

    Other glia: Bergmann glia of the cerebellum, the pituicytes of neurohypophysis, Müller cells of the retina, satellite cells of the sensory ganglia, and olfactory ensheathing cells.

CLINICAL PANEL 6.1   Clinical Relevance of Neuronal Transport

Tetanus

Wounds contaminated by soil or street dust may contain *Clostridium tetani*, which produces a toxin that binds to the plasma membrane of nerve endings, is taken up by endocytosis, and is carried to the spinal cord by retrograde transport. Other neurons upstream take in the toxin by endocytosis—notably Renshaw cells (Chapter 15), which normally exert a braking action on motor neurons through the release of an inhibitory transmitter substance, *glycine*. Tetanus toxin prevents the release of glycine. As a result, motor neurons go out of control, particularly those supplying the muscles of the face, jaws, and spine; these muscles exhibit prolonged, agonising spasms. About half of the patients who show these classic signs of tetanus die of exhaustion within a few days. Tetanus is entirely preventable by appropriate and timely immunisation.

Viruses and Toxic Metals

Retrograde axonal transport has been blamed for the passage of viruses from the nasopharynx to the central nervous system (e.g. herpes simplex virus) and also for the uptake of toxic metals such as lead and aluminium. Viruses, in particular, may be spread widely through the brain by means of retrograde transneuronal uptake.

Peripheral Neuropathies

Defective anterograde transport seems to be involved in certain 'dying back' neuropathies in which the distal parts of the longer peripheral nerves undergo progressive atrophy.

CLINICAL PANEL 6.2 Gliomas

Brain tumours most commonly originate from neuroglial cells, especially astrocytes.

General symptoms produced by expanding brain tumours are indicative of *raised intracranial pressure*. They include headache, drowsiness, and vomiting. Radiologic investigation may reveal displacement of midline structures to the opposite side. Tumours below the tentorium (usually cerebellar) are likely to block the exit of cerebrospinal fluid from the fourth ventricle, in which case ballooning of the ventricular system will add to the intracranial pressure.

Local symptoms depend on the position of the tumour. For example, clumsiness of an arm or leg may be caused by an ipsilateral cerebellar tumour, and motor weakness of an arm or leg may be caused by a contralateral cerebral tumour.

Progression

Expansion of a tumour may cause one or more brain hernias to develop, as shown in Fig. 6.16.

1. *Subfalcine herniation* (in the interval between falx cerebri and corpus callosum) seldom causes specific symptoms.
2. *Uncal herniation* is the term used to denote displacement of the uncus of the temporal lobe into the tentorial notch. Compression of the ipsilateral crus cerebri by the uncus (Fig. 6.17) may give rise to contralateral motor weakness. Alternatively, displacement and compression of the contralateral crus against the sharp edge of the tentorium cerebelli may cause *ipsilateral* motor weakness.
3. *Pressure coning:* a cone of cerebellar tissue (the tonsil) may descend into the foramen magnum, squeezing the medulla oblongata and causing death from respiratory or cardiovascular failure by inactivation of *vital centres* in the reticular formation (Chapter 24).

CLINICAL PANEL 6.3 Multiple Sclerosis

Multiple sclerosis (MS) is the most common neurologic disorder of young adults in the temperate latitudes north and south of the equator. It is more prevalent in women, with a female: male ratio of 3:2. The peak age of onset is around 30 years, the range being 15 to 45 years.

While MS is a *primary demyelinating disease* (the initial feature is the development of plaques (patches) of demyelination in the white matter), demyelinating lesions are commonly found in the grey matter and axonal loss also occurs. The denuded axons also undergo large-scale degeneration, probably initiated by failure of the sodium pump, as described in Chapter 7. Impulse conduction in neighbouring myelinated fibres is also compromised by oedema (inflammatory exudate). Over time, the plaques are progressively replaced by glial scar tissue. Old plaques feel firm (sclerotic) in postmortem slices of the brain.

Common locations of early plaques are the cervical spinal cord, upper brainstem, optic nerve, and periventricular white matter (see Fig. 6.18) including that of the cerebellum. MS is not a systems disease; it is not anatomically selective, and a plaque may involve parts of adjacent motor and sensory pathways.

Presenting symptoms can be correlated with lesion sites as follows.

- *Motor weakness*, usually in one or both legs, signifies a lesion involving the corticospinal tract.
- *Clumsiness* in reaching and grasping usually accompanies a lesion in the cerebellar white matter.
- *Numbness or tingling*, often spreading up from the legs to the trunk, may be caused by a lesion in the posterior white matter of the spinal cord. Tingling ('pins and needles') is attributed to spontaneous firing of partially demyelinated sensory fibres.
- *Diplopia* (double vision) may be produced by a plaque within the pons or midbrain affecting the function of one of the ocular motor nerves.
- A *scotoma* (patch of blindness in the visual field of one eye) is produced by a plaque within the optic nerve.
- *Urinary retention* (failure of the bladder to empty) can be caused by interruption of the central autonomic pathway descending from the brainstem to the lower part of the cord.

The usual course of the disease is one of remissions and relapses, with an overall slow progression and development of multiple disabilities.

Note: Recent research in several laboratories has elicited frequent additional evidence of grey matter degeneration, mainly in the cerebral cortex, leading in many cases to cognitive deficiencies. Several putative causes are under investigation.

✳ Core Information

Neurons

The multipolar neuron of the central nervous system (CNS) comprises soma, dendrites, and axon; the axon gives off collateral and terminal branches. The soma contains rough and smooth endoplasmic reticulum, Golgi complexes, neurofilaments, and microtubules. Microtubules pervade the entire neuron; they are involved in anterograde transport of synaptic vesicles, mitochondria, and membranous replacement material and in retrograde transport of marker molecules and degraded organelles.

The three kinds of chemical neuronal interaction are synaptic (e.g. glutamatergic), nonsynaptic (e.g. peptidergic), and volume (e.g. monoaminergic, serotonergic).

Anatomic varieties of chemical synapse include axodendritic, axosomatic, axoaxonic, and dendrodendritic. Structure includes pre- and postsynaptic membranes, synaptic cleft, and subsynaptic web. Electrical synapses via gap junctions render some neuronal groups electrically coupled, for synchronous activation.

Neuroglia: Astrocytes have supportive, nutritive, and retrieval functions. They are the main source of brain tumours. Oligodendrocytes form CNS myelin sheaths, which are subject to destruction in demyelinating diseases. Microglia are key sentinels monitoring the internal environment and can act as potential phagocytes. Ependymal cells line the ventricular system.

Billions of neurons form a shell, or **cortex**, on the surface of the cerebral and cerebellar hemispheres. In this general context, **nuclei** are aggregates of neurons buried within the white matter.

SUGGESTED READINGS

Benarroch EE. Oligodendrocytes: susceptibility to injury and involvement in neurologic disease. *Neurology.* 2009;72:1779−1785.

Benarroch EE. Neocortical interneurons: functional diversity and clinical correlations. *Neurology.* 2013;81:273−280.

Benarroch EE. Microglia: multiple roles in surveillance, circuit shaping, and response to injury. *Neurology.* 2013;81:1079−1088.

Clarke LE, Barres BA. Emerging roles of astrocytes in neural circuit development. *Nat Rev Neurosci.* 2013;14:311−321.

Gage FH, Kempermann G, Song H, eds. *Adult Neurogenesis.* New York: Cold Spring Harbor Laboratory Press; 2008.

Hirokawa N, Reiko T. Molecular motors in neuronal development, intracellular transport and diseases. *Curr Opin Neurobiol.* 2004;14:564−573.

Howe CH, Mobley WC. Long-distance retrograde neurotrophic signalling. *Curr Opin Neurobiol.* 2005;15:40−48.

Ikegami A, Haruwaka K, Wake H. Microglia: lifelong modulator of neural circuits. *Neuropathology.* 2019;39(3):173−180.

Jessen KR. Glial cells. *Int J Biochem Cell Biol.* 2004;36:1861−1867.

Jiménez AJ, Domínguez-Pinos MD, Guerra MM, Fernández-Llebrez P, Pérez-Fígares JM. Structure and function of the ependymal barrier and diseases associated with ependyma disruption. *Tissue Barriers.* 2014;2:e28426.

Khakh BS, Deneen B. The emerging nature of astrocyte diversity. *Annu Rev Neurosci.* 2019;42:187−207.

Koehler RC, Roman RJ, Harder GR. Astrocytes and the regulation of cerebral blood flow. *Trends Neurosci.* 2009;32:160−169.

Lent R, Azevedo FAC, Andrade-Moraes CH, Pinto AVO. How many neurons do you have? Some dogmas of quantitative neuroscience under review. *Eur J Neurosci.* 2012;35:1−9.

Pannese E. *Neurocytology. Fine Structure of Neurons, Nerve Processes and Neuroglial Cells.* New York: Thieme; 1994.

Stadelmann C, Timmler S, Barrantes-Freer A, Simons M. Myelin in the central nervous system: structure, function, and pathology. *Physiol Rev.* 2019;99(3):1381−1431.

Stassart RM, Möbius W, Nave KA, Edgar JM. The axon-myelin unit in development and degenerative disease. *Front Neurosci.* 2018;12:467.

Stys PK. General mechanisms of axonal damage and its repair. *J Neurol Sci.* 2005;233:3−13.

Sykova E, Nicholson C. Diffusion in brain extracellular space. *Physiol Rev.* 2008;88:1277−1340.

Torrealba F, Carrasco MA. A review on electron microscopy and neurotransmitter systems. *Brain Res Rev.* 2004;47:5−17.

Triarhou LC. *Cellular Structure of the Cerebral Cortex.* Basel: Karger; 2009.

CHAPTER SUMMARY

STUDY GUIDELINES

1. List the different types of ion channels and provide a description of how they function.
2. Describe the resting potential with respect to the major ions involved in its formation.
3. Be able to distinguish and describe the following terms: electrotonic potential, spatial summation, temporal summation, threshold, and trigger point.
4. Discuss the ion channel changes that accompany the development of an action potential and the concepts of all-or-none response and absolute and relative refractory period.
5. Contrast the mechanism or process of action potential development and propagation along an unmyelinated versus a myelinated axon.

Examples of clinical neurophysiology related to the peripheral nervous system await your attention in Chapter 12.

STRUCTURE OF THE PLASMA MEMBRANE

In common with cells elsewhere, the plasma membrane of neurons is a double layer (bilayer) of phospholipids made up of phosphate heads facing the aqueous media of the extracellular and intracellular spaces and paired lipid tails forming a fatty membrane in between (Fig. 7.1). The phosphate layer is water soluble (*hydrophilic*, or *polar*), and the double lipid layer is water insoluble (*hydrophobic*, or *nonpolar*).

Both the extracellular and the intracellular fluids (ECFs and ICFs) are aqueous salt solutions in which many soluble molecules dissociate into positively or negatively charged atoms or groups of atoms called *ions*. Ions and molecules in aqueous solutions are in a constant state of agitation, being subject to *diffusion*, whereby they tend to move from areas of higher concentration to areas of lower concentration. In addition to diffusing down their concentration gradients, ions are influenced by electrical gradients. Positively charged ions such as sodium (Na^+) and potassium (K^+) are called *cations* because, in an electrical field, they migrate to the cathode. Negatively charged ions such as chloride (Cl^-) are called *anions* because these migrate to the anode. Like charges (e.g. Na^+ and K^+) repel one another; unlike charges (e.g. Na^+ and Cl^-) attract one another.

The cell membrane can be regarded as an electric *capacitor* because it comprises outer and inner layers carrying ionic charges of opposite kind, with a (fatty) insulator in between. Away from the membrane the voltage in the tissue fluid is brought to zero (0 mV) by the neutralising effect of Cl^- anions on Na^+ and other cations, and the voltage in the cytosol away from the membrane is brought to zero by the neutralising effect of anionic proteins on K^+ cations.

Ion Channels

Ion channels are membrane-spanning proteins with a central pore that permits passage of ions across the cell membrane. Most channels are selective for a particular ion, such as Na^+, K^+, *or* Cl^-.

Several channel categories are recognised, of which the first three are of immediate relevance.

- *Passive (non-gated) channels* are open at all times, permitting ions to move across the membrane and helping to establish the resting membrane potential of neurons.
- *Voltage-gated channels* contain a voltage-sensitive string of amino acids that cause the channel pore to open or close in response to changes in membrane voltage. Voltage-gated channels are essential to produce an action potential.
- *Channel pumps* are energy-driven ion exporters and/or importers designed to maintain steady-state ion concentrations. The Na^+-K^+ exchange pump is vital to maintain the resting membrane potential.
- *Chemically gated (or transmitter-gated) channels* are used by the nervous system to temporarily alter the membrane potential and these channels abound in the postsynaptic membranes of a synapse. Some are activated directly by transmitter molecules, others indirectly (see Chapter 8).

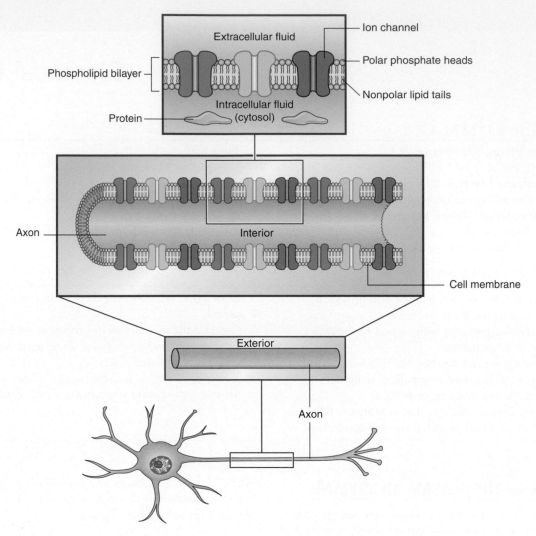

Fig. 7.1 Structure of the neuronal cell membrane. The only membrane proteins shown here are ion channels.

- ***Transduction channels*** are activated by physical stimuli, resulting in depolarisation and the subsequent creation of action potentials so the stimulus can be perceived by the nervous system. Each receptor can transduce a form of energy—for example, changes in length or tension in the muscle, tactile or thermal energy in the skin, chemical energy in the nasal and oral cavities, or electromagnetic energy in the retina. Fig. 7.2 depicts the three passive channels concerned with generating the resting potential.

The existence of distinct channels for Na^+, K^+, and Cl^- ions would result in zero voltage difference across the membrane if passive diffusion of the three ions were equally free. However, the number of Na^+ channels is relatively small, the number of K^+ channels is relatively large, and the number of Cl^- channels is roughly half the number of K^+ channels. In effect the membrane is many times more permeable to K^+ and Cl^- than to Na^+.

Resting Membrane Potential

The membrane potential of the resting (inactive) neuron is generated primarily by differences in concentration of the Na^+ and K^+ ions dissolved in the aqueous environments of the ECF and the cytosol. In Table 7.1, K^+ is 20 times more concentrated in the cytosol than in the ECF, while Na^+ and Cl^- are 10 and 3.8 times more concentrated in the ECF than in the cytosol. Thus, the chemical driving force is outward for K^+ and inward for Na^+ and Cl^-.

In Fig. 7.3 a voltmeter is connected to electrodes inserted into the ECF surrounding an axon. One of the electrodes has been inserted into a glass pipette with a minute tip. On the left side of the figure both electrode tips are in the ECF and there is no voltage difference; a zero value is recorded. On the right side the pipette has pierced the plasma membrane of the axon, allowing the measurement of the ICF of the cytosol. The electrical charge now reveals a *potential* (voltage) difference of -70 mV. In practice the membrane potential ranges from -60 mV to -80 mV in different neurons. These values represent the ***resting membrane potential*** (i.e. when impulses are not being conducted).

Resting Membrane Permeability

Potassium Ions. From what has been mentioned, it is clear that K^+ concentrations on either side of the cell membrane

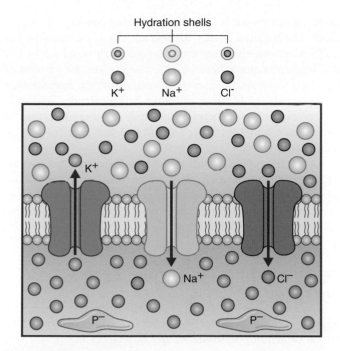

Fig. 7.2 In the resting state, Na$^+$ and Cl$^-$ ions are concentrated external to the membrane, because of the large hydration shell of the Na$^+$ ions, combined with their attraction to Cl$^-$ ions. K$^+$ ions are concentrated on the inside, because of their attraction to protein anions (P$^-$). The *arrows* are directed down the concentration gradients of the respective ions.

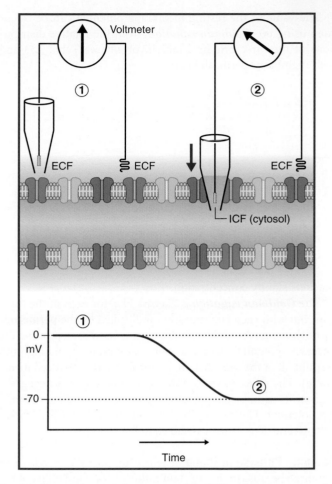

Fig. 7.3 The resting membrane potential. *(1)* The two electrodes of a voltmeter are inserted into the extracellular fluid *(ECF)* surrounding an axon. The left electrode tip occupies a micropipette. There is no voltage difference registering, hence the zero value in the record below. *(2)* The pipette has been lowered *(arrow)*, puncturing the plasma membrane to sample the intracellular fluid *(ICF)* immediately beneath. A voltage difference of −70 mV is recorded.

TABLE 7.1 Ionic concentrations in cytosol and extracellular fluid.

	CONCENTRATION (MMOL/L)		
Ion	Cytosol	Extracellular Fluid	Equilibrium Potential (mV)
K$^+$	100	5	−90
Na$^+$	15	150	+60
Cl$^-$	13	50	−70

would be the same were there no constraint. In fact, there are two electrical constraints at the level of the ion pore: the attraction exerted by the protein anions (P$^-$) on the inside and the repulsion exerted by the K$^+$ cations on the outside. The equilibrium state exists when the outward concentration gradient acting on K$^+$ is exactly balanced by the inward voltage gradient acting on K$^+$; the potential difference at this point is expressed as *E$_K$*, the **potassium equilibrium potential**. This can be expressed by means of the *Nernst equation*, which uses the principles of thermodynamics to convert the concentration gradient of an ion to an equivalent voltage gradient:

$$E_K = \frac{RT}{FZ_K} \ln \frac{[K^+]o}{[K^+]i}$$

where

E_K = equilibrium potential for K$^+$ expressed as millivolts

R = universal gas constant (8.31 J/mol/°absolute)

T = temperature in kelvin (310 at 37°C)

F = Faraday (96,500 C/per mole of charge)

Z_K = valence of K$^+$ (+1)

ln = natural logarithms

$[K^+]_o$ = K$^+$ concentration outside the cell membrane

$[K^+]_i$ = K$^+$ concentration inside the cell membrane

Converting the natural log to log$_{10}$ and resolving the numeric fractions yields

$$E_K = 62 \times \log_{10}(5/100) = -90 mV$$

Repeating the exercise for Na$^+$ and Cl$^-$ yields

$$E_{Na} = +62 mV \text{ and } E_{CL} = -70 mV$$

The value of the resting membrane potential can be calculated using the **Goldman equation**, from the relative distributions of the three principal ions involved (see Table 7.1) and their membrane permeabilities:

$$RP = 62\,log\,\frac{P_{K+}[K^+]o + P_{Na^+}[Na^+]o + P_{Cl^-}[Cl^-]i}{P_{K+}[K^+]i + P_{Na^+}[Na^+]i + P_{Cl^-}[CL^-]o}$$

where
RP = resting potential
62 = RT/F × 2.3 (constant for converting ln to log_{10})
P = the three membrane permeabilities (relative number of channels for each ion)
o and i refer to outside and inside the cell. The concentrations of the negative Cl⁻ ions are shown inverted because − log (X/Y) = log (Y/X).
Brackets signify concentration.

The **Goldman equation** is 'Nernst-like' for each of the three ions, but with each concentration multiplied by the permeability of that ion (the Goldman equation is used to determine the 'reversal' potential across a cell membrane by taking into account all of the ions that are permeable across that cell membrane). The effect of Cl⁻ on the resting potential is negligible, because its equilibrium potential is roughly the same as the resting potential. The sum of the fractions for K⁺ and Na⁺ yields an outcome of −70 mV, as shown in Fig. 7.3.

Sodium−Potassium Pump. The resting potential needs to be stabilised because of the constant influx of Na⁺ and efflux of K⁺ along their concentration gradients. Stability is assured by the **Na⁺−K⁺ pump** making appropriate corrections for the passive flow of the ions. This channel is capable of simultaneously extruding Na⁺ and importing K⁺. Three Na⁺ ions are exported for every two K⁺ ions imported (Fig. 7.4). In both cases the movement is *against* the existing concentration gradient. The required energy for this activity is provided by the ATPase enzyme that converts adenosine triphosphate (ATP) to adenosine diphosphate (ADP). The greater the amount of Na⁺ in the cytosol, the greater the activity of the enzyme. Due to the imbalance of three sodium's being extruded and only two potassium ions being imported, the Na−K pump is electrogenic and contributes slightly to the negative resting membrane potential.

As mentioned in Chapter 6, the axonal degeneration occurring in multiple sclerosis is attributable to failure of the sodium pump along the denuded axolemma. This leads to Na⁺ overload, which in turn promotes excess release of calcium ions (Ca^{2+}) from intracellular stores.

RESPONSE TO STIMULATION: ACTION POTENTIALS

Neurons typically interact at chemical synapses, where the arrival of **action potentials**, or *spikes*, triggers the release of a transmitter substance from vesicles in the presynaptic terminal (see Chapter 8). The transmitter crosses the synaptic cleft and activates *receptors* embedded in the postsynaptic membranes of target neurons. The receptors activate *transmitter-gated* ion channels to alter the level of polarisation of the target neuron. Transmitter-gated channels that cause the membrane potential to become more negative (beyond the resting value of −70 mV, perhaps to −80 mV or more) result in **hyperpolarisation** of the membrane. Channels that cause the membrane potential to become less negative result in **depolarisation** of the membrane.

Electrotonic Potentials

The initial target cell response to excitatory stimulation takes the form of local, *graded* or **electrotonic potentials (ETPs)**. Positive ETPs on multipolar neurons are usually the result of depolarisation via transmitter-gated channels. At a low frequency of stimulation, small, decremental waves of depolarisation extend for 50 to 100 μm along the affected dendrites, typically dying away after 2 or 3 ms (Fig. 7.5). With increasing frequency, the waves undergo stepwise **temporal summation** to form progressively larger waves continuing over the surface of the soma. **Spatial summation** occurs when waves travelling along two or more dendrites converge simultaneously on the soma (Fig. 7.6). About 15 mV of depolarisation, to a value of −55 mV, results in the opening of voltage-gated channels in the most sensitive region of the neuron, the *trigger point* or *trigger zone*, in the initial segment of the axon (Fig. 7.7). When the level of depolarisation (the **generator potential**) reaches the voltage necessary to open the voltage-gated channels (the **threshold**), an action potential is formed.

In the sensory neurons of cranial and spinal nerves, the trigger zone generates what is known as the *receptor potential*. The trigger zone of sensory neurons is exceptionally rich in channels

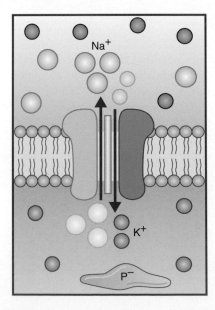

Fig. 7.4 The Na⁺−K⁺ pump. The diagram indicates simultaneous expulsion of three Na⁺ ions for every two K⁺ ions imported.

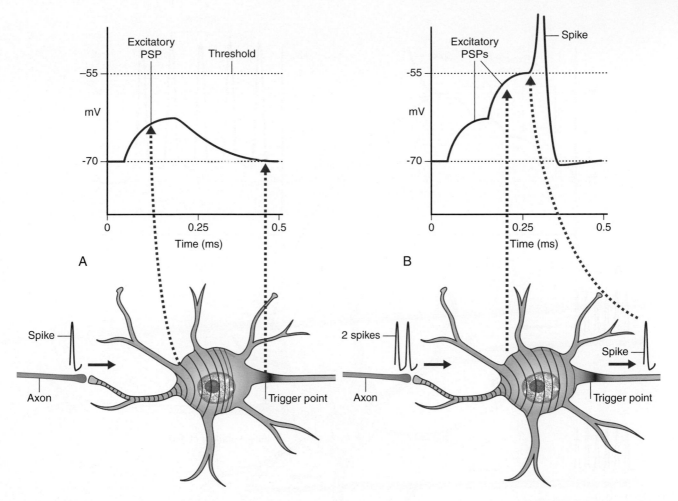

Fig. 7.5 Temporal summation. (A) A sensory axon *(blue)* delivers a single spike to a motor neuron, sufficient to elicit an excitatory postsynaptic potential *(PSP)* that is subthreshold and dies away. (B) The sensory axon delivers multiple spikes that undergo temporal summation to reach threshold in the initial segment of the axon, which responds by generating an action potential (spike) that will pass along the motor axon.

activated by specific sensory stimuli, resulting in a graded, inward depolarising current.

In the case of myelinated nerve fibres the trigger point is easily identified: in multipolar neurons it is immediately proximal to the first axonal myelin segment (axon hillock), and in peripheral sensory neurons it is immediately distal to the final myelin segment.

Inhibitory (hyperpolarising) postsynaptic potentials are elicited by the opening of channels generating an outward current, such as K^+ channels. They too are decremental.

The Shape of Action Potentials

A single action potential is depicted in Fig. 7.8. The *spike* segment of the potential commences when the membrane potential at the axon hillock reaches the threshold value of -55 mV. The rising phase of depolarisation passes beyond zero to include an **overshoot phase** reaching about $+35$ mV. The falling phase returns the membrane potential to an **undershoot phase** of *after-hyperpolarisation* where the membrane potential approaches the Nernst potential for potassium (about

-80 mV) before finally returning to baseline as the voltage-gated K^+ channels close.

Depolarisation of the membrane to threshold, typically via transmitter-gated channels, results in the opening of voltage-gated Na^+ channels (Fig. 7.9). The entry of Na^+ produces further depolarisation, and the positive feedback causes the remaining voltage-gated Na^+ channels in the trigger zone to open, driving the membrane potential into a charge reversal (overshoot) of $+35$ mV and approaching the Nernst potential for Na^+. At this point the Na^+ channels commence a progressive inactivation, while voltage-gated K^+ channels are simultaneously triggered to open. Current flow switches from Na^+ inflow to K^+ outflow, and the membrane potential begins to repolarise. The after-hyperpolarisation phase is explained by the voltage-gated Na^+ channels being completely inactivated prior to the delayed closure of the K^+ channels. Any remaining discrepancy is adjusted by activity of the Na^+-K^+ pump.

Close analyses of the Na^+ channels involved have revealed a dual mechanism of operation (Fig. 7.10). In the resting state

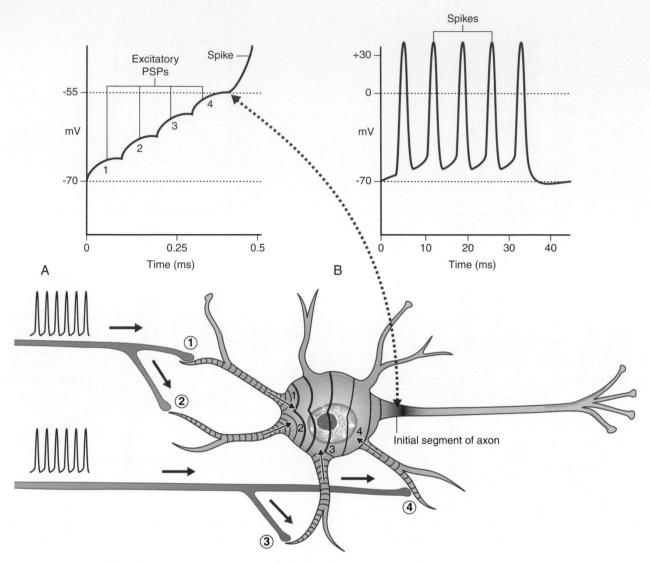

Fig. 7.6 (A) Stepwise summation of excitatory postsynaptic potentials *(PSPs)* triggering a spike. The *dashed arrow* indicates the region enlarged in (A). (B) Multiple spikes are elicited by generator potentials of enough strength.

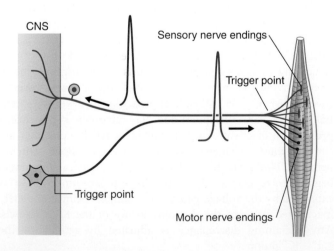

Fig. 7.7 Shape of action potentials for motor and sensory nerves supplying skeletal muscle. *CNS*, Central nervous system.

(−70 mV) an *activation gate* in the midregion of both Na$^+$ and K$^+$ channel pores is closed. The Na$^+$ channel is the first to respond at threshold, by opening its activation gate and allowing Na$^+$ ions to rapidly enter the cell down both the concentration and electrical gradients. At the peak of the action potential (+35 mV), a second gate, *inactivation gate*, in the form of a negatively charged globular protein, closes the Na$^+$ channel while the K$^+$ channel is opening. During repolarisation, when the membrane potential approaches normality (−70 mV), the Na$^+$ channel activation gate closes before the inactivation gate reopens, thus resetting the Na$^+$ channel to its original state. Voltage-gated K$^+$ channels have only a single gating mechanism (activation gate) with slower kinetics.

The action potential response to depolarisation is ***all or none***, a term signifying that if the threshold for activation is reached, all voltage-gated Na$^+$ channels in that region will

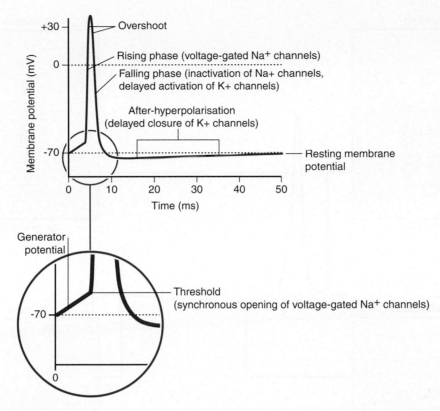

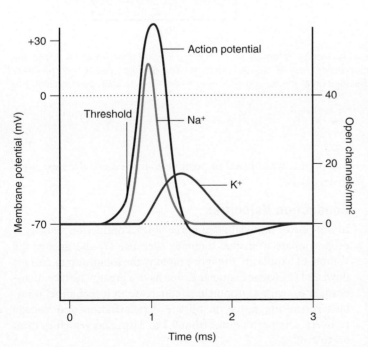

Fig. 7.8 Principal features of the action potential.

Fig. 7.9 Changes in voltage-gated Na$^+$ and K$^+$ conductance responsible for the action potential.

open. In this respect, it is quite unlike the graded transmitter-gated potentials that summate to initiate action potentials. Action potentials are also distinguished from graded potentials in being ***non-decremental***; they are propagated at full strength along the nerve fibre all the way to the nerve endings, which in the case of lower limb neurons may be more than a meter away from the parent somas.

During the rising and early falling phases of the action potential, the neuron passes through an ***absolute refractory period*** during which time it is completely incapable of initiating a second impulse because of the inactivation properties of the voltage-gated Na$^+$ channels (Fig. 7.11). This is followed by a ***relative refractory period***, during which time stimuli in excess of the standard 15 mV depolarisation can elicit a response. It is quite common for the generator potential to reach up to 35 mV, triggering impulses at 50 to 100 impulses per second (expressed as 50 to 100 Hz).

Propagation

Reversal of potential in the trigger zone is propagated (conducted) along the axon in accordance with the electrotonic circuit shown in Fig. 7.12A. The positive internal membrane charge passes in both directions within the axoplasm, while the positive outside charge passes in both directions within the ECF

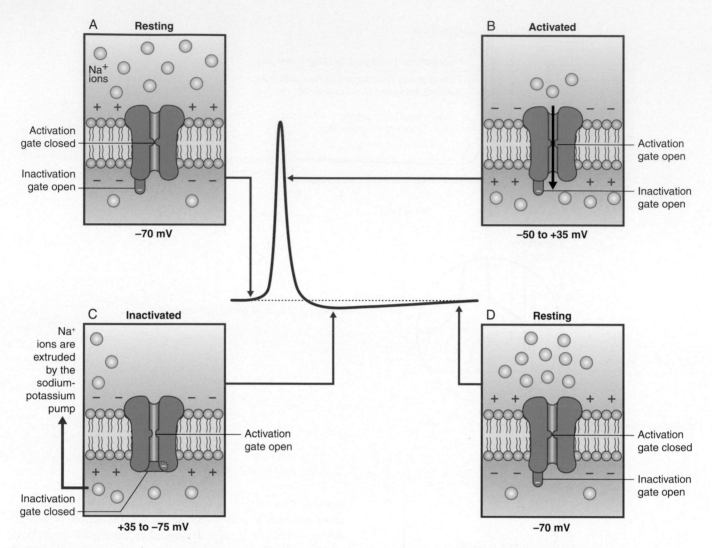

Fig. 7.10 Voltage-gated Na⁺ Channel Behaviour During Various Phases of an Action Potential. (A) During the resting phase prior to onset, the activation gate is closed and the inactivation gate is open. (B) When the threshold level is crossed, the activation gate opens and the channel is open completely. (C) The channel is closed by the inactivation gate. (D) Restoration of the resting potential causes the activation gate to close and the inactivation gate to open, thus resetting the channel.

to neutralise the negative external potential. The membrane immediately proximal is sufficiently refractory to resist depolarisation, whereas that immediately distal undergoes a local response (depolarisation) progressing to firing level. This process continues distally along the stem axon and its branches, thereby conducting the action potential all the way to the nerve terminals.

Whereas conduction along unmyelinated nerve fibres is *continuous*, along myelinated fibres it is **saltatory** ('jumping'). Myelin sheaths are effective insulators overlying the internodal segments of the membrane, whereas Na⁺ channels are most abundant at the nodes. Accordingly, spike potentials are generated at each successive node, with the positive current travelling along the axoplasm of the internode portion of the membrane before exiting at the next node in line. As the current travels back through the ECF to recharge the depolarised patch of

membrane, withdrawal of positive charge causes the next node to depolarise.

Conduction Velocities

In the case of unmyelinated nerve fibres, conduction velocity is proportionate to axonal diameter, because (1) the greater the volume of axoplasm, the more rapid is the longitudinal current flow, and (2) wider diameter axons have a greater surface membrane area, with a proportionate increase in ion channel numbers permitting faster membrane depolarisation and voltage recovery. Diameters range from 0.2 to 2 μm and velocities from 0.5 to 2 m/s.

Myelinated nerve fibres range in external diameter (i.e. including the myelin sheath) from 2 to 25 μm. In addition to the two axonal size benefits mentioned, wider myelinated fibres possess longer internodal myelin segments. The spikes are

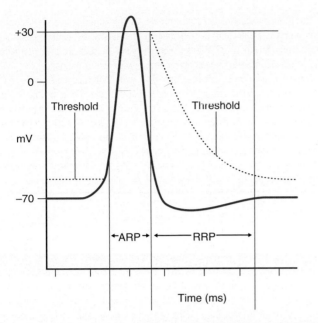

Fig. 7.11 Refractory periods. *ARP*, Absolute refractory period; *CNS*, central nervous system; *RRP*, relative refractory period.

accordingly further apart, with increased conduction velocity, similar to a runner with a longer stride. Conduction velocities for various kinds of peripheral nerve fibres are given in Chapter 9 (Table 9.1).

CLINICAL PANEL 7.1 Local Anaesthetics: How They Work

Locally applied anaesthetics reversibly block nerve conduction by inactivating Na^+ channels—especially voltage-gated Na^+ channels—thereby preventing depolarisation. The more firmly they bind to the protein surround of the ion channels, the longer their duration of action. High lipid solubility is required to access these proteins. When injected close to a peripheral nerve, unmyelinated and finely myelinated (Aδ) fibres are the first to be inactivated, thereby relieving both aching and stabbing pain sensation. If the nerve is mixed, some temporary motor paralysis may follow.

Most local anaesthetics are either *amides* (including bupivacaine and lidocaine) or *esters* (including benzocaine and novocaine). Both groups cause local vasodilation by directly relaxing arteriolar smooth muscle. Because this accelerates their clearance, epinephrine is often included in aesthetic solutions as it causes smooth muscle contraction or vasoconstriction.

BASIC SCIENCE PANEL 7.1 The Node, Paranode, and Juxtaparanode

The junction between myelinating cells surrounding axons within the peripheral and central nervous system (PNS and CNS) consists of three subdomains: *node*, *paranode*, and *juxtaparanode*. The axon between two nodes is called the *internode* and the *node of Ranvier* refers to all three subdomains within the PNS.

Action potentials beginning at the *axon initial segment* are transmitted down myelinated axons in an energy efficient and faster way compared to unmyelinated axons since each *node* 'reinvigorates' this action potential as it jumps from node to subsequent node *(saltatory conduction)* (see Fig. 7.12B). Segregation of voltage-gated sodium channels in the axon initial segment

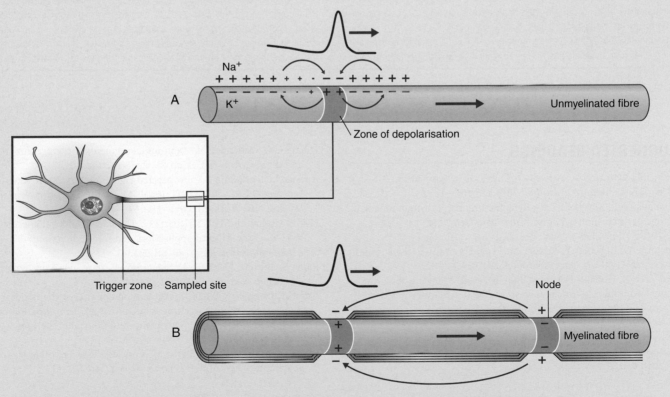

Fig. 7.12 Current flow during impulse propagation, represented as movement of positive charges. (A) Continuous conduction along an unmyelinated fibre. (B) Saltatory conduction along a myelinated fibre.

and the nodes helps to explain their unique physiological characteristics and is accomplished by a host of cytoskeletal and extracellular scaffolding and cell adhesion proteins. *Nodes* are metabolically very active and contain 90% of the organelles found in the whole length of the axon yet comprise only a fraction of an internode.

The *paranode* (axoglial junction) consists of multiple turns of myelin and, by forming a tight connection between the myelin and the axolemma, reduces current flow under the myelin. It also serves to maintain the node of Ranvier; restricts sodium channels to the node; and blocks the currents generated by the node from the internode, critical for maintaining saltatory conduction (see Fig. 9.4). It also separates the voltage-gated sodium channels at the node from potassium channels present at the juxtaparanodes.

The *juxtaparanode* contains most of the voltage-gated potassium channels that promote conduction by maintaining the internodal resting potential, preventing activation of any sodium channels present in the internodal axonal membrane, and preventing reentrant excitation of the nodes.

There are differences between the PNS and CNS subdomains; one such difference is what fills the adjacent nodal space. In the PNS it is occupied by microvilli of the Schwann cells, but in the CNS it is filled with extracellular matrix proteins. Further differences regard scaffolding and cell adhesion proteins, but all their protein—protein interactions make the node, paranode, and juxtaparanode prone to multiple pathological conditions. Aetiologies range from genetic to autoimmune and clinical features comprise a spectrum of disorders that present with PNS or CNS maladies and vary regarding associated disability.

✴ Core Information

Ions are electrically charged atoms or groups of atoms. Na^+ and K^+ are cations; Cl^- and P^- (proteins) are anions. Cell membranes are charged capacitors carrying a resting potential (voltage) of -70 mV.

Ion channels are protein pores that regulate ion movement across the cell membrane that results in current flow and electrical signalling. Passive ion channels for Na^+, K^+, and Cl^- are always open, and the ions diffuse down their concentration gradients through their respective channels. Na^+ channels are relatively scarce, whereas K^+ and Cl^- channels are numerous. K^+ ions are abundant in the cytosol, being attracted by P^- anions in the cytoskeleton and repelled by the Na^+ ions outside. The Na^+–K^+ channel pump maintains the resting steady state of the membrane potential.

The initial response of a multipolar neuron to an excitatory stimulus takes the form of decremental waves of positive electrotonus. Temporal and/or spatial summation of such waves produces a generator potential in the initial segment of the axon. At a threshold value of -55 mV, action potentials are initiated by opening voltage-gated channels and propagate along the nerve fibre. On the other hand, inhibitory stimulation takes the form of negative electrotonic waves that summate to hyperpolarise the membrane, thus taking it farther from threshold and limiting formation of an action potential.

The action potential (spike) is characterised by a rising phase (depolarisation) from baseline up to $+35$ mV, a falling phase (repolarisation) down to baseline followed by an after-hyperpolarisation phase down to -80 mV with return to baseline. Triggering the rapid depolarisation is activation of voltage-gated Na^+ ion channels, whereby the ion channel is briefly (<1 ms) opened completely, allowing massive Na^+ inflow, thus depolarising the membrane potential to $+35$ mV, whereupon the channels are shut by inactivation gates. At the peak of the action potential, voltage-gated K^+ channels are opened with a current switch from Na^+ inflow to K^+ outflow, resulting in repolarisation and the subsequent after-hyperpolarisation of the membrane potential.

For about 1 ms following impulse initiation, the trigger zone in the initial segment is *absolutely refractory* to further stimulation; for the following 3 ms it is relatively refractory.

Action potentials are initiated in an all-or-none manner and propagated at full strength along the fibre and its branches. Propagation is continuous along unmyelinated axons and saltatory (from node to node) along myelinated axons. Saltatory conduction is much faster. The widest diameter fibres have the longest internodal segments and the fastest conduction rates.

SUGGESTED READINGS

Arancibia-Carcamo IL, Attwell D. The node of Ranvier in CNS pathology. *Acta Neuropathol.* 2014;128:161—175.

Chanaday NL, Kavalali ET. Presynaptic origins of distinct modes of neurotransmitter release. *Curr Opin Neurobiol.* 2018;51:119—126.

Debanne D, Inglebert Y, Russier M. Plasticity of intrinsic neuronal excitability. *Curr Opin Neurobiol.* 2019;54:73—82.

Drukarch B, Holland HA, Velichkov M, et al. Thinking about the nerve impulse: a critical analysis of the electricity-centered conception of nerve excitability. *Prog Neurobiol.* 2018;169:172—185.

Gitman M, Barrington MJ. Local anesthetic systemic toxicity: a review of recent case reports and registries. *Reg Anesth Pain Med.* 2018;43:124—130.

Huang CY, Rasband MN. Axon initial segments: structure, function, and disease. *Ann N Y Acad Sci.* 2018;1420:46—61.

Koester J, Siegelbaum SA. Propagated signaling: the action potential. In: Kandel ER, Schwarz JH, Jessell TJ, eds. *Principles of Neural Science*. New York: McGraw-Hill; 2013:148—171.

Lirk P, Hollmann MW, Strichartz G. The science of local anesthesia: basic research, clinical application, and future directions. *Anesthesia & Analgesia.* 2018;126:1381—1392.

Rama S, Zbili M, Debanne D. Signal propagation along the axon. *Curr Opin Neurobiol.* 2018;51:37—44.

Vural A, Doppler K, Meinl E. Autoantibodies against the node of Ranvier in seropositive chronic inflammatory demyelinating polyneuropathy: diagnostic, pathogenic, and therapeutic relevance. *Front Immunol.* 2018;9:1029.

Walter AM, Bohme MA, Sigrist SJ. Vesicle release site organization at synaptic active zones. *Neurosci Res.* 2018;127:3—13.

Transmitters and Receptors

CHAPTER SUMMARY

STUDY GUIDELINES

1. Contrast electrical and chemical synapses and describe the differences between ionotropic receptors and metabotropic receptors.
2. List the three major second messenger systems in the CNS and the functions of a second messenger.
3. List the criteria that must be fulfilled before a substance can be considered a neurotransmitter.
4. List the major types of neurotransmitters and provide an example of each.
5. Describe the steps that occur when a transmitter binds to an ionotropic receptor.
6. Give examples of the various mechanisms used to terminate the action of a neurotransmitter or to recycle them.
7. **Clinical Panel 8.1 and 8.2:** Review the following clinical disorders (stiff person spectrum disorder and Botulinum toxin administration for movement disorders) in regard to pathophysiology and relevance to a chemical synapse.

ELECTRICAL SYNAPSES

Electrical synapses are scarce in the mammalian nervous system. As seen in Fig. 8.1, they consist of *gap junctions* (nexuses) between dendrites or somas of contiguous neurons, where there is cytoplasmic continuity through 1.5-nm channels. No transmitter is involved, and there is no synaptic delay.

The gap junctions are bridged by tightly packed ion channels, each comprising mirror image pairs of *connexons*, which are transmembrane protein groups *(connexins)* arranged hexagonally around an ion pore. Wedge-shaped connexin subunits bordering each ion pore are closely apposed when the neurons are inactive. Action potentials passing along the cell membrane cause the subunits to rotate individually, creating a pore large enough to permit free diffusion of ions and small molecules down their concentration gradients.

The overall function of these gap junctions is to ensure synchronous activity of neurons with a common action. An example is the inspiratory centre in the medulla oblongata, where all the cells exhibit synchronous discharge during inspiration. A second example occurs among neuronal circuits controlling *saccades*, where the gaze darts from one object of interest to another.

CHEMICAL SYNAPSES

Chemical synapses are the primary form of communication in the central and peripheral nervous systems. As seen in Fig. 8.2,

each consists of a pre- and a postsynaptic cell with a synaptic cleft between them of 20—40 nm. Therefore, there is no cytoplasmic continuity between the two cells. The presynaptic cell contains neurotransmitter vesicles, an active zone (proteins for binding and releasing of vesicle contents), and voltage-gated calcium (Ca^{2+}) channels. The postsynaptic cell contains a variable number of receptors that will bind the transmitter released by the presynaptic cell. Due to the numerous steps involved in releasing and binding of neurotransmitters, there is synaptic delay which is typically 1—5 ms (or longer).

Transmitter Release (Fig. 8.2 and Table 8.1)

In resting nerve terminals, synaptic vesicles accumulate near the active zones, where they are tethered to the presynaptic densities by strands of *docking proteins* and actin. With the arrival of action potentials, voltage-gated Ca^{2+} channels located immediately adjacent to the active zone in the presynaptic membrane are opened, leading to instant flooding of the active zone with Ca^{2+} ions. These ions interact with several proteins on both the vesicle and the active zone, leading to vesicle fusion with the presynaptic membrane and neurotransmitter release.

Vesicle fusion begins with the interaction of *vesicle SNARE proteins (v-SNARE)* with a pair of *presynaptic membrane proteins (t-SNAREs)* to form a tight complex. The necessary metabolic components that trigger vesicle fusion are embedded in the active zone. A critical protein for these components is a

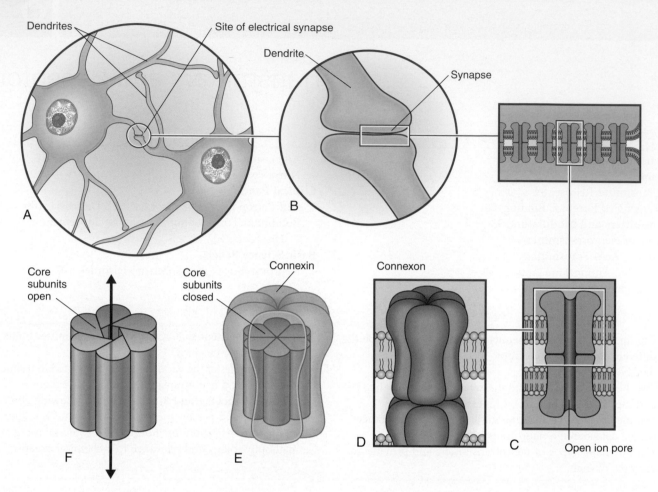

Fig. 8.1 Structure of an electrical synapse. (A) Synaptic contact between two dendrites. (B) Enlargement from (A). (C) The gap junction between the cell membranes is bridged by close-packed ion channels. (D) Each ion channel comprises a mirror image pair of connexons. (E) Each connexon is formed by six identical connexins, each having a wedge-shaped subunit bordering the ion channel. (F) The subunits open the ion channel by synchronous rotation.

large, multidomain protein called *RIM* that binds to Rab3, a GTP-binding protein on synaptic vesicles. Other proteins are also required for vesicle fusion and the release of neurotransmitters. These synaptic components include *synaptic vesicle proteins* (e.g. synaptotagmin, synaptobrevin, synaptophysin, and synapsins), proteins associated with synaptic vesicles (e.g. amphiphysin, dynamin, and CaM kinases), *synaptic plasma membrane proteins* (e.g. syntaxins, neurexins, and SNAP-25), and associated cytosolic proteins (e.g. complexins, SNAPs, and NSF).

Many of the identified synaptic proteins have distinctive roles in the excitation−secretion coupling and synaptic vesicle recovery mechanisms underlying synaptic transmission. Intricate models of the molecular machinery responsible for excitation−secretion coupling and neurotransmission at the synapse have been developed through various techniques. These and other local protein responses to Ca^{2+} entry are extremely rapid, and the time between Ca^{2+} entry and transmitter expulsion is normally less than 1 ms. In the case of small synaptic vesicles such as those containing glutamate or γ-aminobutyric acid (GABA), single spikes are sufficient to yield some transmitter release.

In the case of peptidergic neurons, impulse frequencies of 10 Hz or more are required to induce typically slow (delay of 50 ms or more) transmitter release from the large, dense-cored vesicles. Therefore, the amount of transmitter released from a neuron is not fixed but can be modified by both intrinsic and extrinsic modulatory processes, the most important being the availability of free Ca^{2+} in the presynaptic terminal.

Target Cell Receptor Binding

Transmitter molecules bind with receptor protein molecules in the postsynaptic membrane. The two main categories of receptors are *ionotropic* and *metabotropic*. Each category contains some receptors whose activation leads to the opening of ion pores and others whose activation leads to their closure.

Ionotropic Receptors. Ionotropic receptors are characterised by the presence of an ion channel within each receptor macromolecule (Fig. 8.3). The transmitter binds with its specific receptor facing the synaptic cleft, causing it to change its conformational state, normally opening a closed channel. Ionotropic

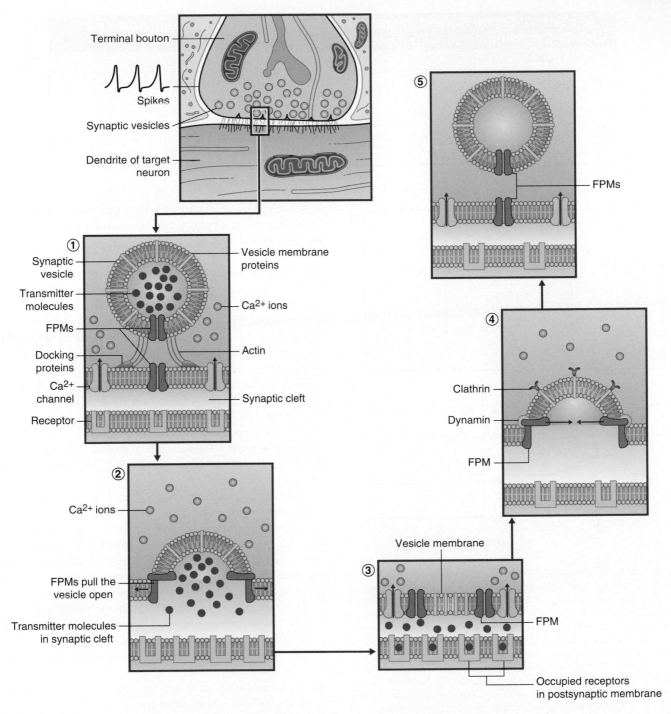

Fig. 8.2 Sequence of events following depolarisation of the presynaptic membrane. (1) Opening of calcium (Ca^{2+}) channels *(arrows)* causes synaptic vesicles to be pulled into contact with the presynaptic membrane by actin filaments. Matching pairs of fusion protein macromolecules *(FPMs)* in the vesicle and presynaptic membrane are aligned. (2) The FPMs separate *(outward arrows)*, permitting transmitter molecules to be released into the synaptic cleft. (3) Vesicle membrane is incorporated into the presynaptic membrane while transmitter is activating the specific receptors. (4) Clathrin molecules assist inward movement of the vesicle membrane. Dynamin molecules *(green)* assist approximation of FPM pairs *(inward arrows)* and pinch the neck of the emerging vesicle. (5) The vesicle is now free for recycling.

receptor channels are said to be *transmitter-gated*, or *ligand-gated*, signifying their capacity to bind a transmitter molecule or a drug substitute. As soon as the transmitter dissociates from the receptor or is broken down, the channel reverts to its original state (closes).

In Fig. 8.3A, the excitatory channel has been opened by the transmitter, causing a major influx of sodium ions (Na^+) and a minor efflux of potassium ions (K^+); the net result is an ***excitatory postsynaptic potential (EPSP)*** that depolarises the membrane. A larger depolarisation can be achieved by opening

TABLE 8.1 **Some Named Proteins Involved in Transmitter Transport and Vesicle Recycling.**

Named Protein	Function
Actin	Brings vesicle into contact with presynaptic membrane
Calmodulin	Expels vesicle content into synaptic cleft
Clathrin	Withdraws vesicle membrane from synaptic cleft
Dynamin	Pinches the neck of the developing vesicle to complete its separation
Ligand	Receptor protein that binds with the transmitter molecule
Synaptophysin	Creates the membrane fusion pore

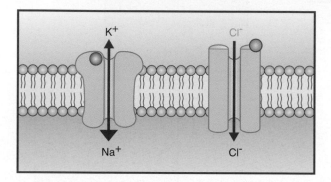

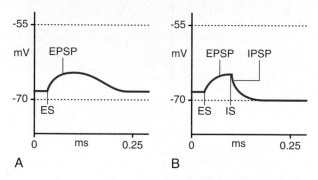

Fig. 8.3 (A) A transmitter-gated excitatory ionotropic receptor. Binding of the transmitter (*red*, representing glutamate; excitatory stimulus, *ES*) has opened the pore of a 'mixed' sodium–potassium cation channel. A large influx of sodium *(Na$^+$)* ions coupled with a small efflux of potassium *(K$^+$)* ions results in a net depolarisation of the membrane, as shown by the excitatory postsynaptic potential *(EPSP)*. (B) A Transmitter-Gated Inhibitory Ionotropic Receptor. Secondary binding of the inhibitory transmitter *(blue*, representing GABA$_A$; inhibitory stimulus, *IS)* has opened the pore of a chloride *(Cl$^-$)* channel. Inward Cl$^-$ conductance has been increased, and the inhibitory postsynaptic potential *(IPSP)* causes the membrane potential to hyperpolarise.

multiple transmitter-gated channels, resulting in summation and possibly reaching the threshold value to trigger an action potential. In Fig. 8.3B, the EPSP is followed immediately by an **inhibitory postsynaptic potential (IPSP)** that hyperpolarises the membrane to −70 mV, the chloride (Cl$^-$) equilibrium potential. A larger hyperpolarisation can be achieved by opening a K$^+$ channel, which has an equilibrium potential of −80 mV.

Ionotropic receptors are called fast receptors because of their immediate but brief effects on ion channels and their changes on the membrane potential.

Metabotropic receptors. Metabotropic receptors are so called because many can generate multiple metabolic effects within the cytoplasm of the neuron. The receptor macromolecule is a transmembrane protein devoid of an ion channel. Its function is initiated by the binding of a transmitter to its extracellular receptor site. This causes a change in the conformational state of the protein, activating one of the attached subunits (α or β *subunit)* that detaches and moves along the intracellular surface of the membrane. The subunits are called **G proteins**, because most bind with guanine nucleotides such as *guanine triphosphate (GTP)* or *guanine diphosphate (GDP)*. Their action on ion channels is usually indirect, via a **second messenger system**. However, some G proteins activate ion channels *directly* (see later).

A G protein with a stimulatory effect is known as **G$_s$ protein**, whereas that with an inhibitory effect is known as **G$_i$ protein**. Because of the numerous steps involved, metabotropic receptors are generally *slow* receptors. Membrane channel effects may continue for hundreds of milliseconds after a single stimulus. Additionally, the creation of intracellular second messengers can alter the excitability properties of neurons.

Three second messenger systems are well recognised:

1. The **cyclic adenosine monophosphate (cAMP) system**, responsible for phosphorylation of proteins.
2. The **phosphoinositol system**, responsible for liberating Ca^{2+} from cytoplasmic stores.
3. The **arachidonic acid system**, responsible for production of arachidonic acid metabolites.

cAMP system. In the examples shown in Fig. 8.4, transmitter–receptor binding (1) releases the α subunit (2) of a G$_s$ protein, leaving it free to link with GTP (3), which in turn facilitates *adenylate cyclase* to convert adenosine triphosphate (ATP) to cAMP (4). The newly formed cAMP serves as the second messenger. Protein kinase A (PKA) in the membrane is stimulated by cAMP (5) to transfer phosphate ions from ATP to an ion channel (6), causing its pore to open and to allow Na$^+$ ions to enter, thus initiating depolarisation of the target neuron. When the G$_s$ protein is switched off, the membrane-attached enzyme *protein phosphatase* (7) catalyses the extraction of phosphate ions, resulting in pore closure.

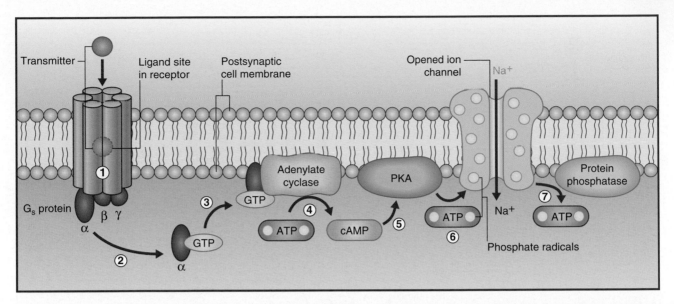

Fig. 8.4 The cyclic AMP *(cAMP)* system. The diagram shows the basic steps along the path from a G_s protein-linked receptor via cAMP to an ion channel. (1) Transmitter is activating the receptor macromolecule. (2) G_s protein α subunit is freed to bind with guanosine triphosphate *(GTP)*. (3) GTP links the unit to adenylate cyclase. (4) Adenylate cyclase catalyses synthesis of cAMP from adenosine triphosphate *(ATP)*. (5) cAMP activates protein kinase A *(PKA)*. (6) PKA transfers phosphate groups from ATP to a sodium ion *(Na$^+$)* channel, causing its pore to open and Na$^+$ ions to rush into the cytosol, causing depolarisation. (7) Following inactivation of the G_s protein, dephosphorylation of the channel by a phosphatase enzyme allows the channel pore to close.

Phosphoinositol system. In the example shown in Fig. 8.5, activation (1) of another kind of G_s protein α subunit (2) causes the effector enzyme *phospholipase C* (PLC) to split a membrane phospholipid (PIP$_2$) (3) into a pair of second messengers: *diacylglycerol* (DAG) and *inositol triphosphate* (IP$_3$). DAG activates protein kinase C (PKC) (4), which initiates protein phosphorylation (5). IP$_3$ diffuses into the cytosol (6), where it opens Ca^{2+}-gated channels, mainly in nearby membranes of smooth endoplasmic reticulum (7). The Ca^{2+} ions activate certain Ca^{2+}-dependent enzymes downstream, resulting in opening and/or closing of ion channels and possibly crossing the nuclear envelope to alter gene expression and protein production (8) (see 'gene transcription effects' below).

Arachidonic acid system. This is described later, in connection with histamine.

Gene transcription effects. It is also well established that the reflex responses to **repetitive** stimuli may be either progressively increased (a state of **sensitisation**, usually induced by noxious stimuli) or diminished (a state of **habituation**, induced by harmless stimuli). Animal experiments that investigate reflex arcs (involving sets of sensory neurons, motor neurons, and interneurons) have shown that a characteristic feature of sensitisation is the development of additional synaptic contacts between the interneurons and the motor neurons with an increase in transmitter synthesis and release, whereas in contrast, a characteristic feature of habituation is a reduction of transmitter synthesis and release. All these changes result from *alterations of gene transcription*. Repetitive noxious stimuli cause cAMP to increase its normal rate of activation of protein kinases involved in the phosphorylation of proteins that

regulate gene transcription. This in turn results in an increased production of proteins (including enzymes) required for transmitter synthesis as well as other proteins for construction of additional channels and synaptic cytoskeletons. Repetitive harmless stimuli merely reduce the rate of transmitter synthesis and release. Both sensitisation and habituation can produce long-term or even permanent changes in how the nervous system responds to these stimuli in the future.

Gene transcription effects are especially important for forming long-term memories (Chapter 33).

TRANSMITTERS AND MODULATORS

Several criteria must be fulfilled for a substance to be accepted as a neurotransmitter:

- The substance must be present within the neurons, together with the molecules and enzymes required to synthesise it (typically in a vesicle).
- The substance must be released following depolarisation of nerve endings that contain it and its release must be induced by the entry of Ca^{2+}.
- The postsynaptic membrane must contain specific receptors that will modify the membrane potential of the target neuron.
- The substance in its pure form must exert the same effect when applied to a target neuron exogenously *(microiontophoresis)*.
- Specific antagonist molecules, whether delivered through the circulation or by iontophoresis, must block the effect of the putative transmitter.

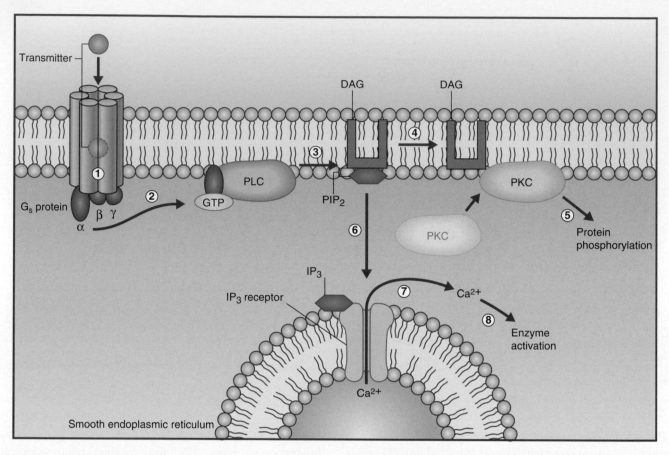

Fig. 8.5 The phosphoinositol system. The steps indicate the dual function of this system. (1) The transmitter activates the receptor macromolecule. (2) The G_s protein α subunit is freed to bind with guanosine triphosphate *(GTP)*, which links it to phospholipase C *(PLC)*. (3) PLC moves along the membrane and splits the membrane phospholipid *(PIP$_2$)* into diacylglycerol *(DAG)* and inositol triphosphate *(IP$_3$)*. (4) DAG attracts the enzyme protein kinase C *(PKC)* to the membrane, where (5) DAG is triggered to phosphorylate several proteins, potentially including ion channels. (6) IP$_3$ activates calcium *(Ca^{2+})* channels in the smooth endoplasmic reticulum. (7) Stored Ca^{2+} is released into the cytosol. (8) Ca^{2+}-dependent enzymes are activated.

• The physiologic mode of termination of the transmitter effect must be identified, whether it is by enzymatic degradation or by active transport into the parent neuron or adjacent neuroglial cells.

Many transmitters limit their own rate of release by negative feedback activation of autoreceptors in the presynaptic membrane, which inhibit further release. Ideally, the existence of specific inhibitory autoreceptors should be established.

The term *neuromodulator* has been subject to several interpretations. The most satisfactory one appears to be derived from electrical engineering terms, amplitude modulation and frequency modulation, signifying superimposition of one wave or signal onto another. Fig. 8.6 represents a sympathetic and a parasympathetic nerve ending, close to a pacemaker cell (modified cardiac myocyte). This neighbourly arrangement of nerve endings is common in the heart and allows the respective transmitters to modulate each other's activity. The sympathetic nerve ending releases norepinephrine (noradrenaline), which has a stimulatory effect. The three modulators shown exert their effects via second messenger systems.

The figure caption also refers to *autoreceptors* and *heteroreceptors*. Receptors for a transmitter that often occur in the

presynaptic and postsynaptic membranes are called ***autoreceptors***. These are activated by high transmitter concentration in the synaptic cleft, and they have a negative feedback effect, inhibiting further transmitter release from the synaptic bouton. ***Heteroreceptors*** occupy the plasma membrane of neurons that do not liberate the specific transmitter. In the example shown, activity at sympathetic nerve endings is accompanied by inhibition of parasympathetic activity through heteroreceptors located on parasympathetic nerve endings.

Fate of Neurotransmitters

The fate of transmitters released into synaptic clefts is highly variable. Some transmitters are inactivated within the cleft, some diffuse away into the cerebrospinal fluid via the extracellular fluid, and some are recycled either by direct uptake by the pre- or postsynaptic cells, or indirectly via glial cells.

The principal transmitters and modulators are shown in Table 8.2. Respective receptor types are listed in Table 8.3.

Amino Acid Transmitters

The most prevalent excitatory transmitter in the brain and spinal cord is the amino acid *L-glutamate* (Fig. 8.7). As an

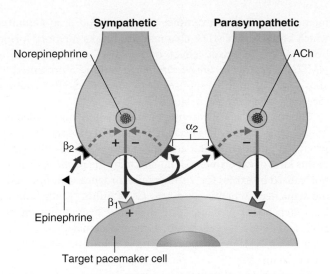

Fig. 8.6 Neuromodulation occurs at nerve endings in the sinoatrial node of the heart, where sympathetic and parasympathetic nerve endings often occur in pairs. In this representation the sympathetic system is the more active, releasing the transmitter norepinephrine, which depolarises cardiac pacemaker cells via β_1 pacemaker membrane receptors. Circulating epinephrine exerts positive modulation on the nerve ending by increasing transmitter release via β_2 presynaptic membrane heteroreceptors. Inhibitory modulation of excess norepinephrine release is expressed via α_2 presynaptic membrane autoreceptors. At the same time, release of the inhibitory transmitter acetylcholine (ACh) from the parasympathetic bouton is inhibited via α_2 heteroreceptors.

TABLE 8.3 Receptor Types Activated by Different Neurotransmitters.

Ionotropic Receptors	Metabotropic Receptors
Acetylcholine (nicotinic)	Acetylcholine (muscarinic)
$GABA_A$	$GABA_B$
Glutamate (AMPA—K)	Glutamate (mGluR)
Glycine	Dopamine (D_1, D_2)
Serotonin ($5\text{-}HT_3$)	Serotonin ($5\text{-}HT_1$, $5\text{-}HT_2$)
	Norepinephrine (noradrenaline) (α_1, α_2), epinephrine (adrenaline)
	Histamine (H_1, H_2, H_3)
	All neuropeptides
	Adenosine

TABLE 8.2 Main Types of Transmitters and Modulators.

Type	Example(s)
Amino acids	Glutamate
	γ-Aminobutyric acid (GABA)
	Glycine
Biogenic amines	Acetylcholine
	Catecholamines* (dopamine, norepinephrine (noradrenaline), epinephrine (adrenaline))
	Histamine*
	Serotonin*
Neuropeptides	Endorphin
	Enkephalin
	Substance P
	Vasoactive intestinal polypeptide
	Many others
Adenosine	—
Gaseous	Nitric oxide

*The five monoamines contain a single amine group. Catecholamines also contain a catechol nucleus.

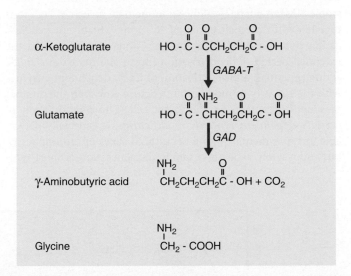

Fig. 8.7 The three amino acid transmitters. Glutamate is derived from α-ketoglutarate by the enzyme GABA transaminase (GABA-T); γ-aminobutyric acid (GABA) is derived from glutamate by glutamic acid decarboxylase (GAD). Glycine is the simplest amino acid.

important example, *all* neurons projecting into the white matter from the cerebral cortex, regardless of their destinations in other areas of the cortex, brainstem, or spinal cord, are excitatory and use glutamate as a transmitter. Glutamate is derived from

α-ketoglutarate; it also provides the substrate for formation of the most common inhibitory transmitter, *GABA*.

GABA is widely distributed in the brain and spinal cord and is the transmitter in approximately one third of all synapses. Millions of GABAergic neurons form the bulk of the caudate and lentiform nuclei, and they are also concentrated in the hypothalamus, periaqueductal grey matter, and hippocampus. Moreover, GABA is the transmitter for the large Purkinje cells, which are the *only* output cells of the cerebellar cortex, projecting to the dentate and other cerebellar nuclei. GABA is synthesised from glutamate by the enzyme *glutamic acid decarboxylase*.

A third amino acid transmitter, *glycine*, is the same molecule that is used in the synthesis of proteins in all tissues. It is the simplest of the amino acids, being synthesised from glucose via serine. It is an inhibitory transmitter largely confined to inter-neurons of the brainstem and spinal cord.

Glutamate. Glutamate acts on both ionotropic and metabotropic receptors. Three ionotropic receptors, named after synthetic agonists that activate them, are *AMPA*, *kainate*, and *NMDA* (referring to amino-methylisoxazole propionic acid, kainate, and N-methyl-D-aspartate, respectively). Kainate receptors are scarce; they only occur in company with AMPA as AMPA—K.

Ionotropic glutamate receptors. Activation of AMPA—K receptor channels by glutamate in the postsynaptic membrane allows an immediate inrush of Na^+ ions together with a small efflux of K^+ ions (Fig. 8.8), generating the early component of the EPSP in the target neuron. Should this component depolarise the target cell membrane from -65 mV to -50 mV, it will generate electrostatic repulsion of magnesium cations (Mg^{2+}) that plug the NMDA receptor ion pore at rest. Similarly, ionotropic NMDA channels allow an immediate inrush of Na^+ ions together with a small efflux of K^+ ions which can generate action potentials. Significantly, Ca^{2+} ions also enter, and the extended period of depolarisation (up to 500 ms from a single action potential) allows activation of Ca^{2+}-dependent enzymes with the capacity to modify the structure and even the number of synaptic contacts in the target cell. The phenomenon of *activity-dependent synaptic modification* is especially detectable in experimental studies of cultured slices of rat hippocampus and is likely to be important in the generation of short-term memory traces. (For example, the anaesthetic drug *ketamine*, which blocks the NMDA channel, also blocks memory formation.) A characteristic effect of repetitive activation of the NMDA receptor is **long-term potentiation**, represented by above-normal EPSP responses even some days after training. (See *long-term depression*, later.)

The role of NMDA receptors in the phenomenon called *glutamate excitotoxicity* has been demonstrated in vascular strokes produced in experimental animals. The mass death of neurons in this kind of experiment is thought to be the result of degradation caused by excess Ca^{2+} influx in accordance with the following sequence: ischemia $\Rightarrow$ excess Ca^{2+} influx $\Rightarrow$ activation of Ca^{2+}-dependent proteases and lipases $\Rightarrow$ degradation of proteins and lipids $\Rightarrow$ cell death. Ischemic damage may be less severe if an NMDA antagonist drug is administered soon after the initial insult.

Metabotropic glutamate receptors. More than 100 different metabotropic glutamate receptors have been identified. All are intrinsic membrane proteins; most occupy postsynaptic membranes and have an excitatory function, whereas others occupy presynaptic membranes where they act as inhibitory autoreceptors.

GABA. Two major classes of GABA receptors are recognised: ionotropic and metabotropic.

Ionotropic GABA receptors. Termed $GABA_A$, these are especially abundant in the limbic lobe. Each is directly linked to a Cl^- ion channel (Fig. 8.9). Following the activation of $GABA_A$

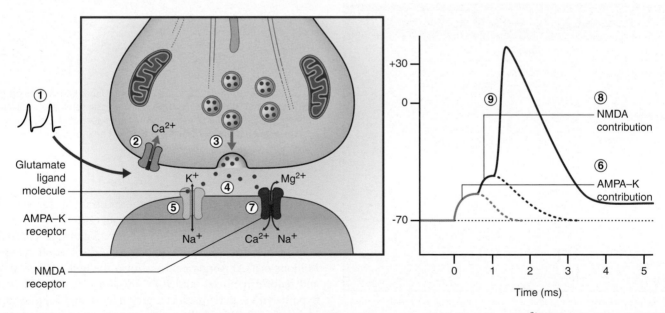

Fig. 8.8 Ionotropic glutamate receptors. (1) On arrival of action potentials at the nerve terminal, (2) calcium *(Ca^{2+})* channels open, and (3) Ca^{2+} ions cause synaptic vesicles to be pulled against the cell membrane. (4) Glutamate molecules undergo exocytosis into the synaptic cleft. (5) Transmitter binding to the amino-methylisoxazole propionic acid—kainate *(AMPA—K)* receptor opens the ion channel permitting a large influx of sodium *(Na$^+$)* and a small efflux of potassium *(K$^+$)*. (6) The resulting excitatory postsynaptic potential *(EPSP)* produces some 20 mV of depolarisation, which (7) permits the glutamate ligand to activate the *N*-methyl-D-aspartate *(NMDA)* receptor by expulsion of its magnesium *(Mg^{2+})* 'plug'. Both Na^+ and Ca^{2+} ions rush into the cell via the NMDA channel while K^+ ions leak out slowly, resulting in further depolarisation. (8) The NMDA-induced EPSP is sufficient to (9) trigger action potentials having an extended repolarisation period because of increased levels of intracellular Ca^{2+}.

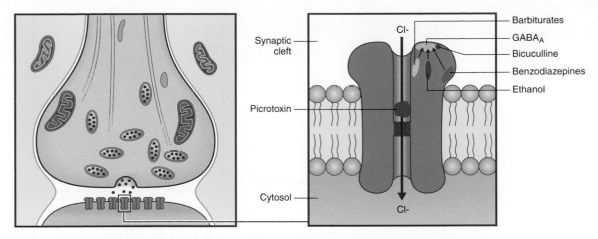

Fig. 8.9 Drugs and the Ionotropic GABA$_A$ receptor. *Green* signifies an agonist effect; *red* signifies an antagonist effect. Barbiturates, benzodiazepines, and ethanol cause hyperpolarisation via the natural receptor. Bicuculline antagonises the receptor, whereas picrotoxin closes the ion pore by direct action locally.

receptors, channel pores are opened and Cl$^-$ ions diffuse down their concentration gradient from the synaptic cleft to the cytosol. Hyperpolarisation up to −70 mV or more is brought about by summation of successive IPSPs (Fig. 8.10). It also results in a decrease in the time constant of the cell, which makes it more difficult for the neuron to reach threshold.

The sedative hypnotic barbiturates and benzodiazepines, such as diazepam, exert their effects by activating the GABA$_A$ receptor. So too does ethanol. (Loss of social control under the influence of ethanol may follow the release of target excitatory neurons normally held in check by tonic GABAergic activity.) Some volatile anaesthetics also bind with the receptor, prolonging the open state of the ion channel.

The chief antagonist at the receptor site is the convulsant drug bicuculline. Another convulsant is picrotoxin, which binds with protein subunits that choke/block the ion pore when activated.

Metabotropic GABA receptors. Termed **GABA$_B$**, metabotropic GABA receptors are relatively uniformly distributed throughout the brain and are also found within peripheral autonomic nerve plexuses. Although most of their G proteins operate via second messengers, a significant number act *directly* on a special class of postsynaptic K$^+$ channels known as *GIRK channels (G protein inwardly rectifying K$^+$ channels)*. As shown in Fig. 8.11, transmitter binding releases. the βγ-subunit, which allows K$^+$ ions to leave through the GIRK channel, thereby producing an IPSP.

The response properties of the target neuronal receptors are slower and weaker than those of GABA$_A$ ionophores, requiring higher-frequency stimulation to be activated. This has led to the belief that they may be extrasynaptic in position rather than facing the synaptic cleft. This is indicated in Fig. 8.12, where the belief is supported by the existence of another type of G-direct channel in extrasynaptic locations. This is a Ca^{2+} channel that is also voltage-gated and therefore

participates in provision of the Ca^{2+} ions needed to draw synaptic vesicles against the presynaptic membrane. Activation of a G−Ca^{2+} ligand site closes Ca^{2+} channels, thereby reducing the effectiveness of action potentials, with an inhibitory effect on the parent neuron and on any nearby glutamatergic neurons.

In clinical disorders that involve excessive tonic muscle reflex responses (the state of *spasticity*, Chapter 16), the muscle relaxant *baclofen*, a GABA$_B$ agonist, is taken orally or sometimes injected into the subarachnoid space surrounding the spinal cord. Baclofen seeps into the cord and inhibits release of glutamate from the terminals of muscle afferents, mainly by diminishing the massive Ca^{2+} entry associated with excessively frequent action potentials.

Recycling of Glutamate and GABA. The two routes for recycling are indicated for glutamate in Fig. 8.13 and for GABA in Fig. 8.14. On the bottom left of each diagram, some transmitter molecules are retrieved from the synaptic cleft by a presynaptic membrane transporter protein and reincorporated directly into a synaptic vesicle. On the right of each diagram, the transmitter molecules are being recycled through an adjacent astrocyte (1). In Fig. 8.13, glutamate is converted to glutamine by *glutamine synthetase* during transit through astrocytes (2). Following intercellular transport into the synaptic bouton (3), glutamate is reassembled by *glutaminase* (4) and then repacked into a synaptic vesicle (5). In Fig. 8.14, GABA is first converted to glutamate by *GABA transaminase* (1), then to glutamine by *glutamine synthetase* (2) during transit. Following its return to the synaptic bouton, glutamine is converted to glutamate (*glutaminase*) (3), which is then converted (*glutamate decarboxylase*) (4) to GABA prior to storage in vesicles (5).

The remarkable autoimmune disorder known as *stiff person syndrome* is caused by blockade of glutamate decarboxylase; see Clinical Panel 8.1.

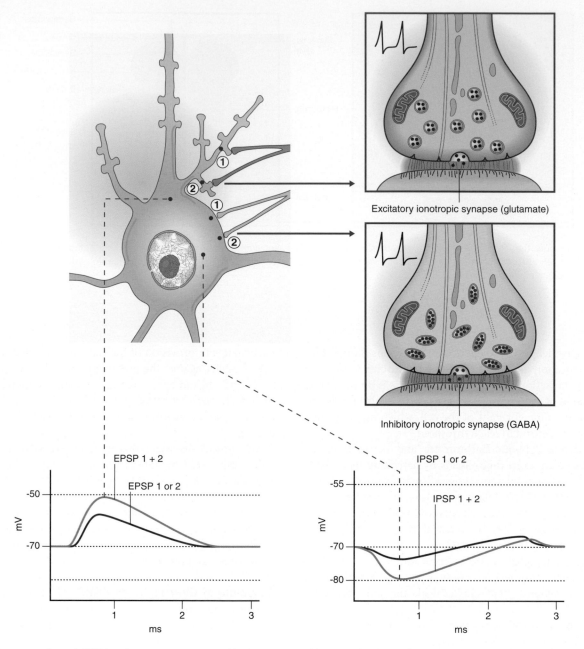

Excitatory ionotropic synapse (glutamate)

Inhibitory ionotropic synapse (GABA)

Fig. 8.10 Glutamatergic and GABAergic synapses on a multipolar neuron with spiny dendrites. Spatial summation of postsynaptic potentials is illustrated for each pair of synapses. *EPSP*, Excitatory postsynaptic potential; *GABA*, γ-aminobutyric acid; *IPSP*, inhibitory postsynaptic potential.

Glycine. Glycine is synthesised from glucose via serine. Its main function as a transmitter is to provide tonic negative feedback on motor neurons in the brainstem and spinal cord. Inactivation of glycine (e.g. by strychnine poisoning) results in painful convulsions (Fig. 8.15).

Recycling. Glycine is rapidly taken up into the synaptic bouton by an axonal transporter and recycled to synaptic vesicles.

Biogenic Amine Transmitters

Acetylcholine. Acetylcholine (ACh) plays a highly significant role as a transmitter. In the central nervous system (CNS) the activity of cholinergic neurons projecting from the basal region of the forebrain to the hippocampus is essential for learning and memory; degeneration of these neurons is consistently associated with the onset of Alzheimer disease. In the peripheral nervous system (PNS) all motor neurons to skeletal muscle are cholinergic; all preganglionic neurons supplying the ganglia of the sympathetic and parasympathetic systems are cholinergic, as is the postganglionic nerve supply of the parasympathetic system to cardiac muscle, the smooth muscle of the intestine and urinary bladder, and the smooth muscles of the eye involved in the accommodation reflex for close-up vision.

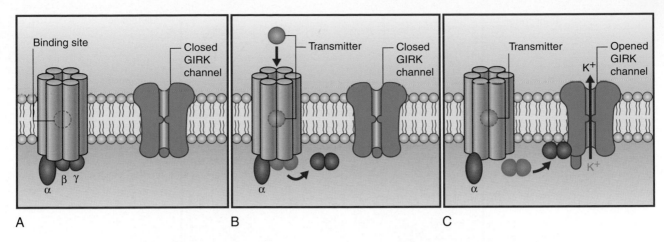

Fig. 8.11 G protein direct opening of a girk channel in a postsynaptic membrane. (A) Inactive state. (B) GABA activation of the receptor causes the G protein βγ subunit to be transferred to the GIRK channel. (C) The βγ subunit causes potassium (K^+) ions to be released, thereby leading to hyperpolarisation of the cell membrane. *GABA*, γ-aminobutyric acid; *GIRK*, G protein inwardly rectifying K^+ channels.

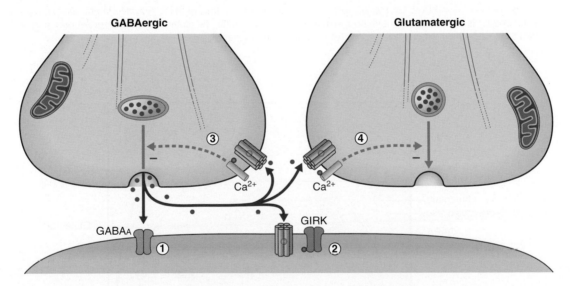

Fig. 8.12 Process following transmitter release from a gabaergic neuron. (1) Transmitter binding with GABA$_A$ receptors has a hyperpolarising effect on the target membrane by opening chloride (Cl^-) channels. (2) Binding with GIRK GABA$_B$ receptors works in the same direction by opening inwardly rectifying potassium (K^+) channels *(GIRKs)*. (3) Binding with GABA$_B$ autoreceptors dampens transmitter release from the parent neuron by closing ligand–G protein-mediated calcium channels (Ca^{2+}). (4) Binding with GABA$_B$ heteroreceptors on neighbouring glutamatergic boutons has the same Ca^{2+} effect. *GABA*, γ-aminobutyric acid.

ACh is formed when an acetyl group is transferred to choline from acetyl coenzyme A (acetyl CoA) by the enzyme *choline acetyltransferase* (Fig. 8.16), which is present only in cholinergic neurons. The choline is actively transported into the neuron from the extracellular space. Acetyl CoA is synthesised in mitochondria that are concentrated in the nerve terminal and provide the enzyme. Following release, ACh is degraded in the synaptic cleft by *acetylcholinesterase (AChE)*, yielding choline and acetic acid. These molecules are largely recaptured and recycled to form fresh transmitters.

Some steps in synthesis, degradation, and recycling of ACh are shown in Fig. 8.17.

Both ligand-gated and G protein-coupled ACh receptors are recognised. Ionotropic ACh receptors are called **nicotinic** because they were first discovered to be activated by nicotine extracted from the tobacco plant. Metabotropic ACh receptors are called **muscarinic** because they are activated by muscarine extracted from the poisonous mushroom *Amanita muscaria*.

Nicotinic receptors. Nicotinic receptors are found in the neuromuscular junctions of skeletal muscle, in all autonomic ganglia, and in the CNS. Activation by ACh causes the ion pore to open, with an immediate inrush of Ca^{2+} and Na^+ ions, resulting in depolarisation of the target neuron.

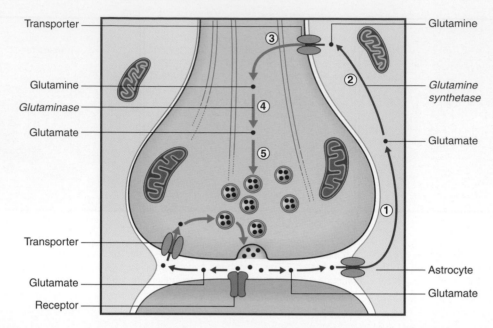

Fig. 8.13 Glutamate reuptake and resynthesis. On the left (bottom), glutamate molecules are being recycled intact. On the right, (1) glutamate is taken up by an astrocyte, and (2) is converted to glutamine by glutamine synthetase. (3) The glutamine is transported back into the nerve terminal, (4) where it is converted to glutamate by glutaminase and (5) returned to a synaptic vesicle.

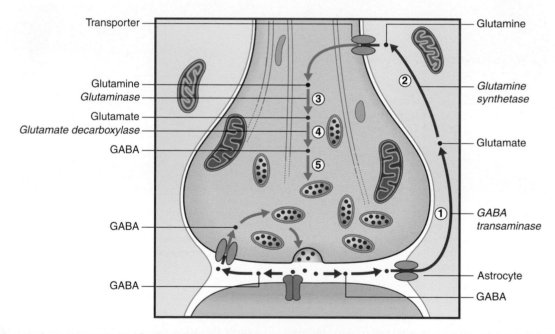

Fig. 8.14 GABA reuptake and resynthesis. On the left (bottom), GABA molecules are being recycled intact. On the right, GABA is taken up by an astrocyte, then (1) GABA is converted to glutamate by GABA transaminase. (2) Glutamate is converted to glutamine by glutamine synthetase. (3) Glutamine is transported back into the nerve terminal and converted to glutamate by glutaminase. (4) Glutamate is converted to GABA by glutamate decarboxylase and (5) returned to a synaptic vesicle. *GABA*, γ-aminobutyric acid.

The nicotinic receptor is considered further in relation to the innervation in skeletal muscle (see Chapter 10).

Muscarinic receptors. The G protein-gated muscarinic receptors are especially numerous in (a) the temporal lobe of the brain, where they are involved in the formation of memories; (b) autonomic ganglia; (c) cardiac muscle fibres, including the modified muscle of the conducting tissue; (d) smooth muscle of the intestine and urinary bladder; and (e) secretory cells

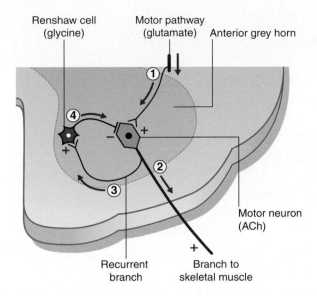

Renshaw cell (glycine)   Motor pathway (glutamate)   Anterior grey horn

Motor neuron (ACh)

Recurrent branch   Branch to skeletal muscle

Fig. 8.15 The negative feedback loop whereby renshaw cells inhibit excessive firing by motor neurons. (1) Fibre from a descending motor pathway is exciting a spinal motor neuron. (2) The motor neuron is stimulating muscle contraction. (3) A recurrent branch stimulates a Renshaw cell. (4) The Renshaw cell provides sufficient inhibition to prevent over activity of the motor neuron. *ACh*, acetylcholine.

of sweat glands. Five subtypes have been identified, numbered M_1 to M_5. In general, M_1, M_3, and M_5 receptors are excitatory and the enzyme cascades, allowing upregulation of phospholipase C and intracellular Ca^{2+} levels; M_2 and M_4 receptors are inhibitory autoreceptors that reduce intracellular cAMP levels and/or increase K^+ efflux, resulting in hyperpolarisation.

Cholinergic effects in the heart and other viscera are described in Chapter 13.

Recycling of acetylcholine. Following hydrolysis in the synaptic cleft, the choline and acetate moieties are recaptured by specific transporters (Fig. 8.17).

Monoamines

Catecholamines. As indicated in Table 8.2, the catecholamines include dopamine, norepinephrine, and epinephrine (adrenaline), and all three are derived from the amino acid tyrosine (Fig. 8.18).

The transmitters are synthesised in nerve terminals, the requisite tyrosine and enzymes having been sent there by rapid transport. A newly synthesised transmitter must be packaged immediately into a synaptic vesicle by a monoamine transporter protein lodged in the vesicular membrane, because the catabolic enzyme ***monoamine oxidase (MAO)*** permeates the cytosol. On release, most of the transmitter molecules bind with one or more specific receptors in the postsynaptic membrane and (where present) with an autoreceptor in the presynaptic membrane. Of the remainder, some are inactivated by ***catechol-O-methyltransferase (COMT)***, an enzyme liberated from the postsynaptic membrane into the synaptic cleft (Fig. 8.19). The rest

are taken up by a specific uptake transporter and are either collected by a vesicular protein transporter or are inactivated by MAO.

Dopamine. Dopamine is of interest in the clinical contexts of Parkinson disease, drug addiction, and schizophrenia. It is synthesised in two steps (Fig. 8.18), being converted from tyrosine to DOPA (dihydroxyphenylalanine) by *amino acid hydroxylase* and from DOPA to dopamine by *dopa decarboxylase*, an enzyme restricted to catecholaminergic neurons. Two principal groups of dopaminergic neurons are found in the midbrain. Specifically, in the substantia nigra and in the ventral part of the tegmentum called the *ventral tegmental area (VTA)*.

The substantia nigra belongs functionally to the basal ganglia (see Chapter 26). A dopaminergic *nigrostriatal pathway* projects from the substantia nigra to the striatum (caudate nucleus and putamen). This pathway controls a motor loop of neurons feeding forward to the motor cortex. Degeneration of neurons in the substantia nigra is a classic feature of *Parkinson disease*, in which normal movements are disrupted by rigidity of the musculature and/or tremor at rest.

The dopaminergic neurons of the VTA project into the forebrain. One group of neurons, called *mesocortical*, projects to the prefrontal cortex. The over-activity of this system has been associated with some clinical features of schizophrenia (see Chapter 33). The other group, called *mesolimbic*, projects to several limbic nuclei including the nucleus accumbens (bedded in the ventral striatum); dopamine liberation within the nucleus accumbens appears to be the basis of the *dopamine rush*, or *dopamine high*, associated with several kinds of drug addiction (see Chapter 33).

Receptors. Dopamine receptors are all G protein-gated (metabotropic). D_1 and D_2 receptors are recognised, and each has more than one subtype. D_1 receptors activate G_s proteins and are excitatory, activating adenylate cyclase with consequent receptor phosphorylation. D_2 receptors activate G_i proteins and are inhibitory; they may inactivate adenylate cyclase and may also promote hyperpolarisation by opening GIRK ion channels and/or inhibiting voltage-gated Ca^{2+} channels. Both kinds are numerous in the striatum, where they are required for the proper execution of learned motor programs including locomotion (see Chapter 26).

Norepinephrine. In the CNS noradrenergic neurons are concentrated in the locus coeruleus located in the floor of the fourth ventricle. From here they project to all parts of the grey matter of the brain and spinal cord (see Fig. 24.8). These neurons are important for regulation of the sleep—wake cycle and the control of mood.

In the PNS norepinephrine is liberated by sympathetic nerve endings, notably throughout the cardiovascular system, where it maintains blood pressure. It is an integral component of the 'fight or flight' response to danger. Formation of norepinephrine takes place in neurons containing *dopamine β-hydroxylase*. This enzyme is remarkable in being restricted to the inner surface of the membrane of synaptic vesicles.

Receptors. All norepinephrine receptors are G protein-gated. They are broadly grouped into α and β sets, with two

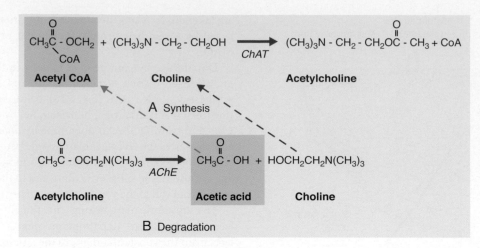

Fig. 8.16 (A) Synthesis of acetylcholine *(ACh)* from acetyl coenzyme A *(acetyl CoA)* and choline catalysed by choline acetyltransferase *(ChAT)*. (B) Degradation of ACh catalysed by acetylcholinesterase *(AChE)*. *Dashed arrows* indicate recycling of acetic acid and choline.

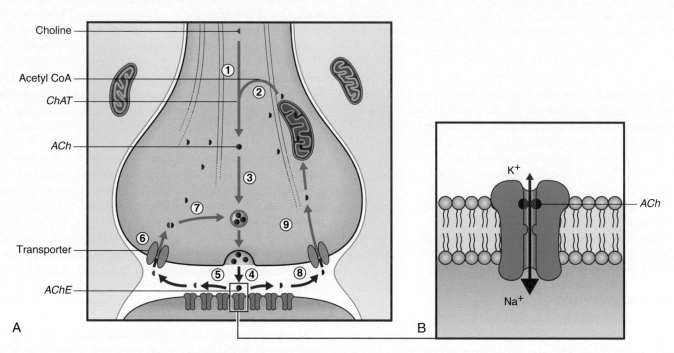

Fig. 8.17 (A) Production and recycling of acetylcholine *(ACh)* molecules in the central nervous system. The postsynaptic membrane shown contains nicotinic receptors (nAChR). (1) Choline taken up from the extracellular fluid is sent to the nerve ending. (2) The choline is acetylated by acetyl coenzyme A *(acetyl CoA)* released by mitochondria, the reaction being catalysed by choline acetyltransferase *(ChAT)*. (3) Completed ACh molecules are taken up by synaptic vesicles. (4) Released ACh bonds briefly with its receptor. (5) Acetylcholinesterase *(AChE)* hydrolyses the transmitter. (6) The choline moiety is transported back into the cytosol. (7) Formation of a fresh molecule of ACh is mediated by the transferase, en route to a synaptic vesicle. (8) The acetate moiety is transported into the cytosol. (9) Mitochondria use the acetic acid to produce fresh acetyl CoA. (B) The Ligand-Gated Nicotinic Receptor, Indicating the Large Inrush of Sodium *(Na$^+$)* Ions and the Small Efflux of Potassium *(K$^+$)* Ions Associated With ACh–Receptor Binding.

principal subtypes within each. Some details are provided in Table 8.4.

Catecholamine recycling. Recycling of dopamine and norepinephrine occurs via specific reuptake transporters (Fig. 8.19). The figure indicates that not all the molecules are recycled into synaptic vesicles within the parent neuron. Any of three other fates are possible: some are metabolised in or near the synaptic cleft by the enzyme *COMT*; others are carried for up to 100 µm by the extracellular fluid, perhaps bonding to isolated specific membrane heteroreceptors on other neurons as

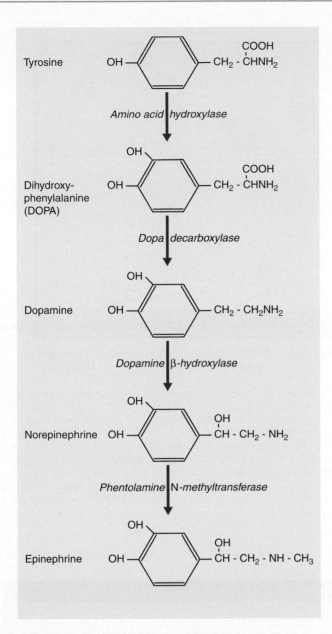

Fig. 8.18 Synthetic pathway of the catecholamine transmitters.

depicted in Fig. 8.6 *(volume transmission)*; and yet others achieve reuptake only to be metabolised by the enzyme *MAO* liberated by nearby mitochondria.

Epinephrine. Neuronal production of epinephrine in the CNS appears to be confined to a group of cells in the upper lateral part of the medulla oblongata. Only these cells contain the enzyme *phentolamine N-methyltransferase* that provides the final link in the catecholamine chain (Fig. 8.18). Some of these neurons project upward to the hypothalamus and others to the lateral grey horn of the spinal cord. Their functions are not yet clear.

In the PNS the *chromaffin cells* of the adrenal medulla release epinephrine as a hormone into the bloodstream. The epinephrine augments sympathetic effects on the circulatory and other systems during the fight or flight response. As shown in Fig. 13.8, the chromaffin cells are modified sympathetic ganglion cells receiving synaptic contacts from preganglionic cholinergic neurons. One function of circulating epinephrine (see Fig. 13.6) is to boost norepinephrine output at sympathetic nerve terminals by activating β_2 heteroreceptors there.

Serotonin. In the medical literature, more has been written about serotonin than about any other neurotransmitter. Depletion of serotonin has a well-established connection with depression. Abnormalities of serotonin metabolism have been implicated in other behavioural disorders, including anxiety states, obsessive–compulsive disorders, and bulimia.

As indicated in Figs 24.1 and 24.5, serotonergic cell bodies occupy the midregion or raphe (seam) of the brainstem. Their axonal ramifications are quite vast, penetrating to every region of the grey matter of the brain and spinal cord.

Serotonin, commonly referred to as *5-HT* (*5-hydroxytryptamine*), is derived from the dietary amino acid tryptophan. It is actively transported across the blood–brain barrier into the brain extracellular fluid and then transported into serotonergic neurons. Formation of serotonin from tryptophan is a two-step process (Fig. 8.20): Tryptophan is converted to 5-hydroxytryptophan by the enzyme *tryptophan hydroxylase* and then to serotonin by *5-hydroxytrytophan decarboxylase*.

Receptors. Seven groups of serotonin receptors have been identified. Ongoing research seeks to refine drug therapy to target individual receptors thought to be responsible for specific disorders, either by overactivity or underactivity, notably in the psychiatric domain.

Table 8.5 provides some details for a selected short list of serotonin receptors. The table includes a reference to receptors on the somas and dendrites of the parent cell. These are targets of recurrent axon collaterals (Fig. 8.21).

Recycling. Recycling follows the same general pattern as for the catecholamines. Here again, the final step of transmitter synthesis takes place within the terminal bouton, and the released molecules may activate either presynaptic autoreceptors on the parent neuron or isolated heteroreceptors on other neurons nearby. There appears to be no degradation enzyme in or near the synaptic cleft comparable with COMT, but MAO is present within the parent bouton (Fig. 8.22).

Monoamines and abnormal emotional or behavioural states. Abnormal monoamine function has been implicated in a great variety of abnormal emotional or behavioural states, including depression, insomnia, anxiety disorders, panic attacks, and specific phobias.

Histamine. Histamine is synthesised from histidine by *histidine decarboxylase* (Fig. 8.23). The somas of histaminergic neurons appear to be confined to the posterior part of the hypothalamus, where they occupy the small *tuberomammillary nucleus* shown in Fig. 34.1. However, their axons extend widely, generally to all parts of the cerebral cortex. The main function of histaminergic neurons is to participate with cholinergic and serotonergic neurons in maintaining the awake state. These neurons are active in the awake state and silent during sleep (see Chapter 24).

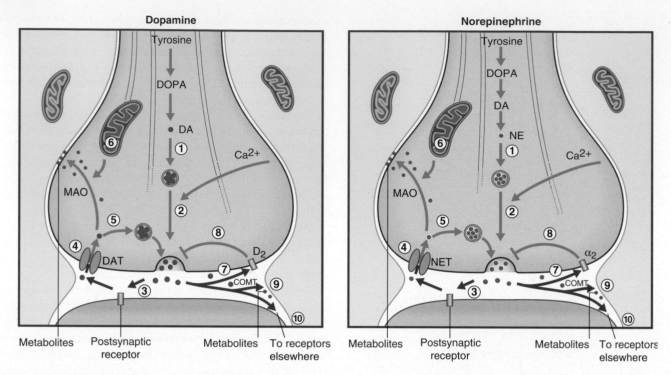

Fig. 8.19 Production and recycling of the main catecholamine transmitter molecules. (1) Transmitter dopamine *(DA)* or norepinephrine *(NE)* molecules are transported into synaptic vesicles. (2) Following depolarisation-induced calcium *(Ca²⁺)* entry to the cytosol, synaptic vesicles are pulled into contact with the presynaptic membrane of the terminal bouton. (3) Liberated transmitter molecules have three possible fates. Most bind with G protein-coupled receptors in the postsynaptic membrane, initiating second messenger events. (4) Specific transmitter reuptake transporters *(DAT, NET)* return transmitter molecules to the cytosol. (5) Some of these molecules are repackaged for further use. (6) Surplus molecules in the cytosol are degraded by mitochondria-derived monoamine oxidase *(MAO)* enzyme. The metabolites float away in extracellular fluid destined to pass through ventricular walls into the cerebrospinal fluid, where some metabolites may be detected. (7) A second group of transmitter molecules within the synaptic cleft are broken down by catechol *O*-methyltransferase *(COMT)*. (8) A third group function as D_2 or α_2 autoreceptors, inhibiting further transmitter release. (9) A second set of metabolites drifting away in the extracellular fluid. (10) Some intact transmitter molecules drifting away to activate receptors elsewhere.

TABLE 8.4	**Main Features of Noradrenergic Receptors.**			
Receptor Type	**Location on Neuron**	**Regions Found**	**Second Messenger**	**Effects**
α_1	Postsynaptic	Smooth muscle, brain	Phosphoinositol	Excitatory. Opens Ca^{2+} channels
α_2	Mainly presynaptic	Brain	G protein direct	Inhibitory. Opens GIRK channels
β_1	Postsynaptic	Heart, brain	Adenylate cyclase +	Excitatory. Opens Ca^{2+} channels
β_2	Postsynaptic	Smooth muscle, liver, brain	Adenylate cyclase ±	Inhibitory to smooth muscle. Glycogen breakdown + in liver. Excitatory in brain

Receptors. H_1, H_2, and H_3 receptors on target neurons have been identified. All three activate G proteins. H_1 and H_2 receptors activate G_s proteins via arachidonic acid production. The acid is processed further to yield prostaglandins and other endoperoxides, some of which modify cAMP activity and others bind directly to ion channels. H_3 receptors are inhibitory autoreceptors.

In clinical practice *antihistamines* are widely prescribed to block H_2 receptors involved in gastric acid secretion and various allergic responses. Drowsiness was a common side effect of such drugs, prior to the production of *cimetidine* (H_2 receptor antagonist) and others that are not able to cross the blood—brain barrier.

Neuropeptides

More than fifty neuropeptides have been isolated. All of them are linear chains of amino acids linked by peptide bonds. Peptide precursor chains (called *propeptides*) are passed through the Golgi complex and budded off in large, dense-cored vesicles that are rapidly transported to the nerve endings, where peptide

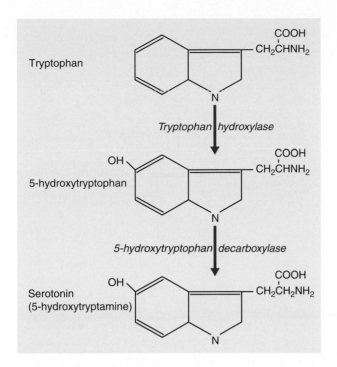

Fig. 8.20 Synthesis of serotonin from tryptophan.

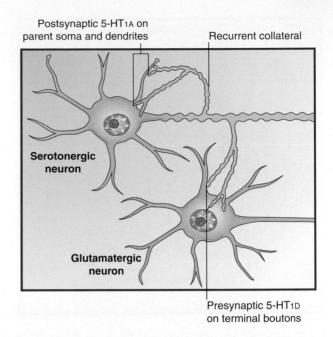

Fig. 8.21 Serotonergic autoreceptors. 5-HT$_{1A}$ autoreceptors reduce both excitability and serotonin synthesis. 5-HT$_{1D}$ autoreceptors reduce serotonin release. (Modified from Nestler EJ, Hyman SE, Malenka RC. Molecular Pharmacology: A Foundation for Clinical Neuroscience, New York: McGraw-Hill; 2001.)

TABLE 8.5	Some Serotonin Receptors of Clinical Interest.			
Receptor Type	Neuronal Location	Second Messenger	Effect	Activity Contributes to
5-HT$_{1A}$	Parent cell somas and dendrites	Inhibits cAMP	Inhibitory	Anxiety, depression, pain
5-HT$_{1D}$	Presynaptic autoreceptors	Inhibits cAMP, opens GIRK channels	Inhibitory	Vasoconstriction. Activation relieves migraine
5-HT$_{2A}$	Target cell somas and dendrites	Stimulates phosphoinositol	Excitatory	Over activity causes hallucinations
5-HT$_{2C}$	Target cell somas and dendrites	Stimulates phosphoinositol	Excitatory	Over activity causes increased appetite
5-HT$_3$	Target cell somas and dendrites in area postrema	No: it is ionotropic	Excitatory	Stimulation causes emesis (vomiting)

formation is completed. As previously illustrated in Fig. 6.8, peptides undergo nonsynaptic release and may travel some distance to reach their receptors.

Receptors. These are all G protein-coupled. In general, they are cotransmitters and their function is to modulate the effect of principal, small-molecule transmitters such as glutamate or ACh. Ca^{2+} channels are relatively scarce outside the synaptic cleft, and peptide release characteristically requires relatively high-frequency action potentials. An example is mentioned in Chapter 13: sweat glands are supplied by cholinergic neurons that have vasoactive intestinal polypeptide (VIP) as a cotransmitter. At low-frequency stimulation, ACh alone is sufficient to provide routine 'insensible perspiration', which is also invisible. *Sweating* for any length of time requires local vasodilation in addition to an abundance

of ACh, and this is provided by VIP, a potent dilator of arterioles.

Within the CNS, naturally occurring *opioid* (opium-like) peptides, called **endorphins**, play a significant role in relation to the control of pain perception, as discussed in Chapter 24.

Adenosine

Adenosine, derived from ATP, is a well-established excitatory cotransmitter with ACh in parasympathetic neurons innervating smooth and cardiac muscle. In the brain, adenosine is an inhibitory cotransmitter with glutamate. Adenosine receptors are G protein-coupled. Those on presynaptic terminals reduce glutamate release, and those on postsynaptic dendrites tend to hyperpolarise by opening K$^+$ and Cl$^-$ membrane channels. Adenosine-containing compounds are sedative. Adenosine

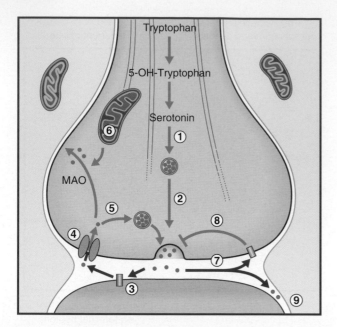

Fig. 8.22 Production and recycling of serotonin transmitter molecules in the central nervous system. (1) Serotonin is transported into synaptic vesicles. (2) Transmitter molecules undergo exocytosis into the synaptic cleft. (3) A postsynaptic serotonin receptor is being targeted. (4) The (therapeutically important) serotonin reuptake transporter returns transmitter to the terminal cytosol. (5) Some transmitter is repackaged into synaptic vesicles. (6) Some is degraded instead by (therapeutically important) monoamine oxidase *(MAO)*. (7) Some activates presynaptic autoreceptors. (8) A 5-HT$_{1D}$ presynaptic autoreceptor is retarding further transmitter release. (9) Some diffuses through the extracellular space, using 'volume transmission' to activate receptors on other neurons.

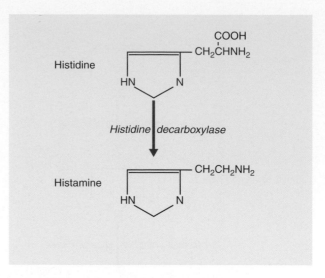

Fig. 8.23 Synthesis of histamine from histidine.

receptor antagonists have the opposite effect: increasing alertness and providing temporary improvement in cognitive function. The antagonists are *methylxanthines*, including *caffeine* found in coffee, *theophylline* in tea, and *theobromine* in cocoa.

Nitric Oxide

Nitric oxide is not a 'classical' transmitter, but it is a lipid- and water-soluble gaseous radical that diffuses briefly and rapidly across cell membranes, including those of neurons. It is synthesised from arginine by the enzyme *nitric oxide synthase* in response to Ca^{2+} entry following depolarisation; it activates guanylate cyclase and increases cAMP in target cells, thereby enabling cAMP to modulate the activity of conventional neurotransmitters. In the autonomic nervous system, it is a powerful smooth muscle relaxant (see Chapter 13). In the brain it appears to be especially relevant to memory formation by eliciting long-term potentiation in glutamatergic neurons in the hippocampus.

CLINICAL PANEL 8.1　Stiff Person Spectrum Disorder (SPS Disorder)

The *SPS disorder* manifests as fluctuating, palpably firm back and abdominal muscles suggesting hyperactivity, but not accompanied by rigidity or spasticity when testing muscle tone. Limb involvement is usually more proximal and typically affects the lower extremities more often than the upper. A hyperlordotic or unusually large, inward arch on the lower back, just above the buttocks can be seen. Painful spasms occur that may be exaggerated as part of the startle response. The discovery of distinctive neurophysiological findings helped to localise the disorder to inhibitory interneurons of the brainstem and spinal motor neurons. Since its original clinical description, more limited forms and asymmetric involvement have been identified and although originally described in a group of men, it is encountered more often in women, but remains rare.

Elucidating the pathogenesis of SPS began with the discovery of an autoantibody to an isoform of glutamic acid decarboxylase *(GAD65)* that supported the target of an immune response against inhibitory CNS interneurons. Further support came from the electrophysiological findings, laboratory studies and the observed symptomatic response to GABAergic

medications (e.g. benzodiazepines and baclofen). However, GAD is localised within nerve terminals and synthesises GABA for neurotransmission, so it is likely that GAD65-antibody is a surrogate maker for an autoimmune disorder mediated by cytotoxic T cells. Other autoantigens associated with GABAergic and glycinergic synaptic transmission have also been identified in patients with SPS.

The GAD65-antibody is not specific for SPS and is found in other neurological disorders and more frequently identified in other autoimmune disorders, diabetes mellitus and thyroid disease most commonly, that can also occur in SPS patients. Unlike onconeuronal antibodies associated with neoplasms and representing a paraneoplastic disorder (see Basic Science Panel 27.1), SPS is uncommonly associated with a neoplasm.

Most of the recommendations for the treatment of GAD65 autoimmune disorders are nonevidence based, except for intravenous immunoglobulin (IVIg) for SPS. Symptom-based management of SPS, targeting GABA transmission (e.g. diazepam and baclofen), is complementary.

CLINICAL PANEL 8.2 Botulinum Toxin Administration for Movement Disorders

Botulinum neurotoxin (BoNT) is produced by nonaerobic Clostridia bacteria and inhibits the release of acetylcholine from the presynaptic terminal. By interfering with the fusion of presynaptic vesicles (containing acetylcholine) with the plasma membrane, it prevents the release of their acetylcholine into the synaptic cleft and their engagement with acetylcholine receptors on the muscle membrane. The result is muscle weakening due to a block of neuromuscular transmission.

BoNTs do not cross the blood—brain barrier and demonstrate selectivity for nerve endings, extreme potency in inhibiting neurotransmitter release. While in time their effects are reversible, once BoNTs enter a nerve, their activity cannot be reversed until it has naturally ceased. These same characteristics and its limited diffusion from the site of an injection have all contributed to its therapeutic effectiveness and its use for an increasing number of neurological and other medical conditions.

The widest application of BoNT (several serotypes are known, but A1 and B1 are most often used clinically) is for treatment of disorders manifested by abnormal, excessive, or inappropriate muscle contractions. It is the treatment of choice for *dystonia* (a movement disorder characterised by involuntary muscle contraction that can affect a part of the body and cause it to twist or take on a prolonged abnormal posture. Examples include *cervical dystonia* where neck muscle contraction causes the head to twist or turn to one side, *blepharospasm* or an episodic closure of the eyelids), and increasingly for spasticity from a prior cortical injury or the sequelae from a stroke. Treatment consists of commercially available BoNT injected into identified target muscles; clinical and symptomatic relief is usually evident in days and persists for 3—4 months. Recovery occurs as affected motor nerve terminals develop sprouts that form new contacts with the sarcolemma soon after inactivation of the motor axon terminal by BoNT. New neuromuscular junctions (NMJ) develop and once reestablished at the original NMJ site, remaining nodal sprouts are eliminated. This process can occur multiple times and without permanent loss of NMJ function allowing repeated treatments.

While the therapeutic effect of BoNT administration is weakening of muscle due to the block of neuromuscular transmission, favourable outcomes may reflect other alterations of motor function. Block of neurotransmission other than cholinergic synapses, reduction in spindle afferent activity reducing excitability of moto neurons, retrograde transport into the spinal cord with effects on Renshaw neuron activity, and alerted plasticity of the brain from peripheral denervation may all contribute to its therapeutic benefits.

BASIC SCIENCE PANEL 8.1 Neuromyelitis Optica Spectrum Disorder

The diagnosis of multiple sclerosis (MS) is based on neurologic history, findings on examination, and exclusion of other disorders. Initially characterised as an unusual presentation of MS, *Devic disease* or *neuromyelitis optica* (*NMO*) presents as optic neuritis with transverse myelitis and is attributed to an inflammatory disorder of the central nervous system that is associated with MS. Similar to MS there was a preponderance of female patients and occurrence in young adults (35—45 years) but differed as it presented as a monophasic disease and recovery was often incomplete with significant residual deficits. Other differences included a preponderance of inflammatory cells within the cerebrospinal fluid (unusual in typical MS) and *oligoclonal bands* (bands of immunoglobulins identified in blood serum or cerebrospinal fluid by immunoelectrophoreis and each one representing antibody proteins (or protein fragments) secreted by plasma cells and reflecting inflammation within the CNS) were absent, but usually identified in MS. Neuroimaging identified other differences; brain MRI did not typically meet criteria for MS based on location of lesions and imaging of the spinal cord showed longitudinally extensive spinal cord lesions.

This clinical presentation became a disease entity, different from MS, with the identification of a serum antibody within the majority (80%) of patients to the water channel called aquaporin-4 (AQP4), found within CNS astrocytes. AQP4—immunoglobulin G (IgG) seropositivity is associated with a high risk of relapses of either myelitis or optic neuritis. Variable presentations, but the same antibody identification has expanded the clinical definition of these *neuromyelitis optica spectrum disorders* (*NMOSD*). The AQP4-IgG can penetrate the blood—brain barrier, react with AQP4 in astrocyte feet, and result in dysfunction of brain water movement, glia scarring, and neuroexcitation. This antibody-initiated complement to injury recruits inflammatory cells and further disrupts the blood—brain barrier. The pathological changes include loss of astrocytic AQP4, myelin sheaths, axonal injury, perivascular deposition of AQP4—IgG, and inflammatory infiltration.

Diagnosis of NMOSD in individuals with a positive AQP4—IgG assay requires two or more clinical attacks with at least one manifesting as optic neuritis, myelitis, or as an *area postrema syndrome* (hiccups, nausea, and/or uncontrollable vomiting for several days; this area is particularly rich in aquaporin-4). An accurate diagnosis is critical as some treatments used in MS (e.g. Fingolimod) may be ineffective or worsen the course of the disease. Initial treatments in NMSOD include steroids or plasmapheresis and preventive therapy using other immunosuppressive drugs is often initiated.

Some patients with a similar clinical presentation as NMOSD, but lacking the AQP4 IgG antibody, are found to have an antibody against *myelin oligodendrocyte glycoprotein* (*MOG*). Further research will determine if they continue to be classified with NMOSD or will become their own disease entity.

✳ Core Information

Electrical synapses are gap junctions designed to ensure synchronous activity in groups of neurons. The gaps are bridged by tightly packed ion channels. Protein subunits forming the individual ion channels are closed when the neurons are silent. The channels open in response to specific stimuli (such as action potentials), allowing instant diffusion of ions directly from one cytosol to another.

At *chemical synapses*, transmitter molecules are expelled into the synaptic cleft and bind to their specific target receptors in the manner already summarised in Table 8.1.

Ionotropic receptors are ligand gated. Each is either excitatory (allowing entry of Na^+ ions) or inhibitory (allowing passage of Cl^- or K^+ ions). *Metabotropic receptors* are transmembrane proteins without an ion pore. Their receptor macromolecule responds to transmitter activation by detaching a G protein subunit that usually binds to guanine triphosphate or guanine diphosphate, which in turn activates the cyclic AMP (cAMP), phosphoinositol, or arachidonic acid system. These *second messengers* interact with intracellular kinases and proteins to alter the membrane potential of the target neuron.

Amino acid transmitters include glutamate, GABA (γ-aminobutyric acid), and glycine. Biogenic amine transmitters and modulators include acetylcholine (ACh) and the monoamines (i.e. the catecholamines (dopamine, norepinephrine, and epinephrine), serotonin, and histamine). Neuropeptides include vasoactive intestinal polypeptide (VIP), substance P, enkephalin, and endorphins. Also prevalent are adenosine and nitric oxide.

- Glutamate activation of target AMPA—K (amino-methylisoxazole propionic acid) receptors produces the early component of the excitatory postsynaptic potential, which in turn opens NMDA (N-methyl-D-aspartate) receptors, producing action potentials through entry of Na^+, and long-term potentiation through entry of Ca^{2+}. Excitotoxicity caused by excessive Ca^{2+} influx may cause target cell necrosis.
- GABA activation of target GABA$_A$ (ionotropic) receptors generates inhibitory postsynaptic potentials by causing Cl^- influx. These receptors are also activated by barbiturates, benzodiazepines, alcohol, and some volatile anaesthetics. Activation of GABA$_B$ (metabotropic)

receptors leads to hyperpolarisation indirectly by depressing cAMP formation and release of K^+ ions through GIRK (G protein inwardly rectifying K^+) channels.

- Glycine released by Renshaw cells provides tonic negative feedback onto motor neurons.
- Acetylcholine target receptors are either nicotinic (causing entry of Na^+ and Ca^{2+}) or muscarinic. The latter include excitatory M_1, M_3, and M_5 receptors and inhibitory M_2 and M_4 autoreceptors.
- Dopamine receptors are all G protein-coupled. D_1 receptors are excitatory via cAMP activation. D_2 receptors are inhibitory via cAMP or Ca^{2+} channel inactivation and/or activation of GIRK channels.
- Norepinephrine is liberated by noradrenergic neurons. The main source within the central nervous system (CNS) is the locus coeruleus; in the peripheral nervous system it is postganglionic sympathetic fibres. Target receptors are all G protein-gated and are grouped into α and β subtypes, some of each being either excitatory or inhibitory.
- Serotonin is synthesised mainly in the raphe nuclei of the brainstem. Seven groups of receptors have been identified. 5-HT$_{1A}$ serves autoinhibition via somatodendritic autoreceptors, 5-HT$_{1D}$ serves autoinhibition via presynaptic receptors, 5-HT$_{2A}$ excites target neurons via phosphoinositol stimulation, and 5-HT$_{2C}$ stimulates excitatory ionotropic channels in the *area postrema* (vomiting centre).
- Histaminergic neurons project from the hypothalamic tuberomammillary nucleus to all parts of the cerebral cortex.
- Neuropeptides include VIP, substance P, enkephalin, and endorphins. In general, they are cotransmitters with a modulatory effect. Their target receptors are all G protein coupled.
- Adenosine is derived from ATP. In the autonomic nervous system, it is an excitatory cotransmitter with ACh. In the CNS it is inhibitory, and adenosine-containing compounds are sedative.
- Nitric oxide is a lipid- and water-soluble gaseous radical synthesised from arginine in response to Ca^{2+} entry following depolarisation. It activates guanylate cyclase and increases cAMP in target neurons, thereby modulating the activity of conventional transmitters.

SUGGESTED READINGS

Alcami P, Pereda AE. Beyond plasticity: the dynamic impact of electrical synapses on neural circuits. *Nat Rev Neurosci.* 2019;20:253—271.

Balint B, Vincent A, Meinck HM, et al. Movement disorders with neuronal antibodies: syndromic approach, genetic parallels and pathophysiology. *Brain.* 2018;141:13—36.

Borodinsky LN, Belgacem YH, Swapna I, et al. Dynamic regulation of neurotransmitter specification: relevance to nervous system homeostasis. *Neuropharmacology.* 2014;78:75—80.

Brosnan JT, Brosnan ME. Glutamate: a truly functional amino acid. *Amino Acids.* 2013;45:413—418.

Budnik V, Ruiz-Cañada C, Wendler F. Extracellular vesicles round off communication in the nervous system. *Nat Rev Neurosci.* 2016;17:160—172.

De Wit J, Ghosh A. Specification of synaptic connectivity by cell surface interactions. *Nat Rev Neurosci.* 2016;17:22—35.

Garry PS, Ezra M, Rowland MJ, et al. The role of the nitric oxide pathway in brain injury and its treatment — from bench to bedside. *Exp Neurol.* 2015;263:235—243.

Ho VM, Lee JA, Martin KC. The cell biology of synaptic plasticity. *Science.* 2011;334:623—628.

Jankovic J. Botulinum toxin: state of the art. *Mov Disord.* 2017;32:1131—1138.

Kaeser PS, Regehr WG. Molecular mechanisms for synchronous, asynchronous, and spontaneous neurotransmitter release. *Annu Rev Physiol.* 2014;76:333—363.

Kavalali ET, Jorgensen EM. Visualizing presynaptic function. *Nat Neurosci.* 2014;17:10—16.

Monday HR, Younts TJ, Castillo PE. Long-term plasticity of neurotransmitter release: emerging mechanisms and contributions to brain function and disease. *Annu Rev Neurosci.* 2018;41:299—322.

Nestler EJ, Hyman SE, Malenka RC. *Molecular Pharmacology: A Foundation for Clinical Neuroscience.* New York: McGraw-Hill; 2001.

Panula P, Nuutinen S. The histaminergic network in the brain: basic organization and role in disease. *Nat Rev Neurosci.* 2013;14:472—487.

Russo AF. Overview of neuropeptides: awakening the senses? *Headache.* 2017;57:37—46.

Shan L, Bao AM, Swaab DF. The human histaminergic system in neuropsychiatric disorders. *Trends Neurosci*. 2015;38:167—177.

Siegelbaum SA, Kandel ER, Sudhof TC. Transmitter release. In: Kandel ER, Schwartz JH, Jessell TM, et al., eds. *Principles of Neural Science*. 5th ed. New York: McGraw-Hill; 2013:260—288.

Skolnick SD, Greig NH. Microbes and monoamines: potential neuropsychiatric consequences of dysbiosis. *Trends Neurosci*. 2019;42:151—163.

Wu Y, Zhong L, Geng J. Neuromyelitis optica spectrum disorder: pathogenesis, treatment, and experimental models. *Mult Scler Relat Dis*. 2019;27:412—418.

STUDY OBJECTIVES

1. In a cross section of a peripheral nerve, be able to identify the different connective tissue sheaths.
2. Describe the anatomic classification of nerve fibres and its relationship to their function.
3. Describe the mechanism of myelination and be able to define internode, paranode, and the node of Ranvier.
4. Describe saltatory conduction and its relationship to myelination.

5. Describe the microscopic changes in a peripheral nerve after nerve injury and their relevance to functional recovery.
6. Contrast peripheral versus central nervous system regeneration.

To further understand the clinical importance of peripheral nerves, we suggest previewing the Clinical Panel Boxes in Chapter 12.

GENERAL FEATURES

The peripheral nerves comprise the cranial and spinal nerves linking the brain and spinal cord to the peripheral tissues. The spinal nerves are formed by the union of **ventral (anterior)** and **dorsal (posterior) nerve roots** at their points of exit from the vertebral canal (Fig. 9.1). The swelling on each dorsal root is a

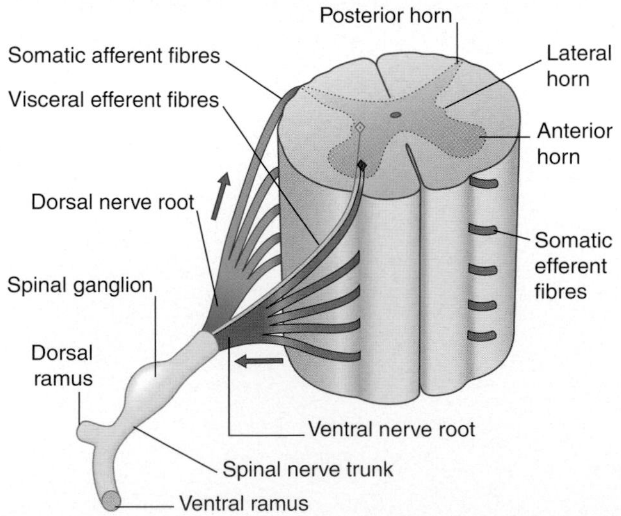

Fig. 9.1 Segment of thoracic spinal cord with attached nerve roots. *Arrows* indicate directions of impulse conduction. *Green* indicates sympathetic outflow.

Labels in figure: Posterior horn; Somatic afferent fibres; Visceral efferent fibres; Lateral horn; Anterior horn; Dorsal nerve root; Somatic efferent fibres; Spinal ganglion; Dorsal ramus; Ventral nerve root; Spinal nerve trunk; Ventral ramus

spinal or dorsal root ganglion. The **spinal nerve** is relatively short (less than 1 cm) and traverses an intervertebral foramen. On emerging from the foramen, it divides into **ventral (anterior)** and **dorsal (posterior) rami**.

The dorsal rami supply the erector spinae muscles and the overlying skin of the trunk. The ventral rami supply the muscles and skin of the side and front of the trunk, including the muscles and skin of the limbs; they also supply sensory fibres to the parietal pleura and parietal peritoneum.

The *cervical, brachial, and lumbosacral plexuses* are derived from ventral rami, which form the *roots* of the plexuses. The term *root* therefore has two different meanings depending on the context. (Details of the plexuses are in standard anatomy texts.)

The neurons contributing to peripheral nerves are partly contained within the central nervous system (CNS) (Fig. 9.2). The cells giving rise to the motor *(efferent)* nerves to skeletal muscles are **multipolar α and γ neurons** of similar configuration to the one depicted in Fig. 6.3; in the spinal cord they occupy the anterior horn of grey matter. Further details are found in Chapter 10. The cells giving rise to posterior nerve roots are **unipolar neurons** whose cell bodies lie in dorsal root ganglia and whose sensory (afferent) central processes enter the posterior horn of grey matter.

The spinal nerves contain **somatic efferent fibres** projecting to the skeletal muscles of the trunk and limbs and **somatic afferent fibres** from the skin, muscles, and joints. They also carry **visceral efferent**, autonomic fibres, and some spinal nerves contain visceral afferent fibres as well.

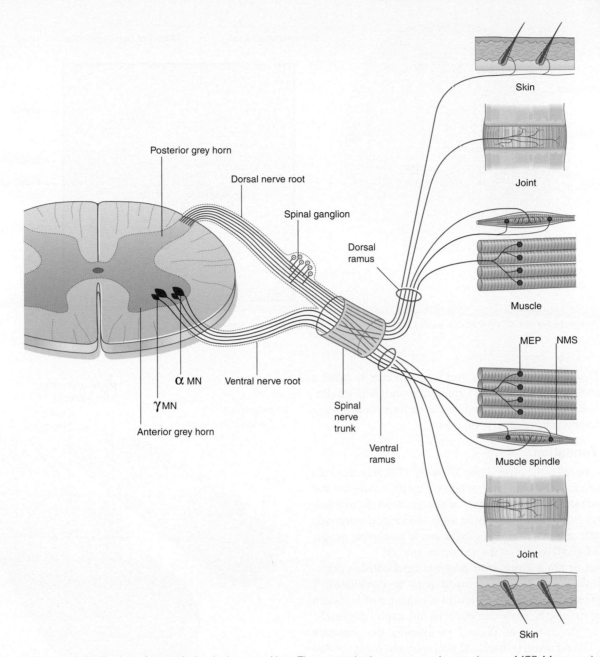

Fig. 9.2 Composition and distribution of a cervical spinal nerve. *Note:* The sympathetic component is not shown. *MEP*, Motor end plate; *MN*, multipolar neurons; *NMS*, neuromuscular spindle.

MICROSCOPIC STRUCTURE OF PERIPHERAL NERVES

Fig. 9.3 illustrates the structure of a typical peripheral nerve. It is not possible to designate individual nerve fibres as motor or sensory based on structural features alone.

Peripheral nerves are invested with **epineurium**, a dense, irregular connective tissue sheath surrounding the fascicles (bundles of nerve fibres) and blood vessels that make up the nerve. Nerve fibres are exchanged between fascicles along the course of the nerve.

Each fascicle is covered by **perineurium**, which is composed of several layers of pavement epithelium arranged in a distinct lamellar pattern and bonded by tight junctions. Surrounding individual Schwann cells is a network of reticular collagenous fibres, the **endoneurium**.

Less than half of the nerve fibres are enclosed in myelin sheaths. The remaining, unmyelinated fibres travel in deep gutters along the surface of Schwann cells.

The term **nerve fibre** is usually used in the context of nerve impulse conduction, where it is equivalent to an *axon*. A **myelinated fibre** consists of an axon ensheathed in concentric layers or lamellae of myelin (the original plasma membrane of a Schwann cell). An **unmyelinated fibre** is embedded in individual nonmyelinating Schwann cells and shares the Schwann cell plasma membrane *(neurolemma)* with other unmyelinated nerve fibres

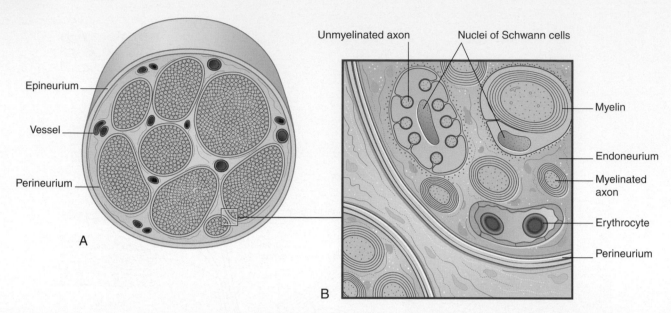

Fig. 9.3 Transverse section of a nerve trunk. (A) Light microscopy. (B) Electron microscopy.

(axons). This collection of axons and Schwann cells is called a *Remak bundle* (Fig. 9.3B). A basal lamina surrounds both myelinated and nonmyelinated fibres and acts as an important conduit in peripheral nervous system (PNS) repair.

Myelin Formation

The *Schwann cell* is the myelinating cell of the PNS. Schwann cells form a continuous chain along nerve fibres in the PNS; in myelinated fibres an individual Schwann cell may be responsible for the myelination of 0.3 to 1 mm of the length of an axon. Modified Schwann cells form *satellite cells* in dorsal root ganglia and in autonomic ganglia and form *teloglia* (Fig. 10.3) at the myoneural junction.

Whether or not a given axon becomes myelinated is determined by the axon itself. If an axon is to be myelinated, it receives the simultaneous attention of a sequence of Schwann cells along its length. Each one encircles the axon completely, creating a 'mesentery' of plasma membrane, the *mesaxon* (Fig. 9.4). The mesaxon is displaced progressively, being rotated around the axon. Successive layers of plasma membrane come into apposition to form the *major* and *minor dense lines* of the myelin sheath (Fig. 9.4) and the cytoplasm is 'squeezed out'. *Paranodal* pockets of cytoplasm persist at the ends of the myelin segments, on each side of the *nodes of Ranvier*, or in the gap between the ends (paranodes) of adjacent Schwann cells.

Myelin Expedites Conduction. In unmyelinated fibres, impulse conduction is *continuous* (uninterrupted) along the axon. Its average speed is only 2 m/s. In myelinated fibres, excitable membrane is confined to the nodes of Ranvier because myelin acts as an electrical insulator. Impulse conduction is called **saltatory** ('jumping') because it leaps from node to node. The speed of conduction is much faster along myelinated fibres, with a maximum of 120 m/s. The number of impulses that can be conducted per second by myelinated fibres is also much greater than that by unmyelinated fibres.

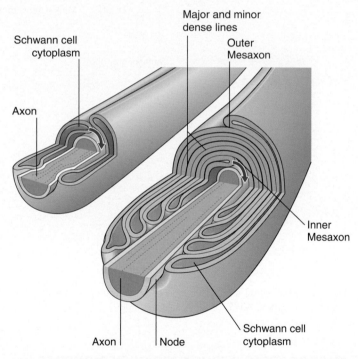

Fig. 9.4 Myelination in the peripheral nervous system. *Arrows* indicate movement of a flange of Schwann cell cytoplasm.

The larger the myelinated fibre, the more rapid the conduction, because larger fibres have longer internodal segments and the nerve impulses take longer 'strides' between nodes. A 'rule of six' can be used to express the ratio between size and speed: a fibre of 10 μm external diameter (i.e. including myelin) will conduct at 60 m/s, one of 15 μm will conduct at 90 m/s, and so on.

In physiologic recordings, peripheral nerve fibres are classified in accordance with conduction velocities and other criteria. Motor fibres are classified into the groups A, B, and C

TABLE 9.1 Classification of Peripheral Nerve Fibres.

Nerve Type	Number	Letter	Diameter (μm)	Conduction Velocity (m/s)
Myelinated				
Large	I	Aα	12–20	70–120
Medium	II	Aβ	6–12	35–70
Small	III	Aγ	3–6	10–40
Small	–	Aδ	2–5	5–35
Unmyelinated	IV	C	0.2–1.5	0.5–2

TABLE 9.2 Locations of Peripheral Nerve Fibre Types.

Fibre Type	Origin
Sensory	
Ia	Muscle spindle annulospiral endings
Ib	Golgi tendon organs
II (Aβ)	Muscle spindle flower spray endings; touch or pressure receptors in skin and elsewhere
III (Aδ)	Follicular endings; fast pain and thermal receptors
IV (C)	Slow pain, itch, touch receptors
Motor	
Aα	α motor neurons supplying extrafusal muscle fibres
Aγ	γ motor neurons supplying intrafusal muscle fibres

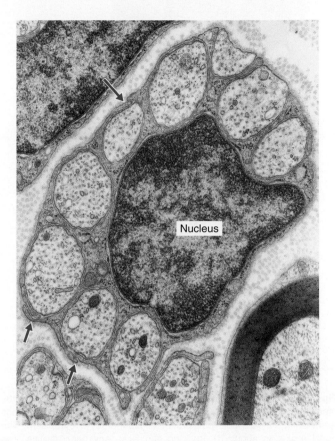

Fig. 9.6 Unmyelinated nerve fibres. Nine unmyelinated fibres are lodged in the cytoplasm of this Schwann cell. Mesaxons (*arrows* indicate examples) are detectable where the axons are fully embedded. Two incompletely embedded axons at top right are covered by the basal lamina of the Schwann cell. (From Pannese E. Neurocytology: Fine Structure of Neurons, Nerve Processes and Neuroglial Cells. New York: Thieme; 1994, with permission of Thieme.)

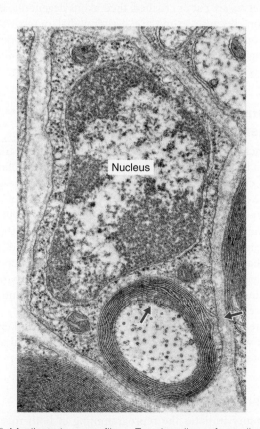

Fig. 9.5 Myelinated nerve fibre. Ten lamellae of myelin form a continuous spiral from the outer to the inner mesaxon of the Schwann cell *(arrows)*. A basal lamina surrounds the Schwann cell. (From Pannese E. Neurocytology: Fine Structure of Neurons, Nerve Processes and Neuroglial Cells. New York: Thieme; 1994, with permission of Thieme.)

in descending order. Sensory fibres are classified into types I to IV, also in descending order. In practice there is some interchange of usage: for example, unmyelinated sensory fibres are usually called C fibres rather than type IV fibres. A commonly used descriptor of the axon myelin relationship is the axon to fibre ratio or the *g-ratio*; this provides information of sheath thickness and relative internodal length. Suboptimal g-ratios have been implicated in several pathological conditions.

Details of diameters and sources of peripheral nerve fibres are given in Tables 9.1 and 9.2.

The electron micrograph in Fig. 9.5 illustrates a myelinated peripheral nerve fibre with attendant Schwann cell. Fig. 9.6

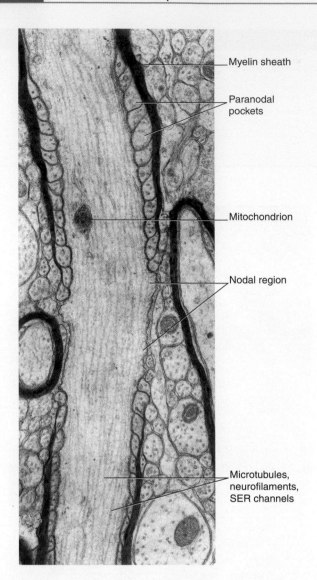

- Myelin sheath
- Paranodal pockets
- Mitochondrion
- Nodal region
- Microtubules, neurofilaments, SER channels

Fig. 9.7 Central nervous system nodal region. The myelin sheaths taper as they approach the nodal region, successive wrappings terminating in paranodal pockets of oligodendrocyte cytoplasm. The nodal region is about 10 μm long and lacks any basal lamina. The longitudinal streaks are created by microtubules, neurofilaments, and elongated sacs of smooth endoplasmic reticulum *(SER)*. (From Pannese E. Neurocytology: Fine Structure of Neurons, Nerve Processes and Neuroglial Cells. New York: Thieme; 1994, with permission of Thieme.)

illustrates a group of unmyelinated fibres embedded in the cytoplasm of a (Remak) Schwann cell. Fig. 9.7 illustrates a nodal region along an axon within the CNS.

Central Nervous System—Peripheral Nervous System Transitional Region

Close to the brainstem and spinal cord, peripheral nerves enter the *CNS—PNS transitional zone* (Fig. 9.8). Astrocyte processes reach out of the CNS into the endoneurial compartments of peripheral nerve rootlets and interdigitate with the Schwann cells. In unmyelinated fibres the astrocytes burrow into the space between axons and Schwann cells. In myelinated fibres,

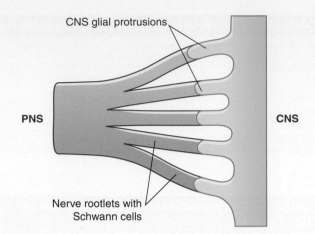

- CNS glial protrusions
- PNS
- CNS
- Nerve rootlets with Schwann cells

Fig. 9.8 Central nervous system *(CNS)*–peripheral nervous system *(PNS)* transitional zone.

nodes are bounded by Schwann cell myelin (showing some transitional features) peripherally and by oligodendrocytic myelin centrally.

DEGENERATION AND REGENERATION

When nerves are cut or crushed, their axons degenerate distal to the lesion, because axons are pseudopodial outgrowths and depend on their parent cells for survival. In the PNS, regeneration is vigorous and is often complete. In the CNS, on the other hand, it is neither vigorous nor complete.

Wallerian (Anterograde) Degeneration of Peripheral Nerves

The principal events in peripheral nerve degeneration are represented in Fig. 9.9A—D and described in the caption. Following a crush or cut injury to a nerve, the axons and myelin sheaths distal to the cut break up into 'ellipsoids' within the first 48 hours, primarily as a result of the Ca^{2+}-activated release of proteases by Schwann cells. The debris is cleared by monocytes that enter the damaged endoneurial sheaths from the blood and become macrophages. In addition to their phagocytic function, the macrophages are mitogenic to Schwann cells and participate with Schwann cells to provide trophic (feeding) and tropic (guidance) factors for regenerating axons.

The result of degeneration (Fig. 9.9D) is a shrunken nerve skeleton with intact connective tissue and perineurial sheaths, and a core of intact, multiplying Schwann cells.

Regeneration of Peripheral Nerves

Nerve injury initiates the reprogramming of both myelinated Schwann cells and nonmyelinated Remak cells to a cell phenotype which promotes repair. These cells provide the molecular cues that promote regeneration and survival of injured neurons.

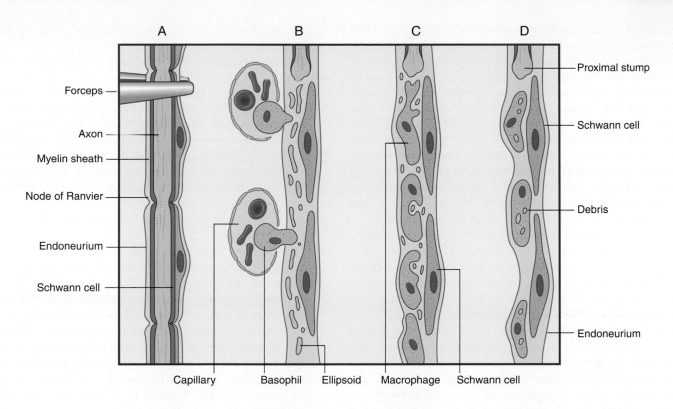

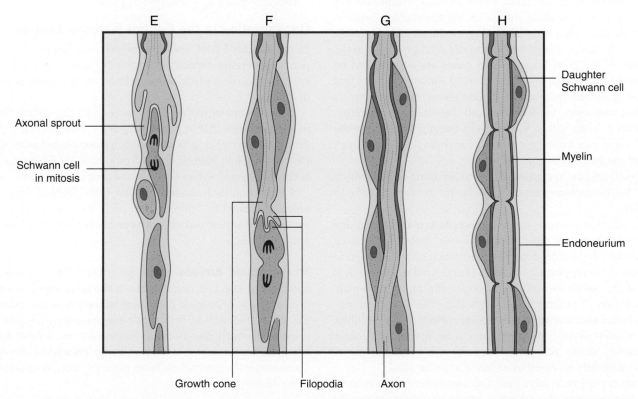

Fig. 9.9 (A—D) Events in the degeneration of a single myelinated nerve fibre. (A) Intact fibre, showing its four components. The fibre is being pinched at its upper end. (B) The myelin and axon have broken up into 'ellipsoids' and droplets. Monocytes are entering the endoneurial tube from the blood. (C) The droplets are being engulfed by monocytes. (D) Clearance of debris is almost complete. Schwann cells and endoneurium remain intact. (E—H) Events in the regeneration of a single myelinated nerve fibre. (E) An axonal sprout has entered the distal stump. The sprout is mitogenic to each Schwann cell it encounters. (F) The growth cone is extending distally along the surface of Schwann cells. (G) Myelination is commencing along the proximal part of the regenerating axon. (H) When regeneration is complete, the fibre has a normal appearance, but the myelin segments are shorter than the originals.

This switch involves dedifferentiation of the Schwann cell and down-regulation of myelin genes; activation of a set of repair-supportive features (including trophic factors) and activation of the innate immune response; promotion of myelin clearance by activation of myelin autophagy in Schwann cells and macrophage recruitment; and the formation of regeneration tracks, called *Büngner bands* (longitudinal bands of Schwann cells contained within the basal lamina tubes), which direct regenerating axons to their targets. Central to this response is the transcription factor *c-Jun*, which is rapidly upregulated in Schwann and Remak cells after injury. Peripheral nerves can regenerate due to the flexible differentiation state of PNS neurons and Schwann cells, which can convert to cells devoted to repair.

The principal events in the regeneration of a peripheral nerve are summarised in Fig. 9.9E−H. Following a clean cut, axons begin to sprout from the face of the proximal stump within a few hours. In the more common crush or tear injuries seen clinically, the axons typically die back for 1 cm or more and sprouting may be delayed for a week. Successful regeneration requires that the axons contact Schwann cells in the distal stump. Failure to make contact leads to the production of a *pseudoneuroma*, consisting of whorls of regenerating axons trapped in scar tissue at the site of the initial injury. Following amputation of a limb, an *amputation pseudoneuroma* can be a source of severe pain.

Two reparative events occur simultaneously within hours of the injury. In the proximal stump, multiple branchlets begin to extend distally, their tips exhibiting swellings called **growth cones**. In the distal stump, Schwann cells send processes in the direction of the growth cones. The cones are surmounted by antenna-like *filopodia*, and these develop surface receptors that become anchored temporarily to complementary *cell surface adhesion molecules* in Schwann cell basement membranes. Filaments of actin within the filopodia become attached to the surface receptors; from these points of anchorage, they can exert onward traction on the growth cones.

Growth cones are mitogenic to Schwann cells, which divide further before wrapping the larger axons with myelin lamellae.

Regeneration in axons initially proceeds at about 1 mm/day in humans, but over time the axons lose their regenerating capacity and the distally denervated Schwann cells also begin to lose their axon-supporting function. (Functional recovery is less likely if the axon does not reinnervate the motor end-plate region within 12 months.) Not surprisingly the functional outlook is better after a crush injury (endoneurium preserved) than after complete severance. At the same time, filopodia of motor and sensory axons 'recognise' Schwann cell basement membranes previously occupied by axons of a similar kind.

When nerve trunks have been completely severed, it is common practice to wait about 3 weeks before attempting repair. By that time the connective tissue sheaths will have thickened a little and will be better able to hold suture material than would freshly injured, oedematous sheaths. Moreover, the trimming of the nerves required before insertion of sutures creates a second axotomy, on the axons emerging from the proximal stump. In animal experiments a second axotomy induces a more vigorous and sustained regenerative response.

Upstream (neuronal cell body) effects of nerve section are as follows:

- Within a few days of axotomy, *Nissl bodies* can no longer be identified by cationic dyes in parent cells in the dorsal root ganglia and spinal grey matter (Fig. 9.10). The phenomenon is known as *chromatolysis* ('loss of colour'). Electron microscopy reveals that the granular endoplasmic reticulum is in fact increased in amount, but it is now dispersed throughout the perikaryon, with accumulations located deep to the plasma membrane.
- The nucleus becomes eccentric because of osmotic changes in the perikaryon.
- Parent motor neurons become isolated from synaptic contacts in the grey matter by the intrusion of neuroglial cells into all the synaptic clefts.
- In monkeys it has been demonstrated that following transection of sensory nerves, 30% to 40% of dorsal nerve root terminals undergo Wallerian degeneration. Because their terminals are in central grey matter, they do not regenerate; however, some of their synaptic sites are taken over by sprouts given off by healthy neighbours. Overall, this observation may account for the usually incomplete recovery of sensory function in patients.

Degeneration in the Central Nervous System

In the damaged CNS axon, regeneration is limited due to the poor regenerative capacity of adult CNS neurons and the presence of a hostile molecular and cellular environment at the site of injury.

Following injury to the white matter, distal degeneration occurs in a manner like that in peripheral nerves. However, clearance of debris by microglial cells and fresh monocytes is much slower. Debris can still be identified after 6 months in the CNS, whereas it is virtually cleared within 6 days in the peripheral nerves.

Chromatolysis is unusual in the CNS. Instead, large-scale necrosis (death) of injured neurons is the rule. Neurons that survive may appear wasted, with permanent isolation from synaptic contacts.

Transneuronal Atrophy. Neurons in the CNS have a trophic (sustaining) effect on one another. If the main input to a group of neurons is destroyed, the group is likely to waste away and die. This is known as *orthograde transneuronal atrophy*. It is comparable with the atrophy that occurs in skeletal muscle when its motor nerve is cut. In some situations, *retrograde transneuronal degeneration* takes place in neurons upstream to those destroyed by a lesion.

End Result of Central Nervous Injury. If the lesion is small, the neuronal debris is ultimately replaced by a glial scar composed of astrocyte processes. A large lesion may result in cystic cavities walled by scar tissue, containing cerebrospinal fluid and haemolysed blood.

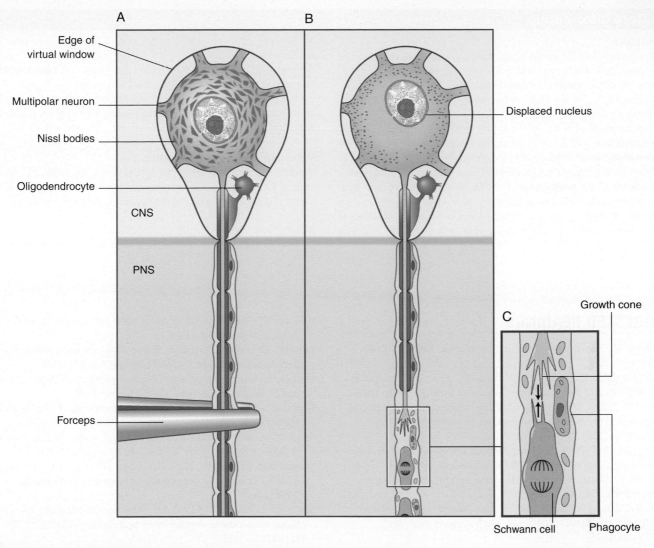

Fig. 9.10 Schematic representation of some events following crush injury to a peripheral nerve. (A) Motor neuron seen through a virtual window in the central nervous system. (B) Chromatolysis is characterised by fragmentation and dispersal of Nissl bodies and displacement of the nucleus. (C) Within the crushed area, clearance of debris permits growth cone filopodia to establish contact with proximal extensions of a Schwann cell *(arrows)*. *CNS*, Central nervous system; *PNS*, peripheral nervous system.

Regeneration in the Central Nervous System

Recent work indicates that it may be possible to overcome some of the barriers to regeneration by reprogramming adult mammalian neurons and removing extracellular growth inhibitors to promote regrowth of axons that project to the brain and spinal cord.

In the CNS, adaptive injury response seen in the PNS is reduced in neurons and there is limited ability of the adult oligodendrocytes to switch phenotype.

Axonal regeneration in the CNS is inhibited by molecules in the environment and by an age-related loss of regenerative potential in CNS axons. However, limited levels of functional recovery have been observed after CNS lesions. Injured motor and sensory pathways do not reestablish their original connections. They regenerate for a few millimetres at most, and synapses that do develop are on other neurons close to the site of injury.

Adult CNS neurons have limited regenerative capacity, as witnessed by their liberal sprouting and invasion of the endoneurial tubes of implanted peripheral nerves.

The principal deterrents to spontaneous regeneration following CNS injury are obstruction by developing glial scar tissue and the formation of a hostile molecular environment.

An active area in neurobiological research is the use of embryonic nervous tissue to replace neurons that have been lost as a result of injury or disease. The mammalian CNS in general seems to lack *trophic factors* required for successful regeneration. Embryonic central neurons have abundant trophic factors and grow well when transplanted (with immunologic precautions) into adult brain tissue. This approach is under investigation in animal models of Parkinson disease, Alzheimer disease, and spinal cord injury, with limited benefits in all three.

✷ Core Information

Structure

Spinal nerve trunks occupy the intervertebral foramina. They are formed by the union of ventral (motor) and dorsal (sensory) **nerve roots**, and they divide into (mixed) **ventral** and **dorsal rami**. The roots of the limb plexuses are ventral rami. The strips of skin supplied by the ventral and dorsal rami comprise the **dermatome**.

Each peripheral nerve is covered externally by a sheath of connective tissue, the **epineurium**. This covers a more organised layer of connective tissue, the **perineurium**. Septa extend into the nerve and subdivide it into several bundles of fibres or fascicles. Myelinated and nonmyelinated axons are surrounded by the collagen of the **endoneurium**. Both fibre types are covered by a basal lamina secreted by the **Schwann cell** that forms an endoneurial tube.

Myelin is formed by the spiral wrapping of the Schwann cell around an axon segment. A myelinated fibre consists of an axon ensheathed by a chain of Schwann cells. An unmyelinated fibre is embedded in individual nonmyelinating Schwann cells and shares the Schwann cell plasma membrane with other unmyelinated axons and known as a **Remak bundle**. Peripheral nerves are richly supplied with blood vessels.

Myelinated nerve fibres enable fast and efficient transduction of electrical signals via **saltatory conduction**. Nerve impulses occur at a rate proportional to the fibre diameter.

Degeneration and Regeneration

The peripheral nervous system (PNS) demonstrates a remarkable regenerative capacity. Regeneration in the central nervous system (CNS) is very limited, but the use of grafts of embryonic neurons has yielded some encouraging results.

SUGGESTED READINGS

Boullerne AI. The history of myelin. *Exp Neurol.* 2016;283(Pt B): 431-45.

Eshed-Eisenbach Y, Peles E. The making of a node: a co-production of neurons and glia. *Curr Opin Neurobiol.* 2013;23:1049—1056.

Glenn TD, Talbot WS. Signals regulating myelination in peripheral nerves and the Schwann cell response to injury. *Curr Opin Neurobiol.* 2013;23:1041—1048.

Harrington AW, Ginty DD. Long-distance retrograde neurotrophic factor signaling in neurons. *Nat Rev Neurosci.* 2013;14:177—187.

He X, Yu Y, Awatramani R, Lu QR. Unwrapping myelination by microRNAs. *Neuroscientist.* 2012;18:45—55.

Jessen KR, Mirsky R, Lloyd AC. Schwann cells: development and role in nerve repair. *Cold Spring Harb Perspect Biol.* 2015; 7(7):a020487.

Khuong HT, Midha R. Advances in nerve repair. *Curr Neurol Neurosci Rep.* 2013;13:1—8.

Lin MY, Manzano G, Gupta R. Nerve allografts and conduits in peripheral nerve repair. *Hand Clin.* 2013;29:331—348.

Pannese E. *Neurocytology: Fine Structure of Neurons, Nerve Processes, and Neuroglial Cells.* New York: Thieme; 1994.

Roberts SA, Lloyd AC. Aspects of cell growth control illustrated by the Schwann cell. *Curr Opin Cell Biol.* 2013;24:852—857.

Salzer JL. Axonal regulation of Schwann cell ensheathment and myelination. *J Peripher Nerv Syst.* 2012;17(suppl 3):14—19.

Stassart RM, Möbius W, Nave KA, Edgar JM. The axon-myelin unit in development and degenerative disease. *Front Neurosci.* 2018;12:467.

Stierli S, Imperatore V, Lloyd AC. Schwann cell plasticity-roles in tissue homeostasis, regeneration, and disease. *Glia.* 2019;67 (11):2203—2215.

Innervation of Muscles and Joints

STUDY GUIDELINES

1. Be able to outline the differences in motor units with respect to movements of all kinds and with respect to the functional significance of their sizes and muscle chemistries.
2. Sketch a motor end plate, indicating the locations of transmitter, receptor, and hydrolytic enzyme.
3. Sketch an intrafusal muscle fibre, indicating the locations of two motor and three sensory nerve endings.
4. Describe the functional significance of coactivation of α and γ motor neurons during voluntary movements.
5. With the essentials of this chapter still in mind, consider a first read through the Electromyography section of Chapter 12.

In gross anatomy the nerves to skeletal muscles are branches of mixed peripheral nerves. The branches enter the muscles about one-third of the way along their length, at **motor points** (Fig. 10.1). Motor points have been identified for all major muscle groups for the purpose of *functional electrical stimulation* by physical therapists, to increase muscle power.

Only 60% of the axons in the nerve to a given muscle are motor points to the muscle fibres that make up the bulk of the muscle. The rest are sensory in nature, although the largest sensory receptors—the neuromuscular spindles—have a motor supply of their own.

MOTOR INNERVATION OF SKELETAL MUSCLE

The nerve of supply branches within the muscle belly, forming a plexus from which groups of axons emerge to supply the muscle fibres (Figs. 10.1 and 10.2). The axons supply single motor end plates placed about halfway along the muscle fibres (Fig. 10.3A).

A **motor unit** comprises a motor neuron in the spinal cord or brainstem together with the *squad* of muscle fibres it innervates. In large muscles (e.g. the flexors of the hip or knee) each motor unit contains 1200 muscle fibres or more, whereas in small muscles (e.g. the intrinsic muscles of the hand) each unit contains 12 muscle fibres or fewer. Small units contribute to the finely graded contractions used for delicate manipulations.

There are three different types of skeletal muscle fibres.

1. *Slow-twitch, oxidative fibres* are small and rich in mitochondria and blood capillaries (hence, red). They exert small forces and are fatigue resistant. They are deeply placed and suited to sustained postural activities, including standing. (Also called *type I* or *slow-twitch, fatigue resistant*.)

2. *Fast, glycolytic (FG) fibres* are large, mitochondria-poor, and capillary-poor (hence, white). They produce brief, powerful contractions. They predominate in superficial muscles. (Also called *type IIb* or *fast-twitch, fatigable*.)

3. *Intermediate (fast, oxidative—glycolytic, FOG) fibres* have properties intermediate between the other two. (Also called *type IIa* or *fast-twitch, fatigue resistant*.)

Every muscle contains all three types of muscle fibres, and the proportion of each within a muscle reflects its function. A given motor unit contains only one type of fibre but the fibres of each motor unit interdigitate with those of other units. A given

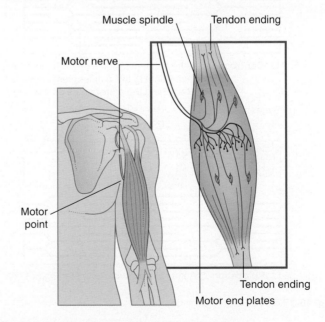

Fig. 10.1 Pattern of innervation of skeletal muscle.

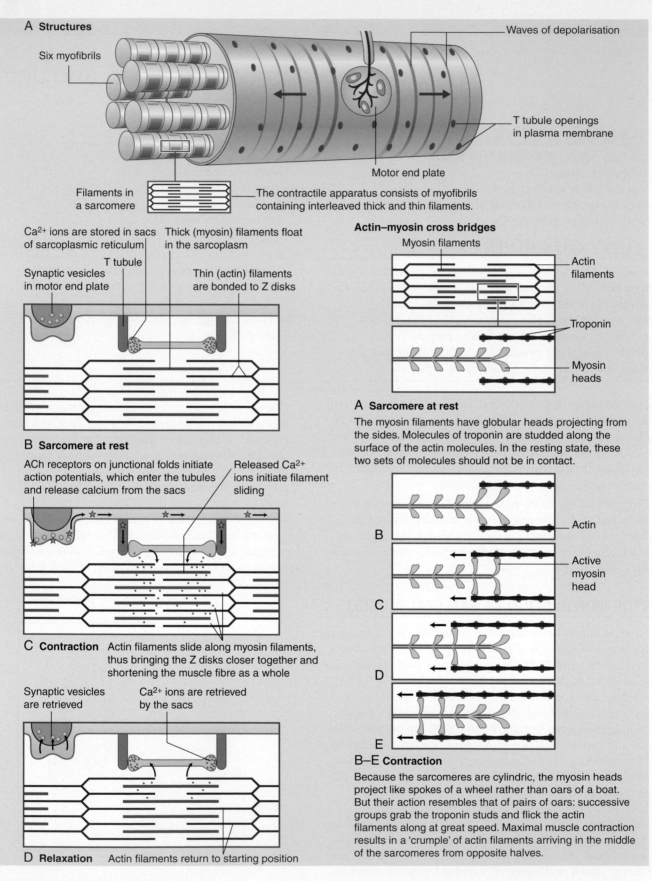

A Structures

Six myofibrils

Waves of depolarisation

T tubule openings in plasma membrane

Motor end plate

Filaments in a sarcomere

The contractile apparatus consists of myofibrils containing interleaved thick and thin filaments.

Ca²⁺ ions are stored in sacs of sarcoplasmic reticulum

Thick (myosin) filaments float in the sarcoplasm

T tubule

Synaptic vesicles in motor end plate

Thin (actin) filaments are bonded to Z disks

B Sarcomere at rest

ACh receptors on junctional folds initiate action potentials, which enter the tubules and release calcium from the sacs

Released Ca²⁺ ions initiate filament sliding

C Contraction   Actin filaments slide along myosin filaments, thus bringing the Z disks closer together and shortening the muscle fibre as a whole

Synaptic vesicles are retrieved

Ca²⁺ ions are retrieved by the sacs

D Relaxation   Actin filaments return to starting position

Actin–myosin cross bridges

Myosin filaments

Actin filaments

Troponin

Myosin heads

A Sarcomere at rest

The myosin filaments have globular heads projecting from the sides. Molecules of troponin are studded along the surface of the actin molecules. In the resting state, these two sets of molecules should not be in contact.

B

Actin

C

Active myosin head

D

E

B–E Contraction

Because the sarcomeres are cylindric, the myosin heads project like spokes of a wheel rather than oars of a boat. But their action resembles that of pairs of oars: successive groups grab the troponin studs and flick the actin filaments along at great speed. Maximal muscle contraction results in a 'crumple' of actin filaments arriving in the middle of the sarcomeres from opposite halves.

Fig. 10.2 Muscle fibre: internal details.

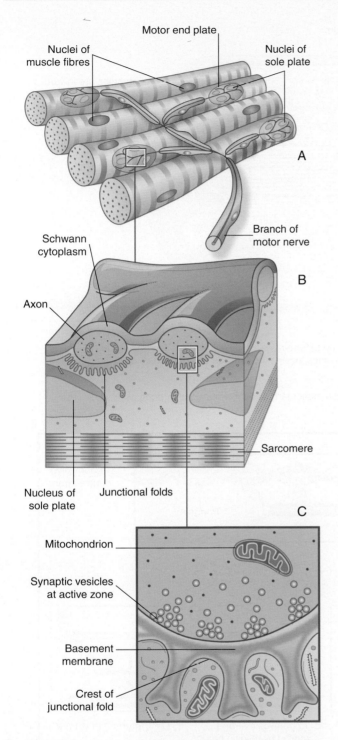

Fig. 10.3 Motor nerve supply to skeletal muscle. (A) Four motor end plates supplied from a single axon. (B) Enlargement from (A). (C) Enlargement from (B), showing active zones.

muscle may be referred to as 'slow' or 'fast' based on the type of muscle fibres it contains.

Motor End Plates

At the *myoneural junction* the axon divides into a handful of branchlets that groove the surface of the muscle fibre (Fig. 10.3B). The underlying sarcolemma is thrown into *junctional folds*. The basement membrane of the muscle fibre traverses the synaptic cleft and lines the folds. The underlying sarcoplasm shows an accumulation of nuclei, mitochondria, and ribosomes known as a *sole plate*.

Each axonal branchlet forms an elongated terminal bouton containing thousands of synaptic vesicles loaded with acetylcholine (ACh). Synaptic transmission takes place at *active zones* facing the crests of the junctional folds (Fig. 10.3C). Vesicular ACh is extruded at great speed by exocytosis into the synaptic cleft. The ACh diffuses through the basement membrane to bind with ACh receptors in the sarcolemma.

Activation of the receptors leads to depolarisation of the sarcolemma. The depolarisation is led into the interior of the muscle fibre by *T tubules*. The sarcoplasmic reticulum liberates Ca^{2+} ions that initiate contraction of the sarcomeres.

The enzyme *acetylcholinesterase* is concentrated in the basement membrane, and about 30% of released ACh is hydrolysed without reaching the postsynaptic membrane. Following hydrolysis, the choline moiety is actively taken back up and returned to the axoplasm.

Terminal boutons also have some dense-cored vesicles containing one or more peptides (Fig. 10.3C). The best known of these is *calcitonin gene-related peptide*, a potent vasodilator.

Details of the muscle fibre contraction process are shown in Fig. 10.4.

Motor Units in the Elderly

The loss of muscle mass and function associated with ageing (sarcopenia) has anatomical sequelae both at cellular and subcellular levels associated with the individual motor unit. The progressive loss of motor neurons with aging is associated with reduced muscle fibre number and size. This is mainly due to loss of motor neurons from the spinal cord and brainstem, often due in part to low-grade peripheral neuropathy arising from vascular disease and/or nutritional deficiency.

Electromyographic records taken from contracting muscles during the seventh and eighth decades of life show giant motor unit potentials. The extra-large potentials result from the takeover of vacated motor end plates of lost motor neurons by collateral sprouts from the axons of adjacent healthy motor units. Details of electromyography and clinical neuromuscular disorders are in Chapter 12. However, the progressive loss of muscle function is related to incomplete reinnervation of the units.

At the intracellular level, key factors include changes in muscle proteins and the loss of the coordinated control between contractile elements. This is coincident with altered protein expression associated with mitochondrial and sarcoplasmic reticulum function.

The changes in skeletal muscle during the process of aging also present in the pathogenesis of acquired and hereditary neuromuscular disorders.

Studies on specific intervention strategies in experimental models have shown promising results, and it is hoped that these advances can soon be translated to clinical practice.

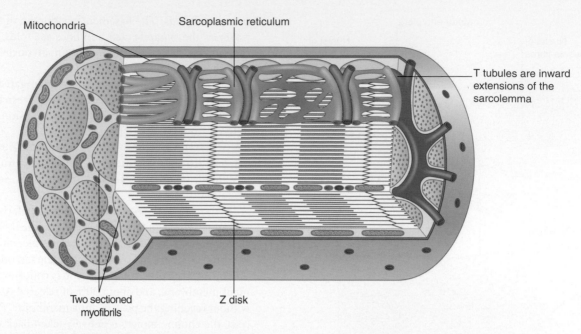

Muscle fibre diagram revealing internal details. T tubules join up to form rings, completing 'triads' of rings around the sarcomeres along with neighbouring pairs of sarcoplasmic sacs, having the function of releasing calcium ions from the sacs when the tubules are depolarised.

Muscle fibre actin comprises a twisted pair of polymerised actin monomers, a double strand of tropomyosin, and a troponin molecular complex at regular intervals.

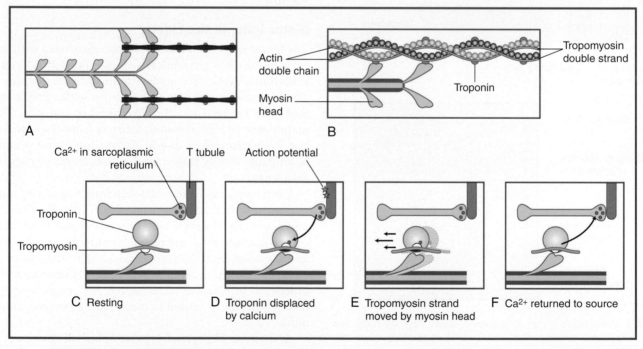

Excitation–contraction coupling:
Calcium liberated by tubule depolarisation causes displacement of troponin, with exposure of actin binding sites to which myosin heads attach and pull the thin fibre towards the centre of the sarcomere. The required energy is provided by ATPase enzyme contained in the myosin heads. Calcium is returned to source and the muscle actively relaxes by using ATPase to detach the myosin heads from the binding sites.

Fig. 10.4 Muscle fibre contraction. This flow diagram shows the sequential events taking place during the contraction of a single striated muscle fibre.

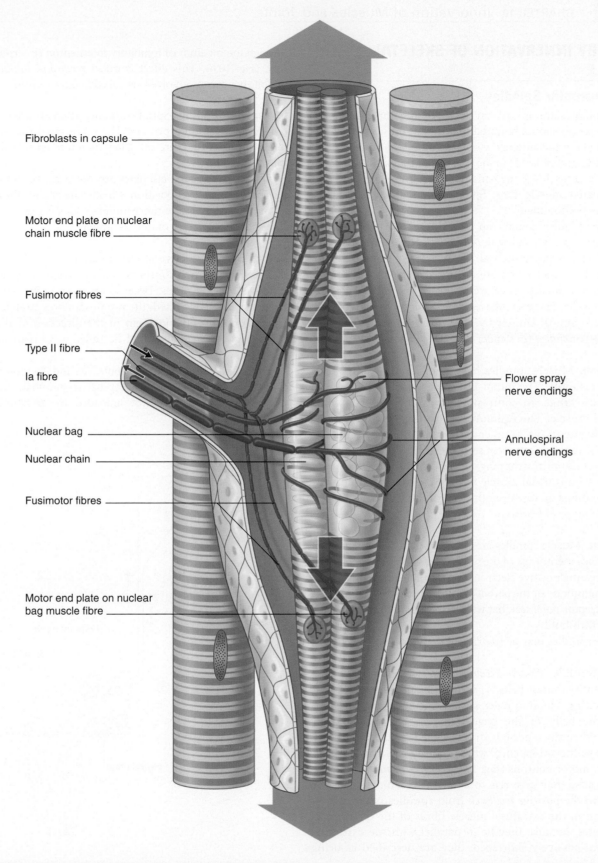

Fibroblasts in capsule

Motor end plate on nuclear chain muscle fibre

Fusimotor fibres

Type II fibre

Ia fibre

Nuclear bag

Nuclear chain

Fusimotor fibres

Motor end plate on nuclear bag muscle fibre

Flower spray nerve endings

Annulospiral nerve endings

Fig. 10.5 Neuromuscular spindle (simplified). *Large arrows* indicate passive stretch of the annulospiral endings produced by lengthening of the relaxed muscle as a whole. *Medium arrows* indicate active stretch of annulospiral endings produced by activity of fusimotor nerve fibres. Active stretch more than compensates for the unloading effect of simultaneous extrafusal muscle fibre contraction. *Small arrows* indicate directions of impulse conduction to and from the spindle when the parent muscle is in use.

SENSORY INNERVATION OF SKELETAL MUSCLE

Neuromuscular Spindles

Muscle spindles are up to 1 cm in length and vary in number from a dozen to several hundred in different muscles. They are abundant (1) in the antigravity muscles along the vertebral column, femur, and tibia; (2) in the muscles of the neck; and (3) in the intrinsic muscles of the hand. All these muscles are rich in slow, oxidative muscle fibres. Spindles are scarce where FG or FOG fibres predominate.

Muscle spindles contain up to a dozen **intrafusal muscle fibres** (Fig. 10.5). (Ordinary muscle fibres are *extrafusal* in this context.) The larger intrafusal fibres emerge from the *poles* (ends) of the spindles and are anchored to connective tissue (perimysium). Smaller ones are anchored to the collagenous spindle capsule. At the spindle *equator* (middle) the sarcomeres are replaced almost entirely by nuclei in the form of *bags* (in wide fibres) or *chains* (in slender fibres).

Innervation. Muscle spindles have both a motor and a sensory nerve supply. The motor fibres, called *fusimotor*, are in the Aγ size range, in contrast to the Aα fibres supplying extrafusal muscle. The fusimotor axons divide to supply the striated segments at both ends of the intrafusal muscles (Fig. 10.5). A single *primary* sensory fibre of type Ia calibre applies *annulospiral* wrappings around the bag or chain segments of the intrafusal muscle fibres. *Secondary, flower spray* sensory endings on one or both sides of the primary fibre are supplied by type II fibres.

Activation. Muscle spindles are *stretch receptors*. Ion channels in the surface membrane of the sensory terminals are opened by stretch, creating positive electronic waves that summate close to the final heminode of the parent sensory fibre. Summation produces a *receptor potential* that will fire off nerve impulses when it reaches threshold.

Muscle spindles may be stretched either *passively* or *actively*.

Passive Stretch. Passive stretch of muscle spindles occurs when an entire muscle belly is passively lengthened. For example, in eliciting a tendon reflex such as the *knee jerk*, the spindles in the belly of the quadriceps muscle are passively stretched when the tendon is struck. Type Ia and type II fibres discharge to the spinal cord, where they synapse on the dendrites of α motor neurons (Fig. 10.6). (*α motor neurons* are so called because they give rise to axons of Aα diameter.) The response to the *positive feedback* from spindles is a twitch of contraction in the extrafusal muscle fibres of the quadriceps. The spindles, because they lie in parallel with the extrafusal muscle, are passively shortened; they are described as being *unloaded*.

Tendon reflexes are *monosynaptic reflexes*. They have a *latency* (stimulus–response interval) of about 15 to 25 ms.

In addition to exciting homonymous motor neurons (i.e. motor neurons supplying the same muscles), the spindle afferents *inhibit* the α motor neurons supplying the antagonist muscles,

through the medium of inhibitory interneuron (interposed) neurons (Fig. 10.6). This effect is called *reciprocal inhibition*. The inhibitory neurons involved are called *Ia interneurons*.

Information Coding. Spindle primary afferents are most active *during* the stretching process. The more rapid the stretch, the more impulses they fire off. They therefore encode the *rate* of muscle stretch.

Spindle secondary afferents are more active than the primaries when a given position is held. The greater the degree of *maintained* stretch, the more impulses they fire off. They therefore encode the *degree* of muscle stretch.

Active Stretch. Active stretch is produced by the fusimotor neurons, which elicit contraction of the striated segments of the intrafusal muscle fibres. Because the connective tissue attachments are relatively fixed, the intrafusal fibres stretch the spindle equators by pulling them in the direction of the spindle poles (Fig. 10.7). (This could be called a 'Christmas cracker' effect.)

During all voluntary movements, Aα and Aγ motor neurons are coactivated by the corticospinal (pyramidal) tract. As a result, the spindles are not unloaded by extrafusal muscle

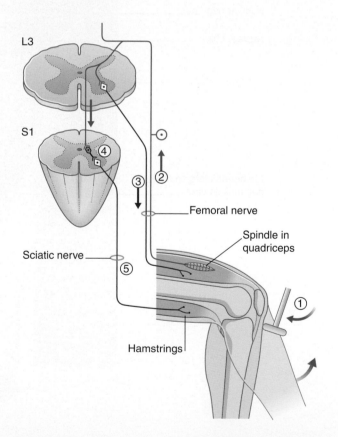

Fig. 10.6 Patellar reflex, including reciprocal inhibition. *Arrows* indicate nerve impulses. (1) A tap to the patellar ligament stretches the spindles in quadriceps femoris. (2) Spindles discharge excitatory impulses to the spinal cord. (3) α motor neurons respond by eliciting a twitch in the quadriceps, with extension of the knee. (4 and 5) Ia inhibitory interneurons respond by suppressing any activity in the hamstrings.

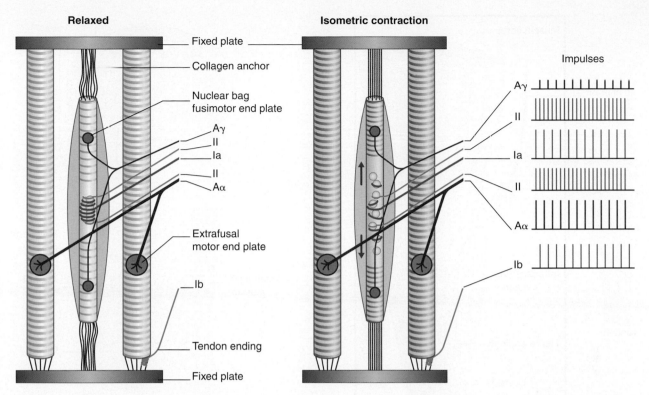

Fig. 10.7 Active stretch of a muscle spindle under isometric conditions. The term *isometric* means 'same length'. Certainly, the extrafusal muscle fibres would remain isometric when pulling with both ends rigidly fixed. The muscle spindle also remains isometric, being anchored to the plate indirectly via connective tissue. But the striated elements of each intrafusal fibre do not remain isometric: they shorten because the spindle equator is elastic and yields to stress. The primary and secondary spindle afferents, applied to the equator, respond to the 'active' stretch produced by fusimotor activity by discharging afferent impulses to the central nervous system, with consequent reinforcement of extrafusal contraction via the gamma loop.

contraction. Through ascending connections, the spindle afferents on both sides of the relevant joints keep the brain informed about contractions and relaxations during any given movement.

Tendon Endings

Golgi tendon organs are found at muscle—tendon junctions (Fig. 10.8). A single Ib calibre nerve fibre forms elaborate sprays that intertwine with tendon fibre bundles enclosed within a connective tissue capsule.

A dozen or more muscle fibres insert into these intracapsular tendon fibres, which are *in series* with the other muscle fibres within a particular muscle. The bulbous nerve endings are activated by the tension that develops during muscle contraction. Because the rate of impulse discharge along the parent fibre is related to the applied tension, tendon endings signal the *force* of muscle contraction.

The Ib afferents exert **negative feedback** on to the homonymous motor neurons, in contrast to the positive feedback exerted by muscle spindle afferents. The effect is called **autogenetic inhibition**, and the reflex arc is disynaptic because of the interpolation of an inhibitory neuron (Fig. 10.9). If need be, there follows *reciprocal excitation* of motor neurons supplying antagonist muscles.

An important function of tendon organ afferents is to dampen (restrict) the inherent tendency of moving limb segments to oscillate (sway to and fro). Dampening introduces an element known to physiologists as *joint stiffness*. Paradoxically, when Ib afferents are allowed too much freedom, as in *Parkinson disease* (Chapter 26), they reinforce the inherent tendency to oscillate and contribute to the characteristic *resting tremor* that is most obvious in the forearm (pronation—supination) and in the fingers ('pill-rolling' of the thumb pad by adjacent fingers).

Free Nerve Endings

Muscles are rich in free-ending nerve fibres, distributed to the intramuscular connective tissue and investing fascial envelopes. They are responsible for pain sensation caused by direct injury or by accumulation of metabolites including lactic acid. See also Clinical Panel 10.1.

INNERVATION OF JOINTS

Free-ending unmyelinated nerve fibres are abundant in joint ligaments and capsules and in the outer parts of intraarticular menisci. They mediate pain when a joint is strained, and they operate an

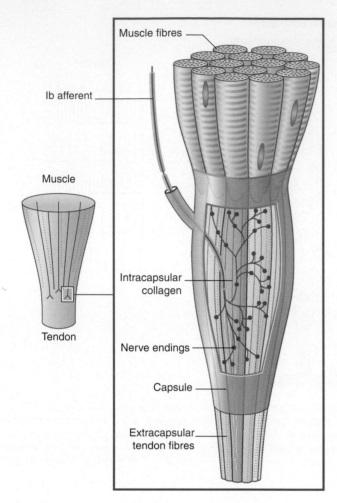

Fig. 10.8 Golgi tendon organ.

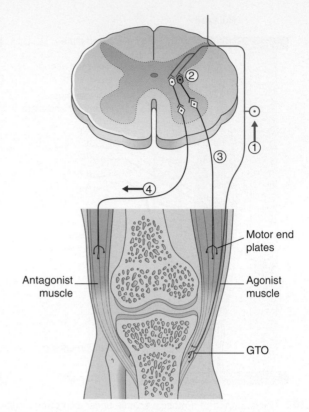

Fig. 10.9 Reflex effects of Golgi tendon organ *(GTO)* stimulation. *(1)* Agonist muscle contraction excites a GTO afferent, which *(2)* excites inhibitory interneuron synapsing on *(4)* a homonymous motor neuron, and *(3)* excites excitatory interneuron synapsing on *(4)* a motor neuron supplying the antagonist muscle.

excitatory reflex to protect the capsule. For example, the anterior wrist capsule is supplied by the median and ulnar nerves; if it is suddenly stretched by forced extension, motor fibres in these nerves are reflexively activated and cause wrist flexion.

Animal experiments have shown that when a joint is inflamed, more free-ending nerve fibres are excited than is the case when a healthy joint capsule is stretched. It seems that some nerve endings are *only* stimulated by inflammation.

Encapsulated nerve endings in and around joint capsules include Ruffini endings that respond to tension, lamellated endings that respond to pressure, and Pacinian corpuscles that respond to vibration (Chapter 11).

CLINICAL PANEL 10.1 Myofascial Pain Syndrome

Myofascial pain syndrome is a common disorder characterised by regional pain and muscle tenderness associated with hypersensitive bands of taut muscle fibres. (A related disorder is *fibromyalgia* that is considered a central pain disorder from a dysfunctional pain modulation system, but there is clinical overlap between the syndromes.) Allowing an examining finger to cross a hypersensitive band elicits pain; hence the clinical term *myofascial trigger point*. The pain is not confined to the dermatomal distribution of the parent sensory nerve, but it may be felt away from the trigger point *(referred pain)* and may be associated with autonomic signs (e.g. erythema and piloerection). Trigger points may develop due to muscle trauma or overuse during occupational or recreational activities, when normal recovery is disturbed. Spontaneously active foci within a muscle are known as *active myofascial trigger points* (MTrPs); currently inactive ones are known as *latent MTrPs*. While the pathophysiology remains unclear, tissue fluid surrounding

active MTrPs contains a greater quantity of several types of molecules associated with inflammation (e.g. bradykinins, prostaglandins, and H⁺ protons) than does that around latent MTrPs.

Over time, pain may become more widespread or severe as a result of sensitisation of dorsal horn neurons. Release of the peptide *substance P* by other branches of sensitised neurons (Clinical Panel 11.1) may initiate the creation of new MTrPs in the same or an adjacent muscle.

The sustained contraction of muscle fibres adjacent to the nodules has been attributed to inactivation of acetylcholinesterase in the basement membrane of their motor end plates. Modes of treatment include the following: sustained passive stretch of the affected muscle(s); sustained pressure in the recumbent position (e.g. by placing a tennis ball beneath the affected area); and mechanical disruption by needling or by injection of a local anaesthetic and/or a steroid into the area.

✳ Core Information

Muscle

A motor unit comprises a motor neuron and the group of muscle fibres it supplies. Each unit contains only one histochemical type of muscle fibre. At the myoneural synapse, the terminal bouton (containing vesicular ACh quanta) is separated from sarcolemmal junctional folds (containing ACh receptors) by a basement membrane containing acetylcholinesterase.

Muscle spindles contain intrafusal muscle fibres activated simultaneously at both ends by γ fusimotor neurons. Sensory fibres of type Ia diameter provide primary annulospiral endings at the equator, and fibres of type II diameter provide secondary endings nearby; both kinds are stretch receptors. Stretch may be passive (e.g. by a tendon reflex) or active (during fusimotor activity). Homonymous motor neurons are monosynaptically excited; antagonists are reciprocally inhibited via Ia interneurons. Spindle primaries signal the rate of muscle stretch; secondaries signal the degree. During voluntary movements, Aα and Aγ motor neurons are coactivated.

Golgi tendon organs signal the force of muscle contraction. They comprise encapsulated tendon tissue innervated by type Ib diameter afferents exerting disynaptic inhibition on homonymous motor neurons and reciprocal excitation of antagonists.

Free intramuscular nerve endings subserve pain sensation.

Joints

Free nerve endings abound in ligaments and capsules and in the outer part of menisci. They mediate pain and operate an articular protective reflex. Encapsulated endings signal joint movement.

SUGGESTED READINGS

Alvarez FJ, Titus-Mitchell HE, Bullinger KL, et al. Permanent central synaptic disconnection of proprioceptors after nerve injury and regeneration. I. Loss of VGLUT1/IA synapses on motoneurons. *J Neurophysiol.* 2011;106:2450—2470.

Banks RW, Hulliger M, Saed HH, et al. A comparative analysis of the encapsulated end-organs of mammalian skeletal muscles and of their sensory nerve endings. *J Anat.* 2009;214:859—887.

Bullinger KL, Nardelli P, Pinter MJ, et al. Permanent central synaptic disconnection of proprioceptors after nerve injury and regeneration. II. Loss of functional connectivity with motoneurons. *J Neurophysiol.* 2011;106:2471—2485.

De Luca CJ, Kline JC, Contessa P. Transposed firing activation of motor units. *J Neurophysiol.* 2014;112:962—970.

Kanning KC, Kaplan A, Henderson CE. Motor neuron diversity in development and disease. *Annu Rev Neurosci.* 2010;33:409—440.

Larsson L, Degens H, Li M, et al. Sarcopenia: aging-related loss of muscle mass and function. *Physiol Rev.* 2019;99(1):427—511.

Liu W, Chakkalakal JV. The composition, development, and regeneration of neuromuscular junctions. *Curr Top Dev Biol.* 2018;126:99—124.

Proske E. Two enigmas in proprioception: abundance and location of muscle spindles. *Brain Res Rec.* 2007;75:495—496.

Sasaki H, Polus BI. Can neck muscle spindle afferents activate fusimotor neurons of the lower limb? *Muscle Nerve.* 2012;45:376—384.

Wang Z, Li LY, Frank E. The role of muscle spindles in the development of the monosynaptic stretch reflex. *J Neurophysiol.* 2012;108:83—90.

Innervation of Skin

STUDY GUIDELINES

1. Define sensory unit, sensory overlap, receptive field, and receptor adaptation.
2. State locations and properties of the three kinds of encapsulated receptor.
3. Sketch a hair follicle with its nerve palisade and rings.
4. Name two kinds of mechanoreceptors used to discriminate textures—for example, to read Braille.
5. Consider a quick preview of the Clinical Panel on peripheral neuropathies in Chapter 12.

From the cutaneous branches of the spinal nerves, innumerable fine twigs enter a *dermal nerve plexus* located at the base of the dermis. Within the plexus, individual nerve fibres divide and overlap extensively with others before terminating at higher levels of the skin. Because of the overlap, the area of anaesthesia resulting from injury to a cutaneous nerve (e.g. superficial radial, saphenous) is smaller than its anatomic territory.

SENSORY UNITS

A given stem fibre forms the same kind of nerve ending at all of its terminals. In physiologic recordings, the stem fibre and its family of endings constitute a *sensory unit*. Together with its parent unipolar nerve cell, the sensory unit is analogous to the motor unit described in Chapter 10.

The territory from which a sensory unit can be excited is its *receptive field*. There is an inverse relationship between the size of receptive fields and sensory acuity; for example, fields measure about 2 cm^2 on the upper arm, 1 cm^2 at the wrist, and 5 mm^2 on the finger pads.

Sensory units interdigitate so that different modalities of sensation can be perceived from a given patch of skin.

NERVE ENDINGS

Our understanding of the pattern and nature of innervation of skin is still rather limited. New advances in microscopical methods are greatly enhancing our understanding of this elaborate organ. There follows a classical account of the main sensory nerve endings in the skin:

Free Nerve Endings (Fig. 11.1A,B)

As they run towards the skin surface, many sensory fibres shed their perineural sheaths and then their myelin sheaths (if any) before branching further in a subepidermal network. The Schwann cell sheaths open to permit naked axons to terminate between collagen bundles *(dermal nerve endings)* or within the epidermis *(epidermal nerve endings)*.New imaging approaches are providing insights into the intricate microanatomy of these endings so the term "free" may be an oversimplification of the axon tissue interface.

Functions

Some sensory units with free nerve endings are *thermoreceptors*. They supply either 'warm spots' or 'cold spots' scattered over the skin. Two kinds of *nociceptors* (pain-transducing units) with free endings are also found. One kind responds to severe mechanical deformation of the skin—for example, pinching with a forceps. The parent fibres are finely myelinated (Aδ). The other kind comprises *polymodal nociceptors;* these are C-fibre units able to transduce mechanical deformation, intense heat (some also intense cold), and irritant chemicals.

C-fibre units are responsible for the axon reflex (Clinical Panel 11.1).

Follicular Nerve Endings (Fig. 11.1A,D)

Just below the level of the sebaceous glands, myelinated fibres apply a *palisade* of naked terminals along the outer root sheath epithelium of the hair follicles. Outside this is a *circumferential* set of terminals.

Each follicular unit supplies many follicles, and there is much territorial overlap. Follicular units are *rapidly adapting*. They fire when the hairs are being bent, but not when the bent position is held. Rapid adaptation accounts for our being largely unaware of our clothing except when dressing or undressing. Hair innervation in other mammals is more complex. Evidence of hair follicle innervation by three types of mechanoreceptors, each relaying specific information to specific brain locations, reflects its important sensory function.

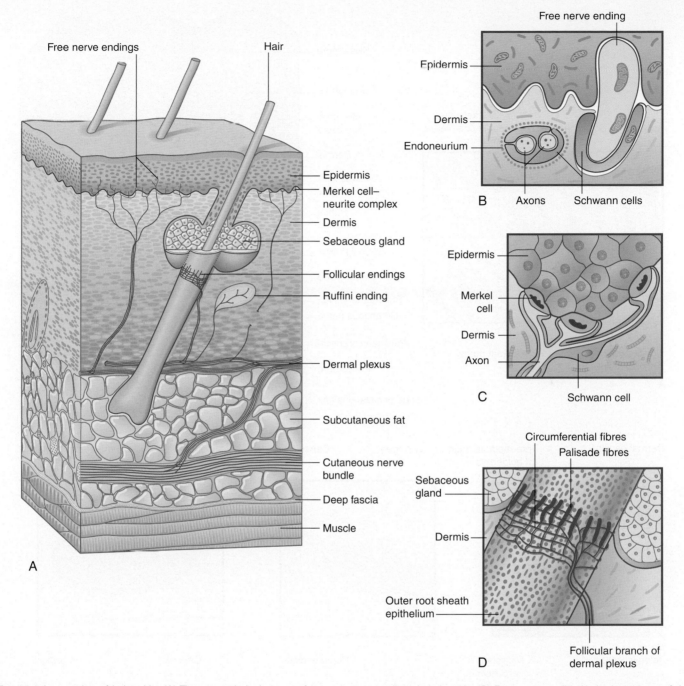

Fig. 11.1 Innervation of hairy skin. (A) Three morphologic types of sensory nerve endings in hairy skin. (B) Free nerve ending in the basal layer of the epidermis. (C) Merkel cell–neurite complex. (D) Palisade and circumferential nerve endings on the surface of the outer root sheath of a hair follicle.

Merkel Cell–Neurite Complexes (Fig. 11.1A,C)

Expanded nerve terminals are applied to **Merkel cells** *(tactile menisci)* in the basal epithelium of epidermal pegs and ridges. These *Merkel cell–neurite complexes* are *slowly adapting*. They discharge continuously in response to sustained pressure, such as while holding a pen or wearing spectacles, and they are markedly sensitive to the *edges* of objects held in the hand.

Encapsulated Nerve Endings

The *capsules* of the three nerve endings to be described comprise an outer coat of connective tissue, a middle coat of perineural

epithelium, and an inner coat of modified Schwann cells *(teloglia).* All three are **mechanoreceptors**, transducing mechanical stimuli.

- **Meissner corpuscles** are most numerous in the finger pads, where they lie beside the intermediate ridges of the epidermis (Fig. 11.2A-C). In these ovoid receptors, several axons zigzag among stacks of teloglial lamellae. Meissner corpuscles are rapidly adapting. Together with the slowly adapting Merkel cell–neurite complexes, they provide the tools for delicate detective work on textured surfaces such as cloth or wood, or on embossed surfaces such as Braille text. Elevations as little as 5 μm in height can be detected!

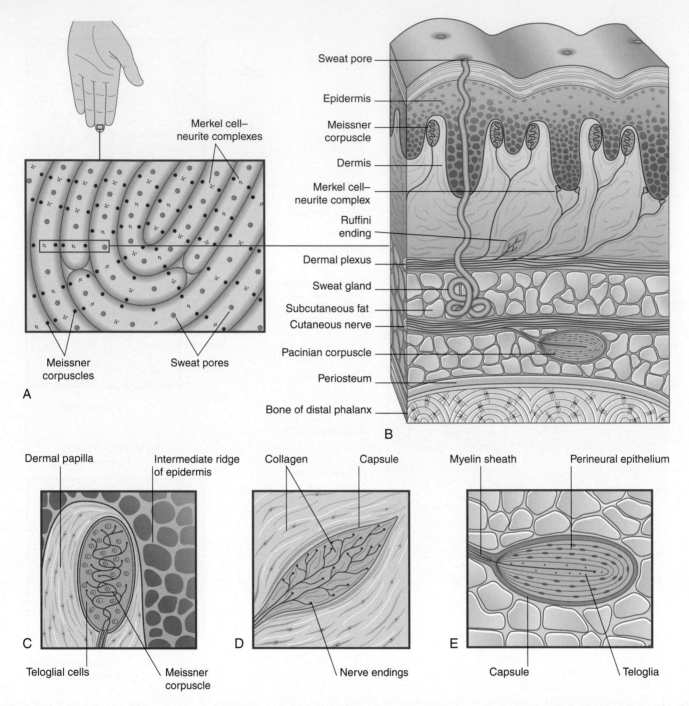

Fig. 11.2 Innervation of glabrous skin. (A) Finger pad showing distribution of two types of sensory nerve endings. (B) Tissue block from (A) showing positions of four types of sensory nerve endings. (C) Meissner corpuscle. (D) Nerve ending of Ruffini. (E) Pacinian corpuscle.

- **Ruffini endings** are found in both hairy and glabrous skin (Figs. 11.1A and 11.2D). They respond to *drag* (shearing stress) and are slowly adapting. Their structure resembles that of Golgi tendon organs, having a collagenous core in which several axons branch liberally.
- **Pacinian corpuscles** (Fig. 11.2B,E) are the size of rice grains. They number about 300 in the hand. They are subcutaneous, close to the underlying periosteum, and numerous along the

sides of the fingers and in the palm. Inside a thin connective tissue sheath are onion-like layers of perineural epithelium containing some blood capillaries. Innermost are several teloglial lamellae surrounding a single central axon that has shed its myelin sheath at the point of entry. Pacinian corpuscles are rapidly adapting and are especially responsive to *vibration*—particularly to bone vibration. In the limbs many corpuscles are embedded in the periosteum of the long bones.

Pacinian corpuscles discharge one or two impulses when compressed and again when released. In the hands they seem to function in group mode: when an object such as an orange is picked up, as many as 120 or more corpuscles are activated momentarily, with a momentary repetition when the object is released. For this reason, they have been called 'event detectors' during object manipulation.

The digital receptors are classified as follows by sensory physiologists.
- Merkel cell—neurite complexes = SA I
- Meissner corpuscles = RA I
- Ruffini endings = SA II
- Pacinian corpuscles = RA II

When three-dimensional objects are being manipulated out of sight, significant contributions to perceptual evaluation are made by muscle afferents (especially from muscle spindles) and articular afferents from joint capsules. The cutaneous, muscular, and articular afferents relay information independently to the contralateral somatic sensory cortex. The three kinds of information serve the function of **tactile discrimination**. They are integrated (brought together at the cellular level) in the posterior part of the contralateral parietal lobe, which is specialised for *spatial sense*, both tactile and visual. Spatial tactile sense is called *stereognosis*. In the clinic stereognosis is tested by asking the patient to identify an object such as a key without looking at it. Cutaneous sensory effects of peripheral neuropathies are described in Chapter 12. Clinical Panel 11.2 gives a short account of *leprosy*.

Skin is a sensory organ that also plays a vital role in homeostasis. These functions are mediated by small cutaneous nerve fibres. There is an increasing awareness of functions of the autonomic nervous system in this important organ. The importance of the early targeting of this system in certain neurodegenerative diseases should be noted as this awareness may enable the development of better early diagnostic markers.

CLINICAL PANEL 11.1 Neurogenic Inflammation: The Axon Reflex

When sensitive skin is stroked with a sharp object, capillary dilatation in direct response to the injury causes a red line to appear in seconds. A few minutes later, arteriolar dilatation causes a red *flare* to spread into the surrounding skin, followed by exudation of plasma from the capillaries that produces a white *wheal*. These phenomena constitute the *triple response*. The wheal and flare responses are produced by *axon reflexes* in the local sensory cutaneous nerves. The sequence of events follows the numbers in Fig. 11.3.

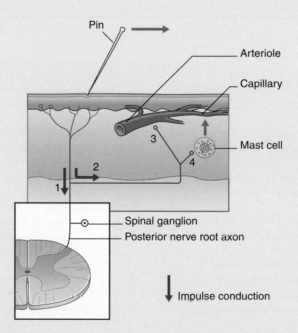

Fig. 11.3 The axon reflex.

1. The noxious stimulus is transduced (converted to nerve impulses) by polymodal nociceptors.
2. As well as transmitting impulses to the central nervous system in the normal, orthodromic direction, the axons send impulses in an *antidromic* direction from points of bifurcation into the neighbouring skin. The nociceptive endings respond to antidromic stimulation by releasing one or more peptide substances, notably substance P.
3. Substance P binds with receptors on the walls of arterioles, leading to arteriolar dilatation—the flare response.
4. Substance P also binds with receptors on the surface of mast cells, stimulating them to release *histamine*. The histamine increases capillary permeability and leads to local accumulation of tissue fluid—the wheal response.

CLINICAL PANEL 11.2 Leprosy

The leprosy bacillus enters the skin through minor abrasions. It travels proximally within the perineurium of the cutaneous nerves and kills off the Schwann cells. Loss of myelin segments ('segmental demyelination') blocks impulse conduction in the larger nerve fibres. Later, the inflammatory response to the bacillus compresses all the axons, leading to Wallerian degeneration of entire nerves and gross thickening of the connective tissue sheaths. Patches of anaesthetic skin develop on the fingers, toes, nose, and ears. The protective function of skin sensation is lost, and the affected parts suffer injury and loss of tissue. Motor paralysis occurs late in the disease cycle as a consequence of bacterial invasion of mixed nerve trunks proximal to the points of origin of their cutaneous branches.

Core Information

Cutaneous nerves branch to form a dermal nerve plexus, where individual afferent fibres branch and overlap. Each stem fibre and its terminal receptors constitute a sensory unit. The territory of a stem fibre is its receptive field.

Sensory units with free nerve endings include thermoreceptors and both mechanical and thermal nociceptors. Follicular units are rapidly adapting touch receptors, active only when hairs are in motion. Merkel cell—neurite complexes are slowly adapting edge detectors.

The encapsulated endings are mechanoreceptors. Meissner corpuscles lie beside intermediate ridges in glabrous skin and are rapidly adapting. Ruffini endings lie near hair follicles and fingernails; they are slowly adapting drag receptors. Pacinian corpuscles are subcutaneous, rapidly adapting event detectors, and vibration receptors.

Coded information from skin, muscles, and joints is integrated at the level of the posterior parietal lobe of the brain, yielding the faculties of tactile discrimination and stereognosis.

The cutaneous innervation is mainly sensory but there is also autonomic innervation. This is mainly sympathetic-associated, but parasympathetic innervation has also been reported in the skin of the face. The associated axons are autonomic C and Aδ fibres, and these play an important role in thermoregulation and wound healing.

The sensory nerves of skin allow sensation of pain, itch, temperature, and touch. Nociceptors (pain), pruriceptors (itch), thermoreceptors (temperature), and some mechanoreceptors (touch) are free nerve endings. Other touch receptors present in the skin are encapsulated. The cell bodies of nerves that innervate the skin are in the trigeminal and dorsal root ganglia. The cutaneous innervation is mainly sensory but there is also autonomic innervation (mainly sympathetic).

SUGGESTED READINGS

Abraira VE, Ginty DD. The sensory neurons of touch. *Neuron.* 2013;79:618—639.

Crawford LK, Caterina MJ. Functional anatomy of the sensory nervous system: updates from the neuroscience bench. *Toxicol Pathol.* 2020;48:174—189.

Eijkelkamp N, Quick K, Wood JN. Transient receptor potential channels and mechanosensation. *Annu Rev Neurosci.* 2013;36:519—546.

Filingeri D, Fournet D, Hodder S, Havenith G. Why wet feels wet? A neurophysiological model of human cutaneous wetness sensitivity. *J Neurophysiol.* 2014;112:1457—1469.

Glatte P, Buchmann SJ, Hijazi MM, Illigens BM, Siepmann T. Architecture of the cutaneous autonomic nervous system. *Front Neurol.* 2019;10:970.

Hays AP. Utility of skin biopsy to evaluate peripheral neuropathy. *Curr Neurol Neurosci Rep.* 2010;10:101—107.

Hosaka M, Yamamoto M, Cho HC, Jang HS, Murakami G, Abe S. Human nasociliary nerve with special reference to its unique parasympathetic cutaneous innervation. *Anat Cell Biol.* 2016;49(2):132—137.

Jeffry J, Kim S, Chen ZF. Itch signaling in the nervous system. *Physiology.* 2011;26:286—292.

Lechner SG, Lewin GR. Hairy sensation. *Physiology.* 2013;28:142—150.

Meftah E-M, Chapman CE. Tactile perception of roughness. *Exp Brain Res.* 2009;3:235—244.

Schepers RJ, Ringkamp M. Thermoreceptors and thermosensitive afferents. *Neurosci Behav Rev.* 2009;33:205—212.

Nolano M, Provitera V, Caporaso G, et al. Cutaneous innervation of the human face as assessed by skin biopsy. *J Anat.* 2013;222(2):161—169.

Tavee JO, Polston D, Zhou L, Shields RW, Butler RS, Levin KH. Sural sensory nerve action potential, epidermal nerve fiber density, and quantitative sudomotor axon reflex in the healthy elderly. *Muscle Nerve.* 2014;49:564—569.

Electrodiagnostic Examination

STUDY GUIDELINES

1. Review the electrical events of action potentials, described in Chapter 7, as it applies to the basic principles described here.
2. Describe the performance of a motor or sensory **nerve conduction study (NCS)** and predict the results if there is an axonal injury or a dysfunction of myelin.
3. Define the relationship between a motor neuron and its corresponding **motor unit action potential (MUAP)**.
4. Describe the origin and relevance of a fibrillation and fasciculation potential.
5. Contrast the expected appearance of a MUAP in a chronic disorder that results in weakness from a muscle versus motor neuron disease.
6. Provide classification rubrics used for neuropathies.
7. Describe the components of a **neuromuscular junction (NMJ)** and sites of involvement/pathogenesis in myasthenia gravis versus congenital myopathies.
8. Explain the significance of a decremental response on repetitive nerve stimulation in **electrodiagnostic (EDX)** testing.
9. Clinical Panel 12.1 and 12.2 and Basic Science Panel 12.1 — Review the following clinical disorders (carpal tunnel syndrome, Guillain-Barré syndrome, myasthenia gravis) regarding their presentation and pathogenesis (mechanism of injury/dysfunction).

The primary concerns of clinical neurophysiology laboratories are two-fold: assessment of the functional state of the peripheral nervous system (PNS) and assessment of cerebral cortical function. PNS assessment entails the use of nerve conduction study (NCS) where stimulation of selected peripheral nerves accesses nerve conduction velocity and waveform appearance, and the use of electromyography (EMG) where waveforms generated by voluntary contraction of selected muscles are recorded. The combination of NCS and EMG is referred to as an electrodiagnostic (EDX) examination.

NERVE CONDUCTION STUDIES

NCS are routinely performed as an extension of the clinical examination of the PNS. Through stimulation of nerves allied to the recording of muscle fibre depolarisations, it is possible to determine whether the disorder involves the nerve, neuromuscular junction, or muscle. NCS can also determine whether the disorder is a focal or diffuse process involving sensory and/or motor axons, and whether it is primarily affecting the myelin or the axons.

Nerve Conduction Studies in the Upper Extremity

A frequent studied nerve in the upper limb is the median nerve. The median nerve is a mixed nerve and has three key advantages for electrophysiologic studies:

1. It is readily accessible for stimulation and/or recording at the elbow as well as at the wrist.
2. For motor NCS the abductor pollicis brevis, supplied by the recurrent branch of the median nerve, is readily available for EMG and/or surface recordings.
3. For sensory NCS the skin of the index finger is ideal for recording action potentials travelling antidromically following median nerve stimulation at the elbow or the wrist. (As noted in Chapter 11, antidromic means 'running against' the normal (orthodromic) direction of impulse conduction.)

Motor Nerve Conduction. Stimulation. A typical stimulating device is one with a cathode and an anode in the form of two blunt prongs and applied to the skin surface overlying the nerve. In Fig. 12.1 it was placed over the median nerve at the wrist (just lateral to the cordlike palmaris longus tendon). The cathode is positioned nearer to the recording site than the anode. When sufficient current passes from cathode to anode, transmembrane ionic movements initiate impulse propagation in both directions along the nerve. Large myelinated nerve fibres lying nearest to the cathode are the first to become depolarised; these include the Aα diameter axons of anterior horn motor neurons. A pulse of 20 to 40 mA with a duration of 0.1 ms is usually sufficient to activate all the motor axons that innervate the abductor pollicis brevis.

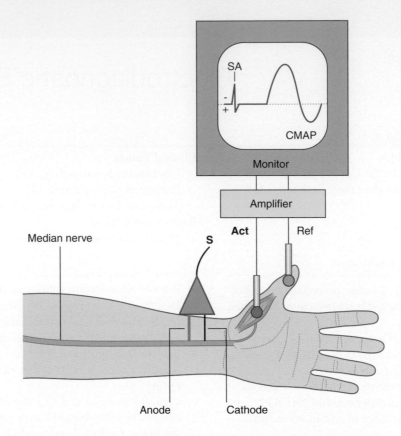

Fig. 12.1 Basic setup for recording a compound motor action potential. The stimulating electrode *(S)* has been placed over the median nerve, and the active recording electrode *(Act)* has been placed over the abductor pollicis brevis muscle and the reference electrode *(Ref)* has been placed distally. *CMAP*, Compound motor action potential; *SA*, stimulus artefact.

Recording. The active electrode is placed over the mid-region of the muscle where the motor end plates are concentrated, the motor point. A second reference electrode is placed over a 'neutral' site a short distance away. The amplifier used to record these evoked motor responses is designed to record the potential differences between these two sites. The setup is arranged so that if the active electrode records a more negative response, this will take the form of an upward deflection on the monitor.

At a low level of stimulation, the only on-screen change in the tracing will be a small stimulus artefact on an otherwise flat tracing. As the current increases a small motor action potential appears. This results from activation of large myelinated motor axons close to the stimulator; the depolarisation wave travelling along each axon will in turn depolarise all of the muscle fibres innervated by that axon. In the case of the intrinsic muscles of the hand, including the abductor pollicis brevis, each motor unit has an innervation ratio of 200 or 300 muscle fibres per motor neuron. In large muscles not specialised for fine movements (e.g., deltoid, gastrocnemius), the minimum deflection on the monitor will be several times larger for two reasons: their motor innervation ratio is 1/1000 or more, and their larger muscle fibres generate action potentials of greater amplitude.

It should be emphasised that the on-screen waveform is not produced by the contraction process itself but by the extracellular potentials generated by depolarisation of the muscle membranes and filtered through the tissues and skin. However, while this distinction needs to be remembered, most disorders of muscle will also affect surface membrane depolarisation and hence lead to abnormalities of the waveform morphology.

Increasing the applied current activates additional axons until all the axons and their motor units are activated by each pulse. The required stimulus is called maximal but, for good measure, the final stimulus is supramaximal at 5% to 10% above maximal to ensure that all axons have been activated. The final waveform observed constitutes the **compound motor action potential (CMAP)**. It represents the summation of the individual muscle fibre potentials of all the motor units of all the motor axons of that nerve (Fig. 12.2).

Routine measurements of the final CMAP are shown in Fig. 12.3. They include the latency (time interval) between stimulus and depolarisation onset, and the amplitude and duration of the negative phase of the waveform. (Inward ion movement

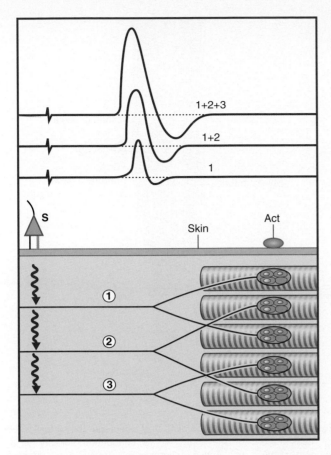

Fig. 12.2 Summation of individual motor units gives rise to the compound motor action potential. Interdigitating pairs of muscle fibres represent motor units. Low *(1)*, medium *(2)*, and maximal *(3)* stimulation yields progressively larger waveforms on the screen, despite being physiologically separate phenomena. *Act*, Active recording electrode; *S*, stimulator electrode.

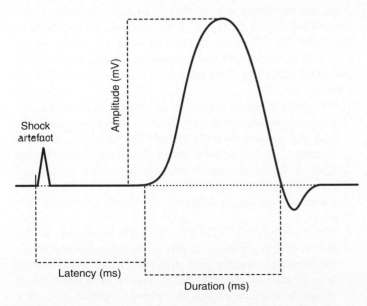

Fig. 12.3 Routine compound motor action potential measurements.

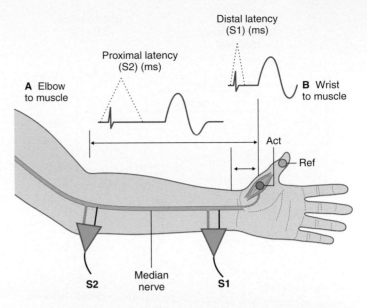

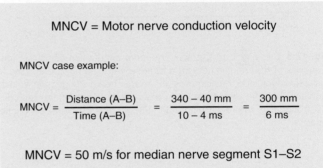

MNCV = Motor nerve conduction velocity

MNCV case example:

$$MNCV = \frac{Distance\ (A–B)}{Time\ (A–B)} = \frac{340 - 40\ mm}{10 - 4\ ms} = \frac{300\ mm}{6\ ms}$$

MNCV = 50 m/s for median nerve segment S1–S2

Fig. 12.4 Calculation of the motor nerve conduction velocity. The nerve is stimulated twice: S1 is the first stimulus and S2 is the second stimulus; the double arrows represent the two length measurements. The time baseline is not included. At the bottom is the calculation performed to determine the motor nerve conduction velocity and in this example, it is normal. *Act*, Active recording electrode; *Ref*, reference electrode.

(K + ions) produces the final, positive phase during collective repolarisation of the muscle fibres.)

Motor nerve conduction velocity. The setup required to determine *motor nerve conduction velocity (MNCV)* for the median nerve is straightforward (Fig. 12.4). Here the nerve has first been activated at the wrist (S1) to generate and store a 'wrist-to-muscle' velocity record. The stimulator has then been placed over the median nerve at the elbow (S2) to provide an 'elbow-to-muscle' record. Speed being the product of distance over time, the elbow-to-wrist conduction velocity is given by subtracting one value from the other, as illustrated by the case example.

Second choice. Normally a confirmatory MNCV is performed on another nerve, and in the upper limb the ulnar nerve is usually the best second choice. The ulnar is the standard second choice: S1 is performed over the nerve at the wrist just

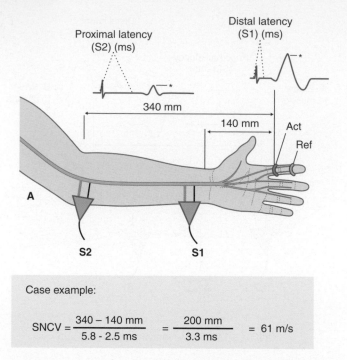

Fig. 12.5 Calculation of the sensory nerve conduction velocity. Digital branches of the median nerve are represented. The basic principles for the calculation are the same as for motor nerve conduction velocity studies. For the asterisks, see main text. *Act*, Active recording electrode; *Ref*, reference electrode; *SNCV*, sensory nerve conduction velocity.

Case example:

$$SNCV = \frac{340 - 140 \text{ mm}}{5.8 - 2.5 \text{ ms}} = \frac{200 \text{ mm}}{3.3 \text{ ms}} = 61 \text{ m/s}$$

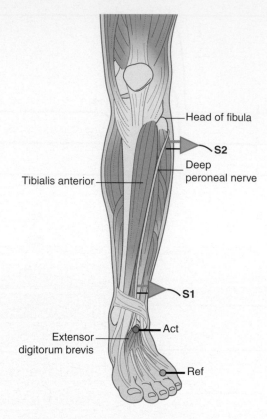

Fig. 12.6 Position for the recording electrodes and stimulator location for measurement of the motor nerve conduction velocity of the peroneal nerve. *Act*, Active recording electrode; *Ref*, reference electrode.

lateral to flexor carpi ulnaris, and S2 is performed where the nerve emerges from behind the medial epicondyle. The active recorder is applied over the hypothenar muscles on the medial margin of the palm.

Sensory Nerve Conduction. For studies of *sensory nerve conduction velocity (SNCV)*, the median is again the nerve of choice (Fig. 12.5). Again, it is large myelinated nerve fibres that will be stimulated, and the site and manner of stimulation at the elbow and wrist will be the same. On this occasion, however, we are selectively recording antidromic stimulation of cutaneous sensory fibres — specifically, of the digital branches of the median nerve to the skin over the index finger, using ring electrodes.

The myelinated nerve fibres to be sampled by the ring electrodes are those supplying the highly sensitive and discriminatory skin of the finger pad (described in Chapter 11). The largest fibres, serving the Meissner and the Pacinian corpuscles and the Merkel cell—neurite complexes, are known to normally conduct at a speed of 60 to 100 m/s and the finest fibres, serving mechanical nociceptors, at 10 to 30 m/s (these nerve fibres do not contribute to these routinely recorded sensory nerve responses). This variation is in marked contrast to that of the relatively uniform fibre size of the axons supplying the small motor units of the abductor pollicis brevis

muscle and conducting at 45 to 55 m/s. One consequence is that when stimulating sensory nerves at increasing distances from the recording site, a change in the waveform shape is normally noted. In Fig. 12.5 the asterisks are intended to highlight the difference in the shape of the distal versus proximal waveforms of the *compound sensory nerve action potential (CSNAP)*. Two important factors involved in the CSNAP are:

1. *Physiologic temporal dispersion.* As runners in a race become progressively separated over distance, the fastest takes the lead and the slowest trails behind. The variable conduction velocities of the sensory axons that contributed to the CSNAP exhibit a similar phenomenon, with consequent elongation of the CSNAP profile over the longer test distance, resulting in temporal dispersion (scattering over time).

2. *Phase cancellation.* The later CSNAP waveform is also flatter. This is explained in part by the phenomenon where the recorded positive and negative phases of individual sensory axon waveforms tend to 'cancel' each other out. It should be emphasised that this phase cancellation is not a physiologic event and the individual axonal waveforms

themselves are not affected by the 'eavesdropper' wrapped around the finger close to the finishing line. The diminishing amount of phase summation of the later CSNAP is the result of this increasing separation of action potentials.

While a similar process of physiologic temporal dispersion results in phase cancellation of the recorded response of the CMAP, it is normally not as evident. This is a result of less variation in conduction velocity of individual axons and characteristics of the motor waveform (duration and amplitude) itself. When temporal dispersion is detected in a CMAP, it is a pathologic sign and indicates demyelination.

Sensory nerve conduction velocity. The basic modes of operation and calculation are the same as shown for the MNCV study. A case example is included in Fig. 12.5, which demonstrates phase cancellation from physiologic temporal dispersion.

Second choice. The ulnar nerve is the standard second choice. Ulnar nerve stimulation is performed at the wrist and elbow as before, with the CMAP recorded over the abductor digiti minimi muscle and a ring electrode slipped onto the little finger to record from the ulnar supplied digital nerves to the finger.

Nerve Conduction Studies in the Lower Extremity

Motor Nerve Conduction. The lower limb nerve most frequently sampled for MNCV is the deep peroneal (fibular) nerve with recordings from the extensor digitorum brevis on the dorsum of the foot (Fig. 12.6). The deep peroneal (fibular) nerve is first stimulated in front of the ankle and then at the level of the neck of the fibula.

A second MNCV is performed on the tibial nerve with recordings from the adductor hallucis, located on the medial side of the foot (Fig. 12.7A).

Sensory Nerve Conduction. For SNCV assessment, the sural nerve is the nerve of choice. It arises from the tibial nerve and receives a contribution from the common peroneal nerve; it supplies the skin along the lateral margin of the foot. The recording electrode is applied to the skin below the lateral malleolus, and the nerve is stimulated antidromically at the levels shown in Fig. 12.7B.

The H Response. Owing to their deep location, conventional means of nerve stimulation are not possible, so nerve conduction in spinal nerve roots can only be assessed indirectly. One method is by activating sensorimotor reflex

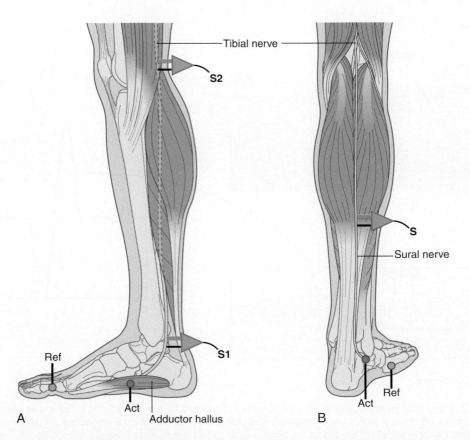

Fig. 12.7 (A) Positions for the recording electrodes and stimulator for measurement of the motor nerve conduction velocity of the tibial nerve. (B) Positions for antidromic recording of the sensory nerve conduction velocity of the sural nerve. *Act,* Active recording electrode; *Ref,* reference electrode.

arcs at appropriate levels. One standard test, named after Hoffmann, who first described it, is known as the **H-response or H-reflex**. This is frequently used to assess overall conduction velocity in the S1 reflex arc — the same neurons that are evaluated clinically by the Achilles reflex (Fig. 12.8).

The tibial nerve is stimulated using a long-duration (1 ms) but minimum-current intensity. The objective here is to excite the largest myelinated afferent fibres, namely those serving annulospiral nerve endings in neuromuscular spindles,

thereby eliciting a monosynaptic, minimal latency twitch in the triceps surae (gastrocnemius and soleus); these are 'preferentially' excited by long-duration stimuli. The minimal latency is in fact quite long—up to 35 ms depending on the patient's overall height—because the S1 segment of the spinal cord lies behind the body of vertebra L1, creating a 130- to 150-cm up and down trip.

At the appropriate stimulation intensity it is possible to preferentially activate the afferent fibres within the tibial nerve, and through the orthodromic transmission of their action potential

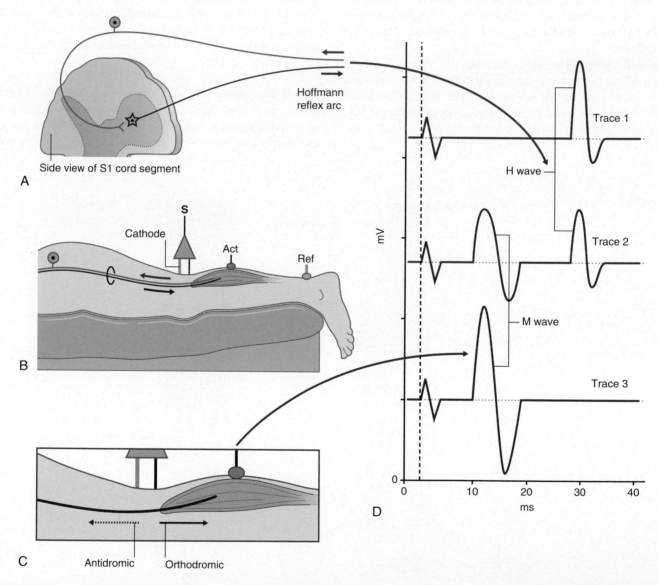

Fig. 12.8 Anatomic background of H and M waves. (A) The H wave is mediated by a monosynaptic reflex arc as shown. (B) Recording of the S1 segment Achilles reflex arc compound motor action potential. The stimulator overlies the tibial nerve; the recording electrode overlies the triceps surae muscle. Both limbs of the reflex arc are within the tibial component of the sciatic nerve. (C) Increasing the current now directly activates axons supplying the muscle as well, yielding the short-latency M wave. (D) Note that the H wave progressively disappears as stimulus intensity increases (moving from trace 1 to trace 3) owing to cancellation of the orthodromic motor impulses in (A) by antidromic impulses newly generated by the cathode, represented by the dashed line in (C). *Act,* Active recording electrode; *Ref,* reference electrode.

in this reflex arc, synapse on α motor neurons, a muscle twitch occurs; this motor response is called the H-reflex (Fig. 12.8A,B). However, increasing the current soon begins to activate α motor neuron axons within the tibial nerve as well, reaching the point where a direct motor response occurs and is recorded, the M wave (Fig. 12.8D). The M wave is produced by direct orthodromic activation of the α motor axons within the tibial nerve. The concurrent antidromic conduction of these same axons accounts for progressive cancelling out of the action potentials descending in the same efferent limb of the H-reflex arc (see Fig. 12.8D).

In the upper limb, the nerve roots of spinal nerve C6 may be tested by stimulating the median nerve and recording from the flexor carpi radialis. C7 roots may be tested by stimulating the posterior cutaneous nerve of the forearm and recording from the triceps brachii muscle.

ELECTROMYOGRAPHY

Electromyography (EMG) is a technique in which an electrode is incorporated into a fine needle and is inserted into a muscle to sample the depolarisation waveforms of muscle fibres produced by voluntary contractions. There are several components to the test that, when combined with the results of NCS, provide valuable diagnostic information.

The test begins, like NCS, with a clinical question, and the individual muscles chosen for EMG are based on the most probable clinical diagnosis provided by the history and physical examination. For example, if there is clinical evidence suggestive of a specific nerve injury, muscles are chosen that are supplied by that nerve. Recordings from adjacent muscles (or from the same muscle on the opposite side) during contraction would also be made to provide control waveforms for comparison. The results are combined with NCS to make a case for or against the provisional diagnosis.

Needle Electrode

The recording electrode occupies the lumen of a fine needle (Fig. 12.9). An insulation sleeve isolates the recording electrode from the barrel of the needle, which functions as a reference electrode. As in the case of NCS, the EMG record is based on the potential difference between the recording and reference electrodes. During muscle contractions, an extracellular record is taken of the low-voltage potentials that originate from the muscle membrane depolarisations.

The needle is passed through the skin and into the muscle in question. It is then pushed, in small increments, into various portions of the muscle, and after each needle movement the effect is observed. The moving needle will normally generate spiky, insertional activity caused by mechanical depolarisation of the muscle membranes by the needle electrode, which cease when the electrode movement stops.

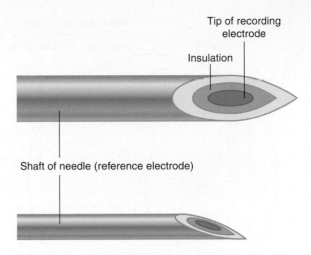

Fig. 12.9 Structure of a conventional concentric electrode. The upper image is a face-on view depicting the insulator separating the active (recording) electrode from the reference electrode.

The Normal Electromyogram

The sensitivity settings on the machine are then adjusted to record the larger amplitude waveforms of voluntary muscle contraction. The patient is asked to slightly contract the muscle, and as they do semirhythmic waveforms appear, representing *motor unit action potentials (MUAPs)*. Each of these individual waveforms represents activation of the muscle fibres that belong to an individual motor unit and those closest to the recoding electrode contribute to the shape of the MUAP.

While the electrode is stationary, all MUAPs that are of similar shape originate from the same individual *anterior horn cell (AHC)* and reflect depolarisation of that cell. The MUAP shape, in normal situations, is like the familiar QRS complex on an electrocardiography (ECG) recording, and measurements are made of their amplitude, duration, and morphology. Each individual MUAP is a sample of the summated depolarisations of the muscle fibres of a single motor unit. We must bear in mind that the electrode can only record from the muscle fibres that are the closest to it and not all fibres of a unit contribute to the observed response. As indicated in Fig. 12.10, overlap of the motor unit territories of individual AHCs permits several motor units to be sampled simultaneously.

The recorded waveforms tell us about the form and function of the motor units and about changes under various pathologic conditions. Each depolarisation of an AHC results in a virtually synchronous depolarisation of all its target muscle fibres. The needle electrode records a summation of the individual muscle fibre depolarisations closest to its exposed tip of the electrode, to provide a MUAP. If the recording electrode remains stationary, the MUAP waveform will remain the same.

On the monitor they 'march across' at a frequency that is the same as the firing rate of the AHCs being sampled. The stronger the voluntary muscle contraction, the greater the number of AHCs that are recruited by the corticospinal tract and the faster are their individual firing rates (Fig. 12.11).

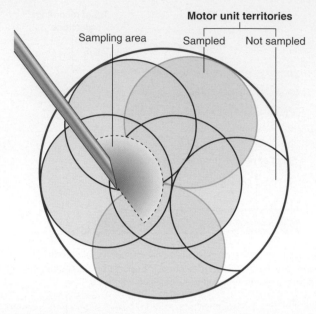

Motor unit territories

Sampling area   Sampled   Not sampled

Fig. 12.10 Sampling motor unit action potentials. This diagram represents the overlap of six motor unit territories. The area *(green)* being sampled includes parts of five units, the sixth being outside of the recording area of the electrode; contributions of individual muscle fibres are greatest close to the recording electrode.

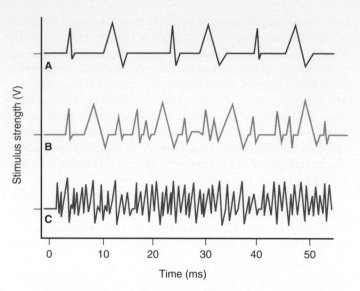

Fig. 12.11 Motor unit activation at increasing strengths of voluntary contraction. (A) In this example, during weak contraction the electrode has picked up activity in two motor unit action potentials (MUAPs), each with its characteristic shape. (B) Stronger contraction has recruited additional MUAPs within reach of the electrode and those originally recruited begin to fire more rapidly. (C) Substantially greater contraction has produced so much overlap of MUAPs that the individual MUAPs can no longer be discerned ('interference pattern').

CLINICAL PANEL 12.1 Entrapment Neuropathies

Peripheral nerves may be 'trapped' beneath ligamentous bridges or stretched at bony angulations, with consequent symptoms depending upon the distribution of the affected nerves. Sensory disturbances caused by compression tend to be early and prominent; motor weakness occurs later and is at times severe.

NCS are helpful to confirm diagnosis, identify the nerve/s involved, assess extent of damage, and monitor progression of the disease. The presence of generalised polyneuropathies are the most frequent predisposing factors involving entrapment syndromes. While entrapment could involve any peripheral nerve, our discussion is limited to the ones most commonly affected.

Upper limb

The most common entrapment neuropathy in the upper limb is carpal tunnel syndrome, which involves the compression of the median nerve in a passageway on the palmar aspect of the wrist. This tunnel is formed by the flexor retinaculum and the carpal bones (Fig. 12.12). Characteristic sensory symptoms are paraesthesia in the affected hand and fingers and bouts of pain, which may extend from the hand up along the arm. These symptoms commonly occur during the night and by day they are commonly brought on by grasping or pinching actions in the workplace. Wringing (flicking) the affected hand may afford some relief. On examination the skin overlying the distal phalanges that is supplied by the median nerve, namely that of the thumb, index, and middle fingers and the lateral half of the ring finger, shows reduced sensory acuity. The thenar eminence may appear flattened as a

result of wasting of the thenar muscles, and these invariably demonstrate marked weakness. Tapping over the nerve at the wrist may elicit paraesthesias in the hand *(Tinel sign)*.

Electrodiagnostic findings include a prolonged distal latency in the motor nerve conduction test (Fig. 12.4) and/or in the sensory nerve conduction test (Fig. 12.5), reflecting compression of the nerve and disruption of normal conduction. Further compression can lead to axonal injury and the resultant CMAP and CSNAP amplitude would be decreased.

Ulnar nerve entrapment may occur at the elbow or at the wrist. At the elbow the nerve may be compressed against the ulna by the fibrous arch linking the humeral and ulnar origins of the flexor carpi ulnaris muscle. The patient may be aware of having a sensitive 'funny bone' in the affected area, and/or of paraesthesia affecting the medial one and a half fingers and the hypothenar skin area. In chronic cases there may be weakness of ulnar innervated muscles, but often the weakness is confined to the hand and this may create diagnostic confusion because compression at the wrist can have the same effect.

Wrist level compression occurs in the interval between the pisiform bone and the hook of the hamate. The sensory effects are confined to the medial one and a half fingers because the palmar branch of the nerve arises in the forearm and is spared. If only the superficial terminal motor branch from the deep ranch of the ulnar nerve to the hypothenar muscle is involved, weakness will be evident during abduction of the little finger against resistance. Involvement of the deep branch of the ulnar nerve

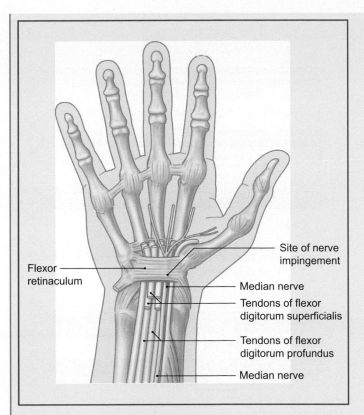

Fig. 12.12 The carpal tunnel is formed by two layers: a carpal arch that arises from the carpal bones and a band of connective tissue that forms its roof, the flexor retinaculum. Within this tunnel are nine tendons and the median nerve. (From Moses KP, Banks JC, Nava PB, Petersen DK. *Atlas of Clinical Gross Anatomy.* 2nd ed. Saunders, an imprint of Elsevier, Inc.; 2013; modified from Fig. 23.3.)

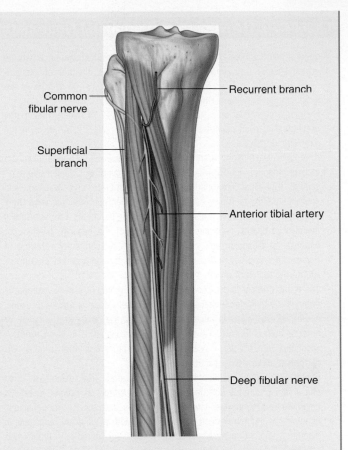

Fig. 12.13 The common peroneal (fibular) nerve as it wraps around the neck of the fibula and before it divides into its superficial and deep divisions. (From Gray AT. *Atlas of Ultrasound-Guided Regional Anesthesia.* 3rd ed. Elsevier, Inc; 2019; modified from Fig. 50.1.)

itself leads to weakness of abduction and adduction of index, middle, and ring fingers.

Electrodiagnostic findings usually include disruption of normal nerve conduction across the site of nerve entrapment (elbow or wrist) and if axonal injury is present, CMAP and CSNAP amplitudes are reduced. Depending on the extent of motor axon injury, EMG abnormalities may also be seen.

Lower limb

Meralgia paresthetica is a condition affecting the lateral cutaneous nerve of the thigh where it passes under the inguinal ligament close to the anterior superior iliac spine. The nerve may be compressed by the ligament during extended periods of physical activity, such as playing football. It may be seen in association with carpal tunnel syndrome during pregnancy due to the presence of increased tissue fluid. Intermittent 'flicks' of pins and needles are experienced on the anterolateral aspect of the thigh, and skin sensitivity may be progressively reduced by degeneration of the nerve.

Nerve conduction studies may demonstrate an absent response in affected individuals and as a purely sensory nerve, there are no motor nerve conduction studies.

Common peroneal (fibular) nerve entrapment is a term used when the common peroneal nerve exhibits signs of compression at the level of the neck of the fibula. Here the nerve passes through a tendinous arch formed by the peroneus longus muscle (Fig. 12.13). However, it is rarely a true entrapment. Usually the problem is one of frequent compression either during sleep or from habitual sitting with the legs crossed, whereby the nerve is pressed against the lateral condyle of the femur of the other knee. Iatrogenic entrapment is a well-known danger associated with application of a plaster cast following fracture of the tibia.

Nerve dysfunction affecting the superficial peroneal branch leads to weakness of eversion of the foot and sensory loss in the skin of the lower leg and dorsum of the foot. Affecting the deep peroneal branch leads to weakness of dorsiflexion of the foot and toes, resulting in foot drop with a characteristic slapping gait. Either branch may 'escape' injury, so further identification of individual affected muscles requires needle EMG.

CLINICAL PANEL 12.2 Peripheral Neuropathies

Peripheral neuropathies are amenable to several classifications, each with its own relevance and all aimed at an accurate diagnosis, direction of interventions or treatment. It is estimated that 5% of individuals (up to 30% in the elderly) may have a neuropathy.

- Histologic classification is touched upon in Fig. 12.14, where neuropathy originates in myelin sheaths of the nerve fibres (Fig. 12.14A,B) or in the axon (Fig. 12.14C,D).
- Anatomic classification identifies nerve numbers and locations. Numbers include mononeuropathy, referring to a single spinal or cranial nerve (e.g., sciatic, trigeminal neuropathy, isolated peripheral nerve trauma), and mononeuropathy multiplex, referring to more than one affected nerve trunk (e.g., right median and radial, left sural, right peroneal). Location labels include plexopathy, referring to involvement of the cervical, brachial, or lumbosacral plexus in an individual case, and radiculopathy, referring to nerve root pathology, most frequently caused by compression of a nerve root in the region of an intervertebral foramen.
- The terms primary and secondary are also anatomic. A primary neuropathy originates within nerve tissue (disease of myelin sheaths and/or of axons; if the process begins in the cell bodies within the dorsal root ganglion or anterior horn cells (AHCs) then the term 'neuronopathy' is often used). A secondary neuropathy is caused by medical illness that affects the peripheral nerves (e.g., diabetes mellitus).
- Etiologic classification identifies causative agents, like toxins (e.g., lead and arsenic), immune disorders including the effects of viruses, metabolic disorders (e.g., diabetes, vitamin deficiencies such as B_{12} in pernicious anaemia, or thiamine deficiency associated with alcoholism), and genetic disorders (e.g., Charcot-Marie-Tooth disease or hereditary motor and sensory neuropathy [HMSN]).
- Time course classification may be acute/subacute when the onset of the disorder is within days or weeks, and chronic when it has been present for more than a year.

Examples of an acute, chronic demyelinative or axonal polyneuropathy are described below:

Guillain—Barré syndrome

Guillain—Barré syndrome (GBS) is an acute, autoimmune, inflammatory neuropathy that affects men slightly more frequently than women and affects all age groups, with an increasing incidence with age. In most cases of GBS there is a preceding history of an upper respiratory or gastrointestinal infection; other antecedent events may include immunisation, or a surgical procedure. The most common antecedent is infection with *Campylobacter jejuni*. The typical presentation is progressive, bilateral, and symmetric weakness accompanied by diminished or absent reflexes, commencing in the feet and hands and ascending to involve the muscles of the trunk, neck, and face and the respiratory muscles; autonomic dysfunction is often present. Rarely, progress may be so rapid as to cause death within a few days from respiratory and/or circulatory collapse; usually the peak of the illness occurs within 2 weeks (by 4 weeks in almost all cases). Aching pain and tenderness occur in affected muscles along with minimal cutaneous sensory loss. Reduced autonomic function may be demonstrated by fluctuating heart rate and blood pressure, and/or retention of urine requiring catheterisation for a few days.

Electrodiagnostic examination reveals reduced conduction velocity, dispersion of motor responses, or conduction block in motor nerves, reflecting varying degrees of disruption of myelin and saltatory conduction. A lumbar puncture is performed in patients suspected of having GBS; diagnosis is supported by an elevated protein level and absence of leucocytes *(albuminocytologic dissociation)*.

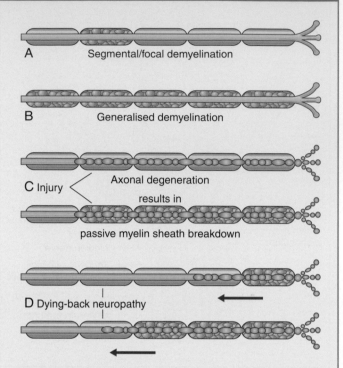

Fig. 12.14 Histologic changes associated with some types of peripheral neuropathy. This figure does not distinguish between sensory and motor nerves. (A) In segmental/focal demyelination, impulse conduction is slowed or blocked, but in a nerve conduction study this will not be apparent if stimulator and recorder are both placed distal to the lesion site. (B) Generalised demyelination results in conduction slowing or block, although the axons may be preserved. (C) Damage to an axon causes the entire distal length of the axon to break up into droplets, and the myelin sheaths follow suit (Wallerian degeneration). (D) In dying-back neuropathy, myelin breakdown is again secondary to axonal degeneration.

Rapid recovery may be spontaneous in relatively mild cases, but many patients require multidisciplinary care for respiratory failure, autonomic dysfunction, and prevention of complications associated with prolonged immobility. Immunomodulatory therapy consisting of either immunoglobin injections or plasmapheresis hastens recovery. Where axons have degenerated in the acute phase, recovery may take more than a year and is often incomplete with residual motor deficits.

Chronic polyneuropathy originating in myelin sheaths

This type of neuropathy is associated with involvement of either the myelin sheath or the Schwann cells. It may be either heritable or acquired, and many of the acquired variants are thought to be immune mediated. Characteristically the myelin sheaths of the peripheral nerves degenerate while the axons remain relatively intact. Because potassium channels are largely 'obliterated' when myelin sheaths are laid down and because saltatory conduction is lost along with the sheaths, nerve conduction is progressively impaired. In addition to involvement of myelin, proteins and ion channels in the nodal region may be the primary area of dysfunction, and these disorders are further referred to as nodopathies.

As might be anticipated, the longer nerves in the lower and upper extremities are more commonly affected (lower > upper extremities and distal > proximal), yielding a '***glove and stocking***' pattern of sensory loss, paraesthesia (paraesthesia refers to sensations of numbness, pins and needles, and/or tingling), and weakness (Fig. 12.15). Initially, demyelination may be segmental/focal, as shown in Fig. 12.14. Progression of motor weakness and wasting become more evident in the muscles of the hands and feet, and joint and vibration sense may also be lost there. (Joint sense refers to the ability to detect passive movement performed by a clinician; vibration sense refers to the ability to feel the 'buzz' of a vibrating tuning fork when applied to a bony prominence; see Chapter 15.)

Chronic polyneuropathy selectively involving Aδ fibres and unmyelinated C fibres

Although the prevalence is unknown, there is increasing clinical awareness of a chronic neuropathy that presents with symptoms of small-fibre nerve dysfunction. Referred to as a ***small-fibre neuropathy***, its symptoms or manifestations have led to other designations, such as 'painful neuropathy' or 'autonomic neuropathy'. The usual pattern is for sensory symptoms to start in the feet and gradually extend proximally with 'positive' (e.g., burning sensation, shooting pain), 'negative' (e.g., numbness, loss of temperature sensation), or autonomic dysfunction (e.g., dry eyes, changes in sweating, orthostasis). As expected, clinical evidence of large nerve fibre involvement (muscle weakness, proprioceptive sensation, or areflexia) is absent and NCS (NCS evaluate axons in the range of 6–12 μm in diameter, but the axons involved in these disorders are less than 6 μm) are normal. Pathologically it is characterised by degeneration of distal terminations of these small-diameter sensory fibres. While it can be the manifestation of an underlying medical illness (diabetes mellitus being the most common) in a substantial number of individuals (up to

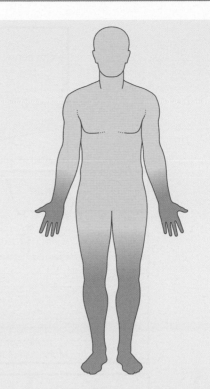

Fig. 12.15 Pattern of 'glove and stocking' paraesthesia.

50% of cases), it remains idiopathic or cryptogenic in aetiology. The pathophysiology, especially in cryptogenic cases, remains unclear, but in cases secondary to another disorder treatment is directed to that disorder and to symptom relief.

CLINICAL PANEL 12.3   Abnormal Motor Unit Action Potentials

In this composite figure, Fig. 12.16, the topmost diagram represents a muscle about to be activated and its depolarisation waves recorded through a needle electrode. (A) The two axons at upper left belong to different anterior horn cells (AHCs); three motor end plates from each unit are shown. (B) One AHC is degenerating. The motor unit action potential (MUAP) has become smaller because of reduced summation. (C) Early reinnervation is taking place by collateral sprouts from the intact motor neuron. Depolarisation waveforms of these muscle fibres are small and their appearance is delayed; their summation results in MUAPs that are characteristically polyphasic, showing multiple positive and negative phases. (D) Several weeks later the reinnervated muscle fibres give normal EMG responses. All six are now synchronously depolarised, yielding a giant motor unit action potential.

Fibrillation potentials (Fig. 12.17)

Fibrillation potentials are a characteristic feature of relaxed muscles in the early stages of denervation. They represent the spontaneous, electrical discharge of individual muscle fibres and are therefore of small amplitude. They take the form of abnormally small potentials, either triphasic or positive ('*positive waves*') in appearance, occurring with great regularity at up to 15 Hz. Fibrillation potentials are not clinically visible and patients are not aware of them. They may be caused either by a neuropathy of any kind that results in

denervation of the motor end plates in the muscle under examination, or by a myopathy as a degenerative change originating in the muscle fibres themselves; for example, in various muscular dystrophies. *Denervation supersensitivity* has been invoked to account for fibrillations in both conditions, which result in spontaneous depolarisations of the individual muscle fibres. Loss of end plate innervation is known to be associated with insertion of numerous new acetylcholine (ACh) receptors into the plasma membrane of denervated muscle fibres at some distance from their original end plates, enough to evoke small, localised action potentials caused by the minute amount of circulating ACh. In primary myopathies the likely explanation is that of a deterioration of the muscle membrane leading to failure of propagation of action potentials originating at the end plate; this appears enough to signal a requirement for additional receptors in the distal portion of the muscle fibre that no longer 'receives' the propagating action potential originating from its end plate.

Fasciculation potentials (Fig. 12.17)

Fasciculation potentials are not infrequent among healthy individuals, being perceived as a localised 'twitching' sensation in a relaxed individual muscle, usually after vigorous exercise. However, in association with motor neuron degeneration from any cause, they are indicative of spontaneous development of action potentials anywhere along the lower motor neuron pathway

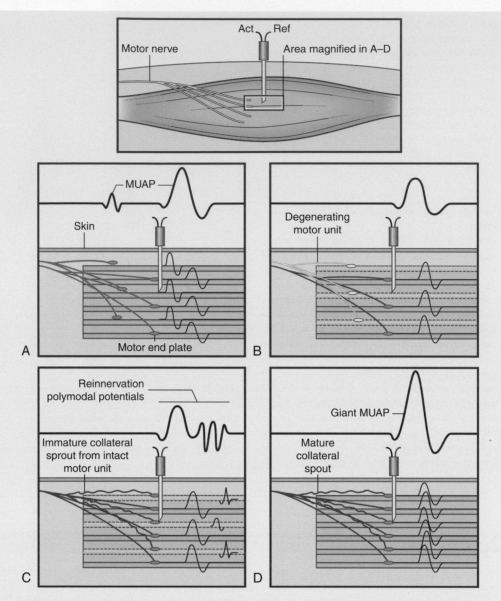

Fig. 12.16 Reinnervation of motor end plates. *MUAP,* Motor unit action potential.

from the AHC to its axon. They are often visible as a twitching and dimpling of the overlying skin. On the EMG record they appear as somewhat mis-shapen MUAPs that appear infrequently and are not under voluntary control.

Prolonged polyphasic and giant MUAPs (Fig. 12.17)
The term polyphasic signifies an abnormally large number of positive and negative phases of a MUAP. Polyphasic MUAPs signify reinnervation of muscle fibres, vacated by earlier degeneration of their nerve supply, by neighbouring healthy axons. Fig. 12.16 provides a basic explanation. In this figure two separate motor neurons are each represented by a single parent axon supplying three muscle fibres. Following interruption of one parent axon, its vacated nerve sheaths exert a chemotropic effect,

inducing the surviving stem and/or branch axons to issue collateral sprouts which eventually reinnervate the 'vacated' end plates of those muscle fibres. The outcome is the production of a giant MUAP by the now enlarged motor unit.

Giant MUAPs are called 'neuropathic' because they often result from chronic motor axon or neuron pathology. As mentioned in Chapter 10, they occur to some degree in the elderly as a result of 'fall out' of spinal motor neurons. Motor neuron disease (Chapter 16) is associated with progressive loss of spinal and cranial nerve motor neurons on a much greater scale; even the neurons that provide reinnervation are eventually lost. Radiculopathy (Chapter 14) resulting from compression of nerve roots and axonal polyneuro-pathy are other causes.

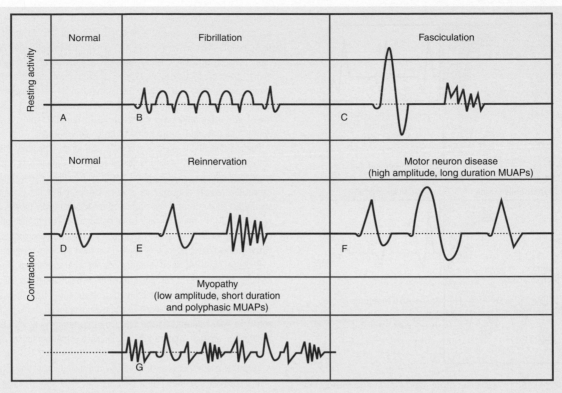

Fig. 12.17 Characteristic waveforms under different conditions. Resting activity: (A) Normal resting muscle is silent. (B) Fibrillation potentials: low-amplitude, high-frequency, and regularly firing pattern. (C) High-amplitude motor unit action potential (MUAP) accompanied by a low-amplitude polyphasic MUAP. (D) Normal MUAP. (E) Reinnervation: normal plus polyphasic MUAP. (F) Normal plus giant MUAP. (G) Low-amplitude, short-duration, and polyphasic MUAPs.

BASIC SCIENCE PANEL 12.1 Myasthenia Gravis and Myasthenic Syndromes

The **neuromuscular junction (NMJ)** converts a motor neuron axon potential into a propagating muscle fibre action potential. This is initiated by acetylcholine released at the *presynaptic (nerve) membrane* that diffuses across the synaptic cleft and binds to *acetylcholine receptors (AChRs)* on the *postsynaptic (muscle) membrane*. Voltage-gated sodium channels on the postsynaptic membrane are activated and a self-propagating potential moves along the muscle membrane, opening voltage-gated calcium channels along the way that increase intracellular calcium and result in muscle contraction.

The NMJ is a large synapse and acetylcholine (ACh) is sequestered within vesicles (~ 10,000 molecules per *vesicle or quanta*) in the presynaptic nerve terminal (hundreds of separate *active zones*) juxtaposed to millions of AChRs in the postsynaptic membrane. Each nerve action potential results in these vesicles releasing their ACh and in an amount that is greater than necessary to initiate an action potential at the postsynaptic membrane. This significant 'safety factor' ensures the effectiveness of the NMJ in initiating a muscle contraction.

The ACh receptors of skeletal muscle normally undergo turnover with a half-life (50% loss rate) of 12 days. New receptors are constantly synthesised in Golgi complexes located near the postsynaptic membrane and inserted into the sarcolemma of the junctional folds; old receptors are removed by endocytosis and degraded by lysosomes.

Dysfunction of the NMJ (presynaptic, synaptic, postsynaptic or the synaptic basal lamina) can lead to a myasthenia disorder, characterised by excessive fatigue upon exertion. Electrodiagnostic (EDX) studies in these cases demonstrate an abnormal response when the nerve of affected muscles is stimulated repetitively, usually at 3Hz. The CMAP response, a summation of the depolarisation of all muscle fibres innervated by that nerve, progressively decreases in size (decremental response). This reflects a failure of

neuromuscular transmission at NMJs and the normal safety factor of transmission cannot overcome.

Myasthenia gravis (MG) is an autoimmune disorder in which the clinical symptoms of weakness and fatigability are caused by antibodies that react with proteins at the postsynaptic neuromuscular junction and, through various mechanisms, interfere with their function. The symptoms and signs are those of variable weakness, expressed by inability to maintain contractions: the eyelids tend to droop, the extrinsic ocular muscles are unable to sustain the gaze, the face tends to sag, and the jaw needs support. Chewing may be difficult, and swallowing may pose a threat of fluid or food inhalation—sometimes with fatal effect. Respiratory muscle weakness may also precipitate pulmonary infection. Limb muscles are affected; if proximal muscle weakness is prominent, it may clinically suggest a muscle disorder and not a disorder of the neuromuscular junction. That the weakness is not caused by nerve paralysis is easily verified by the ability to commence a movement; all that is required is a moment of rest beforehand.

MG is a heterogeneous disorder with complex genetic and environmental risk factors, but is broadly divided into three subgroups based on identified antibodies: the most prominent (about 85% of cases) is *acetylcholine receptor (AChR) antibody—positive MG (AChR-MG)*. AChR antibodies lead to the destruction of the postsynaptic membrane with progressive loss of AChRs and shrinkage of junctional folds (Fig. 12.18). One group, predominantly female, has an onset of AChR-MG before the age of 40 years. The disease starts with ocular muscle weakness; however, generalised muscle weakness subsequently develops, and patients usually have a hyperplastic thymus. The other group, predominantly male, has an onset over the age of 60 years. Weakness is generalised, and while the thymus may be atrophic, thymoma is most commonly seen in this group.

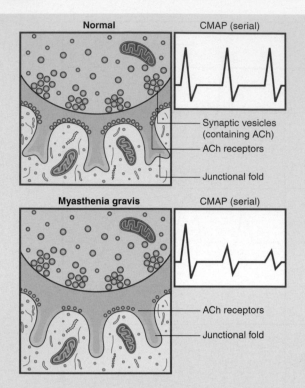

Fig. 12.18 Normal and myasthenic motor end plates and motor unit action potential (compound motor unit action potentials with repetitive stimulation) compared. Note widening of the synaptic cleft in myasthenia gravis (MG) together with reduction of acetylcholine (ACh) receptors and junctional folds. Note that the nerve terminal itself is not affected and the availability and number of vesicles containing ACh are unchanged. *CMAP*, Compound motor unit action potential.

Autoantibodies against *muscle-specific kinase (MuSK)* and *low-density lipoprotein receptor-related protein 4 (LRP4)* are the other two MG subgroups.

Characterisation of these other two subgroups is by the lack of the AChR antibody. The most frequently reported subgroup has an antibody to MuSK that disrupts the clustering of AChRs in the postsynaptic membrane and disrupts synapse efficiency. MuSK-MG has a peak onset in the fourth decade and females predominate. Weakness typically involves the neck, bulbar, and respiratory muscles, often with respiratory crises, and ocular weakness is less common at onset. The third subgroup has an antibody to LRP4 that plays a role in the formation and maintenance of the NMJ and typically presents with a mild generalised syndrome of fatigable weakness.

Confirmation of the diagnosis of MG is through laboratory testing for antibodies. However, EDX testing is useful to test a symptomatic muscle, such as recording from the abductor pollicis brevis with median nerve stimulation. Nerve conduction velocity is normal as is ACh release, but if the nerve is repetitively stimulated at a rate of 3 per second, the CMAPs rapidly dwindle *(decremental response)*. CMAPs return to their baseline after a period of rest (or injection of a short-acting anticholinesterase medication such as edrophonium or neostigmine, which prolongs the binding time of ACh with the surviving receptors).

Because AChR-MG is an autoimmune disorder, treatment is with immunomodulatory drugs (e.g., corticosteroids) or thymectomy (especially in the presence of a thymoma). Symptomatic treatment often includes an oral anticholinesterase medication (e.g., pyridostigmine), which prolongs the action of ACh released at the NMJ by interfering with its catabolism and allowing a greater 'opportunity' to interact with remaining AChRs on the postsynaptic membrane.

Myasthenia disorders can also arise from disruption of the interdependence of the complex of proteins that exist at the NMJ and affecting those in the presynaptic, postsynaptic, synaptic or basal lamina-associated locations. ***Congenital myasthenic syndromes (CMS)*** are those rare genetic disorders characterised by impaired neuromuscular transmission and involving one or more of these sites. All CMS have fatigable muscle weakness (variable regarding location and severity), but age at onset, presenting symptoms, distribution of weakness, prognosis, and response to treatment vary. The clinical diagnosis of a CMS is based on fatigable muscle weakness, abnormal findings on EDX studies (decremental response), and a response to pharmacological treatment. Testing for antibodies to AChR and MuSK are negative and, while limited to some extent, genetic testing is used for further classification.

✳ Core Information

Nerve conduction studies

The functional state of the peripheral nervous system (PNS), assessed by nerve conduction studies (NCS) and electromyography (EMG), clarifies a clinical diagnosis, contributes to a prognosis, and can document the effectiveness of a treatment. For motor NCS, a stimulating electrode is placed on the skin overlying that nerve and a recording electrode over the mid-region (innervation zone) of a muscle it innervates. The surface waveform recorded, *Compound Motor Action Potential (CMAP)*, is produced by summation of individual muscle fibre depolarisation potentials. The stimulus—response latency from two separate stimulation sites along the same nerve enables a motor nerve conduction velocity to be calculated by first subtracting one latency from the other and then dividing by the distance that separates those stimulation points.

Preferred nerve trunks in the upper limb are the median and ulnar nerve and in the lower limb, the deep peroneal and tibial nerves. For sensory NCS, antidromic stimulation of a cutaneous nerve is accompanied by a proximal recording from two sites over the parent nerve trunk; subtraction reveals the sensory nerve conduction velocity (SNCV).

Some spinal nerve roots are accessed by activating their muscle spindle reflex arcs *(H-reflex)* at appropriate levels and represent the electrophysiological correlate of a muscle stretch reflex.

Electromyography

The recording electrode is within a needle inserted into a muscle; voluntary activation of the muscle allows MUAPs to be recorded. Each MUAP shape represents the summated action potentials of muscle fibres belonging to one motor unit. The normal overlap and interdigitating of muscle fibres of different motor unit territories allows sampling of several MUAPs simultaneously when volitionally activated. Abnormal EMG waveforms are associated with dysfunction at different levels of the motor unit (e.g., neuropathies, motor neuron disease, myopathy or neuromuscular junction disorder) and can be a dynamic process.

Denervation of muscle fibres from any cause initially gives rise to *fibrillation potentials* (spontaneous depolarisations of muscle fibres), but reinnervation of those muscle fibres by collateral sprouts from neighbouring intact motor units can result in their resolution.

MUAP shape is a visual representation of the anatomical-physiological characteristics of that motor unit (large-amplitude and polyphasic MUAPs represent denervation and reinnervation, small-amplitude MUAPs represent loss or atrophy of muscle fibres, and an unstable MUAP shape can signify a disorder of neuromuscular transmission).

Peripheral neuropathy classification is in accordance with cause, anatomic location, pathology, and time course. A wide variety of nerve entrapment syndromes are encountered in clinical practice.

Muscle diseases primarily affect skeletal muscle but can involve cardiac and smooth muscle, and are further classified into those that are inherited (e.g., muscular dystrophies, channelopathies, mitochondrial myopathies) or acquired (e.g., inflammatory, metabolic, toxic).

SUGGESTED READINGS

Burden SJ, Huijbers MG, Remedio L. Fundamental molecules and mechanisms for forming and maintaining neuromuscular synapses. *Int J Mol Sci.* 2018;19(2). pii: E490.

Dyck PJB, Tracy JA. History, diagnosis, and management of chronic inflammatory demyelinating polyradiculoneuropathy. *Mayo Clin Proc.* 2018;93(6):777−793.

Evoli A. Myasthenia gravis: new developments in research and treatment. *Curr Opin Neurol.* 2017;30:464−470.

Gasparotti R, Padua L, Briani C, Lauria G. New technologies for the assessment of neuropathies. *Nat Rev Neurol.* 2017;13(4):203−216.

Kincaid JC. Neurophysiologic studies in the evaluation of polyneuropathy. *Continuum (Minneap Minn.).* 2017;23(5):1263−1275.

Naddaf E, Milone M, Mauermann ML, Mandrekar J, Litchy WJ. Muscle biopsy and electromyography correlation. *Front Neurol.* 2018;9:839.

Padua L, Coraci D, Erra C, et al. Carpal tunnel syndrome: clinical features, diagnosis, and management. *Lancet Neurol.* 2016;15(12):1273−1284.

Rodriguez Cruz PM, Palace J, Beeson D. The neuromuscular junction and wide heterogeneity of congenital myasthenic syndromes. *Int J Mol Sci.* 2018;19(6). pii: E1677.

Sener U, Martinez-Thompson J, Laughlin RS, Dimberg EL, Rubin DI. Needle electromyography and histopathologic correlation in myopathies. *Muscle Nerve.* 2019;59(3):315−320.

Slater CR. The structure of human neuromuscular junctions: some unanswered molecular questions. *Int J Mol Sci.* 2017;18(10). pii: E2183.

Terkelsen AJ, Karlsson P, Lauria G, et al. The diagnostic challenge of small fibre neuropathy: clinical presentations, evaluations, and causes. *Lancet Neurol.* 2017;16(11):934−944.

Wijdicks EFM, Klein CJ. Guillain-Barré syndrome. *Mayo Clin Proc.* 2017;92(3):467−479.

Autonomic Nervous System

CHAPTER SUMMARY

STUDY GUIDELINES

1. Resolve the paradox that, despite an outflow restricted to 14 or 15 ventral roots, all 31 spinal nerve trunks acquire sympathetic fibres.
2. Appreciate that the sympathetic ganglia along the abdominal aorta are activated by preganglionic fibres, as is the adrenal medulla.
3. Pay special attention to the autonomic innervation of the eye, discussed both here and in Chapter 23.
4. Appreciate that the four parasympathetic ganglia in the head are functionally similar to intramural ganglia elsewhere.
5. Be aware that the pelvic ganglia are mixed autonomic ganglia.
6. Realise that the preganglionic neurons of both divisions are cholinergic and that the target receptors in all of the autonomic ganglia are nicotinic.
7. Note that at the tissue level, synapses are replaced by looser 'junctions' that permit diffusion of transmitter to outlying receptors.
8. Focus on four kinds of junctional receptors of the sympathetic system and on four actions initiated by muscarinic receptors in the parasympathetic system.
9. Learn from Clinical Panel 13.2 how pharmacologists intercept the recycling and degradation sequence at sympathetic nerve endings. The same principles apply to central nervous system (CNS) drug therapy, notably in psychiatric disorders.
10. Follow Clinical Panel 13.3 to contrast the effects of cholinergic and anticholinergic drugs.
11. Appreciate that visceral afferents utilise autonomic pathways to gain access to the nervous system. They are especially important in the context of thoracic and abdominal pain.

ANATOMY OF THE AUTONOMIC NERVOUS SYSTEM

The autonomic nervous system is the part of the peripheral nervous system responsible for the unconscious regulation of important physiological processes including respiration, heart rate, blood pressure, digestion, and sexual arousal. There are three main divisions to this system: sympathetic, parasympathetic, and enteric nervous systems.

These systems contain both afferent and efferent fibres that provide sensory input and motor output, respectively, to the central nervous system (CNS). The motor outflow from both the sympathetic nervous system (SNS) and the peripheral nervous system (PNS) consists of a two-neuron series: a preganglionic neuron whose neuronal cell body is located in the CNS and a postganglionic neuron with a cell body in the periphery that innervates target tissues.

The autonomic nervous system is distributed to the peripheral tissues and organs by way of outlying autonomic ganglia. Control centres in the hypothalamus and brainstem send central autonomic fibres to synapse upon preganglionic neurons located in the grey matter of the brainstem and spinal cord. From these neurons, *preganglionic fibres* (mostly myelinated) project out of the CNS to synapse upon multipolar neurons in the autonomic ganglia. Unmyelinated *postganglionic fibres* emerge and form terminal networks in the target tissues.

While for the most part it 'functions' at an unconscious or involuntary level, cortical and subcortical areas play an interactive role and are themselves influenced by its activity.

SYMPATHETIC NERVOUS SYSTEM

The sympathetic system is so called because it acts in sympathy with the emotions. In association with rage or fear, or in situations that pose no threat, the sympathetic system prepares the body for 'fight or flight' or for 'rest and digest', respectively. In the 'fight or flight' response the heart rate is increased, the pupils dilate, and the skin sweats. Blood is diverted from the skin and intestinal tract to the skeletal muscles, and the sphincters of the alimentary and urinary tracts are closed.

The sympathetic outflow from the nervous system is *thoracolumbar*. The preganglionic neurons are located in the lateral grey horn of the spinal cord at thoracic and the upper two (or three) lumbar segmental levels. From these neurons, preganglionic fibres emerge in the corresponding ventral nerve roots and enter the ***paravertebral sympathetic chain***. The fibres do one of four things (Fig. 13.1):

1. Some fibres synapse in the nearest ganglion. Postganglionic fibres enter spinal nerves T1 to L2 and supply blood vessels, sweat glands, and erector pili (hair-raising) muscles in the territory of these nerves.

2. Some fibres *ascend* the sympathetic chain and synapse in the *superior or middle cervical ganglion*, or in the **stellate ganglion**. (The stellate consists of the fused inferior cervical and first thoracic ganglia; it lies in front of the neck of the first rib.) Postganglionic fibres supply the head, neck, and upper limbs, and also the heart. Of particular importance is the supply to the dilator muscle of the pupil (Fig. 13.2, Clinical Panel 13.1).

3. Some fibres *descend* to synapse in lumbar or sacral ganglia of the sympathetic chain. Postganglionic fibres enter the lumbosacral plexus for distribution to the blood vessels and skin of the lower limbs.

4. Some fibres *traverse* the chain and emerge as the (preganglionic) **thoracic** and **lumbar splanchnic nerves**.

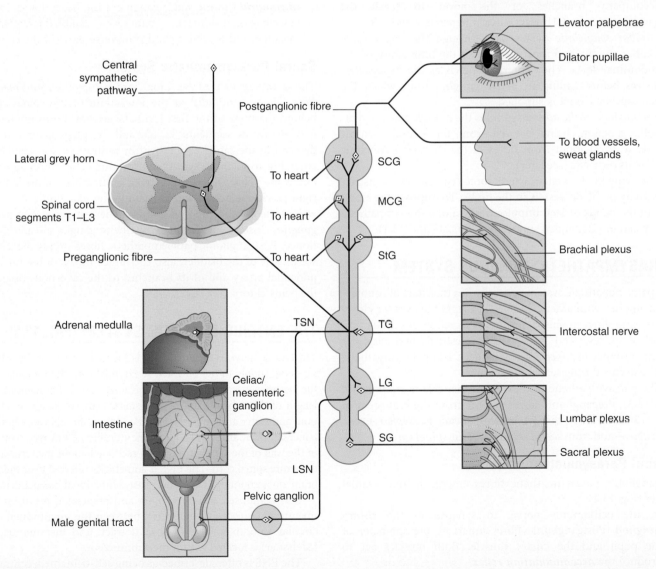

Fig. 13.1 General plan of the sympathetic system. Ganglionic neurons and postganglionic fibres are shown in red. *LG*, Lumbar ganglia; *LSN*, lumbar splanchnic nerve; *MCG*, middle cervical ganglion; *SCG*, superior cervical ganglion; *SG*, sacral ganglia; *StG*, stellate ganglion; *TG*, thoracic ganglia; *TSN*, thoracic splanchnic nerve.

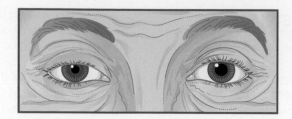

Fig. 13.2 Horner syndrome, patient's right side. Note the moderate ptosis of the eyelid and the moderate miosis (pupillary constriction). The affected pupil reacts to light but recovers very slowly.

The *thoracic splanchnic nerves* (often simply called the splanchnic nerves) pass through the lower eight thoracic ganglia, pierce the diaphragm, and synapse within the abdomen in the **coeliac** and **mesenteric prevertebral ganglia** and in **renal ganglia**. Postganglionic fibres accompany branches of the aorta to reach the gastrointestinal (GI) tract, liver, pancreas, and kidneys. *Lumbar splanchnic nerves* pass through the upper three lumbar ganglia and meet in front of the bifurcation of the abdominal aorta. They enter the pelvis as the **hypogastric nerves** before ending in **pelvic ganglia**, from which the genitourinary tract is supplied.

The *medulla of the adrenal gland* is the homologue of a sympathetic ganglion, being derived from the neural crest. It receives a direct input from fibres of the thoracic splanchnic nerve of its own side (see later).

The sympathetic system exerts tonic (continuous) constrictor activity on blood vessels in the limbs. To improve the blood flow to the hands or feet, impulse traffic along the sympathetic system can be interrupted surgically (Clinical Panel 13.1).

PARASYMPATHETIC NERVOUS SYSTEM

The parasympathetic system generally has the effect of counterbalancing the sympathetic system. It adapts the eyes for close-up viewing, slows the heart, promotes secretion of salivary and intestinal juices, and accelerates intestinal peristalsis. A notable instance of *concerted* sympathetic and parasympathetic activity occurs during sexual intercourse.

The parasympathetic outflow from the CNS is *craniosacral* (Fig. 13.3). Preganglionic fibres emerge from the brainstem in four cranial nerves—the *oculomotor, facial, glossopharyngeal, and vagus*—and from *sacral segments of the spinal cord*.

Cranial Parasympathetic System

Preganglionic parasympathetic fibres emerge in four cranial nerves (Fig. 13.4):
1. In the oculomotor nerve, to synapse in the **ciliary ganglion**. Postganglionic fibres innervate the sphincter of the pupil and the ciliary muscle. Both muscles act to produce the **accommodation reflex**.
2. In the facial nerve, to synapse in the **pterygopalatine ganglion**, which innervates the lacrimal and nasal glands;

and in the **submandibular ganglion**, which innervates the submandibular and sublingual glands.
3. In the glossopharyngeal nerve, to synapse in the **otic ganglion**, which innervates the parotid gland.
4. In the vagus nerve, to synapse in **mural** ('on the wall') or **intramural** ('in the wall') ganglia of the heart, lungs, lower oesophagus, stomach, pancreas, gallbladder, small intestine, and ascending and transverse parts of the colon.

Sacral Parasympathetic System

The sacral segments of the spinal cord occupy the **conus medullaris** (*conus terminalis*) at the lower end of the spinal cord, behind the body of the first lumbar vertebra. From the lateral grey matter of segments S2, S3, and S4, preganglionic fibres descend in the cauda equina within ventral nerve roots. Upon emerging from the pelvic sacral foramina, the fibres separate out as the **pelvic splanchnic nerves**. Some fibres of the left and right pelvic splanchnic nerves synapse on ganglion cells in the wall of the distal colon and rectum. The rest synapse in **pelvic ganglia**, close to the pelvic sympathetic ganglia already mentioned. Postganglionic parasympathetic fibres supply the detrusor muscle of the bladder; also the tunica media of the internal pudendal artery and of its branches to the cavernous tissue of the penis/clitoris (see later).

THE ENTERIC NERVOUS SYSTEM (FIG. 13.5)

The enteric nervous system (ENS) is the name given to the intrinsic nerve supply to the GI tract. It extends from the midregion of the oesophagus all the way to the anal canal. Throughout the length of this tube, it controls peristaltic activity, glandular secretion, and water and ion transfer. In addition, the ENS supplies the pancreas, liver, and gallbladder. The number of intrinsic neurons in the wall of the GI tract has been reckoned about the same as in the entire spinal cord. The ENS is sometimes referred to as the 'gut brain' on account of its size and relative functional independence.

It is composed of two ganglia and associated plexuses: the myenteric (Auerbach) is located between the longitudinal and circular smooth muscle of the GI tract, and the submucosal (Meissner) is located within the submucosa.

The ENS is often described as being self-contained; central to its workings is local reflex activity. This system is intimately integrated with the sensory afferents and both the sympathetic

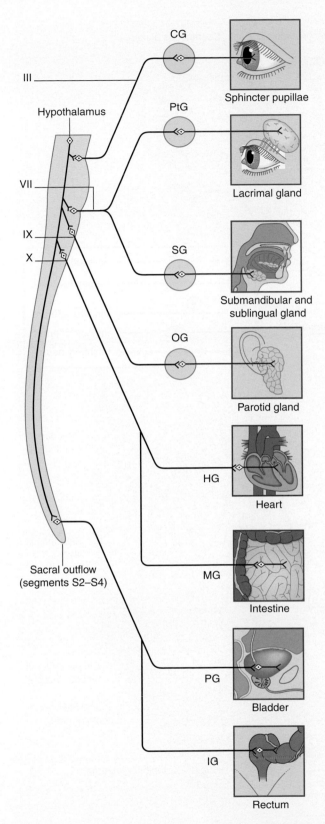

Fig. 13.3 General plan of the parasympathetic system. Ganglionic neurons and postganglionic fibres are shown in *red*. *CG*, Ciliary ganglion; *HG*, heart ganglia; *IG*, intramural ganglia; *MG*, myenteric ganglia; *OG*, otic ganglion; *PG*, pelvic ganglia; *PtG*, pterygopalatine ganglion; *SG*, submandibular ganglion.

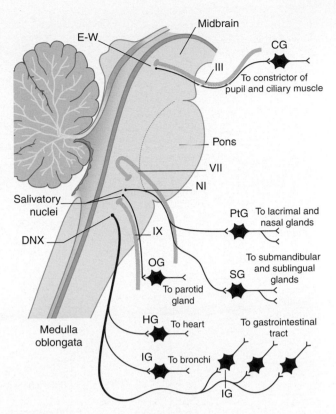

Fig. 13.4 Cranial parasympathetic system. *E-W*, Edinger-Westphal nucleus; *DNX*, dorsal nucleus of the vagus. Other abbreviations as in Fig. 13.3.

and parasympathetic divisions of the autonomic nervous system. The movement of water and electrolytes across the intestinal wall is controlled by the submucosal plexus, while the varied patterns of muscle contraction associated with peristalsis are the responsibility of the myenteric plexus. Enteric neurons are involved in both excitatory and inhibitory communication. A variety of neuronal phenotypes are found in the ENS (bipolar, pseudounipolar, and multipolar forms). Thirty neurotransmitters are similar to those found in the CNS, the most common being cholinergic and nitrergic. The afferent fibres are responsible for numerous reflex activities that regulate everything from heart rate to the immune system. The feedback from the ANS is usually subconscious, eliciting reflex actions in the visceral or somatic portions of the body. The conscious awareness of the viscera is often interpreted as diffuse pain or cramps that may be associated with hunger, fullness, or nausea. This awareness is often a consequence of sudden distention/contractions, chemical irritants, or pathological conditions such as ischemia.

The principal drivers of the muscle and glands belong to the parasympathetic division of the autonomic system. The dorsal (motor) nucleus of the vagus provides the preganglionic parasympathetic supply (1) to all parts with the exception of the distal colon and rectum, which receive their preganglionic supply from the pelvic splanchnic nerves (having parent neurons in the intermediolateral cell column of cord segments S2 to S4). The drivers

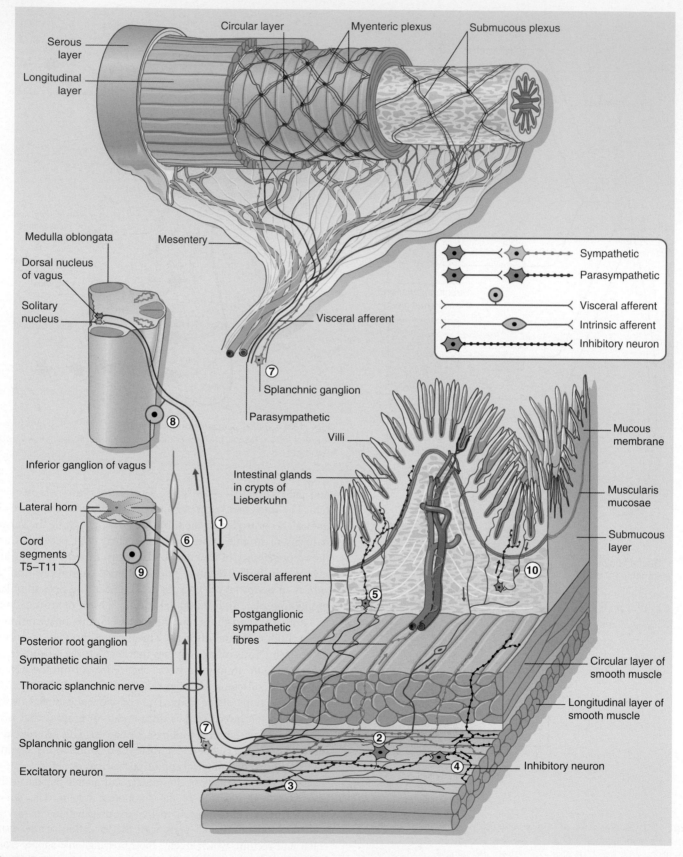

Fig. 13.5 Enteric nervous system. Key to numbers under The Enteric Nervous System section.

throughout are intramural ganglion cells located in both intramural plexuses. The beaded postganglionic fibres of the myenteric plexus (2) initiate peristaltic waves by simultaneously causing the gut to contract in their own location (3) and to relax distally by activating inhibitory neurons (4). Parasympathetic ganglion cells in the wall of the gallbladder cause expulsion of bile. Those in the submucosal plexus (5) and in the pancreas cause glandular secretion.

Peristaltic activity persists even after total extrinsic denervation because of the intrinsic circuitry and the spontaneous excitability of 'pacemaker' patches of smooth muscle (notably in the stomach and duodenum).

The preganglionic sympathetic nerve supply originates in lateral horn cells of cord segments T5 to T11. The fibres traverse the paravertebral sympathetic chain (6) without synapsing here and terminate in the prevertebral, splanchnic ganglia (7) within the abdomen (coeliac, superior, and inferior mesenteric). Their beaded postganglionic fibres supply the smooth muscle of the intestine and of blood vessels, which they relax via β2 receptors.

Visceral afferents reaching the CNS have their unipolar somas in a nodose ganglion of the vagus (8) and in posterior root ganglia at spinal levels T5 to T11 (9). The spinal afferents reach the posterior grey horn via ventral nerve roots. These ventral root afferents are of special clinical importance because they include first-order nociceptive afferents, which synapse centrally upon lateral spinothalamic projection cells providing the principal 'pain pathway' to the brain.

Intrinsic visceral afferent neurons are in the form of bipolar neurons (10). Some participate in local reflex arcs within the myenteric or submucosal plexus. Others (not shown) project as far as the splanchnic ganglia with the potential of exerting more widespread reflex effects.

Transmitters and modulators are numerous among the enteric ganglion cells. The principal excitatory transmitter is acetylcholine (ACh), with substance P cotransmitted as a modulator. The principal inhibitory transmitters are nitric oxide, γ-aminobutyric acid (GABA), and vasoactive intestinal polypeptide (VIP). Large numbers of different peptides have been revealed by means of histochemistry. More often than not, two or more are present within individual cells.

Gut-Brain Axis

The microbiome has been implicated in the pathophysiology and potential treatment of many neurodegenerative diseases. The ENS is an essential component of the gut-brain axis. There is a need to elucidate microbial impact at this important interface.

NEUROTRANSMISSION IN THE AUTONOMIC SYSTEM

Ganglionic Transmission

The preganglionic neurons of the sympathetic and parasympathetic systems are *cholinergic*: the neurons liberate ACh on to the ganglion cells at axodendritic synapses (Fig. 13.6). The receptors on the ganglion cells are *nicotinic*, so named because the excitatory effect can be imitated by locally applied nicotine.

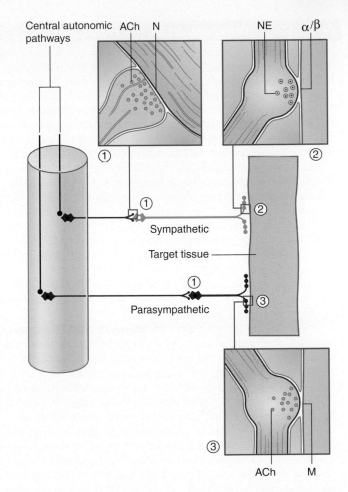

Fig. 13.6 Autonomic transmitters and receptors. *(1)* Axodendritic synapses with nicotinic receptors. *(2)* Neuroeffector junction with adrenoceptors. *(3)* Neuroeffector junction with muscarinic receptors. Ganglionic neurons and postganglionic parasympathetic fibres are shown in *red*, postganglionic sympathetic fibres in *green*. *ACh*, Acetylcholine; *M*, muscarinic receptors; *N*, nicotinic receptors; *NE*, norepinephrine.

Junctional Transmission

Postganglionic fibres of the sympathetic and parasympathetic systems form *neuroeffector junctions* with target tissues (Fig. 13.6). Transmitter substances are liberated from innumerable varicosities strung along the course of the nerve fibres.

The chief transmitter at sympathetic neuroeffector junctions is *norepinephrine (noradrenaline)*, which is liberated from dense-cored vesicles. The postganglionic sympathetic system in general is described as *adrenergic*. An exception to the adrenergic rule is the *cholinergic* sympathetic supply to the eccrine sweat glands over the body surface.

The chief transmitter at parasympathetic neuroeffector junctions is ACh. The postganglionic parasympathetic system in general is *cholinergic*.

Junctional Receptors

The physiologic effects of autonomic stimulation depend upon the nature of the *postjunctional receptors* inserted by target cells into their own plasma membranes. In addition, transmitter

BOX 13.1 Innervation of the Heart

The preganglionic sympathetic supply to the heart arises from neurons in the rostral ventrolateral medulla that send excitatory projections to the lateral grey horn of cord segments T1 to T5. The fibres synapse in all three cervical (most sympathetic fibres to the heart originate from the middle and inferior ganglia) and in the uppermost five thoracic ganglia of the sympathetic chain. Postganglionic adrenergic fibres are distributed to the specialised myocardial cells of nodal and conducting tissues, to the general myocardium (of the left ventricle in particular), and to the coronary arteries.

Experimental evidence indicates that the preganglionic parasympathetic supply originates in neurons occupying the ventrolateral portion of the nucleus ambiguus (and perhaps the dorsal vagal nucleus) in the medulla oblongata. The fibres descend within the trunk of the vagus and synapse within mural ganglia on the posterior walls of the atria and in the posterior atrioventricular groove (Fig. 13.8). Postganglionic cholinergic fibres supply the same tissues as those of the sympathetic system, although the direct supply to ventricles and coronary arteries is minimal.

There is a high level of autonomic interaction where innervation is dense, notably within nodal tissue, in the modes shown in Figs 13.7 and 13.11. Many sympathetic nerve endings also release *neuropeptide Y*, which binds to a specific receptor on cholinergic terminals with adjuvant inhibitory effect on ACh release.

Many parasympathetic endings corelease nitric oxide and VIP, which attenuates the release of ACh by binding with VIP-specific inhibitory autoreceptors on the endings that release it.

An abundance of noradrenergic, noncholinergic (NANC) neurons modulate the activity of parasympathetic ganglion cells. Also found are scattered adrenergic neurons whose preganglionic supply traverses the sympathetic chain and bipolar local circuit neurons.

Autoregulation of myocardial performance by the intramural ganglionic networks of the normal heart is sufficient to withstand the total extrinsic denervation involved in a cardiac transplant.

A fourth set of neurons is afferent in nature. Unipolar somas in the *inferior ganglion (nodose ganglion)* of the vagus provide stretch-sensitive nerve endings close to the endocardium—notably in the right atrium where distension produces reflex slowing of the heart rate by way of a central pathway to the dorsal vagal nucleus via the solitary nucleus (Chapter 24).

Some unipolar somas in spinal dorsal root ganglia send peripheral processes to form chemosensitive endings in the myocardium. Metabolites released by ischemic myocardial cells in response to coronary artery occlusion generate impulse trains that travel along the central processes of these cells to reach the posterior grey horn via *ventral* nerve roots. The central processes synapse upon projection cells of the spinothalamic tract, with consequent perception of referred pain (see main text). A prominent transmitter in the nociceptive neurons is substance P, which is released *at both ends simultaneously*: in the grey matter this peptide is excitatory to spinothalamic projection cells, and in the ischemic tissue it activates specific excitatory receptors on cholinergic endings, thus slowing the heart.

The cardiac pacemaker (sinoatrial node) is on the right side of the body and mainly innervated by the two right-sided sets of autonomic neurons. The atrioventricular node is on the left side and receives a corresponding preponderance.

While the sinoatrial node is highly responsive to emotional states that are believed to have their seat of origin in the right 'emotional' hemisphere (Chapter 33), lateralisation of cardiovascular control is not yet resolved. However, CNS structures, including the anterior insular cortex, anterior cingulate gyrus, amygdala, and hypothalamus, exert their effects. The descending pathways concerned are polysynaptic, prior to reaching the lower autonomic nervous system centres of the medulla and cord. *Sympathetic* overactivity, in response to 'approach' emotions of a sexual or combative nature, may cause the heart to 'miss a beat' (extrasystole) or the 'pulse to race' (tachycardia); there is an interindividual asymmetric left versus right distribution of sympathetic nerves responsible for the observed variable properties on the heart. *Parasympathetic* overactivity, in response to 'withdraw' (aversive) emotions, usually of olfactory or visual origin, may cause bradycardia—or even cardiac arrest.

The atrioventricular node and Purkinje fibres concordantly increase or reduce the speed of transference of action potentials to the ventricles.

Ventricular contractility and *synchrony* throughout the ventricular myocardium are increased by raised sympathetic activity. Both are diminished by the parasympathetic, in this case mainly by autonomic interaction: the scarce cholinergic fibres terminate mainly 'on top' of adrenergic ones without any direct influence on the myocardium.

The coronary arterial tree possesses a considerable degree of autoregulation based on release of myocardial cellular metabolites. However, adrenoceptors are also important. The arterioles (less than 120 μm in diameter) are rich in β_2 receptors responsive to neural norepinephrine at the commencement of exercise and to circulating epinephrine when exercise gets under way. The arteries (more than 120 μm in diameter) contain α_1 receptors exerting a restraining effect, directing blood to the *subendocardial* ventricular myocardium, which is vulnerable on two counts: it is the most distal coronary territory; and it is the most compressed myocardial component during systole, receiving blood only during diastole.

Cholinergic coronary nerve endings are scarce, but they have a significant dilator effect on the main arteries—precisely those most at risk of atherosclerosis! It transpires that released ACh acts *indirectly* by causing release of the potent dilator nitric oxide from the vascular endothelium. Progressive devitalisation of the endothelium by underlying atherosclerotic plaques leads to more or less complete failure of beneficial nitric oxide production.

release is influenced by *prejunctional receptors* in the axolemmal membrane of the nerve terminals.

Sympathetic Junctional Receptors (Adrenoceptors) (Fig. 13.7).

Two kinds of α adrenoceptors and two kinds of β adrenoceptors have been identified for norepinephrine:

1. *Postjunctional α_1 adrenoceptors* initiate contraction of smooth muscle in peripheral small arteries and large arterioles, the dilator pupillae, the sphincters of the alimentary tract and bladder neck, and the vas deferens.
2. *Prejunctional α_2 adrenoceptors* are present on parasympathetic as well as on sympathetic terminals. They inhibit

transmitter release in both cases. On sympathetic terminals they are called *autoreceptors*.

3. *Postjunctional β_1 adrenoceptors* increase pacemaker activity in the heart and increase the force of ventricular contraction (Fig. 13.8, Box 13.1). In response to a severe fall in blood pressure, sympathetic activation of β_1 receptors on the juxtaglomerular cells of the kidney causes secretion of renin. Renin initiates production of the powerful vasoconstrictor *angiotensin II*.
4. *β_2 receptors* respond to circulating epinephrine (adrenaline) (Fig. 13.9) in addition to locally released norepinephrine.

Postjunctional β₂ receptors relax smooth muscle, notably in the tracheobronchial tree and in the accommodatory muscles of the eye. Some postjunctional β₂ receptors are on the surface of hepatocytes in the liver, where they initiate glycogen breakdown to provide glucose for immediate energy needs.

Prejunctional β₂ receptors on adrenergic terminals promote release of norepinephrine.

Most of the norepinephrine liberated at sympathetic terminals is retrieved by an *amine uptake pump*. Some is degraded after uptake by a mitochondrial enzyme, *monoamine oxidase (MAO)*.

The effects of drugs on the sympathetic system are considered in Clinical Panel 13.2 (Fig. 13.10).

Parasympathetic Junctional Receptors. Parasympathetic junctional receptors are called *muscarinic* because they can be mimicked by application of the drug muscarine (Fig. 13.11).

Parasympathetic stimulation produces the following muscarinic effects:

- Slowing of the heart in response to vagal stimulation, and diminished force of ventricular contraction (Box 13.1).

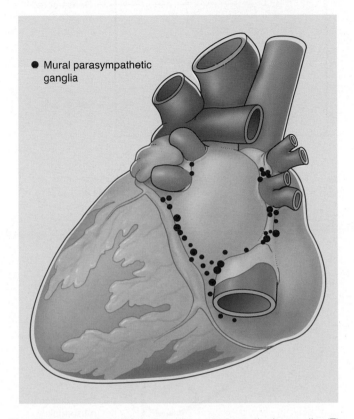

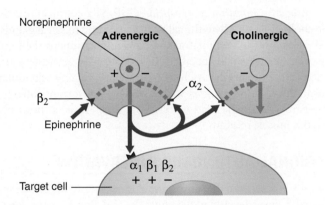

Fig. 13.7 Adrenergic activity at a neuroeffector junction. Release of norepinephrine is promoted by epinephrine and inhibited by prejunctional α₂ receptors, which also inhibit transmitter release from neighbouring parasympathetic varicosities.

Fig. 13.8 Disposition of mural cardiac parasympathetic ganglia. (The assistance of Professor Andrew J. Armour, Centre de Recherche de l'Hôpital du Sacré-Coeur de Montréal, Québec, Canada, is gratefully appreciated.)

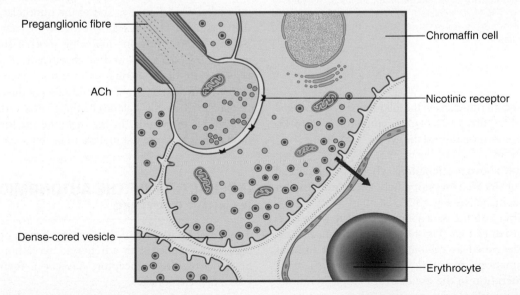

Fig. 13.9 Chromaffin cell of the adrenal medulla receiving a synaptic contact from a preganglionic fibre of the thoracic splanchnic nerve. Acetylcholine *(ACh)* activates nicotinic receptors. In total, 80% of the cells contain large-cored vesicles (represented here) and secrete epinephrine; the *arrow* indicates release into the capillary bed. A total of 20% contain small dense-cored vesicles and secrete norepinephrine.

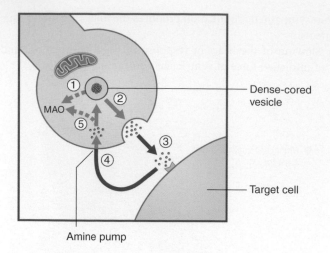

Fig. 13.10 Transmitter release and recycling at adrenergic nerve endings. *MAO*, Monoamine oxidase. Key to numbers in Clinical Panel 13.2.

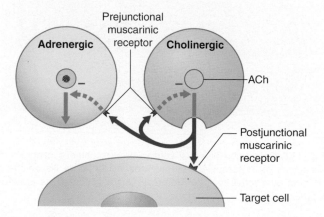

Fig. 13.11 Cholinergic activity at a neuroeffector junction. Release of excess acetylcholine *(ACh)* is inhibited by prejunctional muscarinic receptors, which also inhibit transmitter release from neighbouring sympathetic varicosities.

- Contraction of smooth muscle, with the following effects: intestinal peristalsis (Fig. 13.5, Box 13.2), bladder emptying (Fig. 13.12, Box 13.3), and accommodation of the eye for 'near vision'.
- Glandular secretion.

In addition to the above postjunctional effects, prejunctional muscarinic receptors located on sympathetic varicosities inhibit release of norepinephrine (see Fig. 13.9).

The effects of *drugs* on the parasympathetic system are considered in Clinical Panel 13.3 (Fig. 13.13). Drugs with muscarinic effects are described as *cholinergic*. Drugs that prevent access of ACh to junctional receptors are *anticholinergic*.

A major consideration in the use of drugs either to imitate or to suppress sympathetic or parasympathetic activity is the existence of α, β, and muscarinic receptors in the *CNS*. In psychiatric practice, in particular, drugs are often chosen for their action at their central rather than peripheral receptors.

Other Types of Neurons

Nonadrenergic, noncholinergic (NANC) neurons are found in both divisions of the autonomic system. In sympathetic ganglia, small interneurons liberate *dopamine*—a precursor of norepinephrine. Some of the dopamine is secreted into capillaries; the rest binds with dopamine receptors on the main (adrenergic) neurons and exerts a mild inhibitory effect.

NANC neurons are especially numerous among the ganglion cells in the wall of the alimentary tract and in the pelvic ganglia. More than 50 different *peptide* substances have been identified, either singly or in various combinations, in these neurons. For the most part they act as *modulators*, acting either prejunctionally or postjunctionally to influence the duration of action of classical transmitters. Some are *cotransmitters*, such as those released together with ACh.

Vasoactive intestinal polypeptide (VIP) is a cotransmitter in the cholinergic supply to the salivary glands and to sweat glands. VIP is a powerful vasodilator and conveniently opens the local vascular bed (through specific VIP receptors on arterioles) just when the muscarinic ACh receptors are raising glandular metabolism. *Nitric oxide* is well established as a transmitter in the parasympathetic and enteric systems. It is a powerful smooth muscle relaxant.

REGIONAL AUTONOMIC INNERVATION

Box 13.1 describes the autonomic innervation of the heart, Box 13.2 lower level bladder controls, and Box 13.3 the functional innervation of the genital tract.

Innervation of the Genital Tract (Fig. 13.14, Box 13.3)

The *nervi erigentes* ('erectile nerves') are postganglionic pelvic splanchnic nerve fibres supplying the smooth muscle of the internal pudendal arteries and of the trabecular erectile tissue of the phallus in both sexes. The nervi are activated by central parasympathetic neurons following psychic stimulation of the anterior hypothalamus and/or through a spinal reflex arc in response to direct genital stimulation. Activation produces smooth muscle relaxation, with flooding of the cavernous spaces. In females, Bartholin's glands or the greater vestibular glands act to lubricate the vagina. In the male the urethral and bulbourethral glands lubricate the urethra to facilitate passage of semen.

INTERACTION OF THE AUTONOMIC AND IMMUNE SYSTEMS

The lymphatic tissues of the thymus, lymph nodes, and spleen are richly supplied with adrenergic nerve fibres. So too is the bone marrow. Adrenoceptors have been found on T cells, B cells, and macrophages.

During acute psychologic stress, raised levels of circulating norepinephrine may induce lymphatic tissue to respond by increasing the number of natural killer cells and cytotoxic

BOX 13.2 Lower Level Bladder Controls

The female bladder is selected for this description and also for higher level bladder controls in Chapter 24.

Relevant anatomic details

- The smooth muscle of the detrusor in the body (corpus) of the bladder is an interwoven meshwork of fasciculi that functions as a unit.
- The bladder neck is surrounded by two layers of longitudinal smooth muscle enclosing a layer of circular muscle constituting the ***internal urethral sphincter***.
- The outer longitudinal fibres descend within the mucous membrane of the urethra. When these fibres contract (along with the rest of the detrusor), they shorten and widen the urethral canal.
- The resting urethral canal is kept closed by a rich encircling web of elastic fibres, a highly vascular mucous membrane, a thin circular layer of smooth muscle, and the striated ***external urethral sphincter***. Urologists tend to use the term *rhabdosphincter* to emphasise the *striated* nature of the external sphincter.
- The external urethral sphincter is richly endowed with slow-twitch, fatigue-resistant muscle fibres. It comes into play when abdominal pressure is raised either briefly (e.g., during a cough or sneeze) or for longer (e.g., while a heavy load is being carried). The cell group innervating this rhabdosphincter is the *nucleus of Onuf* in the anterior grey horn at spinal cord levels S2 and S3. Most of the axons travel in the pudendal nerve.

The micturition cycle (see Fig. 13.12)

1. Immediately prior to the act of micturition, the anterior horn motor neurons to the levator ani and other muscles of the pelvic floor are inhibited by axons descending from the micturition centre in the pons (Chapter 24). The neck of the bladder descends passively, and urine trickles into the urethra.
2. Mucosal fibres of the pudendal nerve, sensory to the epithelium of the trigone and urethra, discharge impulses to the posterior grey horn of cord segments S2 to S4.
3. From the sacral cord, second-order sensory neurons discharge to the pontine micturition centre.
4. Sacral parasympathetic neurons serving the bladder are simultaneously activated by the pontine micturition centre and by neurons in the posterior horn at segmental levels S2 to S4.
5. The detrusor responds to postganglionic stimulation by contracting uniformly to expel the urine.
6. The rhabdosphincter, 'slave' to Onuf, contracts to expel urine from the urethral canal.
7. The levator ani contracts to resume its supportive role.
8. Bladder filling recommences, while the bladder wall is rendered *compliant* by tonic inhibitory α_2 action of the sympathetic system on the detrusor muscle and by β_2 receptors on parasympathetic terminals.
9. When the bladder is half-full, the stretch receptor afferents from the detrusor inform higher level neurons in the brainstem, as described in Basic Science Panel 24.1.

Notes on urinary incontinence

Urinary incontinence afflicts about 30% of the female population at some time in their lives. Two types are described.

Stress incontinence is characterised by loss of small amounts of urine caused by a sudden brief rise in intraabdominal pressure, most commonly caused by sneezing or coughing. Its origin is attributed to weakness of the pelvic floor following pregnancy, childbirth, and/or menopause. In males it may be a problem following prostatectomy.

Urge incontinence is caused by *detrusor overactivity* and is characterised by spontaneous expulsion of urine during the filling phase of the micturition cycle despite conscious attempts to inhibit it. (See Basic Science Panel 24.1.)

---

lymphocytes. The consequent reduction of the immune response to pathogens results in increased susceptibility to infections.

VISCERAL AFFERENTS

Afferents from thoracic and abdominal viscera utilise autonomic pathways to reach the CNS. They participate in important reflexes involved in the control of circulation, respiration, digestion, micturition, and coition.

Visceral activities are not normally perceived, but they do reach conscious levels in a variety of disease states. *Visceral pain is of immense importance in the context of clinical diagnosis.*

Visceral Pain

There are three fundamental types of visceral pain:

1. *Pure visceral pain*, felt in the region of the affected organ.
2. *Visceral referred pain*, projected subjectively into the territory of the corresponding somatic nerves.
3. *Viscerosomatic pain*, caused by spread of disease to somatic structures.

Pure Visceral Pain. Pure visceral pain is characteristically vague and deep seated. It is often accompanied by sweating or nausea. It is experienced as the initial pain in association with inflammation and/or ulceration in the alimentary tract; with obstruction of the intestine, bile duct, or ureter; or when the capsule of a solid organ (liver, kidney, or pancreas) is stretched by underlying disease. In marked contrast, the viscera are completely insensitive to cutting or burning.

Visceral Referred Pain. As its severity increases, visceral pain is 'referred' to somatic structures innervated from the same segmental levels of the spinal cord. For example, the pain of myocardial ischemia is referred to the chest wall ('angina pectoris'), pains of biliary or intestinal origin are referred to the anterior abdominal wall, and labour pains are referred to the sacral area of the back.

According to the generally accepted 'convergence–projection' theory of referred pain, the brain falsely interprets the source of noxious stimulation because visceral and somatic nociceptors have some spinothalamic neurons in common; in previous experience these neurons habitually signalled somatic pain.

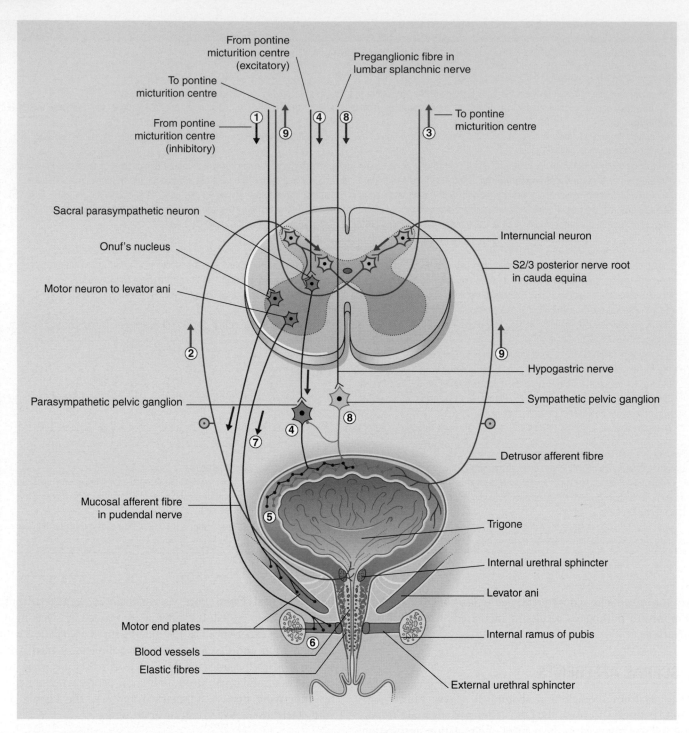

Fig. 13.12 Lower level bladder controls. *GI*, Gastrointestinal. (The assistance of Professor Mary Pat FitzGerald, Consultant Urogynaecologist, Bon Secours Hospital, Galway, Ireland, is gratefully appreciated.) Key to numbers in Box 13.2.

Viscerosomatic Pain. The parietal serous membranes (pleura and peritoneum) receive a rich sensory supply from the overlying intercostal nerves, and they are exquisitely sensitive to acute inflammatory exudates. The extension of an inflammatory process to the surface of stomach, intestine, appendix, or gallbladder gives rise to a severe, steady pain in the abdominal wall directly overlying the inflamed organ. With the onset of acute peritonitis, the abdominal wall is 'splinted' by the muscles in a protective reflex.

Tenderness

Tenderness is *pain elicited by palpation.* In the abdomen, it is sought by pressing the hand and fingers against the abdominal wall. The clinician is in effect clothing the finger pads with the

BOX 13.3 Functional Innervation of the Male Genital Tract (Fig. 13.14)

1. *Erection*. Psychic stimulation of the central *parasympathetic* pathway activates selected preganglionic neurons (P) to pelvic ganglia supplying parasympathetic fibres to the internal pudendal artery, where muscarinic and VIP receptors cause the artery to relax, allowing blood to distend the penile cavernous tissue spaces. Cholinergic fibres also cause the relaxant transmitter nitric oxide to be released from the lining epithelium of the cavernous spaces.

2. *Secretion*. Parasympathetic ganglia in the walls of the prostate and seminal vesicles are stimulated to cause glandular secretion (via muscarinic receptors on the acini). These secretions contribute to 80% of total semen volume.

3. *Emission*. Psychic stimulation of the central *sympathetic* pathway activates preganglionic neurons to pelvic ganglia supplying fibres to α_1 receptors on the smooth muscle of the vas deferens, seminal vesicles, prostate, and internal urethral *(preprostatic)* sphincter. Sperm and glandular contents are expelled into the urethra while the sphincter prevents backfire into the bladder. Simultaneous activation of bladder β_2 receptors prevents detrusor contraction.

4. *Ejaculation*. Entry of semen into the urethra activates somatic afferent nerve endings provided by the pudendal nerve. Through a reflex arc at S2 to S4 segmental levels, somatic motor fibres in the pudendal nerve cause rhythmic contractions of the bulbospongiosus muscles to ejaculate ('throw out') the semen into the vagina.

5. *Detumescence*. Selected central sympathetic fibres activate preganglionic neurons to pelvic sympathetic ganglia supplying fibres to α_1 receptors on pudendal arterioles at points of entry into the cavernous spaces. Arteriolar constriction results in detumescence.

Sympathetic system and psychogenic impotence

In addition to the prevertebral supply of the vas deferens mentioned earlier (3), a second paravertebral sympathetic pathway relays in the sacral sympathetic chain to supply the trabecular tissue, rich in β_2 adrenoceptors. The resting, flaccid state of the penis depends upon tonic activity in this pathway. In this context the corpus cavernosum resembles a well-muscled artery. For erection to take place, the sympathetic supply must be switched off while the parasympathetic, relaxant supply is switched on. Both events may be coordinated at the level of the hypothalamus. Failure to 'switch off' tonic sympathetic activity is regarded as the most common immediate cause of *psychogenic impotence*, defined as impotence in the presence of intact anatomic pathways and necessitating the incorporation of psychosexual therapy for successful treatment. Damage to reflex arcs, such as by spinal cord injury (Chapter 16), may cause *reflexive impotence*.

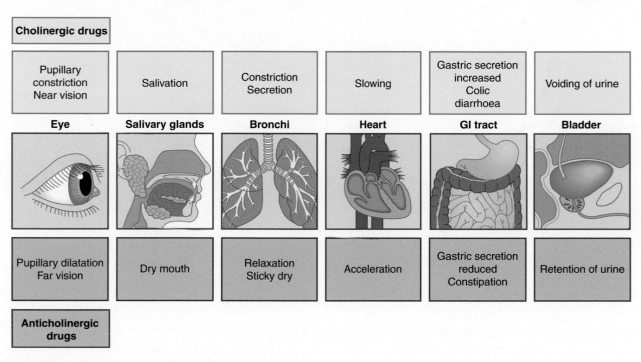

Fig. 13.13 Drugs and the parasympathetic system. *GI*, Gastrointestinal.

patient's parietal peritoneum and using this to seek out an inflamed organ. If the organ is mobile, like the appendix, 'shifting tenderness' may be elicited if the patient is willing to roll from one side to the other.

Pain and the Mind

Although visceral pain has well-established causative mechanisms (inflammation, spasm of smooth muscle, ischemia, and distension),

thoracic or abdominal pain may be experienced in the complete absence of visceral disease. Pain that recurs or persists over a long period (months), and is not accounted for by standard investigational procedures, is more likely to have a *psychologic* rather than a physical explanation. This is not to deny that the pain is real, but to imply that it originates within the brain itself. An example is the abused child whose abdominal pains represent a cry for help. In adults, recurrent and

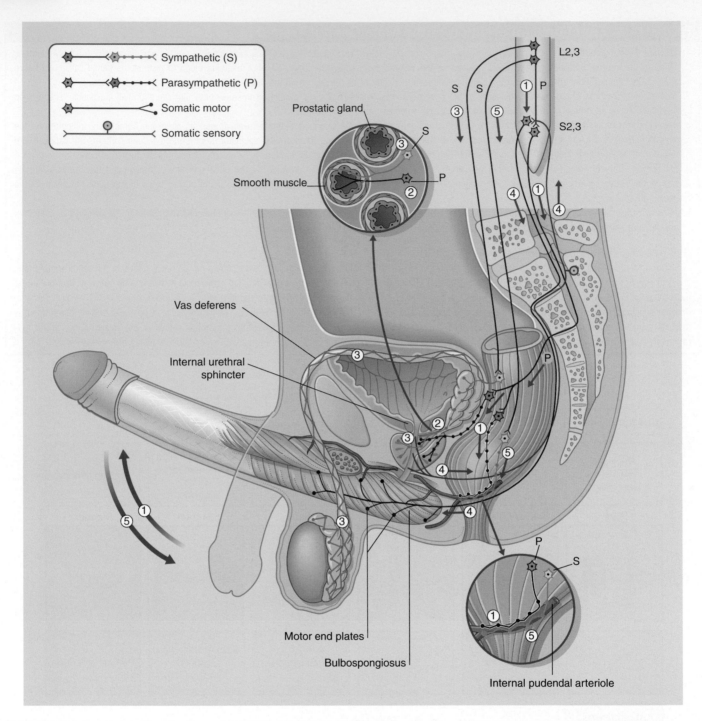

Fig. 13.14 Functional innervation of male genital tract. Key to numbers in Box 13.3.

rather ill-defined pains are a common manifestation of *major depression* (see Chapter 34).

Irritable bowel syndrome (IBS) is a very common disorder usually arising in the third or fourth decade. In this syndrome there *is* evidence of abnormality at the intestinal cellular level, but alterations of bowel behaviour appear to be heightened by a *disorder of the brain—gut axis* (Fig. 13.15, Clinical Panel 13.4).

Note on Vascular Afferents. Two *vascular* sets of unipolar neurons are customarily included in descriptions of the visceral

afferent system. One supplies the carotid sinus and aortic arch with stretch receptors involved in the maintenance of the systemic blood pressure (Chapter 24); the other supplies the carotid body with chemoreceptors and is involved in respiratory control (Chapter 24). There is a progressive tendency to acknowledge *all* vascular afferents as being visceral, because those on peripheral blood vessels are morphologically and functionally the same as those serving the heart. They all contain substance P, are 'silent' in health, and subserve pain in the presence of disease or injury—as witness, the 'dragging' leg pains

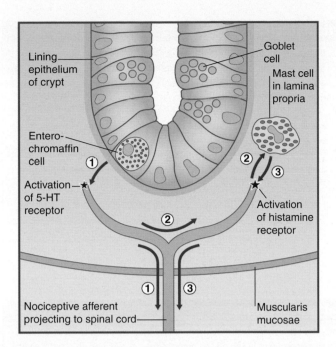

Fig. 13.15 Activation of a nociceptive neuron in the wall of the colon. *(1)* Serotonin liberated by enterochromaffin cells has activated a nociceptive neuron projecting to the posterior horn of the spinal cord. *(2)* Antidromic impulses liberate substance P, which in turn releases histamine from mast cells. *(3)* Histamine reinforces the effect of serotonin. *5-HT*, Serotonin.

accompanying varicose veins, or the stab of pain when a clumsily inserted antecubital venipuncture needle strikes the brachial artery. The pathway to the dorsal nerve roots is still uncertain, but it appears that (to an approximation) perivascular fibres above the elbow and knee send impulses by the sympathetic route (but in the reverse direction), and that more peripheral perivascular fibres send messages in company with cutaneous nerves (and in the same direction). The notion of visceral afferents running in cutaneous nerves is reminiscent of their same service with respect to nerve fibres terminating in Golgi tendon organs at the wrist and ankle.

Diabetic autonomic neuropathy is a serious condition. It has been reported to have a prevalence of 20% to 60% in both type 1 and type 2 diabetes. It is associated with a high mortality rate and the precise pathophysiological mechanisms are not yet fully understood.

The autonomic innervation of skin plays a vital role in thermoregulation. Recent work has suggested that this is often targeted in early stages of neurodegenerative diseases such as **Parkinson's disease**. Various investigative approaches are being developed to better assess functional and structural integrity in this component of the autonomic nervous system. Knowledge of the anatomy and physiology of the autonomic nervous system is still evolving and this is providing opportunities to identify novel diagnostic and therapeutic targets of small fibre neuropathies.

CLINICAL PANEL 13.1   Sympathetic Interruption

Stellate Block

Injection of local anaesthetic around the stellate ganglion — *stellate block* — is a procedure used to test the effects of sympathetic interruption on blood flow to the hand. Both preganglionic and postganglionic fibres are inactivated, producing sympathetic paralysis in the head and neck on that side, as well as in the upper limb. A successful stellate block is demonstrated by (1) a warm, dry hand; (2) *Horner syndrome*, which consists of a constricted pupil resulting from unopposed action of the pupillary constrictor; and (3) *ptosis* (drooping) of the upper eyelid secondary to paralysis of smooth muscle fibres contained in the levator muscle of the upper eyelid (Fig. 13.2).

Dominance of the right stellate ganglion in control of the heart rate is shown by the marked slowing of the pulse following a right, but not a left, stellate block. (See also Box 13.1.)

Functional sympathectomy of the upper limb may be carried out by cutting the sympathetic chain below the stellate ganglion. This is not an anatomic sympathectomy because the ganglionic supply to the limb from the middle cervical and stellate ganglia remains intact. It is a functional sympathectomy because the ganglionic neurons for the limb are deprived of tonic sympathetic drive. Horner syndrome is avoided by making the cut at the level of the

second rib: the preganglionic fibres for the head and neck enter the stellate direct from the first thoracic spinal nerve.

Two relative indications for interruption of the sympathetic supply to one or both upper limbs are painful blanching of the fingers in cold weather *(Raynaud phenomenon)* and *hyperhidrosis* (excessive sweating/perspiration), a condition that typically begins in adolescence and is localised to areas with high concentrations of sweat glands (hands, feet, groin).

The sympathetic supply to the eye is considered further in Chapter 23.

Lumbar Sympathectomy

In the past, to improve blood flow to the lower limb and to treat neuropathic pain, the upper end of the lumbar sympathetic chain was cut to interrupt the preganglionic nerve supply. The usual procedure was to remove the second and third lumbar sympathetic ganglia. However, in males bilateral lumbar sympathectomy can result in persistent, painful erections *(priapism)* because of interruption of a pathway that maintains the resting, flaccid state of the penis. Currently this procedure is rarely performed because there is little evidence that it is effective in the majority of patients. Renal sympathetic nerve ablation (performed via a catheter approach) is increasingly being used to manage hypertension that is resistant to conventional forms of therapy.

CLINICAL PANEL 13.2 Drugs and the Sympathetic System

Considerable scope is offered for pharmacologic interference at sympathetic nerve endings. Drugs that cross the blood–brain barrier (Chapter 4) may exert their effects upon central rather than peripheral adrenoceptors. Potential sites of drug action are numbered in Fig. 13.10.

1. Norepinephrine is loosely bound to a protein in the dense-cored vesicles. It can be unbound by specific drugs, whereupon it diffuses into the axoplasm and is degraded by monoamine oxidase (MAO).
2. Exocytosis into the synaptic cleft can be accelerated. Stimulant drugs such as amphetamine exert their effect by flooding the extracellular space with expelled norepinephrine and dopamine.
3. α or β receptors can be selectively stimulated or blocked. As mentioned in Chapter 7, a receptor can be likened to a lock and a drug that operates the lock is an *agonist*. A drug that 'jams' the lock without operating it is a *blocker*. β agonists are used to relax the bronchial musculature in asthmatic patients. Cardioselective β blockers are used to limit access of norepinephrine to α_1 receptors.

4. The amine uptake mechanism can be blocked in the CNS by the tricyclic antidepressant drugs, or by cocaine. As a result, norepinephrine accumulates in the brain extracellular fluid.
5. Some antidepressant drugs increase the norepinephrine content of synaptic vesicles by inhibiting MAO, which normally degrades some of the transmitter after retrieval.

CLINICAL PANEL 13.3 Drugs and the Parasympathetic System

Possible peripheral effects of cholinergic and anticholinergic drugs are listed in Fig. 13.13. Some success has been achieved in the search for organ-specific or tissue-specific drugs. For example, the contribution of the vagus nerve to acid secretion in the stomach involves activation of a muscarinic receptor (M_1), which is distinct from the receptor type (M_2) found in the heart or on smooth muscle. An M_1-receptor blocker is available to reduce gastric acidity for patients suffering from peptic ulcer.

CLINICAL PANEL 13.4 Irritable Bowel Syndrome

Irritable bowel syndrome (IBS) is considered to be the most prevalent of all gastrointestinal tract disorders, affecting 10% to 15% of the population in most countries. The exact incidence is uncertain because of the absence of a specific test; diagnosis is based upon a constellation of symptoms associated with a suggestive psychosocial history. The disorder is two times more common in women, and onset is most frequent during the third and fourth decades.

The typical clinical picture is one of chronic abdominal pain and altered bowel habits. Some patients may have fewer than three bowel movements per week, others more than three per day. Both groups experience bloating (a feeling of abdominal distension). Sensitivity to visceral sensations may have been triggered by a previous infectious or food allergy gastroenteritis. The typical psychological profile identifies anxiety, sleep disturbance, and somatic symptoms as independent risk factors for the development of IBS. Treatment begins with lifestyle and dietary changes and, if necessary, pharmacologic treatment is instituted and directed to the prominent symptoms (diarrhoea or constipation). Particular attention is made to more worrisome symptoms (e.g., rectal bleeding, weight loss, anaemia) that may indicate a more serious underlying condition and the necessity for further evaluation. The overall situation is generally accepted as one of *dysfunction of the gut–brain axis.*

Box 33.1 shows the position of the *emotional nociceptive area* within the cingulate gyrus. This area is activated by aversive (unpleasant) painful stimulation of any body part, as revealed by positron emission tomography (PET). In IBS patient volunteers it is activated by balloon distension of the distal colon at a lower balloon volume than in healthy controls. Heightened sensitivity to intestinal events seems to some extent to be *centrally* rather than peripherally generated. It is now believed that the preganglionic neurons of the parasympathetic system synapse mainly on *interneurons* in the intestinal wall, rather than on the 'traditional' postganglionic motor neurons shown in Fig. 13.5. The central drive of the parasympathetic system may be an expression of stress, and because interneurons may activate nociceptive afferents as well as motor neurons, heightened sensitivity may be maintained or even increased through this feedback loop.

At a peripheral level, biopsies taken from the ileum and colon indicate that heightened sensitivity may be the outcome of an immune response generated by earlier gastrointestinal infection or food allergy, as evidenced by proliferation of enterochromaffin cells in the wall of intestinal crypts and/or mast cells in the lamina propria (Fig. 13.15). The peptide granules of enterochromaffin (chromate-staining) cells collectively contain more serotonin (5-HT) than does the entire brain. 5-HT liberated in response to intestinal distension has a double effect: it activates $5\text{-}HT_3$ receptors on smooth muscle cells, thereby promoting peristaltic contractions; and it activates nociceptors on nearby visceral afferents, thereby causing mast cells to liberate histamine, which in turn may potentiate the local effect of 5-HT.

Following investigations to rule out organic disease, reassurance alone may be sufficient to restore equilibrium, although many patients benefit from psychotherapy. Drug treatments are essentially symptomatic and include $5\text{-}HT_3$-receptor antagonists or M_3-receptor anticholinergics for diarrhoea and $5\text{-}HT_3$-receptor agonists or cholinergics for constipation.

Core Information

The autonomic nervous system contains three neuron chains of effector neurons: central neurons project from hypothalamus/brainstem to brainstem/spinal cord preganglionic neurons. These send preganglionic fibres to autonomic ganglion cells, which in turn send postganglionic fibres to target tissues.

Sympathetic preganglionic outflow to the sympathetic chain of ganglia is thoracolumbar. Some fibres synapse in the nearest ganglia. Some ascend to the superior cervical, middle cervical, or stellate ganglion, whence postganglionic fibres innervate the head, neck, upper limbs, and heart. Some descend to synapse in lumbar or sacral ganglia, whence postganglionic fibres enter the lumbosacral plexus to supply lower limb vessels. Some pass through the chain and synapse instead in central abdominal ganglia (for the supply of gastrointestinal and genitourinary tracts) or in the adrenal medulla.

Parasympathetic preganglionic outflow is craniosacral. Cranial nerve distributions are the oculomotor nerve via the ciliary ganglion to the sphincter pupillae and ciliaris; the facial nerve via the pterygopalatine ganglion to lacrimal and nasal glands; the facial nerve via the submandibular ganglion to submandibular and sublingual glands; the glossopharyngeal nerve via the otic ganglion to the parotid gland; and the vagus nerve via ganglia on or in walls of the heart, bronchi, and alimentary tract to muscle tissue and glands. Sacral nerves S2 to S4 deliver preganglionic fibres to intramural ganglia of the distal colon and rectum, and to pelvic ganglia for supply of the bladder and internal pudendal artery.

The enteric nervous system (ENS) is the name given to the intrinsic nerve supply to the gastrointestinal tract. The ENS is sometimes referred to as the 'gut brain' on account of its size and relative functional independence.

All preganglionic neurons are cholinergic. They activate nicotinic receptors in the ganglia. All postganglionic fibres end at neuroeffector junctions. In the sympathetic system these are generally adrenergic, liberating norepinephrine, which may activate postjunctional α_1 adrenoceptors on smooth muscle, prejunctional α_2 adrenoceptors on local nerve endings, postjunctional β_1 adrenoceptors on cardiac muscle, or postjunctional β_2 adrenoceptors, which are more responsive to epinephrine. Epinephrine is liberated by adrenomedullary chromaffin cells and resultant activation of β_2 adrenoceptors on smooth muscle causes relaxation.

Parasympathetic postganglionic fibres are cholinergic. The cholinoceptive receptors on cardiac and smooth muscle and glands are muscarinic.

Visceral Afferents

Nociceptive afferents from thoracic and abdominal viscera and from blood vessels use autonomic pathways to reach the CNS. Pure visceral pain is vague and deep seated. Visceral referred pain is experienced in somatic structures innervated from the same segmental levels. Viscerosomatic pain arises from chemical/thermal irritation of one of the serous membranes: the pain is severe and steady, and accompanied by protective contraction of body wall muscles.

SUGGESTED READINGS

Axelrod FB. Genetic autonomic disorders. *Semin Pediat Neurol.* 2013;20:3–11.

Cortelli P, Giannini G, Favoni V, et al. Nociception and autonomic nervous system. *Neurol Sci.* 2013;34:41–46.

Ferreira JN, Hoffman MP. Interactions between developing nerves and salivary glands. *Organogenesis.* 2013;9:199–205.

Gibbins I. Functional organization of autonomic neural pathways. *Organogenesis.* 2013;9:169–175.

Glatte P, Buchmann SJ, Hijazi MM, Illigens BM, Siepmann T. Architecture of the cutaneous autonomic nervous system. *Front Neurol.* 2019;10:970.

Koike H, Watanabe H, Sobue G. The spectrum of immune-mediated autonomic neuropathies: insights from the clinicopathological features. *J Neurol Neurosur Psy.* 2013;84:98–106.

Schneider S, Wright CM, Heuckeroth RO. Unexpected roles for the second brain: enteric nervous system as master regulator of bowel function. *Annu Rev Physiol.* 2019;81:235–259.

Spallone V. Update on the impact, diagnosis and management of cardiovascular autonomic neuropathy in diabetes: what is defined, what is new, and what is unmet. *Diabetes Metab J.* 2019;43(1):3–30.

Waxenbaum JA, Varacallo M. *Anatomy, Autonomic Nervous System.* StatPearls [Internet]. Treasure Island, FL: StatPearls Publishing; 2019. Available from http://www.ncbi.nlm.nih.gov/books/NBK539845. Accessed 20 April, 2020.

Nerve Roots

CHAPTER SUMMARY

STUDY GUIDELINES

1. Describe the fate of immature neurons during embryonic development within the developing spinal cord (some send out ventral roots, others project along the marginal zone to form fibre tracts) and of the neural crest.
2. Outline the anatomy of a typical spinal nerve.
3. Explain the clinical implications of the mature vertebral canal relationship between the spinal column and respective spinal cord level; for example, a collapsed T11 vertebra would crush spinal cord segment L1.
4. Contrast the clinical presentation of an injury to S2 to S4 ventral roots of the cauda equina (containing preganglionic parasympathetic fibres vital for bladder and bowel control)

or the corresponding posterior roots (contain visceral afferents vital for reflexes).
5. Provide an illustration of how the normal extradural venous plexus could facilitate the spread of an adjacent neoplasm.
6. Discuss how the sense of numbness/tingling in the fingers in later life may result from compression of posterior nerve roots.
7. Explain why for the most common and lowest two levels of disk prolapse, the next spinal nerve is the one likely to be caught.
8. Be able to illustrate the structures traversed during, and the rationale for the site chosen to perform, a lumbar puncture (spinal tap).

DEVELOPMENT OF THE SPINAL CORD

The Notochord

By day 17 of embryonic development a small aggregate of cells come together to form a thin rostral/caudal strip known as the *notochord*. This chord of cells induces the process of *neurulation*, in which a flattened region of the embryo known as the *neural plate* rolls up to form the *neural tube*. The notochord regresses in the adult except for a small portion contributing to the nucleus pulposus of the intervertebral disk.

Cellular Differentiation

The neural tube of the embryo consists of a pseudostratified epithelium surrounding the neural canal (Fig. 14.1A). Dorsal to the sulcus limitans the epithelium forms the *alar plate*; ventral to the sulcus it forms the *basal plate*.

The neuroepithelium contains germinal cells that synthesise DNA before retracting to the innermost *ventricular zone*, where they divide. The daughter nuclei move outward, synthesise fresh DNA, then retreat and divide again. After several such cycles, postmitotic cells round up in the *intermediate zone*. Some of the postmitotic cells are immature neurons; the rest are *glioblasts*, which

after further division become astrocytes or oligodendrocytes. Some of the glioblasts form an ependymal lining for the neural canal.

The microglial cells of the central nervous system (CNS) are derived from basophil cells of the blood.

Enlargement of the intermediate zone of the alar plate creates the dorsal horn of grey matter. The dorsal horn receives central processes of dorsal root ganglion cells (Fig. 14.1B). As explained in Chapter 1, the ganglion cells are derived from the neural crest.

Partial occlusion of the neural canal by the developing dorsal grey horn gives rise to the dorsal median septum and to the definitive central canal of the cord (Fig. 14.1C).

Enlargement of the intermediate zone of the basal plate creates the ventral grey horn and the ventral median fissure (Fig. 14.1C). Axons emerge from the ventral horn and form the ventral nerve roots.

In the outermost *marginal zone* of the cord, axons run to and from the spinal cord and brain.

Ascent of the Spinal Cord (Fig. 14.2)

The spinal cord occupies the full length of the vertebral canal until the end of the twelfth postconceptual week. The sixth to eighth weeks are marked by the regression of the caudal end of the neural tube, to become a neuroglial thread, the *filum terminale*.

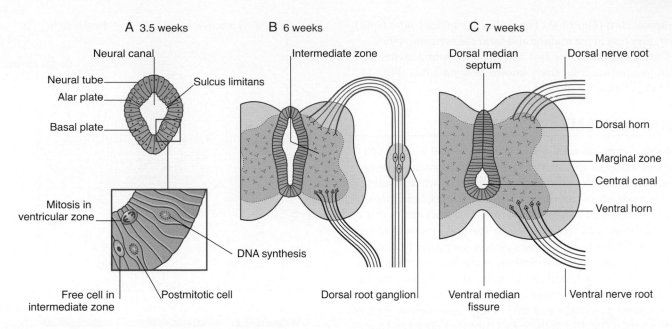

Fig. 14.1 (A–C) Cellular differentiation in the embryonic spinal cord.

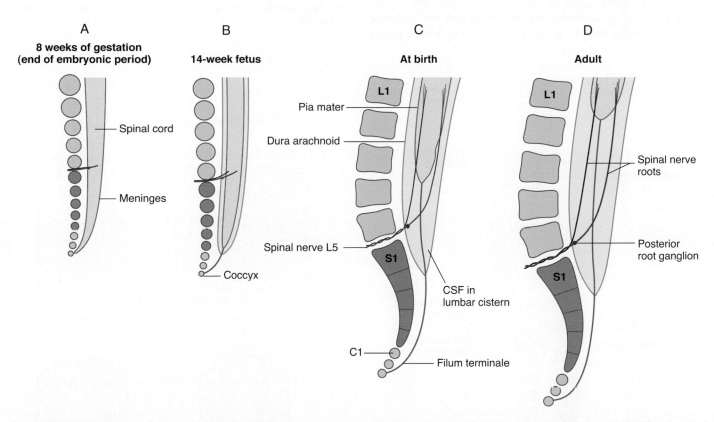

Fig. 14.2 (A, B) Regression of coccygeal segments of the spinal cord creates the filum terminale. (C, D) Ascent of the spinal cord. *CSF,* Cerebrospinal fluid. (*Note:* Recent evidence indicates that, as represented here, the number of embryonic coccygeal vertebrae does not exceed three or four.)

After the 12th week, the vertebral column grows rapidly and drags the spinal cord upward. The tip of the spinal cord is at the third lumbar (L3) at birth. The adult level (L1 or L2) is attained 2 months postnatally.

As a consequence of the greater ascent of the lower part of the cord compared to the upper part, the spinal nerve roots show an increasing disparity between their segmental levels of attachment to the cord and the corresponding vertebral levels (Fig. 14.3).

Neural Arches

During the fifth week, the mesenchymal vertebrae surrounding the notochord give rise to **neural arches** for the protection of the spinal cord (Fig. 14.4). The arches are initially *bifid* (split). Later, they fuse in the midline and form the vertebral spines.

Conditions where the two halves of the neural arches have failed to unite are collectively known as *spina bifida* (Figs. 14.5 and 14.6, Clinical Panel 14.1).

ADULT ANATOMY

The spinal cord has an almost circular sectional profile. An H-shaped column of grey matter is located in its centre. The grey matter contains neurons. The surrounding white matter is mainly made up of myelinated axons. The peripheral nervous system is described as being segmental, this is related to that of the body in general. As outlined in the previous section, segmentation of the body becomes evident very early in development. This segmentation is obvious in the body wall but rather obscure in the head, neck and limbs. The vertebrae are also based on this embryonic segmentation. Each body segment has an associated pair (right and left) of segmental nerves. Each of these nerves is attached to the spinal cord via a dorsal and a ventral root. The unipolar sensory neuron cell bodies are located outside of the spinal cord in the dorsal root ganglion. These, along with the spinal cord, are located within the vertebral canal. The roots join to form a spinal nerve which passes

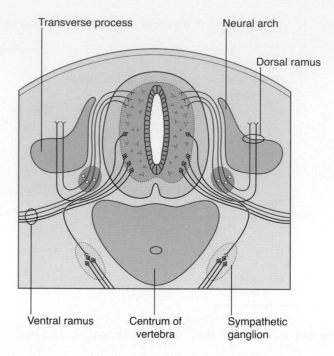

Fig. 14.4 Normal bifid stage of neural arch development in an embryo of 8 weeks.

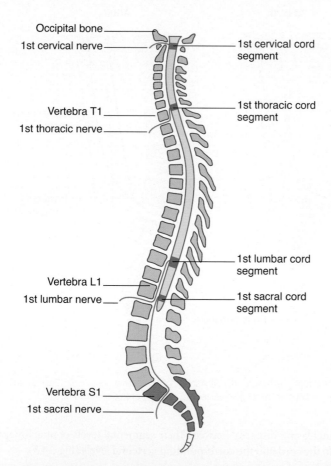

Fig. 14.3 Segmental and vertebral levels compared. Spinal nerves 1 to 7 emerge above the corresponding vertebrae; the remaining spinal nerves emerge below.

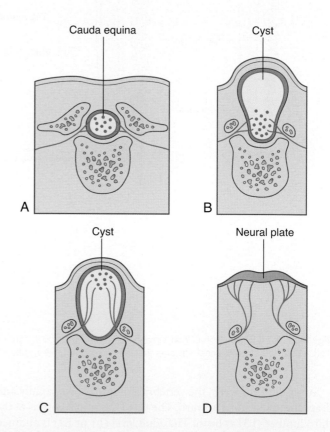

Fig. 14.5 Varieties of spina bifida. (A) Spina bifida occulta. (B) Meningocele. (C) Meningomyelocele. (D) Myelocele.

through the intervertebral foramen from the vertebral canal and then divides into a ventral and dorsal primary ramus. The ventral ramus runs forwards around the body wall and supplies the voluntary muscles of its segment with motor innervation. It also supplies the overlying skin. The dorsal ramus passes backwards and supplies the skin and muscles of the back in its segment. The strips of skin supplied by the ventral and dorsal rami are in line with one another and comprise the dermatome of that particular segmental nerve, extending as a band around the body surface from the midline posteriorly to the midline anteriorly. At all levels of the vertebral column the dorsal rami have a similar arrangement. In the neck and at levels of outflow to the limbs the arrangement of the ventral rami is modified. The nerves that supply the limbs are the ventral rami of those segments from which the limb buds grow out in the embryo. These branch, combine, and rebranch in a complex way. The networks

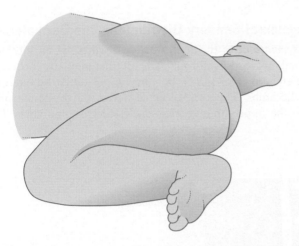

Fig. 14.6 Lumbar meningomyelocele (from a photograph). The 'frog leg' posture is characteristic of combined femoral and sciatic nerve paralysis, with preservation of hip flexion by the iliopsoas.

so formed are the plexuses of the limbs. The named peripheral nerves that emerge run into and through the limbs to their destinations. These peripheral nerves supply a relatively constant group of muscles and a defined area of skin, which together constitute the distribution of the nerve. In peripheral nerve disorders, testing for loss or modification of sensation and loss or weakness of motor function in the various nerve distributions gives vital clues to the identification of the nerve involved.

The spinal cord and nerve roots are sheathed by pia mater and suspended in the cerebrospinal fluid contained in the subarachnoid space. The pial **denticulate ligament** pierces the arachnoid and anchors the cord to the dura mater on each side. Outside the dura is the **extradural (epidural) venous plexus** (Fig. 14.7), which communicates with the vertebral red marrow and empties into the segmental veins (deep cervical, intercostal, lumbar, and sacral). These veins are valveless, and reflux of blood from the territory of segmental veins is a *notorious* cause of cancer spread from the prostate, lung, breast, and thyroid gland. For example, nerve root compression from collapse of an invaded vertebra may be the presenting sign of cancer in one of these organs.

The respective ventral and dorsal nerve roots join at the intervertebral foramina, where the dorsal root ganglia are located (see Fig. 14.7). The arachnoid mater blends with the perineurium of the spinal nerve and the dura mater blends with the epineurium. The nerve roots carry extensions of the subarachnoid space into the intervertebral foramina.

Below cord level, nerve roots seeking the lower lumbar and sacral intervertebral foramina constitute the **cauda equina** ('horse's tail'). The cauda equina is suspended in the lumbar subarachnoid cistern (Figs. 14.8 to 14.10), which reaches to the level of S2. At its upper end the cauda comprises nerve roots L3 to S5 of both sides for *a total of 32 roots* (excluding the insignificant coccygeal roots).

In the centre of the cauda equina is the filum terminale, which provides longitudinal support to the spinal cord. It is a

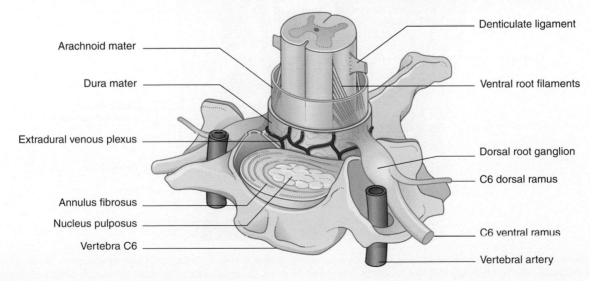

Arachnoid mater

Dura mater

Extradural venous plexus

Annulus fibrosus

Nucleus pulposus

Vertebra C6

Denticulate ligament

Ventral root filaments

Dorsal root ganglion

C6 dorsal ramus

C6 ventral ramus

Vertebral artery

Fig. 14.7 Relationships of the sixth cervical spinal nerve.

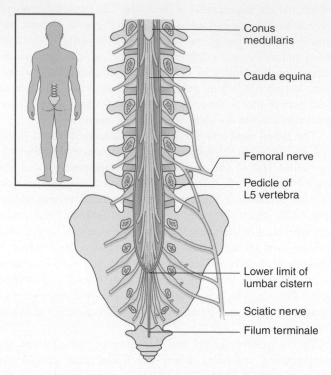

Fig. 14.8 The cauda equina in the lumbar cistern. Contributions to the femoral and sciatic nerves are shown on the right side.

thread of fibrous tissue, a modification of pia mater. It is about 20 cm in length and descends from the apex of the conus medullaris. It has two parts: an upper portion or filum terminale internum (15 cm) and a lower portion or filum terminale externum (5 cm) which closely adheres to the dura mater and is attached to the back of the first segment of the coccyx.

DISTRIBUTION OF SPINAL NERVES

Each spinal nerve gives off a *recurrent* branch that provides mechanoreceptors and pain receptors for the dura mater, posterior longitudinal ligament, and intervertebral disk. The synovial *facet* joints between successive articular processes are each supplied by the nearest three spinal nerves. Pain caused by injury to or disease of any of the above structures is referred to the cutaneous territory of the corresponding posterior rami (Fig. 14.11).

Segmental Sensory Distribution: The Dermatomes

A **dermatome** is the strip of skin supplied by an individual spinal nerve dorsal root. The dermatomes are orderly in the embryo (Fig. 14.12), but they are distorted by outgrowth of the limbs (Fig. 14.13). Spinal nerves C5 to T1 are drawn into the upper limb so that the C4 dermatome abuts T2 at

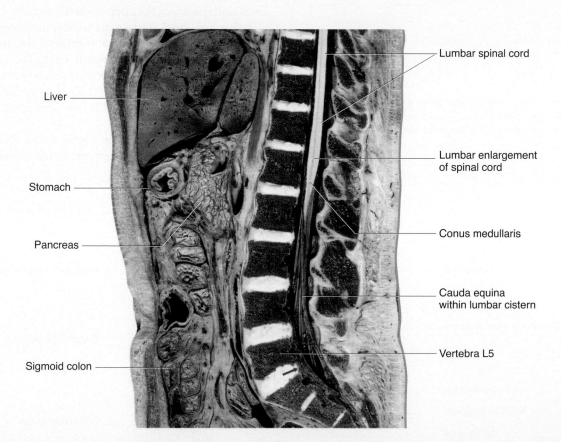

Fig. 14.9 Midline sagittal section of embalmed cadaver displaying thoracic, lumbar, and sacral spinal cord and cauda equina. *Arrow* indicates most frequent intervertebral disk to prolapse. (Reproduced with permission from Liu S. et al., eds. *The Atlas of Human Sectional Anatomy*. Jinan: Shantung Press of Science and Technology; 2003.)

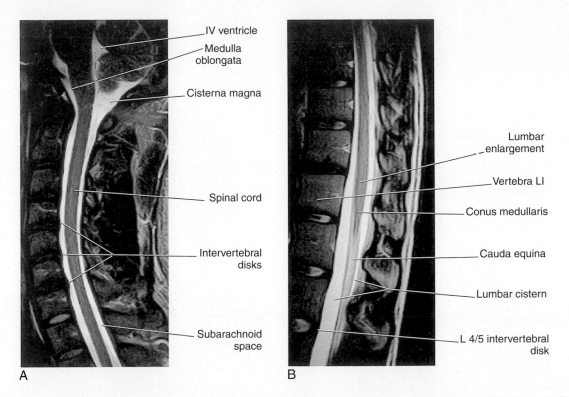

Fig. 14.10 Sagittal magnetic resonance imaging scans of the vertebral canal, weighted so as to enhance cerebrospinal fluid. (A) The brainstem, cerebellum, and cervical spinal cord are outlined. (B) The lumbosacral spinal cord and cauda equina are outlined. (From a series kindly provided by Professor J. Paul Finn, Director, Magnetic Resonance Research, Department of Radiology, David Geffen School of Medicine at UCLA, CA.)

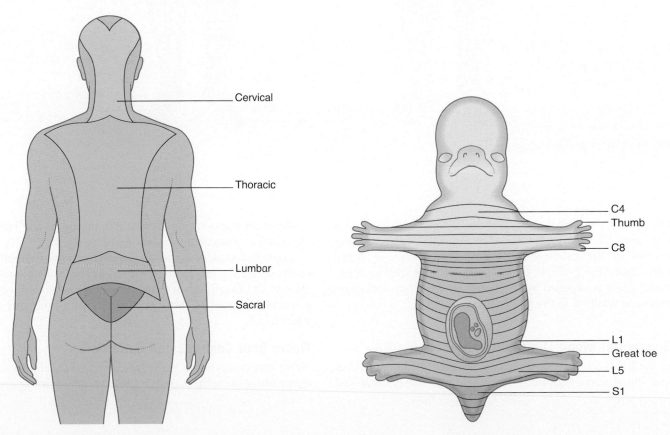

Fig. 14.11 Cutaneous distribution of posterior rami of spinal nerves.

Fig. 14.12 Embryonic dermatome pattern.

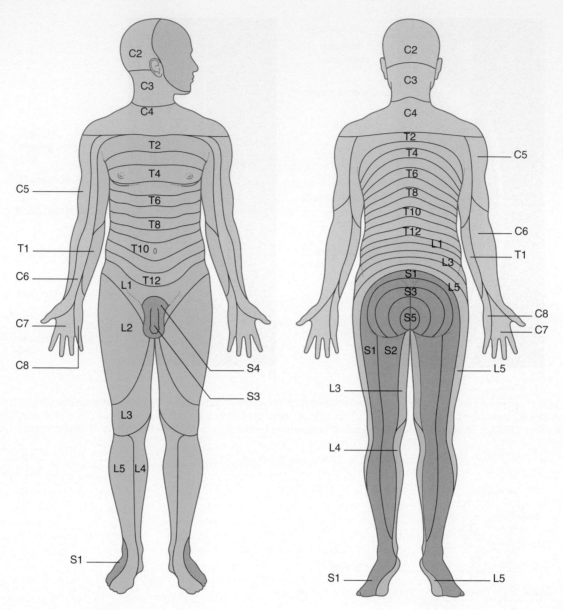

Fig. 14.13 Adult dermatome pattern.

the level of the sternal angle. Nerves L2 to S2 are drawn into the lower limb. Maps like those in Fig. 14.13 fail to portray *overlap* in the cutaneous distribution of successive dorsal nerve roots. For example, on the trunk the skin over an intercostal space is supplied by the nerves immediately above and below, in addition to the proper nerve.

Segmental Motor Distribution

In the limbs the individual muscles are supplied by more than one spinal nerve because of interchange in the brachial and

lumbosacral plexuses. The segmental supply of the limbs is expressed in terms of *movements* in Fig. 14.14.

Segmental sensory inputs and segmental motor outputs are combined during execution of *withdrawal* or *avoidance reflexes* (Box 14.1). (The prevalent term, *flexor reflex*, is too limited; e.g., a stimulus applied to the lateral surface of a limb may elicit adduction.)

Nerve Root Compression Syndromes

Nerve root compression within the vertebral canal is most frequent where the spine is most mobile, namely at lower cervical

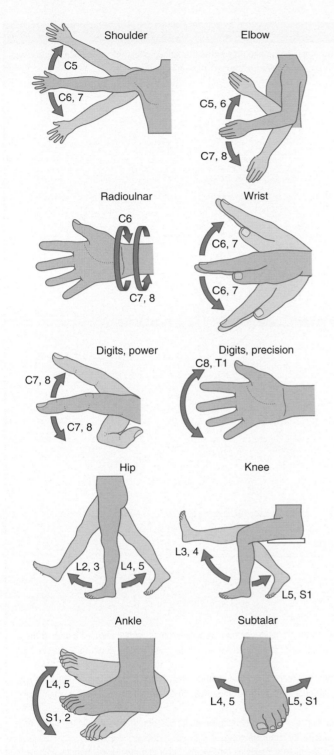

Fig. 14.14 Segmental control of limb movements. (Modified from Last RJ. *Anatomy: Regional and Applied.* 5th ed. Edinburgh: Churchill Livingstone; 1973; and Rosse C, Clawson DK. *The Musculoskeletal System in Health and Disease.* Hagerstown: Harper & Row; 1980.)

and lower lumbar levels (Clinical Panel 14.2). The effects of root compression may be expressed in five different ways:

1. *Pain* perceived in the muscles supplied by the corresponding spinal nerve(s).
2. *Paraesthesia* (numbness or tingling) along the respective dermatome(s).
3. *Cutaneous sensory loss* — more likely if two successive dermatomes are involved, because of overlap.
4. *Motor weakness.*
5. *Loss of a tendon reflex* if the segmental level is appropriate (Table 14.1).

Note: Peripheral nerve entrapment syndromes are considered in Chapter 12.

Lumbar Puncture (Spinal Tap)

The procedure involved in removing a sample of cerebrospinal fluid from the lumbar cistern is described in Core Information. This procedure should not be performed if there is any reason to suspect the presence of raised intracranial pressure. (It *is* performed as a diagnostic test for the syndrome of *pseudotumor cerebri*, but only when there is no evidence of a CNS mass or other contraindication.)

Anaesthetic Procedures

A *spinal anaesthesia* is often given in preference to a general anaesthesia prior to surgical procedures, such as prostate surgery in the elderly. A local anaesthetic is injected into the lumbar cistern to block impulse conduction in the lumbar and sacral nerve roots. Care is taken that the anaesthetic does not reach a high level in the subarachnoid space, for fear of paralyzing the intercostal and phrenic nerve root fibres serving respiration.

Anaesthesia and Childbirth. In skilled hands, pain-free labour can be assured by blocking the lumbar and sacral nerve roots extradurally. For *epidural anaesthesia* the local anaesthetic is carefully introduced into the extradural space by the lumbar route. For *caudal anaesthesia* (rarely performed), the extradural space is approached in an upward direction, through the sacral hiatus. In both procedures the anaesthetic diffuses through the dural sheath of the nerve roots where they leave the vertebral canal. Labour may be prolonged because of interruption of excitatory reflex arcs linking the perineum to the uterus through the lower end of the spinal cord.

Recent developments in MRI imaging approaches provide exciting clinical tools to visualise the anatomy of nerve roots in vivo that may afford a means of monitoring disease progression and treatment effects (Fig. 14.16).

BOX 14.1 Lower Limb Withdrawal Reflex

Fig. 14.15 depicts a lower limb *withdrawal reflex* with *crossed extensor thrust*. (A) The right foot is about to enter the stance phase of locomotion. (B) Contact with a sharp object initiates a withdrawal reflex, together with the crossed extensor response required to support the entire body weight.

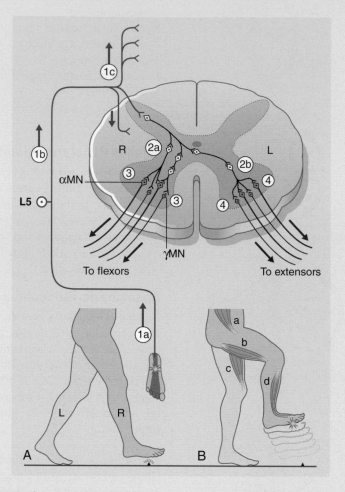

Fig. 14.15 Withdrawal reflex. *MN*, Motor neuron.

Sequence of events

1. Plantar nociceptors send impulse trains along tibial—sciatic afferent fibres (a) having parent posterior root ganglion somas within the L5-S1 intervertebral foramen. The impulses ascend the cauda equina (b) and enter segment L5 of the spinal cord. Some impulses are dispatched up and down the Lissauer tract (c) to activate segments L2 to L4 and S1.
2. In all five segments, primary nociceptive afferents excite flexor reflex interneurons in the base of the posterior horn (2a). Several interneurons may be interposed, in series, between entering afferents and target motor neurons. Axons of medially placed interneurons cross the midline in the grey commissure, allowing impulse trains to activate contralateral interneurons (2b).
3. On the stimulated side, α and γ motor neurons in cord segments L3 to S1 contract iliopsoas (a), hamstrings (b), and ankle dorsiflexors (d). At the same time (not shown here), ipsilateral 1a inhibitory interneurons are recruited to silence the antigravity motor neurons.
4. On the contralateral side, α and γ motor neurons in cord segments L2 to L5 contract the gluteus maximus (not visible here) and quadriceps femoris (c).
   Note: Not shown in the figure are *spinothalamic tract* relay neurons (see Chapter 15). These neurons receive inputs from nociceptive afferent fibres in the Lissauer tract, and they relay impulses to brain sites able to decode the location and nature of the initial stimulus.

TABLE 14.1 Segmental Levels of Tendon Reflexes.	
Segmental Level	**Reflex**
C5, 6	Biceps
	Brachioradialis ('supinator reflex')
C7	Triceps
L3, 4	Knee jerk
S1	Ankle jerk

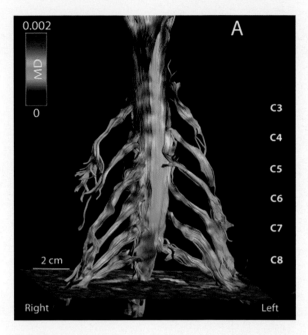

Fig. 14.16 Fibre tractography. From Stam M, Haakma W, Kuster L, et al. Magnetic resonance imaging of the cervical spinal cord in spinal muscular atrophy. *Neuroimage Clin.* 2019;24:102002.

CLINICAL PANEL 14.1 Spina Bifida

Among the more common congenital malformations of the CNS are several conditions included under the general heading *spina bifida*. The 'bifid' effect is produced by failure of union of the two halves of the neural arches, usually in the lumbosacral region (see Fig. 14.5).

Spina bifida occulta (A) is usually symptom free, being detected incidentally in lumbosacral radiographs.

In *spina bifida cystica*, a meningeal cyst protrudes through the vertebral defect. In 10% of these cases the cyst is a *meningocele* containing no nervous elements (B). In 90%, unfortunately, the cyst is a *meningomyelocele*, containing either spinal cord or cauda equina (C); the lower limbs, bladder, and rectum are paralyzed, as in the case illustrated in Fig. 14.6, and meningitis is likely to supervene sooner or later. To make matters worse, an *Arnold—Chiari malformation* (Chapter 5) is almost always present as well.

The most severe form of spina bifida is *myelocele* (D), where the neural folds have remained open and cerebrospinal fluid leaks onto the surrounding skin. The clinical outlook is very poor.

CLINICAL PANEL 14.2 Nerve Root Compression

Cervical Roots

The intervertebral disks and synovial joints of the neck are subject to degenerative disease *(cervical spondylosis)* in 50% of 50 year olds and in 70% of 70 year olds. Although any or all of the joints may deteriorate, problems are most frequent in relation to the C6 vertebra, which provides the fulcrum for flexion/extension movements of the neck. Spinal nerve C6 (above) or C7 (below) may be pinched by extruded disk material or by bony outgrowths *(osteophytes)* beside the synovial joints (Fig. 14.17). Sensory, motor, and reflex disturbances may result in accordance with the data in Figs. 14.12 and 14.13, and Table 14.1.

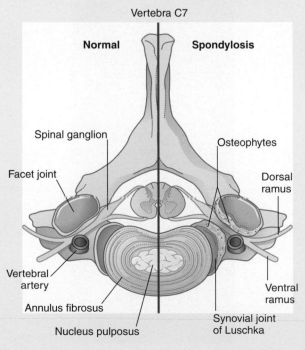

Fig. 14.17 Spondylosis on the right side of the C7 vertebra. Osteophytes are pinching the C7 spinal nerve trunk.

Lumbosacral Roots

The term **lumbar spinal stenosis** signifies narrowing of the lumbar vertebral canal as a result of encroachment by a prolapsing intervertebral disk or by bony osteophytes. Fully 95% of all disk prolapses occur immediately above or below the last lumbar vertebra. The typical herniation is *posterolateral*, with compression of the nerve roots passing to the *next* intervertebral foramen (Fig. 14.18).

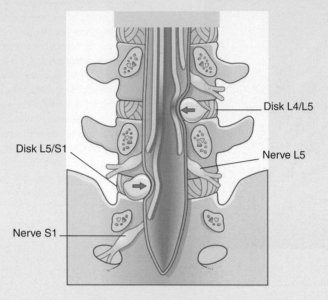

Disk L4/L5

Disk L5/S1

Nerve L5

Nerve S1

Fig. 14.18 Nerves Compressed (*arrows*) by Posterolateral Prolapse of the Two Lowest Intervertebral Disks.

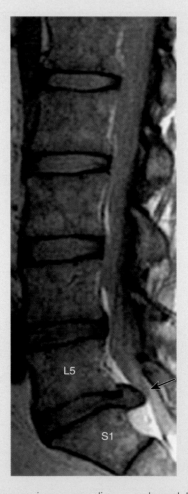

L5

S1

Fig. 14.19 Sagittal magnetic resonance image revealing a prolapsed L5/S1 intervertebral disk pressing against the cauda equina *(arrow)*. (Kindly provided by Professor Robert D. Zimmerman, Department of Radiology, Weill Cornell Medical College, NY.)

Symptoms include backache, caused by rupture of the annulus fibrosus, and pain in the buttock/thigh/leg, caused by pressure on posterior root fibres contributing to the sciatic nerve. The pain is increased by stretching the affected root; for example, by having the straightened leg raised by the examiner.

An L4—L5 disk prolapse produces pain/paraesthesia over the L5 dermatome. Motor weakness may be detected during dorsiflexion of the great toe (later, of all toes and of the ankle) and during eversion of the foot. Abduction of the hip may also be weak (this movement is tested with the patient lying on one side).

With an L5—S1 prolapse (the commonest of all) (Fig. 14.19), symptoms are felt in the back of the leg/sole of the foot (S1 dermatome). Plantar flexion may be weak and the ankle jerk reduced or absent.

✴ Core Information

The neuroepithelium of the embryonic cord undergoes mitotic activity in the inner ventricular zone. Daughter cells move into the intermediate zone and become either neuroblasts or glioblasts. The developing dorsal horn receives central processes of neural crest-derived spinal ganglion cells. The ventral horn issues axons that form ventral nerve roots. The outer marginal zone contains the axons of developing nerve pathways. The caudal end of the cord develops separately from the caudal cell mass, which links up with the neural tube. After the 12th week, rapid growth of the vertebral column drags the cord up the vertebral canal; the lower tip of the cord is at the L2 to L3 level at birth and at the L1 to L2 level 8 weeks later. The result is a progressive disparity between segmental levels of nerve root attachment to the cord and intervertebral levels of exit of spinal nerves. The neural arches are dorsal projections of vertebral mesenchyme; the initial bifid arrangement is normally lost by fusion of the projections to form spines.

The mature cord and nerve roots are sheathed by pia mater and suspended in the subarachnoid space, anchored to dura by the denticulate ligament. The extradural space contains valveless veins that drain vertebral bone marrow into segmental veins and provide potential avenues for spread of cancer cells. Below the level of the cord the cauda equina comprises paired nerve roots L3 to S5 of both sides.

As it emerges from the intervertebral foramen (occupied by the posterior root ganglion), each spinal nerve gives a recurrent branch supplying ligaments and dura mater.

Segmental sensory distribution is shown by the regular dermatomal pattern of skin innervation by the posterior roots (via the mixed peripheral nerves). Segmental motor supply is expressed in the form of movements performed by specific muscle groups. Nerve root compression, for example by a prolapsed disk, may be expressed segmentally by muscle pain, dermatomal paraesthesia, cutaneous sensory loss, motor weakness, or loss of a tendon reflex.

Lumbar puncture (spinal tap) is performed by carefully passing a needle between spines at the L3—L4 or L4—L5 level, but should not be performed if raised intracranial pressure is suspected. A spinal anaesthesia is given by injecting local anaesthetic into the lumbar cistern, an epidural anaesthesia is given into the lumbar epidural space, and a caudal anaesthesia is given through the sacral hiatus.

SUGGESTED READINGS

Gebremariam L, Koes BW, Peul WC, et al. Evaluation of treatment effectiveness for the herniated cervical disc: a systematic review. *Spine*. 2012;37:E109—E118.

McNamee J, Flynn P, O'Leary S, et al. Imaging in cauda equina syndrome — a pictorial review. *Ulster Med J*. 2013;82:100—108.

Sharma H, Lee SWJ, Cole AA. The management of weakness caused by lumbar and lumbosacral nerve root compression. *J Bone Joint Surg Br*. 2012;94:1442—1447.

Stam M, Haakma W, Kuster L, et al. Magnetic resonance imaging of the cervical spinal cord in spinal muscular atrophy. *Neuroimage Clin*. 2019;24:102002.

Toledano M, Bartleson JD. Cervical spondylotic myelopathy. *Neurol Clin*. 2013;31:287—305.

Wright BLC, Lai TF, Sinclair AJ. Cerebrospinal fluid and lumbar puncture: a practical review. *J Neurol*. 2012;259:1530—1545.

Spinal Cord: Ascending Pathways

STUDY GUIDELINES

1. Recognise that the mature spinal cord is not segmented internally.
2. Recall that the ventral horn cells take the form of columns rather than laminae.
3. Recognise that 'unconscious sensation' remove simply means that the ascending afferent impulse activity concerned does not generate any kind of perception.
4. Recognise that 'conscious proprioception' is more sensitive than either vision or the vestibular labyrinth in telling us when we are going off balance.
5. Explain why muscles tell us more than joints do about the position of our limbs in space.
6. Illustrate why it is clinically important to remember that one of the two 'conscious' pathways crosses the midline at all levels of the spinal cord, whereas the other crosses in the brainstem.
7. Explain the meaning of the term 'dissociated sensory loss' and why it can occur.

GENERAL FEATURES

The arrangement of grey and white matter at different levels of the spinal cord is shown in Fig. 15.1. White matter consists mainly of axons and dendrites, and is divided into ventral, lateral, and dorsal funiculi (*L. funiculus*, 'rope'), which are further divided into fasciculi (*L. fascis*, 'bundle'). The *cervical* (**C5 to T1**) and *lumbosacral* (**L1 to S2**) *enlargements* are produced by expansions of the grey matter required to innervate the upper and lower limbs at those levels. White matter is most abundant in the upper reaches of the cord, which contain the sensory and motor pathways serving all four limbs. For example, within the dorsal funiculus, the gracile fasciculus carries information from the lower limb and is present at the cervical as well as lumbosacral segmental levels, whereas the cuneate fasciculus carries information from the upper limb and is not seen at the lumbar level.

Although, as mentioned, it is convenient to refer to different levels of the spinal cord in terms of numbered segments corresponding to the sites of attachment of the paired nerve roots, the cord shows no evidence of segmentation internally. The nuclear groups seen in transverse sections are in reality a series of discontinuous cell columns, most of them spanning several segments (Fig. 15.2).

Types of Spinal Neurons

The smallest neurons (soma diameters of 5 to 20 μm) are *interneurons*, and their cell bodies are contained within the cord.

While the processes of some interneurons are confined within a single segment, others send their axons into the white matter surrounding the grey matter and ascend or descend two or more segments, interconnecting different spinal cord segments. These latter processes are termed *propriospinal fibres* and form the *fasciculi proprii.* Many of these smallest neurons participate in spinal reflexes. Others are intermediate cell stations interposed between fibre tracts descending from the brain and motor neurons projecting to cells controlling locomotion. Others are so placed as to influence sensory transmission from lower to higher levels of the central nervous system (CNS).

Medium-sized neurons (soma diameters of 20 to 50 μm) are found in most parts of the grey matter. Most are *relay (projection) cells* receiving inputs from dorsal root afferents and projecting their axons to the brain. The projections are in the form of *tracts*, a tract being defined as a functionally homogeneous group of fibres. As will be seen, the term 'tract' is often used loosely because many projections originally thought to be 'pure' contain more than one functional class of fibre.

The largest neurons of all are the α **motor neurons** (soma diameters of 50 to 100 μm) that innervate skeletal muscles. Scattered among them are smaller γ **motor neurons** supplying muscle spindles. In the medial part of the ventral horn are **Renshaw cells**, which exert a tonic inhibition upon α motor neurons.

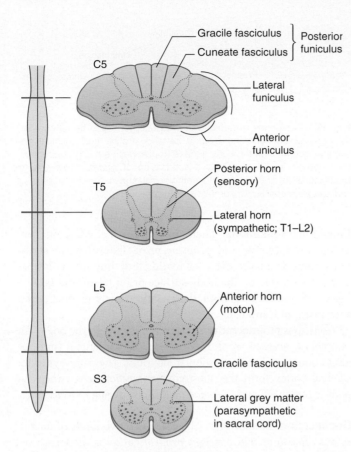

Fig. 15.1 Representative transverse sections of the spinal cord. (From Vedantam A, Bruera E, Hess KR, Dougherty PM, Viswanathan A. Somatotopy and organization of spinothalamic tracts in the human cervical spinal cord. *Neurosurgery* 2019;84(6):E311–E317; Yuengert R, Hori K, Kibodeaux EE, et al. Origin of a non-Clarke's column division of the dorsal spinocerebellar tract and the role of caudal proprioceptive neurons in motor function. *Cell Rep.* 2015;13(6):1258-1271.)

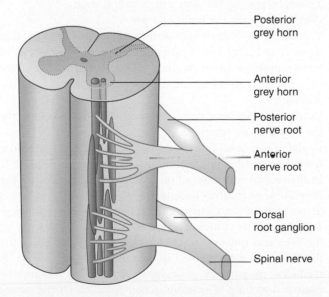

Fig. 15.2 Two segments of the spinal cord, showing cell columns in the ventral grey horn.

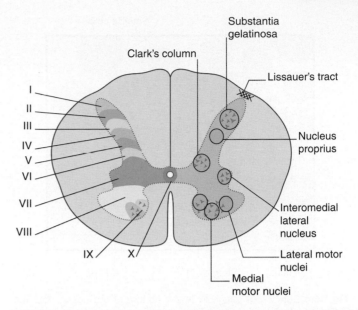

Fig. 15.3 Laminae (I to X) and named cell groups at midthoracic level.

Spinal reflex arcs originating in muscle spindles and tendon organs have been described in Chapter 10 and are part of the withdrawal reflex as described in Chapter 14.

On the basis of cytoarchitectonic characteristics (e.g., neuronal size, staining characteristics, receptors, and connectivity), the spinal cord grey matter is divided into 10 layers, the **laminae of Rexed**, that serve a descriptive but not necessarily functional purpose. Their configuration differs at various levels of the spinal cord; at some spinal cord levels, specific cell columns are recognised within the laminae, whereas in others, they are less clear (Fig. 15.3).

Spinal Ganglia

The spinal or dorsal root ganglia are located on the dorsal root in the intervertebral foramina, where the ventral and dorsal roots come together to form the spinal nerves. Thoracic ganglia contain about 50,000 unipolar neurons and spinocerebellar pathways serving the limbs contain about 100,000. These neurons are described as unipolar (or more correctly pseudounipolar). Their axons are morphologically indistinguishable from their dendrites because their somas are attached by a short **stem axon**. The individual ganglion cells are invested with modified Schwann cells called **satellite cells** (Fig. 15.4).

Central Terminations of Dorsal Root Afferents (Fig. 15.5). In the **dorsal root entry zone** close to the surface of the cord, the afferent fibres become segregated into medial and lateral divisions. The medial division comprises medium and large fibres that divide within the dorsal funiculus into ascending and descending branches. The branches swing into the dorsal grey horn and may synapse in the nucleus dorsalis (also known as the dorsal nucleus of Clarke). The largest ascending fibres run all the way to the dorsal column nuclei (gracilis/cuneatus) in the medulla oblongata, forming the bulk of the gracile and cuneate fasciculi.

The lateral division comprises small (Aδ and C) fibres, which upon entry divide into short ascending and descending branches within the **Lissauer tract** and synapse upon neurons

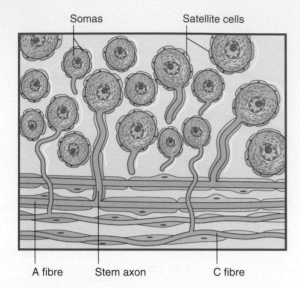

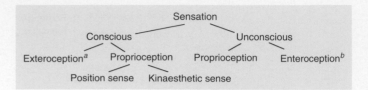

Fig. 15.6 Categories of sensation. Exteroceptors[a] can be categorised as *telereceptors* receiving from a distance (retina and cochlea) and somatic receptors on the body surface (touch, pain, etc.). Enteroceptors[b] (*Gr. enteron*, 'gut') are strictly a subdivision of *interoceptors*, a term signifying all of the viscera. In pathological states they may produce conscious visceral/viscerosomatic sensations.

Conscious Sensations. There are two types of conscious sensation: *exteroceptive* and *proprioceptive*. Exteroceptive sensations come from the external world; they impinge either on somatic receptors on the body surface or on telereceptors serving vision and hearing. Somatic sensations include touch, pressure, heat, cold, and pain.

Conscious proprioceptive sensations arise within the body. The receptors concerned are those of the locomotor system (muscles, joints, bones) and of the vestibular labyrinth. The pathways to the cerebral cortex form the substrate for *position sense* when the body is stationary, and for *kinaesthetic sense* during movement.

Unconscious Sensations. There are also two kinds of unconscious sensations. *Unconscious proprioception* is the term used to describe afferent information reaching the cerebellum through the spinocerebellar pathways. This information is essential for smooth motor coordination. The second is *interoception*, although it is a little-used term referring to unconscious afferent signals involved in visceral reflexes.

Sensory Testing

Routine assessment of *somatic exteroceptive sensation* includes tests for the following:
- Touch, by grazing the skin with a cotton swab
- Pain, by applying the point of a pin
- Thermal sense, by applying warm or cold test tubes to the skin

In alert and cooperative patients, active and passive tests of conscious proprioception can be performed. Active tests examine the patient's ability to execute set-piece activities with the eyes closed:
- In the erect position, stand still, and with feet together 'toe the line' without swaying.
- In the seated position, bring the index finger to the nose from the extended position of the arm (finger-to-nose test).
- In the recumbent position, place the heel of the foot on the opposite knee (heel-to-knee test).

Passive tests of conscious proprioception include the following:
- *Joint sense.* The clinician grasps the thumb or great toe by the sides and moves it while asking the patient to name the direction of movement (up or down). Joint sense is mediated in part by articular receptors but mainly by passive stretching of neuromuscular spindles. (If the nerves supplying a joint are anaesthetised or if the joint is completely replaced by a prosthesis, joint sense is only

Fig. 15.4 Dorsal root ganglion. In the bottom of the figure, note the T-shaped bifurcation of stem fibres, which explains why the neurons are described as 'pseudounipolar'.

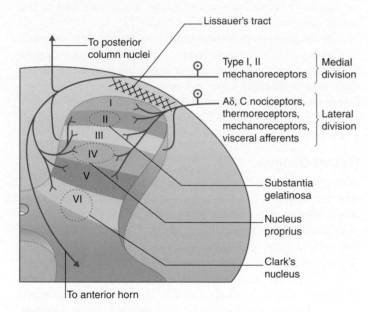

Fig. 15.5 Targets of primary afferent neurons in the dorsal grey horn.

of the substantia gelatinosa; some fibres synapse upon dendrites of cells belonging to the nucleus proprius. The nucleus proprius gives rise to the spinothalamic tract.

ASCENDING SENSORY PATHWAYS

Categories of Sensation

In accordance with the flowchart in Fig. 15.6, neurologists speak of two kinds of sensation, conscious and unconscious. Conscious sensations are perceived at the level of the cerebral cortex. Unconscious sensations are not perceived and they are relayed to the cerebellum.

slightly impaired.) Alternatively, activation of spindles by means of a vibrator creates the illusion of movement when the relevant joint is stationary.

- *Vibration sense.* The clinician assesses the patient's ability to detect the vibrations of a tuning fork applied proximal to the nail bed of the fingernail or toenail.

SOMATIC SENSORY PATHWAYS

Two major pathways are involved in somatic sensory perception. They are the *dorsal column—medial lemniscal pathway* and the *spinothalamic (ventrolateral) tract*. They have the following features in common (Fig. 15.7):

- Both comprise a first-order, second-order, and third-order set of sensory neurons.
- The somas of the first-order neurons, or *primary afferents*, are found in the dorsal root ganglia.
- The somas of the second-order neurons are located in the CNS grey matter on the same side as the first-order neurons.
- The second-order axons *cross the midline* and then ascend to terminate in the thalamus.

- The third-order neurons project from the thalamus to the somatosensory cortex (Brodmann areas 3, 1, and 2).
- Both pathways are *somatotopic*: an orderly map of body parts can be identified experimentally in the grey matter at each of the three loci of fibre termination.
- Synaptic transmission from primary to secondary neurons and from secondary to tertiary neurons can be modulated (inhibited or enhanced) by other neurons.

Dorsal Column—Medial Lemniscal Pathway

The first-order afferents include the largest somas in the dorsal root ganglia. Their peripheral processes collectively receive information from the largest sensory receptors: Meissner and Pacini corpuscles, Ruffini endings and Merkel cell—neurite complexes, neuromuscular spindles, and Golgi tendon organs. The central processes from cells supplying the lower limb and lower trunk give branches to the spinal cord grey matter before ascending as the *fasciculus gracilis* to reach the nucleus gracilis in the medulla oblongata (Fig. 15.8). The corresponding fibres from the upper limb and upper trunk form the *fasciculus cuneatus* to reach the nucleus cuneatus.

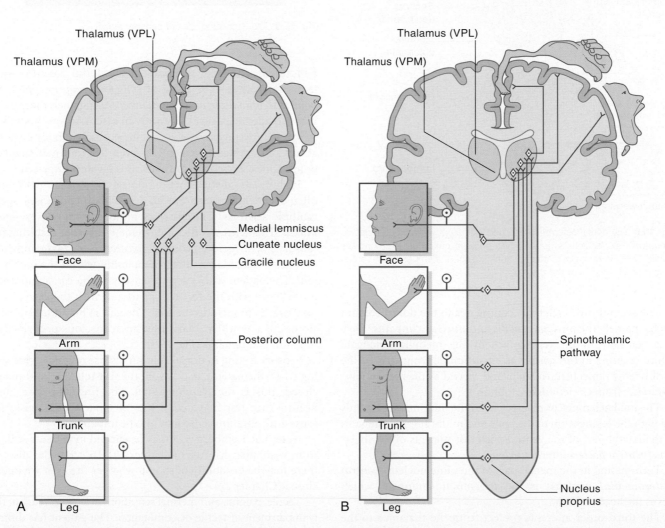

Fig. 15.7 Basic plans of the (A) dorsal column—medial lemniscal pathway and (B) spinothalamic tract. *VPL,* Ventral posterolateral nuclei of the thalamus; *VPM,* ventral posteromedial nuclei of the thalamus.

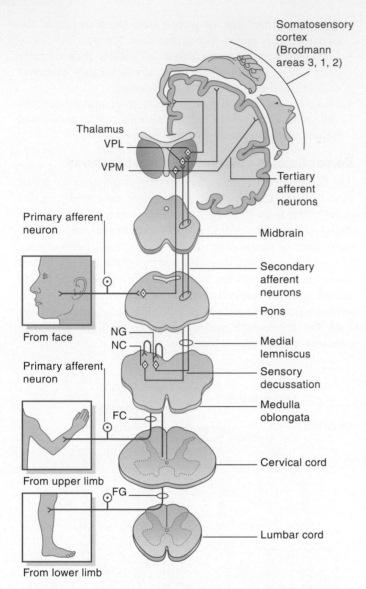

Fig. 15.8 The dorsal column—medial lemniscal pathway. *FC*, Fasciculus cuneatus; *FG*, fasciculus gracilis; *NC*, nucleus cuneatus; *NG*, nucleus gracilis; *VPL*, ventral posterolateral nuclei of the thalamus; *VPM*, ventral posteromedial nuclei of the thalamus.

The second-order afferents commence in the dorsal column nuclei, namely the **nucleus gracilis** and **nucleus cuneatus**. They pass ventrally in the tegmentum of the medulla oblongata before crossing in the **sensory decussation**. Having crossed the midline, the fibres turn rostrally and ascend as the **medial lemniscus** (*L.*, from *Gr. lēmniskos*, 'ribbon').

The medial lemniscus diverges from the midline as it ascends through the tegmentum of the pons and midbrain. It terminates in the lateral part of the ventral posterior nucleus of the thalamus (**ventral posterolateral nucleus**).

Terminating in the medial part of the same nucleus (**ventral posteromedial nucleus**) is the *trigeminal lemniscus*, which serves the head region.

The third-order afferents project from the thalamus to the somatosensory cortex (Brodmann areas 3, 1, and 2) (see Chapter 28 for details).

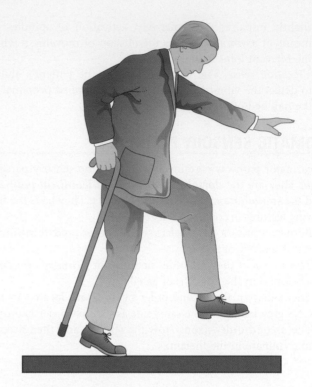

Fig. 15.9 The 'stomping' gait of sensory ataxia.

Functions. The chief functions of the dorsal column—medial lemniscal pathway are those of *conscious proprioception, two-point discrimination, and vibration sense.* Together, these modalities provide the parietal lobe with an instantaneous body image so that we are constantly aware of the position of body parts both at rest and during movement. Without this informational background, the execution of movements is severely impaired.

In humans, disturbance of dorsal column function most often occurs in association with demyelinating diseases, such as multiple sclerosis. The classic symptom is known as *sensory ataxia*. This term signifies a movement disorder resulting from sensory impairment, in contrast to *cerebellar ataxia*, in which a movement disorder results from a lesion within the motor system. The patient with a severe sensory ataxia can stand unsupported only with the feet well apart and with the gaze directed downwards to include the feet. The gait is broad based, with a stomping action that maximises any conscious proprioceptive function that remains (Fig. 15.9).

Sensory testing in dorsal column disease reveals severe swaying when the patient stands with the feet together and the eyes closed; this is the *Romberg sign*. The finger-to-nose and/or heel-to-knee test may reveal loss of kinaesthetic sense. Joint sense and vibration sense may also be impaired.

Note: The Romberg sign may be elicited in patients suffering from vestibular disorders (Chapter 19). In cerebellar disorders there may be instability of station whether the eyes are open or closed (Chapter 27).

Tactile, painful, and thermal sensations are preserved, but there is impairment of tactile discrimination. The patient has difficulty in discriminating between single and paired stimuli applied to the skin (*two-point discrimination test*), in identifying numbers traced on to the skin by the examiner's finger, and in distinguishing between objects of similar shape but of different textures.

Spinothalamic Tract

The spinothalamic tract consists of second-order sensory neurons projecting from the nucleus proprius (also known as the proper sensory nucleus) of the dorsal grey horn to the contralateral thalamus (Fig. 15.10). The cells of origin receive excitatory and inhibitory synapses from neurons of the substantia gelatinosa; these have important 'gating' (modulatory) effects on sensory transmission, as explained in Chapter 24.

Axons from those neurons within the dorsal grey horn cross the midline in the ventral commissure at all segmental levels. Having crossed, they run upward in the anterolateral part of the cord and form a somatotopic organisation; those from the lower spinal cord segments are more dorsal and lateral, while more rostral levels are more ventral and medial. The spinothalamic tract is joined by trigeminal afferents from the head region, and

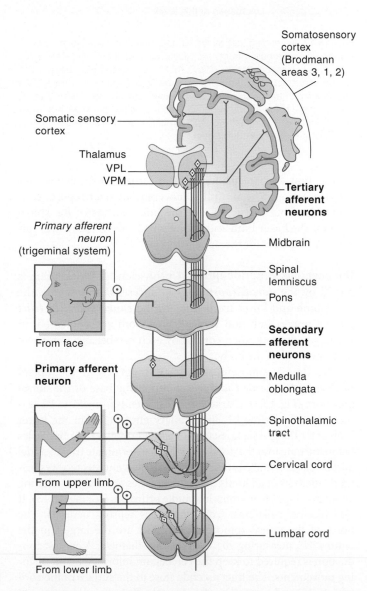

Fig. 15.10 The spinothalamic tract. *VPL*, Ventral posterolateral nuclei of the thalamus; *VPM*, ventral posteromedial nuclei of the thalamus.

they accompany the medial lemniscus to the ventral posterior nuclei of the thalamus, terminating immediately behind the medial lemniscus. The third-order sensory neurons project from the thalamus to the somatosensory cortex (Brodmann areas 3, 1, and 2) (Chapter 28).

Functions. The 'functions' of the spinothalamic tract have been confirmed by careful testing of patients who experienced a surgical procedure known as spinal *cordotomy*, whereby the spinothalamic tract was interrupted on one or both sides for the relief of intractable pain. Today, this surgery is seldom performed, as medical means for relieving intractable pain continue to improve. Considerable information was actually gained during the surgery. In a *percutaneous cordotomy* the patient is sedated and a needle is passed between the atlas and the axis into the subarachnoid space. Under radiological guidance the needle tip is advanced into the anterolateral region of the cord. A stimulating electrode is passed through the needle. If the placement is correct, a mild current will elicit paraesthesia (tingling) on the opposite side of the body. The tract is then destroyed electrolytically. Afterwards, the patient is insensitive to *pinprick*, *heat*, or *cold* applied to the opposite side (Fig. 15.11). Sensitivity to *touch* is also reduced. The effect commences several segments below the level of the procedure because of the oblique passage of spinothalamic fibres across the white commissure.

Cordotomy was sometimes performed for patients terminally ill with cancer. It is not used for benign conditions because the analgesic (pain-relieving) effect wears off after about a year. This functional recovery may be the result of nociceptive transmission either in the uncrossed fibres of the spinoreticular system (see later) or in the C-fibre collaterals sent to the dorsal column nuclei by some axons of the lateral root entry stream.

The spinothalamic tract is primarily responsible for localisation of and intensity of pain and temperature (and touch) sensation, and is at times referred to as the *neospinothalamic tract*. Other indirect tracts (one is the *paleospinothalamic tract* that projects to other thalamic nuclei) transmit the other characteristic responses to pain sensation: arousal, affective, motor, and autonomic components. As a group those tracts demonstrate less somatotopic organisation; form less discrete collections of fibres; are often polysynaptic; and develop connections with the reticular formation of the brainstem, limbic, hypothalamic, and autonomic centres. All of these tracts travel within the same area of the spinal cord and together are referred to as the **anterolateral pathway**.

A rare but classical condition illustrating dissociated sensory loss is illustrated in Clinical Panel 15.1.

Spinoreticular Tract

The spinoreticular tract is the phylogenetically oldest somatosensory pathway. The reticular formation of the brainstem has scant regard for the midline, being often bilaterally distributed in terms of its ascending and descending connections. Spinoreticular fibres originate in laminae V to VII and accompany the spinothalamic tract as far as the brainstem (Fig. 15.12). Postmortem studies of nerve fibre degeneration following cordotomy procedures indicate that at least half of the spinoreticular fibres may be uncrossed.

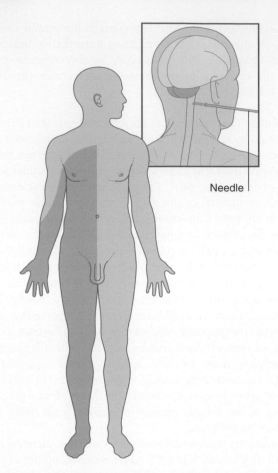

Fig. 15.11 Usual extent of analgesia (shaded) following left side cordotomy at the c1–c2 segmental level.

Accurate estimations based on axonal degeneration are difficult because some spinothalamic fibres give off collaterals to the reticular formation as they pass by.

The spinoreticular tract terminates at all levels of the brainstem and is not somatotopically organised. Neuronal activity is projected rostrally to the thalamus in the central tegmental tract (CTT) (Chapter 24). Briefly, the spinoreticular system has two interrelated functions:

1. Arouse the cerebral cortex, that is, to induce or maintain the waking state.
2. Relay to the anterior cingulate gyrus (a part of the limbic lobe) information about the nature of a stimulus producing an emotional response that may be pleasurable (e.g., to stroking) or aversive (e.g., to pinprick).

In summary, the phylogenetically old spinoreticular tract through the reticular formation is concerned with the arousal and affective (emotional) aspects of somatic sensory stimuli. In contrast, the direct spinothalamic tract (the 'neospinothalamic' tract) is analytical, encoding information about modality, intensity, and location.

Spinocerebellar Pathways

Four fibre tracts run from the spinal cord to the cerebellum:
- Dorsal spinocerebellar
- Cuneocerebellar
- Ventral spinocerebellar
- Rostral spinocerebellar

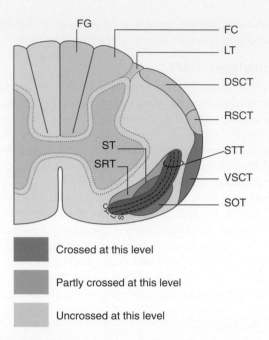

Fig. 15.12 Ascending pathways at the upper cervical level. *DSCT*, Dorsal spinocerebellar tract; *FC*, fasciculus cuneate; *FG*, fasciculus gracile; *LT*, Lissauer tract; *RSCT*, rostral spinocerebellar tract; *SOT*, spinoolivary tract; *SRT*, spinoreticular tract; *ST*, spinotectal tract; *STT*, spinothalamic tract (somatotopic laminar organization, with the *S*, sacral fibres being most superficial and *C*, cervical fibres are most deeply located, *T*, thoracic, and *L*, lumbar, are interposed as shown); *VSCT*, ventral spinocerebellar tract.

The first two are principally concerned with unconscious proprioception. The ventral spinocerebellar tract reports continuously about the activity of the interneurons of the spinal cord for the lower limb and the assumed role of the rostral spinocerebellar tract for the upper limb.

Unconscious Proprioception. Unconscious proprioception is served by the ***dorsal (posterior) spinocerebellar tract*** for the lower limb and lower trunk, and by the ***cuneocerebellar tract*** for the upper limb and upper trunk. Both are uncrossed, in keeping with the known control by each cerebellar hemisphere of its own side of the body.

The dorsal spinocerebellar tract originates in the ***dorsal nucleus of Clarke*** or ***Clarke's column*** at the base of the dorsal grey horn (Fig. 15.3). Clarke's nucleus extends from T1 to L2 segmental levels. Below L2, the primary afferents from the lower limb enter the gracile fasciculus to ascend to upper lumbar levels before turning into the dorsal grey horn to terminate in the caudal part of Clarke's nucleus (Fig. 15.12). Clarke's nucleus receives primary afferents of all kinds from the muscles and joints, including an intense input from muscle spindle primaries (see Fig. 15.13). It also receives collaterals from cutaneous sensory neurons. The fibres of the dorsal spinocerebellar tract are the largest in the entire CNS, measuring 20 μm in external diameter. Very fast conduction is required to keep the cerebellum informed about ongoing movements. The tract ascends close to the surface of the cord (Fig. 15.12) and enters the inferior cerebellar peduncle.

The ***cuneocerebellar tract*** arises from the ***accessory cuneate nucleus*** (also termed ***lateral or external cuneate nucleus***),

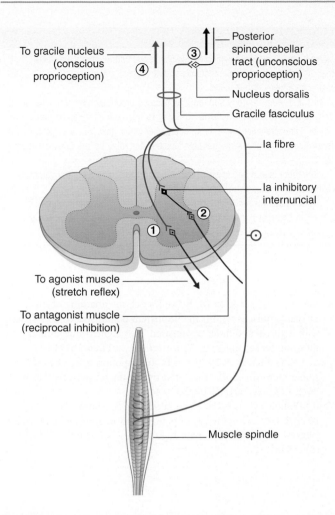

Fig. 15.13 Functional anatomy of a spindle primary afferent from the lower limb. *(1)* Stretch reflex; *(2)* Ia interneuron serving reciprocal inhibition; *(3)* unconscious proprioception; *(4)* kinaesthesia.

which lies above and outside the cuneate nucleus. The primary afferent inputs are of the same nature as those for the dorsal spinocerebellar tract and they reach the accessory cuneate nucleus through the cuneate fasciculus. The cuneocerebellar tract also contributes to the inferior cerebellar peduncle.

Information from Reflex Arcs. The main function of the ***ventral (anterior) spinocerebellar tract*** is to monitor the state of activity of spinal reflex arcs. The component fibres cross the midline at spinal levels and run close to the surface of the lateral funiculus as far as the midbrain (Fig. 15.12). They then join the *superior* cerebellar peduncle and re-cross the midline within the cerebellar white matter. (The *rostral spinocerebellar tract* arises from lower cervical spinal cord segments C7 to C8, ascends uncrossed and enters the cerebellum via the inferior and/or superior cerebellar peduncles. It is assumed to provide the same function as the ventral spinocerebellar system but for the upper limbs.)

OTHER ASCENDING PATHWAYS

The ***spinotectal tract*** runs alongside the spinothalamic tract (Fig. 15.12), which it resembles in origin and functional composition. It ends in the superior colliculus, where it joins crossed visual inputs involved in turning the eyes/head/trunk towards sources of sensory stimulation *(visuospinal reflex)*.

The ***spinoolivary tract*** sends tactile information to the *inferior olivary nucleus* in the medulla oblongata. The inferior olivary nucleus has an important function in *motor learning* through its action on the contralateral cerebellar cortex (Chapter 27). Spinoolivary discharge can modify cerebellar activity in response to environmental change; for example, while climbing a surprisingly steep stairway. This feature is called *motor adaptation*. On the other hand, learning to perform routine motor programs automatically is a function of the basal ganglia (Chapter 26).

CLINICAL PANEL 15.1 Syringomyelia

Syringomyelia (Fig. 15.14) is a disorder of uncertain aetiology, characterised by the development of a *syrinx* (fusiform cyst) in or beside the central canal, usually in the cervical region (Fig. 15.1). Initial symptoms arise from the obliteration of spinothalamic fibres decussating in the white commissure.

The early clinical picture is one of **dissociated sensory loss** (or a **commissural syndrome**): Sensitivity is lost to painful and thermal stimuli whereas sensitivity to touch and proprioception is retained because the dorsal column—medial lemniscal pathway is preserved. The sensory loss is described as a 'vested' loss of sensation because of the pattern of loss. There is usually a 'sacral sparing' of loss as the syrinx grows because of the morphology of the spinothalamic tract. Neck and arm fibres are located more medially than trunk and leg fibres. Typically, the patient develops ulcers on the fingers arising from painless cuts and burns. The joints of the elbow, wrist, and hand may become disorganised over time, or even dislocated, owing to loss of warning sensation from the stretched joint capsules. Progressive expansion of the syrinx may compromise conduction in the long ascending and descending pathways.

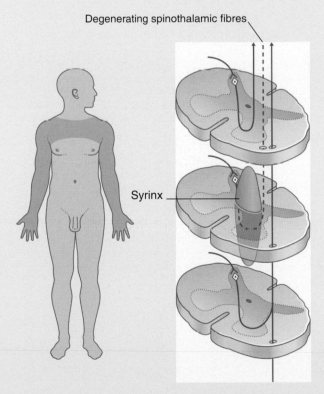

Fig. 15.14 Syringomyelia. Shading shows distribution of analgesia.

Core Information

The unipolar neurons of the spinal ganglia are first-order (primary) sensory neurons. They receive information from specific receptors in the skin, muscles, or joints. They serve all categories of somatic and visceral sensation, conscious and unconscious.

Conscious proprioception and discriminative touch are served by large central processes that ascend to the dorsal column nuclei in the medulla where the second-order neurons project via the sensory decussation to the contralateral thalamus; the third-order neurons project to the somatosensory cortex.

Discriminative painful, thermal, and more crude tactile sensations are served by fine processes that enter the Lissauer's tract and end in the dorsal grey horn; the second-order neurons project across the midline at all segmental levels, coalescing at the spinothalamic tract, which is similarly relayed by the thalamus. The spinoreticular tract projects to the brainstem reticular formation of both sides; it has an arousal function and is concerned with qualitative aspects of stimuli. Together with the spinothalamic and spinotectal tracts, they form the anterolateral pathway of the spinal cord.

The first-order neurons serving unconscious proprioception from the lower body end in the Clarke's nucleus, for relay to the ipsilateral cerebellum by the dorsal spinocerebellar tract. From the upper body, they run via the cuneate fasciculus to the accessory cuneate nucleus for relay by the cuneocerebellar tract.

Information about activity in spinal reflex arcs is relayed by the ventral and rostral spinocerebellar tract.

The spinotectal tract (tactile function, crossed) runs to the superior colliculus for integration with visual information. The spinoolivary tract projects to the inferior olivary nucleus.

SUGGESTED READINGS

Barnes SJ, Finnerty GT. Sensory experience and cortical rewiring. *Neuroscientist.* 2010;16:186−198.

Dhnad A, Aminoff MJ. The neurology of itch. *Brain.* 2014; 137:313−322.

Greitz D. Unraveling the riddle of syringomyelia. *Neurosurg Rev.* 2006;29(4):251−263.

Lallemend F, Ernfors P. Molecular interactions underlying the specification of sensory neurons. *Trends Neurosci.* 2012;35:373−381.

McGlone F, Wessberg J, Olausson H. Discriminative and affective touch: sensing and feeling. *Neuron.* 2014;82:737−755.

Romanowski CA, Hutton M, Rowe J, et al. the anatomy of the medial lemniscus within the brainstem demonstrated at 3 Tesla with high resolution fat suppressed T1-weighted images and diffusion tensor imaging. *Neuroradiol J.* 2011;24(2):171−176.

Stecina K, Fedirchuk B, Hultborn H. Information to cerebellum on spinal motor networks mediated by the dorsal spinocerebellar tract. *J Physiol.* 2013;591:5433−5443.

Yam MF, Loh YC, Tan CS, Khadijah Adam S, Abdul Manan N, Basir R. General pathways of pain sensation and the major neurotransmitters involved in pain regulation. *Int J Mol Sci.* 2018;19 (8):2164.

Spinal Cord: Descending Pathways

STUDY GUIDELINES

1. Reproduce the tracts descending the spinal cord and recall that each is strategically placed for access to its particular set of motor neurons, in accordance with the layout in Fig. 16.7.
2. Identify target neurons selected by the lateral corticospinal tract.
3. Describe how the reticulospinal tracts are concerned with automatic movements and with postural fixation.
4. Summarise the Clinical Panels dealing with upper and lower motor neuron disease and spinal cord injury and contrast upper versus lower motor neuron symptoms.

ANATOMY OF THE VENTRAL GREY HORN

Cell Columns

Each of the columns of motor neurons in the ventral grey horn supplies a group of muscles with similar functions (Table 16.1). The individual muscles are supplied from cell groups (neurons) within the columns. Axial (trunk) muscles are supplied from the medially placed motor columns, proximal limb segment muscles from the mid-region, and distal limb segment muscles from the lateral columns (Fig. 16.1). Columns supplying extensor muscles lie anterior to those supplying flexors. The autonomic nervous system is represented by the intermediolateral cell column.

Cell Types

Large α *motor neurons* supply the extrafusal fibres of skeletal muscles. Interspersed among them are small γ *motor neurons* that supply the intrafusal fibres of neuromuscular spindles.

TABLE 16.1 The Somatomotor Cell Columns.

Cell Column	Muscles
Ventromedial (all segments)	Erector spinae
Dorsomedial (T1–L2)	Intercostals, abdominals
Ventrolateral (C5–C8, L2–S2)	Arm/thigh
Dorsolateral (C6–C8, L3–S3)	Forearm/leg
Retrodorsolateral (C8, T1, S1–S2)	Hand/foot
Central (C3–C5)	Diaphragm

Tonic and Phasic Motor Neurons. The α motor neurons have large dendritic trees receiving some ten thousand excitatory boutons from propriospinal neurons and from supraspinal pathways descending from the cerebral cortex and brainstem. (The term *supraspinal* refers to any pathway descending to the cord from a higher level.) The somas of α motor neurons receive some five thousand inhibitory boutons, mainly from propriospinal sources.

Two principal types of α motor neurons are recognised: tonic and phasic. Tonic α motor neurons innervate slow oxidative (red) muscle fibres; they are readily depolarised and have relatively slow conducting axons with small spike amplitudes. Phasic α motor neurons innervate fast glycolytic (white) muscle fibres. The phasic neurons are larger, have higher thresholds, and have rapidly conducting axons with large spike amplitudes. Tonic neurons are usually the first recruits when voluntary movements are initiated, even if the movement is to be fast.

Renshaw Cells. The axons of the α motor neurons give off recurrent branches, which form excitatory cholinergic synapses upon inhibitory interneurons called *Renshaw cells* in the medial part of the ventral horn. The Renshaw cells form inhibitory, *glycinergic* synapses upon the α motor neurons. This is a classic example of *negative feedback*, or *recurrent inhibition*, through which the discharges of α motor neurons are self-limiting (cf. Clinical Panel 8.1).

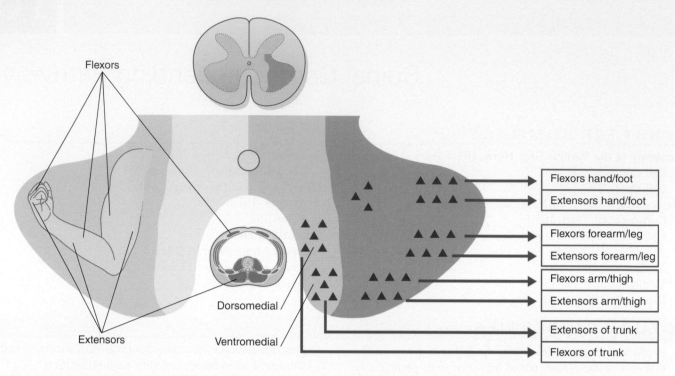

Fig. 16.1 Cell columns in the ventral grey horn of the spinal cord: somatotopic organisation.

Segmental-Level Inputs to α Motor Neurons. At each segmental level, α motor neurons receive powerful inputs from muscle spindles, Golgi tendon organs, and joint capsules. Note that any inhibitory effect produced by activity in dorsal nerve root fibres requires interpolation of inhibitory interneurons because all primary afferent neurons are excitatory in nature.

Segmental-level inputs to a flexor α motor neuron include the following:

- Type Ia and type II afferents from spindles in the flexor muscles provide the afferent limb of the monosynaptic stretch reflex (e.g. the biceps reflex).
- Type Ia afferents from spindles in extensor muscles exert reciprocal inhibition upon the flexor motor neurons via Ia inhibitory interneurons. Type Ib afferents from Golgi tendon organs in the flexor muscles exert autogenic inhibition upon the flexor motor neurons.
- Type Ib afferents from Golgi tendon organs in extensor muscles exert reciprocal excitation of flexors via excitatory interneurons. Afferents from the flexor aspect of relevant synovial joints are stimulated when the capsule becomes taut in extension. They initiate an articular protective reflex, as described in Chapter 10.
- In execution of the withdrawal reflex described in Chapter 14, large numbers of excitatory 'flexor reflex' interneurons are activated over several spinal segments on the same side as the stimulus, as well as inhibitory interneurons supplying motor neurons to antagonist muscles.
- Renshaw cells.

A reciprocal list can be drawn up for extensor motor neurons, with substitution of extensor thrust inputs for flexor reflex interneurons.

DESCENDING MOTOR PATHWAYS

Important pathways descending to the spinal cord are:
- Corticospinal (pyramidal tracts)
- Reticulospinal (extrapyramidal tracts)
- Vestibulospinal
- Tectospinal
- Raphespinal
- Aminergic
- Autonomic

Corticospinal Tract

The corticospinal tract is the great voluntary motor pathway. About 30% of its fibres take their origin from the primary motor cortex in the precentral gyrus. Other sources include the supplementary motor area on the medial side of the hemisphere. About 30% originate from the premotor cortex on the lateral side and 40% of the corticospinal tract originate from the somatosensory cortex and the parietal lobe (Fig. 16.2). The contributions from the two sensory areas mentioned terminate in the sensory nuclei of the brainstem and spinal cord, where they modulate sensory transmission.

The corticospinal tract descends through the corona radiata and posterior limb of the internal capsule to reach the brainstem. It continues through the crus (cerebral peduncle) of the midbrain and the basilar pons to reach the medulla oblongata (Fig. 16.3). Here it forms the **pyramid** (hence the synonym, *pyramidal tract*).

During its descent through the brainstem, the corticospinal tract gives off fibres that activate motor cranial nerve nuclei, notably those serving the muscles of the face, jaw, and tongue.

These fibres are called ***corticobulbar*** (Fig. 16.4). (The term '*corticonuclear*' is also used because the term 'bulb' is open to different interpretations.)

At the ***spinomedullary junction*** (Fig. 16.5):
- About 80% (70% to 90%) of the fibres cross the midline in the ***pyramidal decussation***.

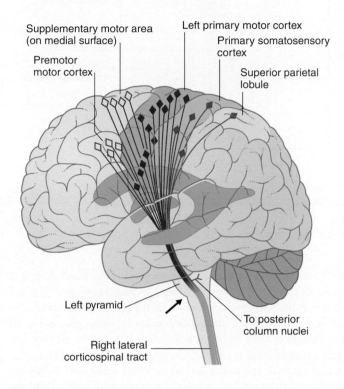

Fig. 16.2 Pyramidal tract visualised from the left side. The supplementary motor area is on the medial surface of the hemisphere. The *arrow* indicates the level of pyramidal decussation. Nonmotor neurons are shown in *blue*.

- These fibres descend on the contralateral side of the spinal cord as the ***lateral corticospinal tract*** (crossed corticospinal tract).
- About 10% of the fibres that do not decussate enter the ***ventral corticospinal tract/anterior corticospinal tract,*** which occupies the ventral/anterior funiculus and terminate at cervical and upper thoracic levels. These fibres cross in the white commissure and supply motor neurons serving muscles in the anterior and posterior abdominal walls.
- The other 10% of uncrossed fibres join the lateral corticospinal tract on the same side.

The corticospinal tract is stated to have about one million nerve fibres. The average conduction velocity is 60 m/s, indicating an average fibre diameter of 10 μm (see 'rule of six' in Chapter 9). About 3% of the fibres are extra-large (up to 20 μm); they arise from ***giant neurons (cells of Betz)***, located mainly in the leg area of the motor cortex (see Chapter 29). All corticospinal fibres are excitatory and appear to use glutamate as their transmitter substance.

Targets of the Lateral Corticospinal Tract

Distal limb motor neurons. In the ventral grey horn, lateral corticospinal tract axons may directly synapse upon the dendrites of α and γ motor neurons supplying limb muscles, notably in the upper limb, but typically do so via interneurons within the spinal cord grey matter. Individual axons within the lateral corticospinal tract may activate either 'large' or 'small' motor units. A ***motor unit*** consists of a ventral horn cell and all the muscle fibres it innervates. Neurons of small motor units selectively innervate a small number of muscle fibres and play a role in performing delicate and precise movements such as those required to play the piano. Ventral horn cells controlling a muscle such as the gluteus maximus individually excite

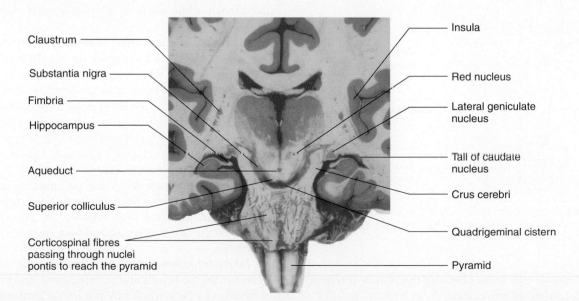

Fig. 16.3 Coronal section of embalmed brain following treatment with copper sulphate (mulligan stain), showing unstained corticospinal fibres displacing nuclei pontis en route to the pyramid. (Illustration kindly provided by Professor David Yew, University of Hong Kong.)

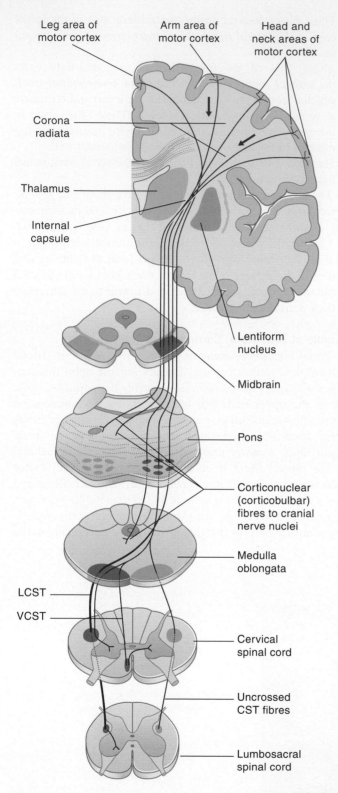

Fig. 16.4 The pyramidal tract. *Note:* Only the motor components are shown; the parietal lobe components are omitted. *LCST,* Lateral corticospinal tract; *VCST,* ventral corticospinal tract.

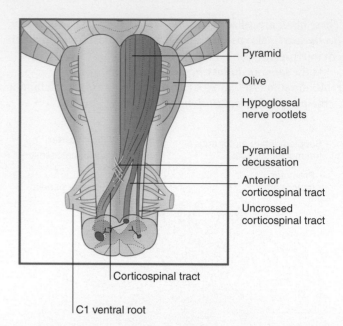

Fig. 16.5 Ventral view of medulla oblongata and upper spinal cord, showing the three spinal projections of the left pyramid.

hundreds of muscle cells at once because this muscle is responsible for gross, unrefined movements.

A unique property of these *corticomotoneuronal* fibres of the lateral corticospinal tract is the concept of fractionation, relating to the variable activity of interneurons, whereby small groups of neurons can be selectively activated to perform a specific function. It is most obvious in the case of the index finger, which can be flexed or extended quite independently, although three of its long tendons arise from muscle bellies devoted to all four fingers. Fractionation is essential for the execution of skilled movements such as buttoning a coat or tying shoelaces. Following damage to the corticomotoneuronal system anywhere from the motor cortex to the spinal cord, skilled movements are lost and seldom recover completely.

As mentioned already in Chapter 10, the α and γ motor neurons are coactivated by the lateral corticospinal tract during a given movement, so that spindles in the prime movers signal active stretch while those in the antagonists signal passive stretch.

Renshaw cells. The number of possible functions served by lateral corticospinal tract synapses on Renshaw cells is large because some of the cells synapse mainly upon Ia inhibitory interneurons and others upon other Renshaw cells. Probably the most important function is to permit *cocontraction* of prime movers and their antagonists in order to fix one or more joints, such as when a chopping or shoveling action is required of the hand. Cocontraction is achieved by the inactivation of Ia inhibitory interneurons by Renshaw cells.

Excitatory interneurons. In the intermediate grey matter and the base of the ventral horn, motor neurons supplying axial (vertebral) and proximal limb muscles are mainly recruited indirectly by the lateral corticospinal tract, by way of excitatory interneurons.

Ia inhibitory interneurons. Also located in the intermediate grey matter are the Ia inhibitory interneurons, and these are the *first* neurons to be activated by the lateral corticospinal tract during voluntary movements. Activity of the Ia interneurons causes the antagonist muscles to relax before the prime movers

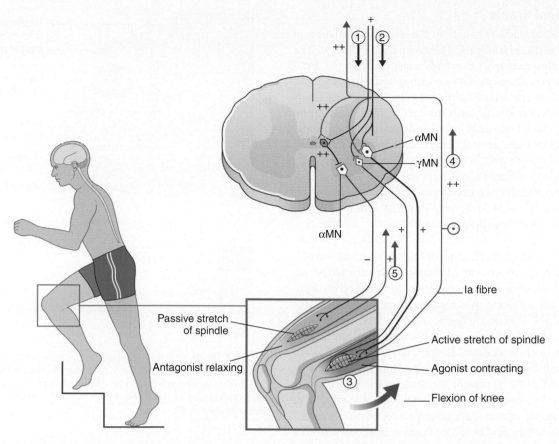

Fig. 16.6 Sequence of events in a voluntary movement (flexion of the knee). *(1)* Activation of Ia interneurons to inhibit antagonist α motor neurons (αMN); *(2)* activation of agonist α and γ motor neurons; *(3)* activation of extrafusal and intrafusal muscle fibres; *(4)* feedback from actively stretched spindles increases excitation of agonist α motor neurons and inhibition of antagonist α motor neuron; *(5)* Ia fibres from passively stretched antagonist spindles will find the respective α motor neurons refractory. *Note:* The sequence γ motor neuron—Ia fibre—α motor neuron is known as the *γ loop.*

(agonists) contract. In addition, it renders the antagonists' motor neurons refractory to stimulation by spindle afferents passively stretched by the movement. The sequence of events for voluntary flexion of the knee is shown in Fig. 16.6 and its caption.

(*Note on terminologies:* During quiet standing, the knees are 'locked' in slight hyperextension and the quadriceps is inactive, as indicated by the patellae being 'loose'. Any tendency of one or both knees to go into flexion is counteracted by a twitch of quadriceps in response to passive stretching of dozens of muscle spindles there. Because the flexion movement is resisted in this way, the reflex concerned is called a *resistance reflex.* During voluntary flexion of the knee, on the other hand, the movement is helped along in the manner described in the caption to Fig. 16.6, through an *assistance reflex.* The *change of sign*, from negative to positive, is called *reflex reversal.*)

Presynaptic inhibitory neurons serving the stretch reflex. Consider a sprinter. At each stride, gravity pulls the body out of the air onto a knee extended by the quadriceps muscle. At the moment of impact, all of the muscle spindles in the contracted quadriceps are thrown into active stretch. The obvious danger is that the quadriceps may rupture. Golgi tendon endings (see Chapter 10) offer some protection through autogenic inhibition, but the main protection seems to be through presynaptic

inhibition by the lateral corticospinal tract of spindle afferents close to their contact points with motor neurons. At the same time, preservation of the ankle jerk is advantageous in this situation, giving immediate recruitment of calf motor neurons for the next take-off. The extent of suppression of the stretch reflex by the lateral corticospinal tract in fact appears to depend upon the particular motor program being executed.

Presynaptic inhibition of first-order afferents. In the dorsal grey horn, there is some suppression of sensory transmission into the spinothalamic tract during voluntary movement. This is brought about by the activation of inhibitory interneurons synapsing upon primary afferent nerve terminals.

Modulation is more subtle at the level of the gracile and cuneate nuclei, where pyramidal tract fibres (after crossing) are capable of either enhancing sensory transmission during slow, exploratory movements or reducing it during rapid movements.

Upper and Lower Motor Neurons

In the context of disease, clinicians refer to the corticospinal (and corticobulbar) neurons as ***upper motor neurons*** (Clinical Panel 16.1) and those of the brainstem and spinal cord as ***lower motor neurons*** (Clinical Panel 16.2).

Reticulospinal Tracts

The reticulospinal tracts originate in the reticular formation of the pons and medulla oblongata. They are partially crossed. The **pontine reticulospinal tract** descends ipsilaterally in the anterior funiculus, and the **medullary reticulospinal tract** descends, partly crossed, in the lateral funiculus (Fig. 16.7). Both tracts act, via interneurons shared with the corticospinal tract, upon motor neurons supplying axial (trunk) and proximal limb muscles. Information from animal experiments indicates that the pontine reticulospinal tract acts upon extensor motor neurons and the medullary reticulospinal tract acts upon flexor motor neurons. Both pathways exert reciprocal inhibition. The reticulospinal system is involved in two different kinds of motor behaviour: *locomotion* and *postural control*.

Locomotion. Walking and running are rhythmic events involving all four limbs. Movements of the two sides are reciprocal with respect to flexor and extensor contractions and relaxations. In lower animals, locomotion is regulated by a hierarchical system in which the lowest members are interneurons on both sides at cervical and lumbosacral levels, activating the flexors and extensors of the individual limbs. They are called *pattern generators*. Coordinating the pattern generators for the individual limbs is a further generator situated in the intermediate grey matter at the upper end of the spinal cord; it is capable of initiating rhythmic movements after section of the neuraxis at the spinomedullary junction. Locomotion is initiated from a *locomotor centre* located in the lower midbrain of humans and in the pons in laboratory animals. In anaesthetised cats, electrical stimulation of the locomotor centre with pulses of increasing frequency produces walking movements, then trotting, and finally galloping.

Although the basic locomotor patterns are inbuilt, they are modulated by sensory feedback from the terrain. Overall control of the motor output resides in the premotor cortex, which has direct projections to the brainstem neurons that give rise to the reticulospinal tracts. The tracts are used to steer the animal as it walks or runs and to override the spinal generators, such as when scaling a wall.

Human locomotion is less 'spinal' than that of quadrupeds. However, the general neuroanatomic framework has been conserved during higher evolution, and the basic physiology seems to be in place as well. In particular, a bilaterally organised motor system controlling proximal and axial muscles *must* exist to account for the return of near-perfect locomotor function following removal of an entire cerebral hemisphere during childhood or adolescence. Such people never recover manual skill on the contralateral side, and this reinforces the belief among physical therapists that two distinct pathways are involved in motor control: *pyramidal* and *extrapyramidal*. The latter term denotes the reticulospinal tract and its controls upstream in the cerebral cortex and basal ganglia.

Higher-level locomotor controls are described in Chapter 24.

Posture. Definitions of *posture* vary with the context in which the term is used. In the general context of standing, sitting, and recumbency, posture may be defined as *the position held*

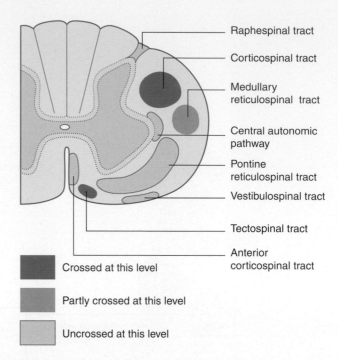

Crossed at this level

Partly crossed at this level

Uncrossed at this level

Raphespinal tract
Corticospinal tract
Medullary reticulospinal tract
Central autonomic pathway
Pontine reticulospinal tract
Vestibulospinal tract
Tectospinal tract
Anterior corticospinal tract

Fig. 16.7 Descending pathways at the upper cervical level. *Notes:* The ventral corticospinal tract/anterior corticospinal tract crosses partially at the lower cervical level and engages ventral horn cells supplying postural muscles of the trunk. Some 10% of corticospinal tract fibres descend ipsilaterally.

between movements. In the local context of a single hand or foot, the term signifies *postural fixation*, the immobilisation of proximal limb joints by cocontraction of the surrounding muscles, leaving the distal limb parts free to do voluntary business. As will be noted in Chapter 29, there is reason to believe that the human premotor cortex is programmed to select appropriate proximal muscle groups by way of the reticulospinal tracts, to set the stage for any particular movement of the hand or foot.

The interpolation of interneurons between the two main motor pathways acting upon motor neurons serving axial and proximal limb muscles means that either pathway may be in command for a particular movement sequence—the extrapyramidal (reticulospinal) pathway for routine tasks such as walking along a clear path and the pyramidal pathway for tasks requiring close attention such as picking one's way along a path strewn with rubble.

Tectospinal Tract

The tectospinal tract is a crossed pathway descending from the tectum of the midbrain to the medial part of the ventral grey horn at cervical and upper thoracic levels. It is strategically placed for access to axial motor neurons (Fig. 16.7). This tract is an important motor pathway in the reptilian brain, being responsible for orienting the head/trunk towards sources of visual stimulation (superior colliculus) or auditory stimulation (inferior colliculus). It is likely to have similar automatic functions in humans.

Vestibulospinal Tract

The vestibulospinal tract is an important uncrossed pathway whereby the tone of appropriate antigravity muscles is automatically increased when the head is tilted to one side. It descends in the anterior funiculus (Fig. 16.7), and its function is to keep the centre of gravity between the feet. It originates in the vestibular nucleus in the medulla oblongata. (*Note:* As explained in Chapter 19, there are in fact two vestibulospinal tracts on each side. The unqualified term refers to the lateral vestibulospinal tract.)

Raphespinal Tract

The raphespinal tract originates in and beside the raphe nucleus situated in the midline in the medulla oblongata. It descends on both sides within the dorsolateral tract of Lissauer. Its function is to modulate sensory transmission between first order and second order neurons in the dorsal grey horn, particularly with respect to pain (see Chapter 24).

Aminergic Pathways

Aminergic pathways descend from specialised cell groups in the pons and medulla oblongata (see Chapter 24). The principal neurotransmitters involved are *norepinephrine* and *serotonin*, both of which are classified as biogenic amines. The aminergic pathways descend in the outer parts of the ventral and lateral funiculi and are distributed widely in the spinal grey matter. In general terms, they have inhibitory effects on sensory neurons and facilitatory effects on motor neurons.

Central Autonomic Pathways

Central sympathetic and parasympathetic fibres descend laterally to the intermediate grey matter (Fig. 16.7). Sympathetic fibres originate from autonomic control centres in the hypothalamus while parasympathetic fibres originate from several nuclear groups in the brainstem. These sympathetic central fibres terminate in the intermediolateral cell columns that give rise to the preganglionic sympathetic fibres. The intermediolateral cell columns reside in the lateral horn, which exists from T12 through to L2. The central sympathetic pathway is required for normal *baroreceptor reflex* activity. (For example, if the spinal cord is crushed in a neck injury, the patient loses consciousness if raised from the recumbent position within the first week or so because a fall of blood pressure in the carotid sinus on sitting up normally causes a compensatory increase in sympathetic activity to maintain blood flow to the brain.)

Central parasympathetic fibres synapse on specific sacral nuclei, which control the function of various pelvic structures (e.g. the *Onuf nucleus,* which controls bladder voiding). The fibres concerned originate in the reticular formation, mainly at the level of the pons (see Chapter 24). The pontine micturition centre has a tonic inhibitory action on the sacral parasympathetic system. Severe injury to the spinal cord or cauda equina results in reflex voiding when the bladder is only half full (Clinical Panel 16.3).

Note on the Rubrospinal Tract. In humans, the rubrospinal tract is one of several motor control pathways and it has fewer axons than the corticospinal tract. The tract is thought to be responsible for large muscle movement, and it extends primarily into the cervical spinal cord, suggesting that it functions in upper limb, but not in lower limb, control. It is believed to primarily facilitate extensor motor neurons and inhibit flexor motor neurons in the upper extremities. It is small and rudimentary in humans, but in some primates over time, the rubrospinal tract can assume almost all the duties of the corticospinal tract when the corticospinal tract is cut.

It originates in the magnocellular red nucleus of the midbrain, crosses to the other side of the midbrain, and descends in the lateral part of the brainstem tegmentum. In the spinal cord it travels through the lateral funiculus of the spinal cord anterior to or overlapping the corticospinal tract.

BLOOD SUPPLY OF THE SPINAL CORD

Arteries

Close to the foramen magnum, the two vertebral arteries give off *anterior* and *posterior spinal* branches. The anterior branches fuse to form a single *anterior spinal artery* in front of the ventral median fissure (Fig. 16.7). Branches are given alternately to the left and right sides of the spinal cord. The posterior spinal arteries descend along the line of attachment of the dorsal nerve roots on each side. The two posterior spinal arteries supply the posterior one third of the spinal cord.

The three spinal arteries (Fig. 16.8) are assisted by several *radiculospinal branches* from the vertebral arteries and from intercostal arteries. They are distinguishable from the small *radicular arteries* that enter every intervertebral foramen to

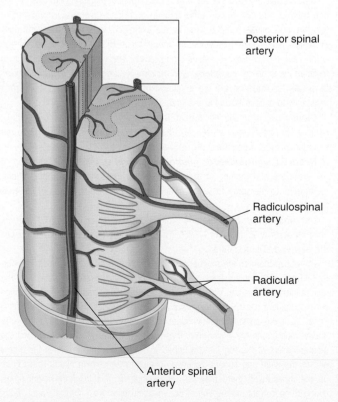

Posterior spinal artery

Radiculospinal artery

Radicular artery

Anterior spinal artery

Fig. 16.8 Arteries of the spinal cord and spinal nerve roots.

nourish the nerve roots. The largest radiculospinal artery is the *artery of Adamkiewicz*, which arises from a lower intercostal artery or upper lumbar artery on the left side and supplies the lumbar enlargement and conus medullaris.

Vascular disorders of the spinal cord are quite rare and are currently most often attributed to atherosclerotic disease or surgery of the aorta. As part of atherosclerosis, a branch of the anterior spinal artery may become occluded, causing necrosis of the anterior half of the cord on one side. The clinical picture may eventually resemble a 'one-sided amyotrophic lateral sclerosis' owing to the destruction of ventral horn motor neurons and diminished function in the lateral corticospinal tract on the same side. However, arterial disease should be suspected because of the relatively abrupt onset of symptoms and because concurrent damage to the spinothalamic tract produces loss of pain and thermal sense on the opposite side, below the level of the lesion.

There are distinct spinal cord syndromes of vascular origin, the most common of which is the *anterior spinal artery syndrome* that can occur as a complication of surgical repair of the aorta or acutely from an aortic dissection. When a vascular surgeon is attempting to deal with an abdominal aortic aneurysm, the artery of Adamkiewicz must be identified and isolated. If a clamp is placed across the aorta and the artery happens to arise below that level, the patient is at risk of a spinal cord infarction. In this setting, the anterior spinal artery syndrome is suspected when there is acute onset of symmetric lower extremity weakness, bilateral spinothalamic sensory deficit below the midthoracic level (relative hypovascularity at this level of the spinal cord making it susceptible to hypoperfusion), normal position sense, and autonomic sphincter dysfunction. The weakness may initially be flaccid and tendon reflexes may be absent, but later, hyperreflexia and a Babinski sign develop.

Veins

The venous drainage of the cord is by anterior and posterior spinal veins, which drain outwards along the nerve roots. Any obstruction to the venous outflow is liable to produce oedema of the cord, with progressive loss of function.

CLINICAL PANEL 16.1   Upper Motor Neuron Disease

Upper motor neuron disease is a clinical term used to denote interruption of the corticospinal tract somewhere along its course. If the lesion occurs above the level of the pyramidal decussation, the signs will be detected on the opposite side of the body; if it occurs below the decussation, the signs will be detected on the same side.

Sudden interruption of the corticospinal tract is characterised by the following features:

The affected limb(s) show an initial flaccid (floppy) paralysis with loss of tendon reflexes. Normal muscle tone, defined as resistance to passive movement (e.g. flexion/extension of the knee by the examiner), is lost. After several days or weeks, some return of voluntary motor function can be expected. At the same time, muscle tone increases progressively. The typical long-term effect on muscle tone is one of **spasticity**, with abnormally brisk reflexes **(hyperreflexia)**. Classically, spasticity in the leg is 'clasp knife' in character; after initial strong resistance to passive flexion of the knee, the joint gives way.

Clonus can often be elicited at the ankle/wrist. It consists of rhythmic contraction of the flexor muscles 5 to 10 times per second in response to the examiner's sudden dorsiflexion of the ankle.

Babinski sign (extensor plantar response) consists of dorsiflexion of the great toe and fanning of the other toes in response to a scraping stimulus applied to the sole of the foot. The normal response is flexion of the toes (Fig. 16.9).

The **abdominal reflexes** are absent on the affected side. A normal abdominal reflex consists of brief contraction of the abdominal muscles when the overlying skin is scraped.

The above features are most commonly observed after a vascular *stroke* interrupting the corticospinal tract on one side of the cerebrum or brainstem. The usual picture here is one of initial flaccid **hemiplegia** ('half-paralysis'), followed by a permanent spastic **hemiparesis** ('half-weakness'). As illustrated in Clinical Panel 35.3, the spasticity following a stroke characteristically affects the antigravity muscles. In the lower limb, these are the extensors of the knee and the plantar flexors of the foot; in the upper limb, they are the flexors of the elbow and of the wrist and fingers. Following complete transection of the spinal cord, on the other hand, there may be a *paraplegia in flexion* of the lower limbs, owing to concurrent interruption of the vestibulospinal tract (Clinical Panel 16.3).

Some of the 'positive' signs listed above cannot be explained based on interruption of the corticospinal tract alone. In the rare cases in which the human pyramid has been transected surgically, spasticity and hyperreflexia have not been prominent later on, although a Babinski sign has been present.

Spasticity and hyperreflexia are largely explained by the fact that stretch reflexes in spastic muscle groups are hyperactive. Electromyography (EMG) records of spastic muscles show enhanced motor unit activity in response to relatively slow rates of stretch, such as slow passive elbow extension. However, this is not the sole basis of explanation. In patients with spastic hemiparesis, the ankle flexors show increased tone (resistance to passive dorsiflexion) even with very slow rates of stretch that are too slow to elicit any EMG response. The resistance takes several weeks to become

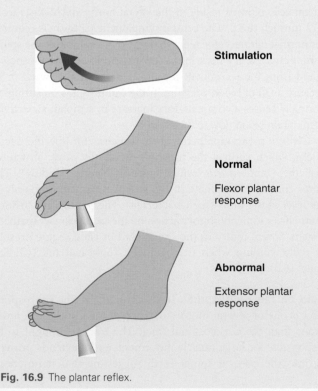

Stimulation

Normal

Flexor plantar response

Abnormal

Extensor plantar response

Fig. 16.9 The plantar reflex.

pronounced. It is called *passive stiffness* and may be caused by progressive accumulation of collagen within the muscles affected. In addition, biochemical changes within paretic muscle lead to increasing change of fast-twitch to slow-twitch fibres, accounting for progressively greater difficulty in execution of rapid movements.

Why Are Motor Neurons Hyperexcitable?

In paraplegic patients, spasticity and hyperreflexia are often accompanied by increased *cutaneomuscular reflex* excitability, through polysynaptic propriospinal pathways. Pulling on a pair of trousers may be enough to produce spasms of the hip and knee flexors, sometimes accompanied by autonomic effects (sweating, hypertension, emptying of the bladder). Where the requisite technical facilities exist, the situation can be dramatically improved by perfusion of the lumbar cerebrospinal fluid cistern with minute amounts of *baclofen*, a γ-aminobutyric acid (GABA) mimetic (imitative) drug (oral administration has a similar, but less dramatic effect). The first inference is that the drug diffuses through the pia—glial membrane of the spinal cord, activates GABA receptors located on the surface of primary afferent nerve terminals, and dampens impulse traffic by means of presynaptic inhibition. The second inference is that the resident population of GABA neurons in the substantia gelatinosa has fallen silent in these cases through loss of tonic supraspinal 'drive'. The normal source of supraspinal drive seems to derive in part from the corticospinal tract, and in part from cortico-reticulospinal fibres that reach the spinal cord via the tegmentum of the brainstem rather than via the pyramids.

Fig. 16.10 shows the distribution of inhibitory nerve endings derived from Renshaw cells. Not only do they normally have a tonic breaking action on α and γ motor neurons at their own segmental level, they also tonically inhibit heteronymous motor neurons (i.e. those serving other muscle groups). For example, they act simultaneously upon motor neurons controlling knee and ankle movements, as part of the executive arm of central motor programs regulating successive muscle engagements and disengagements during locomotion. Locomotion is controlled by reticulospinal rather than corticospinal neurons, and any reduction in reticulospinal drive will render motor neurons hyperexcitable, and accounts for the

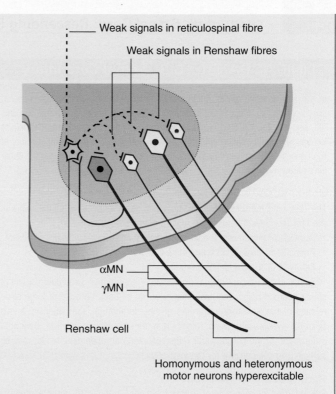

Weak signals in reticulospinal fibre

Weak signals in Renshaw fibres

αMN
γMN

Renshaw cell

Homonymous and heteronymous motor neurons hyperexcitable

Fig. 16.10 Impaired renshaw cell activity in spasticity. *MN*, Motor neurons.

frequent occurrence of ill-timed contractions produced by heteronymous motor neurons.

How Do Voluntary Movements Recover?

Multiple explanations are discussed in the final Clinical Panel in the final chapter.

CLINICAL PANEL 16.2 Lower Motor Neuron Disease

Disease that primarily affects the lower motor neurons may be seen in neurodegenerative diseases and genetic disorders or may be caused by toxins or a variety of infectious agents, notably the poliomyelitis virus. The term **motor neuron disease**, or **MND**, is used to describe this group of disorders, but the most common type is a symptom complex characterised by the prominence of the degeneration of upper and lower motor neurons (other nonmotor neuron cells are also affected) in late middle age.

During the first year or two, initial symptoms often appear in a single limb and progress in a segmental pattern; but eventually, the disease becomes widespread and involves bulbar and respiratory muscles. Clinical evidence of lower motor neuron involvement includes the following manifestations:

1. *Weakness* of the muscles affected, together with
2. *Wasting* that is not merely disuse atrophy, but results from loss of a trophic (nourishing) factor produced by motor neurons and conveyed to muscle by axonal transport.
3. *Loss of tendon reflexes* (areflexia) in the wasted muscles.
4. *Fasciculations*, which are visible twitches of small groups of muscle fibres in the early stage of wasting. They arise from spontaneous discharge of motor neurons with activation of motor units, as described in the context of EMG in Clinical Panel 12.3.
5. *Fibrillations*, which are minute contractions detectable only by needle EMG, also described in Clinical Panel 12.3.

Sooner or later, the signs of upper motor neuron disease appear, and limbs become weaker, but increased muscle tone and brisk reflexes also appear. (However, the findings so typical of upper motor neuron disease in stroke may

be less marked as the disease process disrupts the intrinsic connections within the spinal cord.) While other disorders that involve either upper or lower motor neurons are considered, the clinical and electrodiagnostic (see Chapter 12) evidence of upper and lower motor neuron involvement are characteristic of the condition called **amyotrophic lateral sclerosis (ALS)**. Motor cranial nerve nuclei in the pons and medulla oblongata may be involved from the start (*progressive bulbar palsy*, see Chapter 18) or only terminally. Median survival is 3 years, and death is from respiratory impairment and its related complications.

ALS is now considered a heterogeneous disorder and is best considered a syndrome because it may not have a single pathogenesis. It is considered a multisystem neurodegenerative disease, and degeneration of nonmotor system neurons results in other symptoms (e.g. behavioural, extrapyramidal, and sensory). More than 20 genes have so far been implicated, but their identification in sporadic cases where a family history is lacking suggests they may result in various phenotypes within individuals.

The first gene identified, superoxide dismutase 1 *(SOD1)*, encodes copper/zinc superoxide dismutase, and mutations are identified in 15% to 20% of familial cases of ALS. (However, a hexanucleotide expansion repeat in a noncoding region of the chromosome 9 open-reading frame 72 gene [*C9ORF72*] may soon eclipse its importance.) Currently the best studied of the ALS-related genes, the pathogenic mechanism of *SOD1* mutations may not be related to the gene's assumed 'function' of neutralising superoxides within the cytoplasm. Misfolding of *SOD1* with a gain-of-function can disrupt mitochondrial function and have a downstream effect that leads to oxidative stress and excitotoxicity. Clearly, the search for etiologic clues in ALS remains intense.

CLINICAL PANEL 16.3 Spinal Cord Injury

In the industrialised world, automobile accidents are the commonest cause of spinal cord injury. More than half of the victims are between 16 and 30 years old, and the cervical cord is most commonly affected. Injury at the thoracic or lumbar segmental level results in *paraplegia* (paralysis of lower limbs). Injury at the cervical level causes *tetraplegia (quadriplegia)*, in which the extent of upper limb paralysis depends on the number or level of cervical segments involved.

Spinal Shock

The following features are found below the segmental level of the injury in the first few days following a complete cord transection:

- Paralysis of movement. The limbs are flaccid and tendon reflexes are absent.
- Anaesthesia (loss of all forms of sensation).
- Paralysis of the bladder and rectum.

Spinal shock is currently attributed to a generalised hyperpolarisation of spinal neurons below the level of the lesion, perhaps because of large-scale release of the inhibitory transmitter glycine. In addition, the patient develops *postural hypotension* when raised from the recumbent position, owing to interruption of the baroreceptor reflex. (Wearing an abdominal binder may be sufficient to compensate for the lost reflex.)

Return of Spinal Function

Several days or weeks later, reflex functions of the cord become progressively restored, and 'upper motor neuron signs' appear. Muscle tone becomes excessive (spastic). Tendon reflexes become abnormally brisk. A Babinski sign can be elicited on both sides. Ankle clonus is commonly seen when a patient's leg is lifted as it is placed in a wheelchair and the leg comes into contact with the footplate.

If extensor spasticity in the lower limbs is dominant, the patient develops *paraplegia in extension*; if flexor spasticity is dominant, the patient develops *paraplegia in flexion*. An extended posture may permit *spinal standing*; it is promoted by appropriate passive placement of the limbs, and it is the rule following cord injury that is either incomplete or low. A flexed posture is promoted by repetitive mass flexor reflexes involving the ankles, knees, and hips; mass reflexes can follow any cutaneous stimulation of the legs if the flexor reflex interneurons of the cord are already sensitised by afferent discharges from a pressure sore or from an infected bladder.

The condition of the bladder is of great importance because of the twin dangers of infection and bladder stone formation. For the initial *atonic* bladder, a sterile catheter is intermittently inserted to ensure unobstructed drainage. Later, the bladder may become *automatic*, emptying itself every 4 to 6 hours through a reflex arc involving the sacral autonomic centre in the conus medullaris.

In animals, much of the damage done to the cord by injury has been shown to be secondary to local shifts in electrolyte concentrations and to vascular changes, including arterial spasm and venous thrombosis. Modest success is being achieved in counteracting these effects. Another line of experimental research is to implant *embryonic* spinal grey matter at the site of injury. These grafts often survive and establish local synaptic connections, but the goal of functional recovery has not yet been attained.

Considerable interest has been aroused by observations in several spinal rehabilitation centres, to the effect that patients with complete cord transections can be trained to activate spinal locomotor generators, as described in Chapter 24.

✷ Core Information

Fibres of the corticospinal tract governing voluntary movement originate in motor, premotor, and supplementary motor areas of the cerebral cortex; fibres governing sensory transmission during movement originate in the parietal lobe. The corticospinal tract includes corticobulbar fibres innervating motor cranial nerve nuclei. The corticospinal tract innervates ventral horn cells supplying trunk and limb muscles; 80% of these fibres cross in the pyramidal decussation and enter the lateral corticospinal tract; 10% descend ipsilaterally in the ventral/anterior corticospinal tract prior to crossing at lower levels; and 10% remain entirely ipsilateral. The corticospinal tract targets include α and γ motor neurons via the Ia inhibitory interneurons and Renshaw cells.

Clinically, the corticospinal tract is an *upper motor neuron*. Damage (e.g. in hemiplegia from stroke) is characterised by initial flaccid paralysis, later by spasticity, brisk reflexes, clonus, and the Babinski sign. *Lower motor neuron* (ventral horn cell) disease is characterised by muscle weakness, wasting, fasciculation, and loss of related segmental reflexes. Spinal cord transection is characterised by initial flaccid paraplegia/tetraplegia with areflexia, atonic bladder, and (permanent) anaesthesia below the segmental level involved;

and later by spasticity, hyperreflexia, clonus, the Babinski sign, and automatic bladder.

Reticulospinal tracts are activated by the premotor cortex. For locomotion, they originate in a midbrain locomotor centre and travel to pattern generators in the cord. For postural fixation, they originate in the pons and medulla and supply motor neurons via interneurons.

The tectospinal tract descends (crossed) from colliculi to the ventral horn; it operates to direct the gaze towards visual/auditory/tactile stimuli. The (lateral) vestibulospinal tract (uncrossed) increases antigravity tone on the side to which the head is tilted. The raphespinal tract descends from the medullary raphe nucleus to the dorsal horn via the Lissauer tract; it modulates sensory transmission, especially for pain.

A central sympathetic pathway from the hypothalamus/brainstem to the lateral horn includes the efferent limb of the baroreceptor reflex. A central parasympathetic pathway activates the bladder and rectum.

The cord receives spinal branches from the vertebral arteries, assisted by radiculospinal arteries at segmental levels. Venous drainage is into segmental veins.

SUGGESTED READINGS

Alstermark B, Isa T. Circuits for skilled reaching and grasping. *Annu Rev Neurosci*. 2012;35:559—578.

Arber S. Motor circuits in action: specification, connectivity, and function. *Neuron*. 2012;74:975—989.

Bican O, Minagar A, Pruitt AA. The spinal cord: a review of functional anatomy. *Neurol Clin*. 2013;31:1—18.

Davis-Dusenbery BN, Williams LA, Klim JR, Eggan K. How to make spinal motor neurons. *Development*. 2014;141:491—501.

Guertin PA. Central pattern generator for locomotion: anatomical, physiological, and pathophysiological considerations. *Front Neurol*. 2013;3:183.

Lemon RN, Landau W, Tutssel D, Lawrence DG. Lawrence and Kuypers (1968a, b) revisited: copies of the original filmed material from their classic papers in Brain. *Brain*. 2012;135:2290—2295.

Miri A, Azim E, Jessell TM. Edging toward entelechy in motor control. *Neuron*. 2013;80:827−834.

Peng J, Charron F. Lateralization of motor control in the human nervous system: genetics of mirror movements. *Curr Opin Neurobiol*. 2013;23:109−118.

Riddle CN, Baker SN. Convergence of pyramidal and medial brain stem descending pathways onto macaque cervical spinal interneurons. *J Neurophysiol*. 2010;103:2821−2832.

Rothwell JC. Overview of neurophysiology of movement control. *Clin Neurol Neurosurg*. 2012;114:432−435.

Rubin MN, Rabinstein AA. Vascular disease of the spinal cord. *Neurol Clin*. 2013;31:153−181.

Santillan A, Nacarino V, Greenberg E, Riina HA, Gobin YP, Patsalides A. Vascular anatomy of the spinal cord. *J Neurointerv Surg*. 2012;4:67−74.

Schieber MH. Comparative anatomy of the corticospinal system. *Handbook Clin Neurol*. 2007;82:15−37.

Soteropoulos DS, Edgley SA, Baker SN. Lack of evidence for direct corticospinal contributions to control of the ipsilateral forelimb in monkey. *J Neurosci*. 2011;31:11208−11219.

CHAPTER SUMMARY

STUDY GUIDELINES

1. This chapter largely deals with the identification of structures in transverse sections of the brainstem. A separate study guide is provided for the sections.
2. Four brainstem decussations should recall those described in Box 3.1.

3. Note that in magnetic resonance images, brainstem orientation is the reverse of the anatomic convention.

GENERAL ARRANGEMENT OF CRANIAL NERVE NUCLEI

In the thoracic region of the developing spinal cord, four distinct cell columns can be identified in the grey matter on each side (Fig. 17.1A,B). From the basal plate the *general somatic efferent (GSE) column* supplies the striated muscles of the trunk and limbs and the *general visceral efferent (GVE) column* supplies preganglionic neurons of the autonomic system. From the alar plate, neurons in the *general visceral afferent (GVA) column* receive afferents from thoracic and abdominal organs. A *general somatic afferent (GSA) column* receives afferents from the body wall and the limbs.

In the brainstem these four cell columns can be identified; but they are fragmented, and not all contribute to each cranial nerve. Their connections are as follows.

- *GSE column.* Supplies the striated musculature of the orbit (via the oculomotor, trochlear, and abducens nerves) and tongue (via the hypoglossal nerve).
- *GVE column.* Gives rise to the cranial parasympathetic system introduced in Chapter 13. The target ganglia are the ciliary, pterygopalatine, submandibular, and otic ganglia in the head and neck and the vagal ganglia in the neck, thorax, and abdomen.
- *GVA column.* Receives afferents from the visceral territory of the glossopharyngeal and vagus nerves.
- *GSA column.* Receives afferents from the skin and mucous membranes, mainly over the trigeminal nerve from the skin and mucous membranes of the oronasofacial region, and the dura mater.

Three additional cell columns (Fig. 17.1C,D) serve branchial arch tissues and the inner ear, as follows.

- *Special visceral (branchial) efferent (SVE) column.* Supplying efferents to the branchial arch musculature of the face, jaws, palate, larynx, and pharynx (via facial, trigeminal, glossopharyngeal, vagus, and cranial accessory nerves). These striated muscles have visceral functions in relation to food and air intake (hence, *visceral*).
- *Special visceral afferent (SVA) column.* Receives afferent fibres from the taste buds that develop from endodermal lining of branchial arches.
- *Special somatic afferent (SSA) column.* Receives afferents from the vestibular (balance) and cochlear (hearing) organs of the inner ear.

Fig. 17.2 shows the position of the various nuclei in a dorsal view of the brainstem.

In this chapter, details of the internal anatomy of the brainstem accompany nine representative transverse sections and their captions. Connections (direct or indirect) with the *right* cerebral hemisphere have been highlighted in accordance with information to be provided.

BACKGROUND INFORMATION

As stated earlier, exteroceptive and conscious proprioceptive information is transferred (by anterolateral and dorsal column—medial lemniscal pathways) from the trunk and limbs to the contralateral cerebral hemisphere. It was also explained that corticospinal fibres of the pyramidal tract arising from motor areas of the cerebral cortex synapse on the contralateral

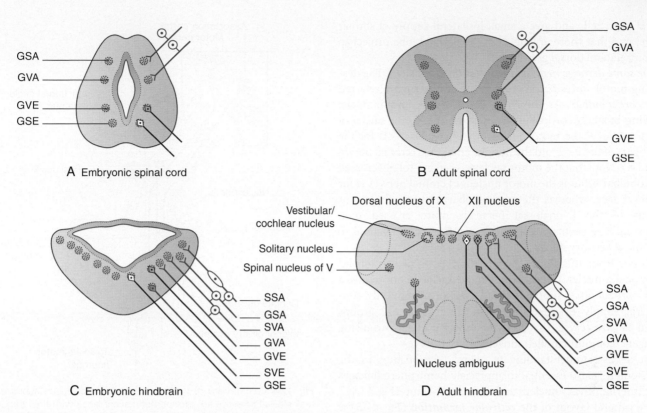

Fig. 17.1 Cell columns of the spinal cord and brainstem. (A) Embryonic spinal cord. (B) Adult spinal cord. (C) Embryonic hindbrain. (D) Adult hindbrain. *Afferent cell columns: GSA*, General somatic afferent; *GVA*, general visceral afferent; *SSA*, special somatic afferent; *SVA*, special visceral afferent. *Efferent cell columns: GSE*, General somatic efferent; *GVE*, general visceral efferent; *SVE*, special visceral efferent.

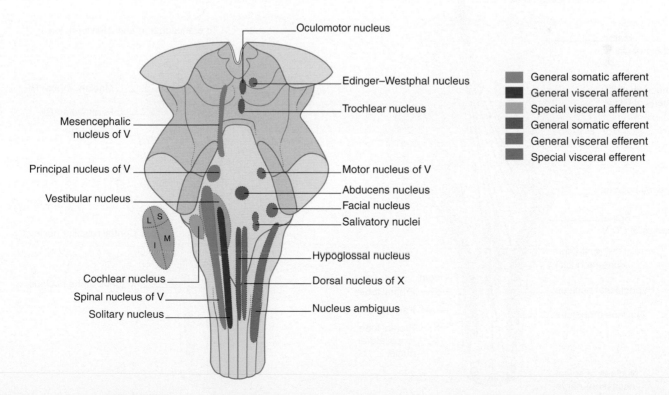

Fig. 17.2 Dorsal view of adult brainstem, showing position of cranial nerve cell columns. *L*, Lateral; *S*, superior; *I*, inferior; *M*, medial vestibular nuclei (the vestibular nuclei are projected to the side for clarity).

ventral horn cells and give a small ipsilateral supply of similar nature, and that those arising from the parietal lobe project to the contralateral dorsal grey horn.

The same arrangement holds true for the brainstem. The descending motor fibres terminating in the brainstem are referred to as *corticobulbar*. As shown in Fig. 17.3, the motor nuclei receiving bilateral corticobulbar input are the motor nuclei of cranial nerve V, the motor nuclei of cranial nerve VII for the upper part of the face, and the nucleus ambiguus (cranial nerves IX and X). Note that the motor nucleus receiving totally crossed corticobulbar input is the motor nucleus of cranial nerve VII for the lower face, whereas the corticobulbar input to the motor nucleus of the hypoglossal nerve is more crossed than uncrossed. The corticobulbar input is entirely contralateral to the somatic sensory nuclei.

Absent from this figure are the three pairs of extraocular motor ocular nuclei. Why? Because these nuclei do not receive a direct corticobulbar supply. Instead their predominantly contralateral supply originates from the brainstem cell groups known as *gaze centres* that have the function of synchronising conjugate (conjoint parallel) movements of the eyes.

For a basic understanding of neural relationships in the brainstem, it is also essential to appreciate hemisphere linkages to the inferior olivary nucleus and to the cerebellum (Fig. 17.4).

The general layout of the **reticular formation** (Fig. 17.5) is borrowed from a figure in Chapter 24 devoted to this topic. It

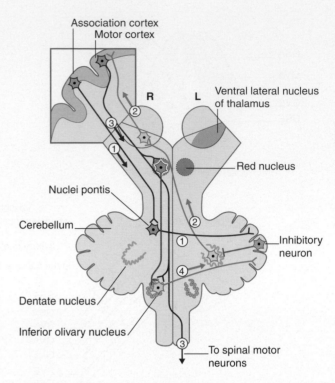

Fig. 17.4 Ventral view of the four principal motor decussations of the brainstem. Pathways are numbered in accordance with their sequence of activation in voluntary movements: *(1)* corticopontocerebellar; *(2)* dentatothalamocortical; *(3)* corticospinal; *(4)* olivocerebellar. Also shown is the rubro-olivary connection.

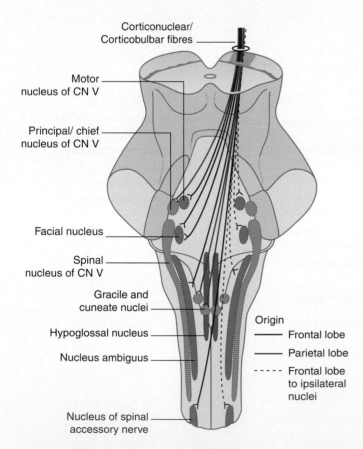

Fig. 17.3 Dorsal view of brainstem, showing distribution of corticobulbar fibres from the right cerebral cortex.

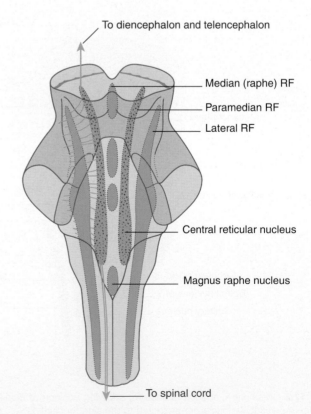

Fig. 17.5 Layout of the reticular formation *(RF)*.

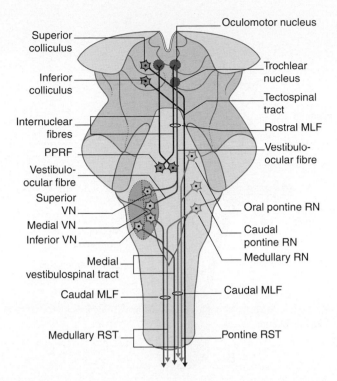

Fig. 17.6 Main fibre composition of the medial longitudinal fasciculus *(MLF)*. *PPRF*, Paramedian pontine reticular formation; *RN*, reticular nucleus; *RST*, reticulospinal tract; *VN*, vestibular nucleus.

may be consulted when reading under this heading in successive descriptions.

Fig. 17.6 depicts the main components of the ***medial longitudinal fasciculus (MLF)***. This fibre bundle extends the entire length of the brainstem, originating from different structures and serving different functions at different levels of the brainstem. This figure, too, may be consulted during study of the brainstem sections to be described, following inspection of the C1 segment of the spinal cord.

Study Guide

This presentation departs from the traditional method used in this textbook which is to describe photographs or diagrams at successive brain levels in ascending order without highlights. In the present approach:

1. The various nuclei and pathways are highlighted and labelled on the side having primary affiliation with the right cerebral hemisphere.
2. The nuclei and pathways are colour coded by systems, for example red for motor, blue for sensory, and green for connections of the cerebellum and reticular formation.
3. Colour coding makes it possible to study individual systems in vertical, 'multiple window' mode. The descriptive text related to the brainstem sections enables a logical sequence of study whereby afferent pathways can be followed from caudal levels rostrally to the thalamus (commencing with Fig. 17.10) and efferent pathways can be followed caudally from rostral levels (commencing with (see Fig. 17.19). It must be emphasised that, following study in the vertical mode, a

horizontal approach must be undertaken, with the location of the various systems identified at each level. This is because occlusion of a small artery supplying arterial blood to the brainstem or a tumour developing in the brainstem will most likely affect the function of more than one neuronal system that is either present at the lesion site or is projecting axons through the affected organ. At each level, miniature replicas of the diagrams in Fig. 17.7 are inserted to assist left–right orientation.

Special note: Readers unfamiliar with the internal anatomy of the brainstem may be disconcerted by the amount of new information contained in the series of sections to be described. It may be reassuring to know that *all* the information will come up again in later chapters. Therefore, a sensible approach would be to initially browse through the sections and then recheck the location of individual items during later reading.

Overview of Three Pathways in the Brainstem

Fig. 17.8 shows the *dorsal column–medial lemniscal* and *anterolateral pathways* already described in Chapter 15. Recall that the latter comprises the *neospinothalamic tract* serving pain and temperature and the *reticulospinal tract* serving dull aching pain. This pathway terminates in the reticular nuclei of the brainstem that subsequently give rise to axons contributing to the *central tegmental tract* (CTT), which terminates in the intralaminar nuclei of the thalamus. The third component of the anterolateral system is the *spinotectal tract* that terminates in the midbrain (at the level of the superior colliculus) and is responsible for the coordination of head and eye movements.

The *corticospinal tract*, discussed in Chapter 16, is shown in Fig. 17.9. Also included are corticobulbar projections to the facial and hypoglossal nuclei.

C1 SEGMENT OF THE SPINAL CORD (FIG. 17.10)

Blue

The *gracile* and *cuneate fasciculi* constitute the dorsal column of the spinal cord. Their axons are ipsilateral central processes of dorsal root ganglion cells whose peripheral processes receive information from the large tactile nerve endings in the skin, including Meissner and Pacinian corpuscles, and from neuromuscular spindles and Golgi tendon organs. The fasciculi terminate ipsilaterally in the gracile and cuneate nuclei (see Fig. 17.12).

Unlike the dorsal column, the anterolateral tract contains *crossed* axons. As indicated in Fig. 15.10, the second-order neurons traverse the ventral white commissure at all segmental levels before ascending to the thalamus.

The *dorsolateral tract of Lissauer* contains fine first-order sensory fibres that divide and span several cord segments prior to synapsing in the dorsal grey horn.

The *spinal (descending) tract* of the trigeminal nerve contains nociceptive and thermoceptive first-order neurons about to synapse in the dorsal grey horn of segments C2 and C3.

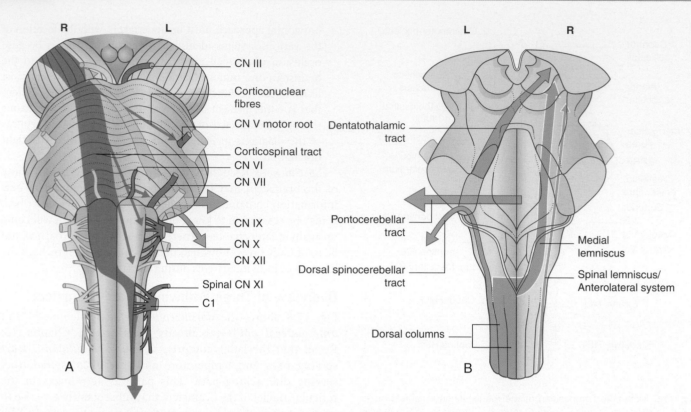

R   L

— CN III

— Corticonuclear fibres

— CN V motor root

Dentatothalamic — tract

— Corticospinal tract
— CN VI
— CN VII

— CN IX

Pontocerebellar tract

— CN X

— CN XII

Dorsal spinocerebellar tract

— Medial lemniscus

— Spinal lemniscus/ Anterolateral system

— Spinal CN XI

— C1

Dorsal columns —

A

B

L   R

Fig. 17.7 (A) Ventral and (B) dorsal view of brainstem, showing disposition of some major pathways. *L*, Left; *R*, right.

Red

The large red area on the left side of the cord represents the (crossed) *lateral corticospinal tract*. The *ventral corticospinal tract* has not yet crossed.

Anterior motor neurons projecting from the ventral grey horn occupy the ventral root of spinal nerve C1 and the uppermost root of the spinal accessory nerve.

The *lateral vestibulospinal tract* (uncrossed) descends in the ventral funiculus to activate antigravity muscles ipsilaterally. *The medial vestibulospinal tract* (partly crossed) descends in the caudal MLF to activate head-righting reflexes.

Lateral to the ventral grey horn is the autonomic projection from the hypothalamus. Its functions include activation of sacral parasympathetic neurons causing contraction of the bladder and rectum.

Green

The *dorsal spinocerebellar tract* (from the posterior thoracic/Clarke nucleus) conveys high-speed unconscious proprioception from the ipsilateral trunk and limbs, notably from muscle stretch receptors.

The *pontine reticulospinal tract* is descending ipsilaterally   to supply motor neurons innervating antigravity muscles.   The *medullary reticulospinal tract* supplies flexor motor neurons.

SPINOMEDULLARY JUNCTION (FIG. 17.11)

Blue

The *gracile* and *cuneate fasciculi* continue to occupy the dorsal white column, with the *spinal tract and nucleus* of the trigeminal

nerve alongside. The position of the *spinal lemniscus* is also unchanged.

Red

The dominant feature in this diagram is the *decussation of the pyramids*. Observe the right pyramid: 80% of its fibres cross the midline by decussating with its opposite numbers, to form the left *lateral corticospinal tract*; 10% form the ipsilateral *ventral corticospinal tract* which will cross lower down; and 10% remain ipsilateral among the fibres of the right lateral corticospinal tract.

Within the lateral tegmentum is the *lateral vestibulospinal tract*. The red spots in the medial longitudinal fasciculi represent the *medial vestibulospinal tract*, which descends bilaterally within them.

Green

The *dorsal spinocerebellar tract* is nearing its point of departure into the inferior cerebellar peduncle. The *paramedian* and *lateral reticular formation* occupy the tegmentum.

MIDDLE OF THE MEDULLA OBLONGATA (FIG. 17.12)

Blue

The left dorsal column of the spinal cord ascends to the midmedulla before turning ventrally. The *gracile fasciculus* synapses in the *gracile nucleus* and the cuneate fasciculus in the *cuneate nucleus*. Second-order neurons give rise to *internal arcuate fibres*, which cross over in the *sensory decussation* and then ascend (to the ventroposterolateral (VPL) nucleus of the

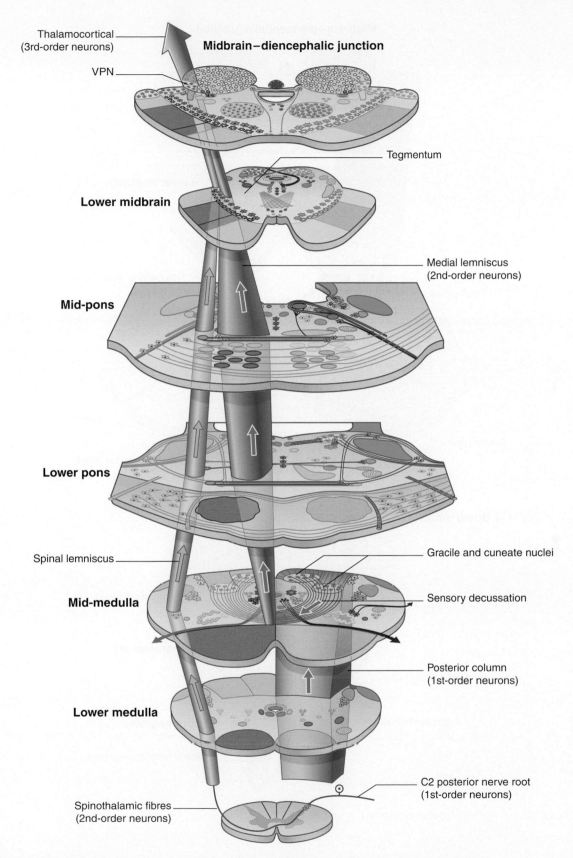

Thalamocortical
(3rd-order neurons)

VPN

Midbrain–diencephalic junction

Tegmentum

Lower midbrain

Medial lemniscus
(2nd-order neurons)

Mid-pons

Lower pons

Spinal lemniscus

Gracile and cuneate nuclei

Mid-medulla

Sensory decussation

Posterior column
(1st-order neurons)

Lower medulla

C2 posterior nerve root
(1st-order neurons)

Spinothalamic fibres
(2nd-order neurons)

Fig. 17.8 Dorsal column–medial lemniscal and anterolateral pathways. *VPN,* Ventral posterior nucleus of the thalamus.

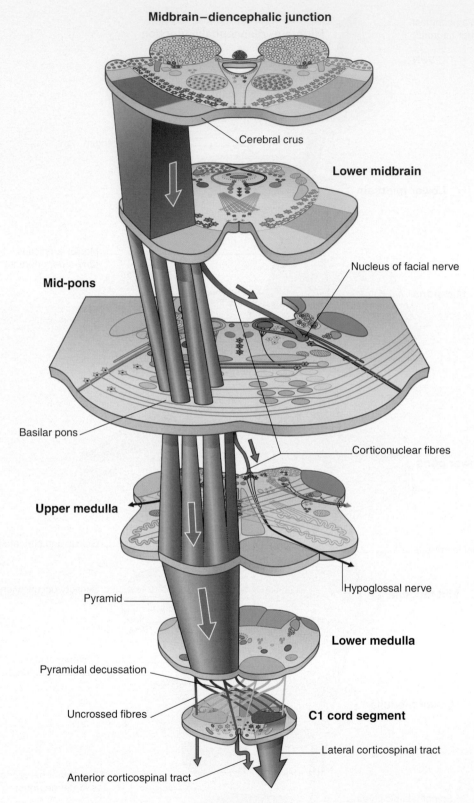

Midbrain–diencephalic junction

Cerebral crus

Lower midbrain

Nucleus of facial nerve

Mid-pons

Basilar pons

Corticonuclear fibres

Upper medulla

Hypoglossal nerve

Pyramid

Lower medulla

Pyramidal decussation

Uncrossed fibres

C1 cord segment

Lateral corticospinal tract

Anterior corticospinal tract

Fig. 17.9 Corticospinal tract; two corticobulbar projections. *L,* Left; *R,* right.

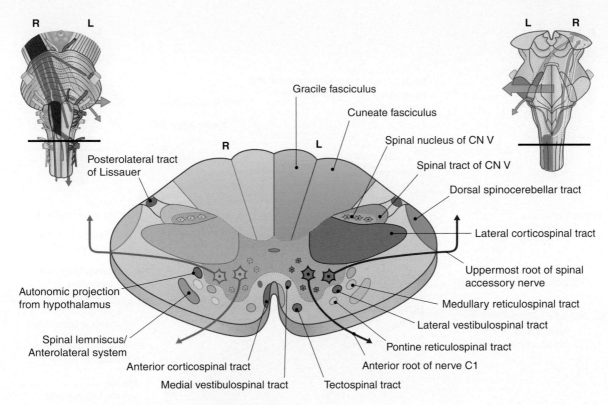

Gracile fasciculus

Cuneate fasciculus

Spinal nucleus of CN V

Spinal tract of CN V

Dorsal spinocerebellar tract

Lateral corticospinal tract

Uppermost root of spinal accessory nerve

Medullary reticulospinal tract

Lateral vestibulospinal tract

Pontine reticulospinal tract

Anterior root of nerve C1

Tectospinal tract

Medial vestibulospinal tract

Medial vestibulospinal tract

Anterior corticospinal tract

Spinal lemniscus/ Anterolateral system

Autonomic projection from hypothalamus

Posterolateral tract of Lissauer

Fig. 17.10 C1 segment of the spinal cord. *L,* Left; *R,* right.

thalamus) as the *medial lemniscus*. The anterolateral system (ALS) contains the neospinothalamic, spinoreticular, and spinotectal tracts. The *vestibulospinal tract* is descending from the vestibular nucleus to the spinal cord.

Red

The *pyramid* contains the corticospinal tract prior to the pyramidal decussation; the *hypoglossal nerve* emerges at its lateral edge. Lateral to the XII nucleus is the *dorsal nucleus of vagus nerve*. The 'cranial' accessory nerve has emerged from the nucleus ambiguus; it will be incorporated into the vagus below the jugular foramen. The *dorsal longitudinal fasciculus (DLF)* contains autonomic fibres descending from the hypothalamus to the spinal cord.

Green

The projections from *inferior* and *accessory olivary nuclei* to the contralateral cerebellar cortex are shown. The paramedian and lateral reticular formation and the inferior cerebellar peduncle are seen again now.

UPPER PART OF THE MEDULLA OBLONGATA (FIG. 17.13)

Blue

In the mid-region the *medial lemnisci* are continuing their ascent to the thalamus. Laterally, we see the *spinal lemniscus,*

the *spinal tract and nucleus of the trigeminal nerve*, the *solitary tract and nucleus* (STN in Fig. 17.15) and the *medial and lateral nuclei of the vestibular nerve*. Sensory fibres of the glossopharyngeal nerve synapse in the *spinal nucleus of the trigeminal nerve* and in the *solitary nucleus*.

Red

The *pyramids* are in the same position as before. On the anatomic right side, the *vagus nerve* is emerging anterior to the *inferior cerebellar peduncle*. On the left side the motor components of the *glossopharyngeal nerve* derive from the *inferior salivatory nucleus* and the *nucleus ambiguus*.

Green

The *principal* and *accessory olivary nuclei* are sending fibres across to the contralateral inferior cerebellar peduncle. Dorsal to these are the *chemoreceptive area* (sensitive to HCO_3 levels in the cerebrospinal fluid), the *lateral reticular nucleus, pontine reticulospinal tract*, and *paramedian reticular formation*. Occupying the midline region are the *magnus raphe nucleus* and the *medial* and *dorsal longitudinal fasciculi*.

PONTOMEDULLARY JUNCTION (FIG. 17.14)

Blue

Previously seen are the medial and spinal lemnisci, and the spinal tract and nucleus of the trigeminal nerve. Newly seen are the *lateral* and *trigeminal lemnisci*. As explained in Chapter 20, the

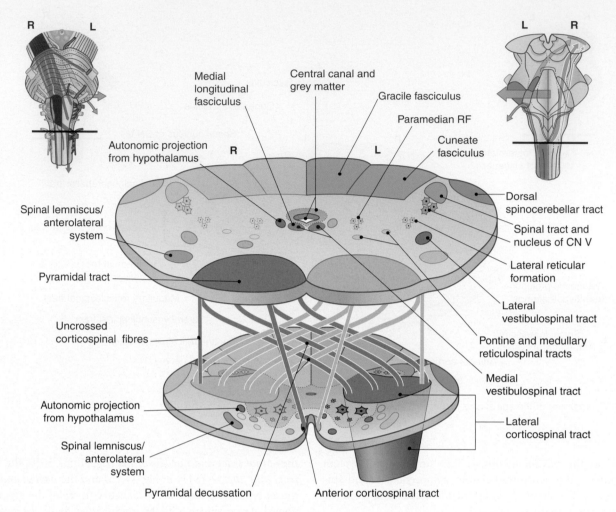

Fig. 17.11 Spinomedullary junction. *L*, Left; *R*, right; *RF*, reticular formation.

lateral lemniscus is an auditory fibre bundle ascending to the inferior colliculus, having crossed in the *trapezoid body* from the *superior olivary nucleus*. This nucleus receives auditory information from the *dorsal* and *ventral cochlear nuclei*, where the cochlear nerve terminates.

Red

Reflex balance pathways here are the *medial* and *lateral vesti-bulospinal tracts (VST in the figure)*. The medial tract descends to the spinal cord within the *MLF*. Also seen are the *corticospinal tract* and the emerging *abducens* and *facial nerves*. The *DLF* contains autonomic fibres descending to the spinal cord.

Green

At top are the *superior cerebellar peduncles* which project from the dentate nucleus of the cerebellum to the contralateral thalamus. Caudal to these are the *inferior cerebellar peduncles*. More

centrally are the *pontine reticulospinal tract* and the *paramedian reticular formation*.

MID-PONS (FIG. 17.15)

Blue

Medial, *lateral*, and *trigeminal lemnisci* are progressing towards the thalamus. We have reached the upper end of the *vestibular*, *spinal trigeminal*, and *solitary nuclei* and are at the level of the *trapezoid body*. The *nervus intermedius* contains gustatory fibres from taste buds found in the anterior two-thirds of the tongue. These fibres terminate centrally in the solitary nucleus.

Red

The *facial nerve* is J-shaped, like a bended knee (genu), where it winds around the nucleus of the *abducens nerve* before passing

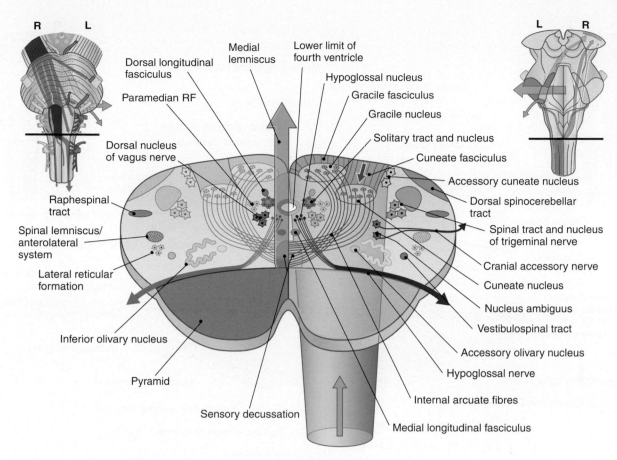

Fig. 17.12 Middle of the medulla oblongata. *L,* Left; *R,* right; *RF,* reticular formation.

through the tegmentum, where it is joined by the *nervus intermedius*. In addition to taste, this nerve contains parasympathetic secretomotor fibres that will synapse on autonomic ganglia innervating the lacrimal and submandibular/sublingual glands (among others).

Green

Dorsally, the arrows indicate imminent intersection of the *superior cerebellar peduncles* in the roof of the fourth ventricle. At a lower level, the *inferior peduncles* are entering the cerebellum.

In the basilar pons, millions of *corticopontine fibres* descend from the cerebral cortex to synapse upon millions of individual neurons collectively called the nuclei *pontis*. These give rise to transverse fibres that separate the corticospinal tracts into bundles (fascicles), on their way to forming the *middle cerebellar peduncle* on the contralateral side.

Alongside the abducens nucleus is the *pontine gaze centre/ paramedian pontine reticular formation*, a node of reticular formation that activates the contraction of the lateral rectus muscle in the orbit, thereby causing abduction of the ipsilateral eyeball.

In the midline, the *pontine raphe nucleus* projects serotonergic fibres throughout the pons and cerebellum.

UPPER PONS (FIG. 17.16)

Blue

The *sensory root of the left trigeminal nerve* terminates in the *pontine sensory nucleus*. From here, axons project across the midline and turn rostrally as the *trigeminal lemniscus*. Three lemnisci previously seen are the *spinal, lateral,* and *medial lemnisci*. The *mesencephalic tract of the trigeminal nerve* (Mes. t. V in the figure) contains processes of pseudounipolar neurons in the midbrain, as explained in Chapter 21.

Red

The *locus coeruleus*, in the floor of the rostral end of the fourth ventricle, is the largest group of noradrenergic neurons in the brain. It distributes fine, beaded axons to all parts of the cerebral and cerebellar hemispheres. The *motor nucleus of the trigeminal nerve* innervates the masticatory muscles. Previously seen are the *corticospinal fibre bundles* and the *DLF*.

Green

Next to the superior cerebellar peduncle (SCP in the figure), the *pedunculopontine nucleus* is part of the locomotor centre (see

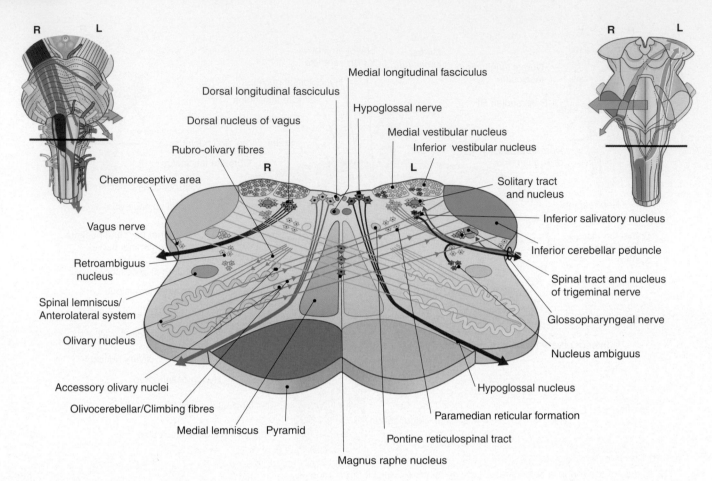

Fig. 17.13 Upper medulla oblongata. *DLF*, Dorsal longitudinal fasciculus; *ICP*, inferior cerebellar peduncle; *L*, left; *MLF*, medial longitudinal fasciculus; *R*, right; *RF*, reticular formation; *VST*, vestibulospinal tracts.

Chapter 24). Previously seen are the corticopontine and ponto-cerebellar fibres.

LOWER MIDBRAIN (FIG. 17.17)

Blue

The *medial*, *spinal*, and *trigeminal (V) lemnisci* are still ascending, whereas most of the fibres in lateral lemniscus are now synapsing in the inferior colliculus, i.e. the lower centre for hearing.

The *mesencephalic nucleus of the trigeminal nerve* (it is labeled as Mesencepahlic nucleus of CN V in the figure) is the *only* pseudounipolar cell group within the central nervous system (CNS). It conveys centrally proprioceptive information from muscles innervated by the mandibular division of the trigeminal nerve.

Red

The *trochlear nerve* is the *only* cranial nerve to decussate (as shown); as well as the *only* cranial nerve to emerge from the dorsal surface of the brainstem. The *DLF* contains autonomic fibres traveling to the spinal cord. The crus of the midbrain contains *corticobulbar* and *corticospinal fibres*; the former activate motor cranial nerve nuclei. The *tectospinal tract* is

commencing its descent, having crossed from the contralateral superior colliculi. It participates in visuospinal reflexes whereby the head and trunk are turned in the direction of visual stimuli.

Green

The *fronto-* and *parieto-temporo-occipital pontine fibres* are travelling from the corresponding association areas of the cerebral cortex to reach the ipsilateral nuclei pontis.

Brown/Grey

The anterior tegmentum is occupied by *compact* and *reticular* elements of the *substantia nigra*. The compact part, comprising pigmented dopaminergic neurons, is the source of the *nigrostriatal pathway* to the corpus striatum. The nigrostriatal pathway loses both pigment and cells in patients suffering from *Parkinson disease* (see Chapter 26). The reticular part contains γ-aminobutyric acid (GABA) releasing neurons.

UPPER MIDBRAIN (FIG. 17.18)

The four components of the crus cerebri and the substantia nigra are in the same relative positions as seen in the previous

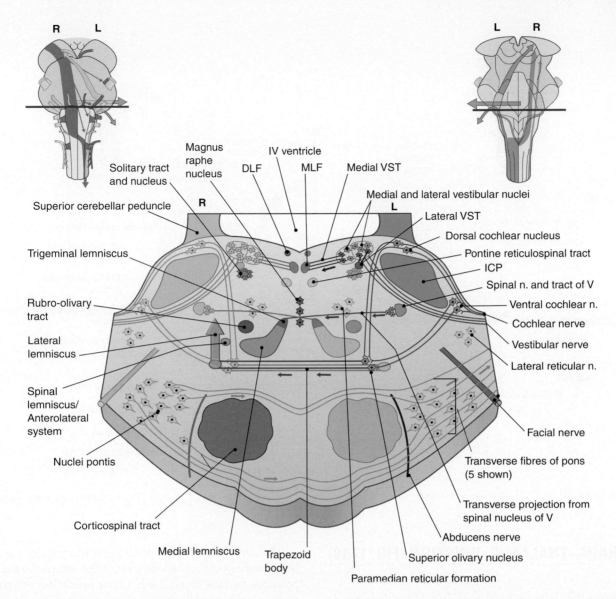

Fig. 17.14 Pontomedullary junction. *DLF,* Dorsal longitudinal fasciculus; *ICP,* inferior cerebellar peduncle; *L,* left; *MLF,* medial longitudinal fasciculus; *n.,* nerve; *R,* right; *VST,* vestibulospinal tracts.

figure. So too are the midbrain raphe nucleus and the ventral tegmental and interpeduncular nuclei.

Blue

The *medial, spinal,* and *trigeminal lemnisci* continue to move dorsally as they near the thalamus. The *spinotectal tract* has emerged from the spinal lemniscus to enter the superior colliculus.

Red

Dorsally, the two *tectospinal tracts* have emerged from the superior colliculus and have undergone decussation. The spinotectal and tectospinal tracts participate in the *spinovisual reflex* whereby the eyes and head turn in the direction of tactile and visual stimuli.

The *oculomotor nerves* have pierced the *red nuclei* and *substantia nigra* to reach the *interpeduncular fossa.* The *Edinger–Westphal nucleus* contribute preganglionic parasympathetic fibres into the CN III nerves; they activate the ciliary ganglion whose postganglionic fibres cause contraction of the pupillary sphincter and the ciliary muscle.

Green

Most *dentatothalamic fibres* travel uninterrupted to the contralateral thalamus. A minority synapse in the red nucleus from which the *rubro-olivary* fibres project caudally within the *central tegmental tract to the ipsilateral inferior olivary nucleus.*

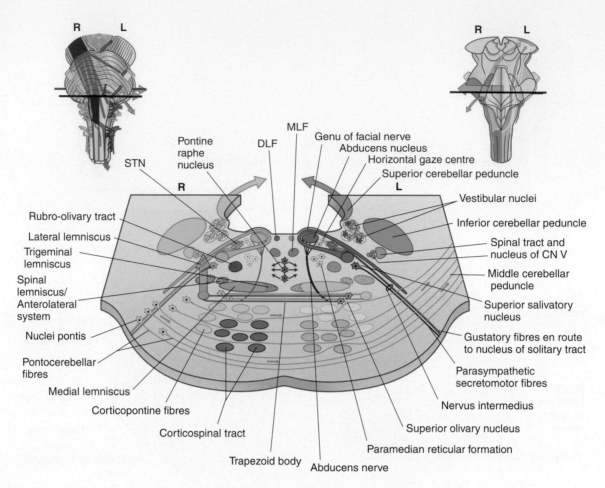

Fig. 17.15 Mid-pons. *DLF*, Dorsal longitudinal fasciculus; *L*, left; *MLF*, medial longitudinal fasciculus; *R*, right; *S. t. n.*, Solitary tract and nucleus.

MIDBRAIN—THALAMIC JUNCTION (FIG. 17.19)

Blue

Ascending to the ventral posterior nucleus of the thalamus are three lemnisci *(medial, spinal, trigeminal)*. Entering the *medial (auditory) geniculate nucleus (MGN)* of the thalamus is the *inferior brachium*, which arose from the *inferior colliculus*. The *lateral (visual) geniculate nucleus (LGN)* receives the superior brachium (not seen here).

Red

The *subthalamic nucleus* receives an input from the centromedian nucleus of the thalamus and projects to the lentiform nucleus. It may become overactive in Parkinson disease (see Chapter 26). The red nucleus and the contents of the crus cerebri are unchanged.

Green

In the dorsal tegmentum the *pretectal nucleus* participates as a part of the visual system. It receives an input from the optic tract and projects to both Edinger—Westphal nuclei, giving rise to bilateral pupillary constriction when a light is shone into one eye (see Chapter 23).

Near the midline are the centres for upward and downward gaze. Rarely, a *pinealoma* (pineal gland tumour) may signal its presence by causing *paralysis of upward gaze*.

The superior cerebellar peduncle is heading for the ventral lateral nucleus of the thalamus, which lies anterior to the ventral posterior nucleus. From there, a final projection will reach the motor cortex and will coordinate ongoing movements.

Green

The *habenular nuclei* are connected across the midline and project via the *fasciculus retroflexus* to the *interpeduncular nucleus*, which participates in the sleep—wake cycle (see Chapter 34).

ORIENTATION OF BRAINSTEM SLICES IN MAGNETIC RESONANCE IMAGES (FIG. 17.20)

Fig. 17.20 shows brainstem slices in magnetic resonance images. Their orientation is the opposite of those in the preceding sections. In photographs and drawings, the convention is to represent anterior structures below. As already mentioned in Chapter 2, in magnetic resonance imaging scans, anterior structures are represented above.

Epilogue

Fig. 17.21 offers an unlabelled overview of the brainstem sections. Gentle skimmers may opt to photocopy lightly and to crayon pathways.

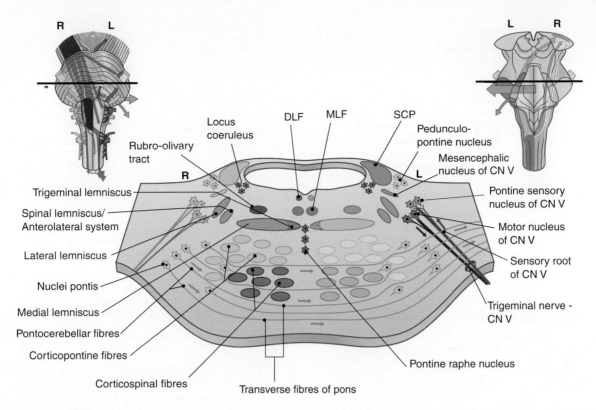

Fig. 17.16 Upper pons. *DLF,* Dorsal longitudinal fasciculus; *L,* left; *MLF,* medial longitudinal fasciculus; *R,* right; *SCP,* superior cerebellar peduncle.

Labels (Fig. 17.16):
- Locus coeruleus
- DLF
- MLF
- SCP
- Pedunculo-pontine nucleus
- Mesencephalic nucleus of CN V
- Rubro-olivary tract
- Trigeminal lemniscus
- Spinal lemniscus/Anterolateral system
- Lateral lemniscus
- Nuclei pontis
- Medial lemniscus
- Pontocerebellar fibres
- Corticopontine fibres
- Corticospinal fibres
- Transverse fibres of pons
- Pontine raphe nucleus
- Trigeminal nerve - CN V
- Sensory root of CN V
- Motor nucleus of CN V
- Pontine sensory nucleus of CN V

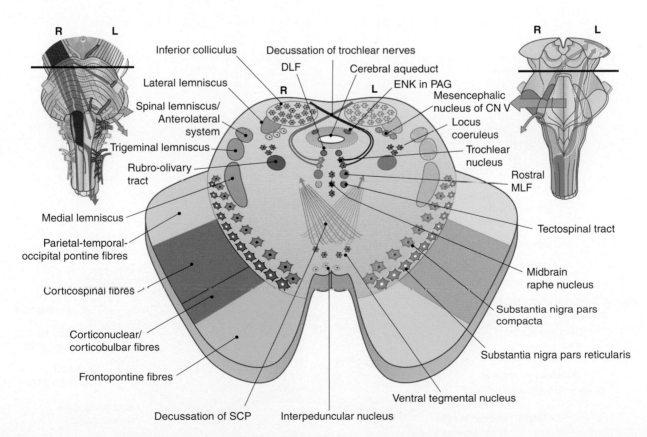

Fig. 17.17 Lower midbrain. *DLF,* Dorsal longitudinal fasciculus; *ENK,* enkephalin; *L,* left; *Mes. n. V,* mesencephalic nucleus of the trigeminal nerve; *MLF,* medial longitudinal fasciculus; *PAG,* periaqueductal grey; *R,* right.

Labels (Fig. 17.17):
- Inferior colliculus
- Decussation of trochlear nerves
- DLF
- Cerebral aqueduct
- ENK in PAG
- Mesencephalic nucleus of CN V
- Lateral lemniscus
- Locus coeruleus
- Spinal lemniscus/Anterolateral system
- Trochlear nucleus
- Trigeminal lemniscus
- Rostral MLF
- Rubro-olivary tract
- Medial lemniscus
- Tectospinal tract
- Parietal-temporal-occipital pontine fibres
- Midbrain raphe nucleus
- Corticospinal fibres
- Substantia nigra pars compacta
- Corticonuclear/corticobulbar fibres
- Substantia nigra pars reticularis
- Frontopontine fibres
- Ventral tegmental nucleus
- Decussation of SCP
- Interpeduncular nucleus

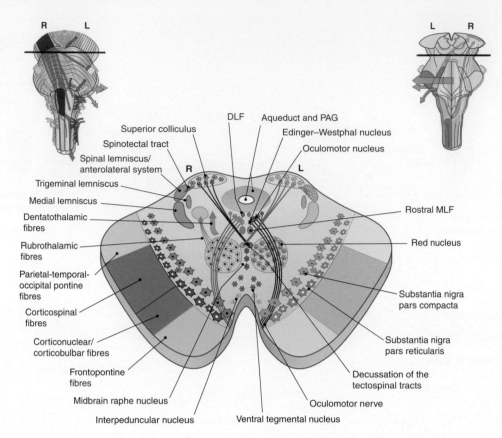

Fig. 17.18 Upper midbrain. *DLF,* Dorsal longitudinal fasciculus; *L,* left; *MLF,* medial longitudinal fasciculus; *PAG,* periaqueductal grey; *R,* right.

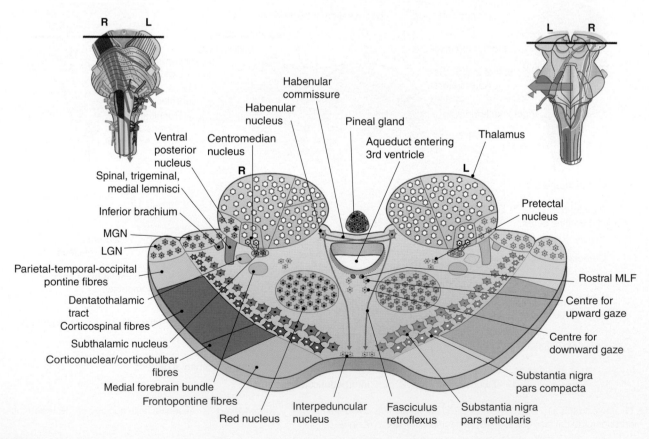

Fig. 17.19 Midbrain–thalamic junction. *L,* Left; *LGN,* lateral geniculate nucleus; *MGN,* medial geniculate nucleus; *R,* right.

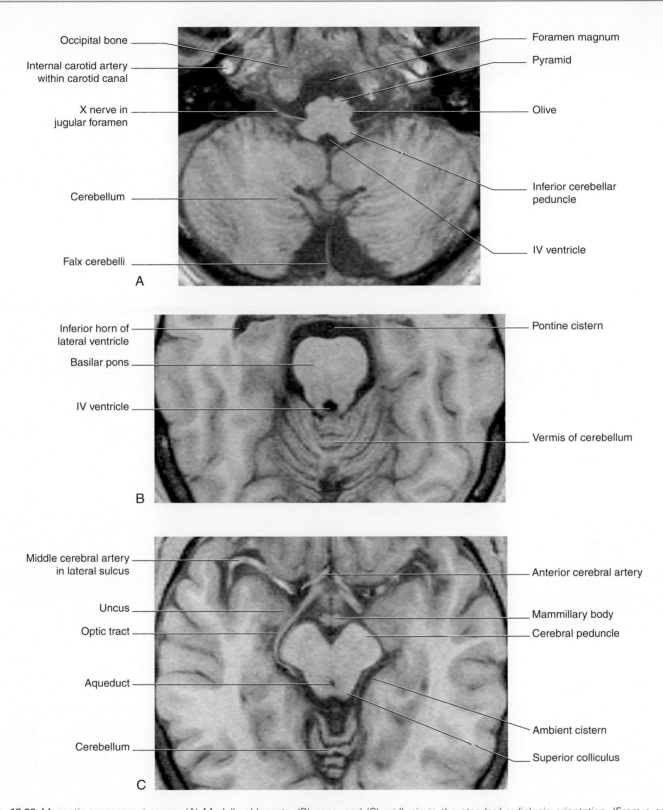

Fig. 17.20 Magnetic resonance images. (A) Medulla oblongata, (B) pons, and (C) midbrain in the standard radiologic orientation. (From a series kindly provided by Professor J. Paul Finn, Director, Magnetic Resonance Research, Department of Radiology, David Geffen School of Medicine at UCLA, California.)

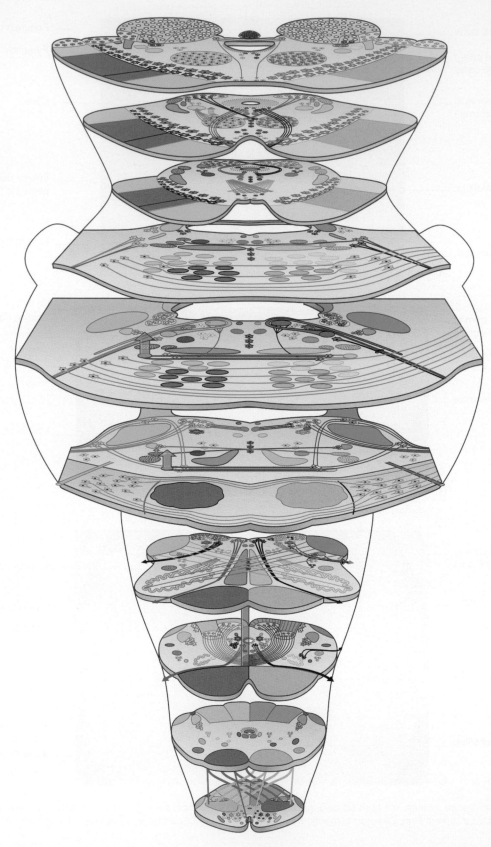

Fig. 17.21 Brainstem review.

✴ Core Information

Cell Columns

Cranial nerve cell columns and their representations are as follows.

- *GSE*, represented in the medulla by the hypoglossal nucleus, in the pons by the abducens nucleus, and in the midbrain by the oculomotor and trochlear nuclei.
- *SVE*, supplying muscles of branchial arch origin, represented in the medulla by the nucleus ambiguus and in the pons by trigeminal and facial motor nuclei.
- *GVE*, represented in the medulla by the dorsal motor nucleus of vagus, in the medulla and pons by the inferior and superior salivatory nuclei, and in the midbrain by the Edinger—Westphal nucleus.
- *GVA*, represented in the medulla by the inferior solitary nucleus.
- *SVA*, represented in the pons by the superior solitary nucleus.
- *GSA*, represented by trigeminal sensory nuclei: spinal in the medulla, principal sensory in the pons, and mesencephalic in the midbrain.
- *SSA*, represented at the pontomedullary junction by the cochlear and vestibular nuclei.

Ascending Pathways

The gracile and cuneate nuclei send internal arcuate fibres across the midline to form the medial lemniscus, which ascends through the pons and midbrain to reach the thalamus. The spinal trigeminal nucleus project their fibres across the midline to form the trigeminothalamic tract. The dorsal spinocerebellar and cuneocerebellar tracts send their fibres into the ipsilateral inferior cerebellar peduncle, where they mingle with olivocerebellar fibres crossing from the inferior and accessory olivary nuclei. The (crossed) ventral spinocerebellar tract enters the superior cerebellar peduncle; its fibres cross a second time within the cerebellar white matter.

- The spinal lemniscus is formed of the ventral and lateral spinothalamic tracts. It is accompanied first by trigeminothalamic fibres, later by the lateral lemniscus, and by fibres crossing from the principal trigeminal nucleus completing the trigeminal lemniscus.
- The cochlear nuclei project fibres across the trapezoid body to form the lateral lemniscus, which ascends to the inferior colliculus. Some fibres synapse instead in a superior olivary nuclear relay to the ipsilateral inferior colliculus. Third-order neurons of the inferior colliculus project via the inferior brachium to the medial geniculate body. The medial and superior vestibular nuclei send fibres to the oculomotor nucleus to participate in the vestibuloocular reflex.
- The upper part of the central tegmental tract contains fibres of the ascending reticular activating system.

- In the ventral tegmentum of the midbrain can be found the pigmented (compact) substantia nigra giving rise to the nigrostriatal pathway and the ventral tegmental nucleus giving rise to the mesocortical and mesolimbic pathways. The nonpigmented (reticular) nigral neurons are inhibitory.

Descending Pathways Other Than Reticulospinal

Corticobulbar fibres from motor areas of the cerebral cortex are distributed preferentially to contralateral motor cranial nerve nuclei excepting the ocular motor slaves of gaze centres. Corticobulbar fibres from sensory areas synapse in the contralateral trigeminal and dorsal column nuclei and dorsal grey horn of the spinal cord.

- Prior to the initiation of a voluntary movement on the left side of the body, the left cerebellar hemisphere is notified by discharges from association areas found in the right cerebral cortex, along the corticopontocerebellar pathway. The left cerebellum responds via the dentatothalamocortical pathway, to the right primary motor cortex. Then the right pyramidal tract discharges and on its way caudally projects information to the cerebellum a second time via collaterals to the right red nucleus, which in turn activates the right olivocerebellar tract.
- Corticospinal fibres pass through the middle three fifths of the cerebral crus/peduncle and through the basilar pons (where they are segregated into bundles by transverse fibres), finally creating the pyramid of the medulla before four fifths enter the pyramidal decussation.
- The lateral vestibular nucleus gives rise to the lateral vestibulospinal tract that has an antigravity function. The medial and inferior vestibular nuclei contribute to the medial vestibulospinal tract involved in head-righting reflexes. The tectospinal tract belongs to the spinovisual reflex arc. The DLF contains ipsilateral central autonomic fibres.
- A sleep-related pathway from the septal area reaches the interpeduncular nucleus by way of the habenular nucleus and fasciculus retroflexus.

Reticular Formation

In the uppermost midbrain can be found the upward and downward gaze centres. (The lateral gaze centres adjoin the abducens nucleus in the pons.) The midbrain also contains an upgoing 'arousal' projection from the cuneiform nucleus, a descending pain-suppressant projection from the periaqueductal grey matter, and a locomotor generator, the pedunculopontine nucleus.

The pons contains the noradrenergic, cerulean nucleus, along with the oral and caudal pontine reticular nuclei, which transmit ipsilateral pontine reticulospinal tracts to extensor motor neurons. The medullary reticulospinal tract is partly crossed and supplies flexor motor neurons. Three respiratory reticular nuclei also occupy the medulla.

SUGGESTED READINGS

Literature references to individual brainstem nuclei and pathways are to be found in the relevant chapters.

Horn-Bochtler AKE, Büttner-Ennever JA. Neuroanatomy of the brainstem. In: Urban PP, Caplan LR, eds. *Brainstem Disorders*. Berlin: Springer; 2011:1—34.

Kautcherov Y, Huang X-F, Halliday G, et al. Organization of human brainstem nuclei. In: Paxinos G, Mai JK, eds. *The Human Nervous System*. 2nd ed. Amsterdam: Elsevier; 2004:267—320.

Noback CR, Strominger NL, Demarest RJ. *The Human Nervous System: Structure and Function*. Baltimore: Williams & Wilkins; 1996.

Parraga RG, Possatti LL, Alves RV, Ribas GC, Ture U, de Oliveira E. Microsurgical anatomy and internal architecture of the brainstem in 3D images: surgical considerations. *J Neurosurg*. 2016;124(5): 1377—1395.

Soria G, De Notaris M, Tudela R, et al. Improved assessment of *ex vivo* brainstem neuroanatomy with high-resolution MRI and DTI at 7 Tesla. *Anat Rec (Hoboken)*. 2011;294(6):1035—1044.

Watson C, Bartholomaeus C, Puelles L. Time for radical changes in brain stem nomenclature—applying the lessons from developmental gene patterns. *Front Neuroanat*. 2019;13:10.

The Lowest Four Cranial Nerves

STUDY GUIDELINES

Comments on the last four cranial nerves in ascending order:

1. The hypoglossal nerve is the motor to the tongue. The spinal accessory nerve is the motor to the sternocleidomastoid and trapezius muscles.
2. The cranial accessory nerve supplies the intrinsic muscles of the larynx and pharynx and all palatine muscles, except the tensor veli palatini (supplied by the mandibular branch of the trigeminal nerve). It is *distributed* by the vagus.
3. The vagus nerve proper is the principal preganglionic parasympathetic nerve. It is also the principal visceral afferent nerve.

4. The main features of the glossopharyngeal nerve are as follows: (1) it provides the afferent limb of the gag reflex; (2) it tells us when we have an inflamed throat; (3) it signals (tastes) bitterness from the posterior one-third of the tongue; (4) its carotid branch carries afferents from the carotid sinus, monitoring blood pressure, and from the carotid body, monitoring blood gases; and (5) it gives a clinically significant branch to the middle ear.

HYPOGLOSSAL NERVE

The hypoglossal nerve (cranial nerve (CN) XII) contains somatic efferent fibres supplying all the extrinsic and intrinsic muscles of the tongue, except for the palatoglossus, which is supplied by the pharyngeal plexus (CN X). Its nucleus lies close to the midline in the floor of the fourth ventricle and extends almost the full length of the medulla (Fig. 18.1D). The nerve emerges as a series of rootlets in the interval between the pyramid and the olive (pre-olivary sulcus). It crosses the subarachnoid space and leaves the skull through the hypoglossal canal. Just below the skull it lies close to the vagus and spinal accessory nerves (Fig. 18.2). It descends on the superficial aspect of the carotid sheath to the level of the angle of the mandible, and then passes forwards on the surface of the hyoglossus muscle where it gives off its terminal branches.

Afferent impulses from about 100 muscle spindles in the same side of the tongue travel from the hypoglossal to the lingual nerve and are then relayed to the mesencephalic nucleus of the trigeminal nerve.

Phylogenetic Note

In reptiles the lingual muscles, the geniohyoid muscle, and the infrahyoid muscles develop together from the rostral mesodermal somites. The somatic efferent neurons supplying this *hypobranchial muscle sheet* form a continuous ribbon of cells extending from the lower medulla to the third cervical spinal segment. In mammals the hypoglossal nucleus is located more rostrally, and its rootlets emerge separately from the cervical rootlets. However, the caudal limit of the hypoglossal nucleus remains linked to the cervical motor cell column by the *supraspinal nucleus*, from which the thyrohyoid muscle is supplied via the first cervical ventral root. In rodents some of the intrinsic muscle fibres of the tongue receive their motor supply indirectly, from axons that leave the most caudal cells of the hypoglossal nucleus and emerge in the first cervical nerve to join the hypoglossal nerve trunk in the neck. Whether this arrangement holds for primates is not yet known.

Corticobulbar (Corticonuclear/Supranuclear) Supply to the Hypoglossal Nucleus

The hypoglossal nucleus receives inputs from the reticular formation, whereby it is recruited for stereotyped motor routines in eating and swallowing. For delicate functions including articulation, most of the fibres from the motor cortex cross over in the upper part of the pyramidal decussation; the majority of the

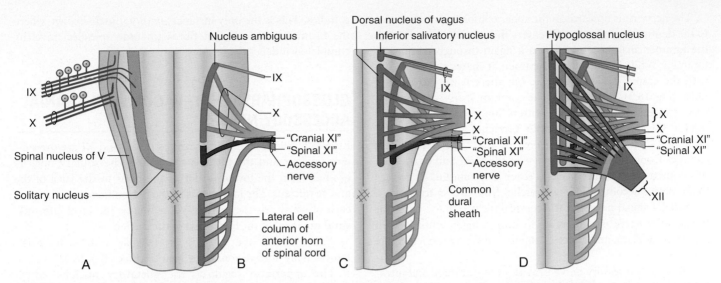

Fig. 18.1 (A) Sensory nuclei (left) and motor nuclei (right) serving cranial nerves IX to XII. (B) The Special visceral efferent cell column giving contribution to the glossopharyngeal and the cranial accessory nerves. (C) The general visceral efferent cell column contributing to the glossopharyngeal and vagus nerves. (D) The somatic efferent cell column giving rise to the hypoglossal nerve.

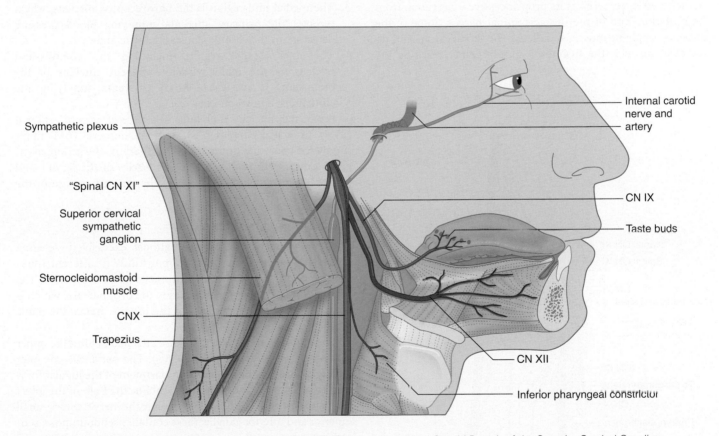

Fig. 18.2 Semischematic Illustration of the Lowest Four Cranial Nerves and the Internal Carotid Branch of the Superior Cervical Ganglion.

corticobulbar input fibres to the hypoglossal nucleus are more crossed, but a few remain uncrossed and supply the ipsilateral hypoglossal nucleus.

Corticobulbar/corticonuclear/supranuclear, nuclear, and infranuclear lesions of the hypoglossal nerve are described together with lesions of the accessory nerve (see Clinical Panels 18.1–18.3.)

SPINAL ACCESSORY NERVE

The spinal accessory nerve (cranial nerve XI) is a purely motor nerve attached to the uppermost five spinal segments of the spinal cord. The nucleus of origin is a column of α and γ motor neurons in the basolateral ventral grey horn.

The nerve runs upwards in the subarachnoid space, posterior to the denticulate ligaments. It enters the cranial cavity through the foramen magnum and leaves it again through the jugular foramen. While in the jugular foramen, it shares a dural sheath with the cranial accessory nerve, but there is no exchange of fibres (Fig. 18.3). Upon leaving the cranium, it crosses the transverse process of the atlas and enters the sternocleidomastoid muscle (SCM), in company with branches from the ventral rami of C2 and C3 spinal nerves of the cervical plexus. It emerges from the posterior border of the SCM and crosses the posterior triangle of the neck to reach the trapezius. It pierces the trapezius accompanied by branches from the ventral rami of C3 and C4 spinal nerves of the cervical plexus. In the posterior triangle the nerve is vulnerable to injury, being embedded in prevertebral fascia and covered only by investing cervical fascia and skin.

The spinal accessory nerve provides the extrafusal and intrafusal motor supply to the SCM and trapezius. The branches from the cervical plexus are proprioceptive in function to the SCM and to the cranio-cervical part of the trapezius. The thoracic part of the trapezius, which arises from the spines of all the thoracic vertebrae, receives its proprioceptive innervation from the posterior rami of the thoracic spinal nerves. Some of the afferents supplying muscle spindles in the thoracic trapezius do not meet up with the fusimotor supply before reaching the spindles. This is the only instance, *in any muscle known*, where the fusimotor and afferent fibres to some spindles travel by completely independent routes.

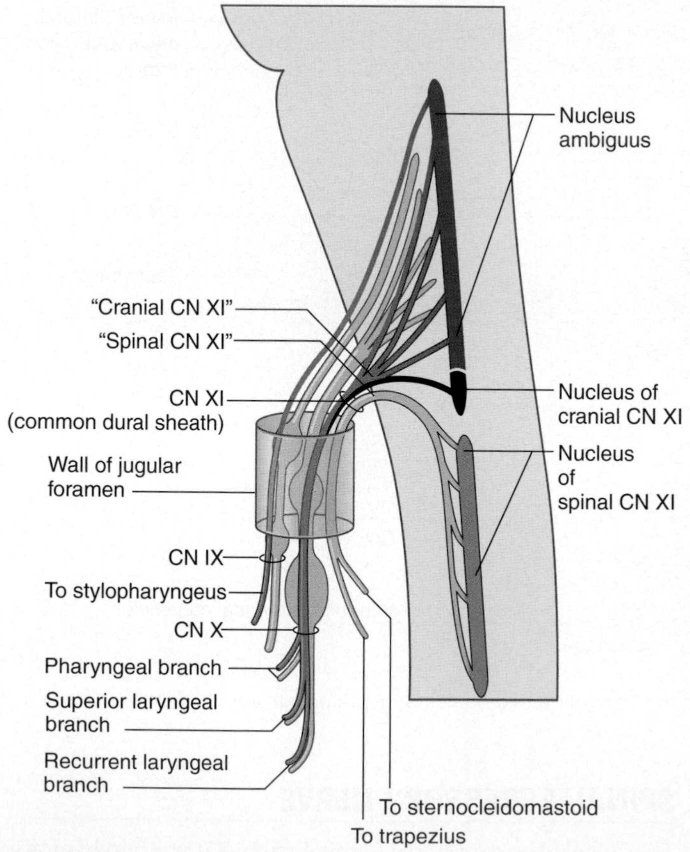
Nucleus ambiguus
"Cranial CN XI"
"Spinal CN XI"
CN XI (common dural sheath)
Nucleus of cranial CN XI
Wall of jugular foramen
Nucleus of spinal CN XI
CN IX
To stylopharyngeus
CN X
Pharyngeal branch
Superior laryngeal branch
Recurrent laryngeal branch
To sternocleidomastoid
To trapezius

Fig. 18.3 Course and distribution (in *red*) of special visceral efferent fibres derived from the nucleus ambiguus.

GLOSSOPHARYNGEAL, VAGUS, AND CRANIAL ACCESSORY NERVES

Especially relevant to cranial nerves IX, X, and XI are the solitary nucleus and the nucleus ambiguus. The solitary nucleus extends from the lower border of the pons to the level of the gracile nucleus. The lower ends of the two solitary nuclei fuse to each other across the median plane, hence the term **commissural nucleus** for the lower part of the nucleus.

Anatomically, the nucleus is divisible into eight parts. Functionally, four *regions* have been clarified (Fig. 18.4):

1. The uppermost region is the **gustatory nucleus**, which receives primary afferents supplying taste buds in the tongue and palate.
2. The lateral mid-region is the **dorsal respiratory nucleus** that carries afferents from the carotid body (see Chapter 24).
3. The medial mid-region is the **baroreceptor nucleus**, which receives the primary afferents supplying blood pressure detectors in the carotid sinus and aortic arch.
4. The most caudal region, including the commissural nucleus, is the major **visceral afferent nucleus** of the brainstem. It receives primary afferents supplying the alimentary and respiratory tracts.

From the nucleus ambiguus the *special visceral efferent* (SVE), branchial efferent (BE), or branchiomeric (BM) fibres supply the constrictor muscles of the pharynx, the stylopharyngeus, levator veli palatini, intrinsic muscles of the larynx, and (via the recurrent laryngeal nerve) the striated muscle of the upper one-third of the oesophagus.

Glossopharyngeal Nerve

The glossopharyngeal nerve is almost exclusively sensory. It carries no less than five different kinds of afferent fibres travelling to five separate afferent nuclei in the brainstem. The largest of its peripheral territories is the oropharynx, which is bounded in front by the back of the tongue, hence the name for the nerve.

The glossopharyngeal rootlets are attached behind the upper part of the olive (post-olivary sulcus). The nerve accompanies the vagus through the anterior compartment of the jugular foramen (the posterior compartment contains the bulb of the internal jugular vein). Within the foramen the nerve shows small superior and inferior ganglia; these contain pseudounipolar sensory neurons.

Immediately below the skull the glossopharyngeal is in the company of three other nerves (see Fig. 18.2): the vagus, the spinal accessory, and the internal carotid (sympathetic) branch of the superior cervical ganglion. Together with the stylopharyngeus, it passes between the superior and middle constrictor muscles to reach the mucous membrane of the oropharynx.

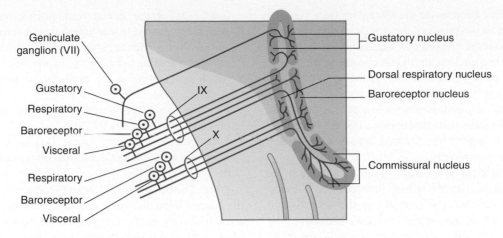

Fig. 18.4 Functional composition of the solitary nucleus (NTS).

Functional Divisions and Branches

- Before emerging from the jugular foramen, the IX nerve gives off a *tympanic branch*, which ramifies on the tympanic membrane and is a potential source of referred pain (see later). The central processes of the tympanic branch synapse in the spinal nucleus of the trigeminal nerve (see Fig. 18.1).
- Some fibres of the tympanic branch are parasympathetic fibres originating in the inferior salivary nucleus. They pierce the roof (tegmen tympani) of the middle ear as the lesser petrosal nerve, leave the skull through the foramen ovale, and synapse in the otic ganglion. Postganglionic fibres supply secretomotor fibres to the parotid gland (see Fig. 13.3).
- The BE supply to the stylopharyngeus comes from the nucleus ambiguus.
- Branches serving 'common sensation' (touch) supply the mucous membranes bounding the oropharynx (throat), including the posterior one-third of the tongue. The neurons synapse centrally in the spinal nucleus of the trigeminal nerve. The glossopharyngeal branches provide the afferent limb of the *gag reflex*—contraction of the pharyngeal constrictors in response to touching the posterior wall of the oropharynx. (The gag reflex is unpleasant because of accompanying nausea. To test the integrity of the CN IX, it is usually sufficient to test sensation on the pharyngeal wall.) Generalised stimulation of the oropharynx elicits a complete swallowing reflex through a linkage between the commissural nucleus and a specific swallowing centre nearby (Chapter 24).
- Gustatory neurons supply the taste buds contained in the posterior third of the tongue; they terminate centrally in the gustatory nucleus of the nucleus tracts solitarii (NTS) (Fig. 18.4).
- An important *carotid branch* descends to the bifurcation of the common carotid artery. This branch contains two different sets of afferent fibres. One set ramifies in the wall of the carotid sinus (at the commencement of the internal carotid artery), terminating in *stretch receptors* responsive to systolic

blood pressure; these *baroreceptor neurons* terminate centrally in the medial part of the nucleus solitarius (Fig. 18.4).

Note: the important carotid *baroreceptor reflex* is described in Chapter 24.

- The second set of afferents in the carotid branch supplies glomus cells in the carotid body. These nerve endings are *chemoreceptors* monitoring carbon dioxide and oxygen levels in the blood. The central terminals enter the dorsal respiratory nucleus (Fig. 18.4).

Note: carotid chemoreceptor reflex arcs are described in Chapter 24.

Vagus and Cranial Accessory Nerves

The vagus is the main parasympathetic nerve. Its preganglionic component has a large area of distribution that includes the heart, the lungs, and the alimentary tract from the oesophagus through the proximal two-thirds of the transverse colon (Chapter 13). At the same time, the vagus is the largest visceral afferent nerve; afferents outnumber parasympathetic motor fibres by four to one. Overall, the vagus contains the same seven fibre classes as the glossopharyngeal nerve, and they will be listed in the same order.

The rootlets of the vagus and cranial accessory nerves are in series with the glossopharyngeal nerve, and the three nerves travel together into the jugular foramen. At this point the cranial accessory nerve shares a dural sheath with the spinal accessory, but there is no exchange of fibres (see Fig. 18.3). Just below the foramen, the cranial accessory is incorporated into the vagus. The vagus itself shows a small, jugular (superior) and a large, nodose (inferior) ganglion; both are sensory.

Functional Divisions and Branches

- An *auricular branch* supplies skin lining the outer ear canal, and a *meningeal branch* ramifies in the posterior cranial fossa. Both branches have their cell bodies in the jugular ganglion; the central processes enter the spinal trigeminal nucleus.

- The parasympathetic neurons for the alimentary tract from the lower oesophagus to the proximal two-thirds of the transverse colon originate from the dorsal motor nucleus of the vagus.
- SVE neurons of the nucleus ambiguus constitute the motor elements in the pharyngeal and laryngeal branches of the vagus. They supply the pharyngeal and laryngeal muscles already noted and all palatine muscles except the tensor veli palatini (supplied by the mandibular branch of the trigeminal nerve). They also supply the striated musculature of the upper third of the oesophagus.
- General visceral afferent fibres from the heart and from the respiratory and alimentary tracts have their cell bodies in the nodose ganglion and synapse centrally in the commissural nucleus. They serve important reflexes including the *Bainbridge reflex* (cardiac acceleration brought about by distension of the right atrium), the *cough reflex* (stimulation of a coughing centre (Chapter 24) by irritation of the tracheobronchial tree), and the *Hering–Breuer reflex*

(inhibition of the dorsal respiratory centre by pulmonary stretch receptors). In addition, afferent information from the stomach (in particular) is forwarded to the hypothalamus and influences feeding behaviour (Chapter 34).
- A few taste buds on the epiglottis project to the gustatory nucleus.
- *Baroreceptors* in the aortic arch project to the medial part of the solitary nucleus (NTS).
- *Chemoreceptors* in the aortic bodies and corresponding receptors at the carotid bifurcation are also innervated by the NTS.

Note: The official term 'cranial accessory nerve' seems inappropriate. Given its course and distribution, 'vagal accessory' is an appropriate name for this nerve. Moreover, it shares no fibres or functions with the spinal accessory nerve.

Corticobulbar/corticonuclear (supranuclear), nuclear, and infranuclear lesions of the IX, X, and XI nerves are described in the Clinical Panels.

CLINICAL PANEL 18.1 Supranuclear Lesions of the Lowest Four Cranial Nerves

Supranuclear lesions of all four nerves are commonly seen following vascular strokes damaging the pyramidal tract in the cerebrum or brainstem.

Effects of Unilateral Supranuclear Lesions

1. The corticobulbar innervation of the hypoglossal nucleus is more crossed than uncrossed. The usual picture following a hemiplegic stroke is as follows: during the first few hours or days, the tongue, when protruded, deviates towards the paralysed side because of the stronger push of the healthy genioglossus. Later the tongue does not deviate on protrusion. However, normal hypoglossal nerve function on the affected side is *not* restored. Electrophysiological testing has revealed that tongue movement, in response to electrical stimulation of the crossed monosynaptic corticonuclear supply to the hypoglossal nucleus, is both delayed and weaker than normal. This, together with comparable deficiency in the corticonuclear supply to the facial nerve (which includes a motor supply to the lips), accounts for the *dysarthria* (slurred speech) that persists after a hemiplegic stroke.
2. Damage to the corticobulbar innervation of the nucleus ambiguus may cause temporary interference with phonation and swallowing.
3. On testing the power of the trapezius by asking the patient to shrug the shoulders against resistance, the muscle on the affected side is relatively weak. This accords with expectation. But on testing sternocleidomastoid muscle (SCM) by asking the patient to turn the head against resistance applied to the side of the jaw, the SCM on the *unaffected* side appears to be relatively weak. Given that electrical stimulation applied to the supranuclear supply for SCM has shown that the crossed supply is strong

and monosynaptic and the uncrossed is weak and disynaptic, there appears to be an 'SCM paradox'.

However, the most parsimonious explanation is that the prime mover for the 'no' headshake is not the contralateral SCM but the *ipsilateral inferior oblique (obliquus capitis inferior)*, a muscle within the suboccipital triangle passing from the spine of the axis to the transverse process of the atlas. Supplementary ipsilateral muscles include the splenius capitis and longissimus capitis. All three are typical spinal muscles and would be expected to share in the general muscle weakness on the affected side.

During the head rotation test, the functionally intact contralateral (healthy side) SCM does contract strongly. However, the three ipsilateral head rotators also have a *tilting* action at the atlanto–occipital joint. The laterally placed insertion of the SCM has strong leverage potential and is well placed to counter the tilting action of the ipsilateral muscles inserting onto the skull.

Effects of Bilateral Supranuclear Lesions

The supranuclear supply to the hypoglossal nucleus and nucleus ambiguus may be compromised *bilaterally* by thrombotic episodes in the brainstem in patients suffering from arteriosclerosis of the vertebrobasilar arterial system. The motor nuclei of the trigeminal nerve (to the masticatory muscles) and of the facial nerve (to the facial muscles) may also be affected. The characteristic picture, known as *pseudobulbar palsy*, is that of an elderly patient who has spastic (tightened) oral and pharyngeal musculature, with consequent difficulty with speech articulation, chewing, and swallowing. The gait is slow and shuffling because of involvement of corticospinal fibres descending to lower limb motor neurons.

CLINICAL PANEL 18.2 Nuclear Lesions of the X, XI, and XII Cranial Nerves

Lesions of the hypoglossal nucleus and nucleus ambiguus occur together in *progressive bulbar palsy*, a variant of progressive muscular atrophy (Chapter 16) in which the cranial motor nuclei of the pons and medulla are attacked at the outset. The patient quickly becomes distressed by a multitude of problems: difficulty in chewing and articulation (mandibular and facial

nerve nuclei) and difficulty in swallowing and phonation (hypoglossal and cranial accessory nuclei).

Unilateral lesions at nuclear level may be caused by occlusion of the vertebral artery or of one of its branches (see Clinical Panel 19.2). The distribution of motor weakness is the same as for infranuclear lesions (see Clinical Panel 18.3).

CLINICAL PANEL 18.3 Infranuclear Lesions of the Lowest Four Cranial Nerves

Jugular Foramen Syndrome

The last four cranial nerves, and the internal carotid (sympathetic) nerve nearby, are at risk of entrapment by a tumour spreading along the base of the skull. The tumour may be a primary one in the nasopharynx or a metastatic one within lymph nodes of the upper cervical chain. In the second case the primary tumour may be in an air sinus or in the tongue, larynx, or pharynx. In either case a mass can usually be felt behind the ramus of the mandible. The symptomatology varies with the number of nerves caught up in the tumour and the degree to which they are compromised.

Symptoms

- Pain in or behind the ear, attributable to irritation of the auricular branches of the IX and X nerves. Whenever an adult complains of constant pain in one ear, without evidence of middle ear disease, a cancer of the pharynx must be suspected.
- Headache from irritation of the meningeal branch of the vagus.
- Hoarseness owing to paralysis of laryngomotor fibres.
- Dysphagia (difficulty in swallowing) owing to paralysis of pharyngomotor fibres.

Signs (see Fig. 18.5)

Horner syndrome (ptosis of the upper eyelid, with some pupillary constriction) from interruption of the sympathetic internal carotid plexus.

Infranuclear paralysis of the hypoglossal nerve, with wasting of the affected side of the tongue and deviation of the tongue to the affected side on protrusion.

When the patient is asked to say 'Aahh', the uvula is pulled away from the affected side by the unopposed healthy levator veli palatini muscle.

Sensory loss in the oropharynx on the affected side.

On laryngoscopic examination, inability to adduct the vocal cord to the midline.

Interruption of the spinal accessory nerve produces weakness and wasting of the SCM and trapezius.

A jugular foramen syndrome may also be caused by invasion of the jugular foramen from above—for instance, by a tumour extending from the cerebellopontine angle (Chapter 22). In this case the sympathetic and spinal accessory nerves will be out of reach and unaffected.

Isolated Lesion of The Spinal Accessory Nerve

The surface marking for the spinal accessory nerve in the posterior triangle of the neck is a line drawn from the posterior border of the SCM one-third of the way down to the anterior border of the trapezius two-thirds of the way down. It may be injured in this part of its course by a stab wound or during a surgical procedure for removal of cancerous lymph nodes. The trapezius is selectively paralysed, whereupon the scapula and clavicle sag noticeably because the trapezius normally helps to carry the upper limb. Shrugging of the shoulder is weakened because the levator scapulae must work alone. Progressive atrophy of the muscle leads to characteristic scalloping of the contour of the neck (see Fig. 18.6).

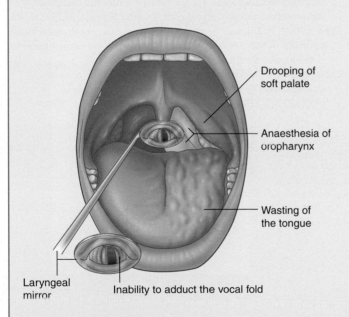

Drooping of soft palate

Anaesthesia of oropharynx

Wasting of the tongue

Laryngeal mirror

Inability to adduct the vocal fold

Fig. 18.5 Left-sided jugular foramen syndrome. A laryngeal mirror is being used to inspect the vocal folds during an attempt to cough.

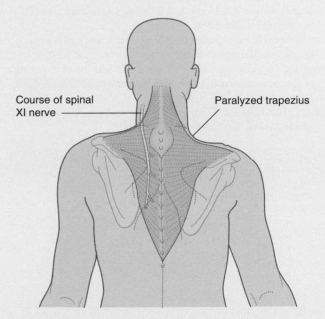

Course of spinal XI nerve

Paralyzed trapezius

Fig. 18.6 Visible effects of right-sided spinal xi paralysis: scalloping of the neck and drooping of the shoulder.

✳ Core Information

Hypoglossal Nerve

The hypoglossal nerve (CN XII) contains somatic efferent neurons supplying extrinsic and intrinsic muscles of the tongue, except the palatoglossus, which is supplied by the pharyngeal plexus (CN X). Its nucleus is close to the midline and is innervated by reticular neurons for automatic/reflex movements and by (mainly crossed) corticobulbar neurons for speech articulation. CN XII emerges lateral to the pyramid in the pre-olivary sulcus, exits through the hypoglossal canal, and descends on the carotid sheath where cervical proprioceptive fibres join the hypoglossal nerve to the lingual muscle spindles. Supranuclear lesion of CN XII is characterised by a slight deviation of the tongue to the contralateral side of the lesion on protrusion of the tongue. Nuclear/infranuclear paralysis is characterised by atrophy and fasciculation of the tongue as well as deviation of the tongue to the ipsilateral side of the lesion.

Spinal Accessory Nerve

The spinal accessory nerve (CN XI) is purely motor. From motor neurons of spinal segments C1 to C5, the axons join and enter the foramen magnum and exit through the jugular foramen; they pierce and supply the SCM, then pass deep to the trapezius and supply it. Proprioceptive connections are received from the cervical and thoracic spinal nerves. Corticobulbar/supranuclear lesions are characterised by weakness of the contralateral trapezius and contralateral head rotators, nuclear/infranuclear lesions by ipsilateral wasting of the two muscles, and drooping of the scapula.

Glossopharyngeal Nerve

The glossopharyngeal nerve (CN IX) emerges posterior to the olive (post-olivary sulcus) and exits the jugular foramen, where it shows two pseudounipolar cell ganglia and gives off a tympanic branch that is partly sensory to the middle ear and partly parasympathetic to the parotid gland via the otic ganglion. IX then passes between superior and middle constrictors to enter the oropharynx, where it supplies general sensation to the mucous membrane including the posterior third of tongue (hence the name), and taste fibres to the posterior one-third of the tongue and the circumvallate papillae. A carotid branch supplies the carotid sinus and carotid body.

Vagus and Cranial Accessory Nerves

The vagus nerve (CN X) and cranial XI rootlets emerge posterior to the olive and unite in the jugular foramen. Cranial CN XI fibres arise in the distal part of the nucleus ambiguus and utilise the laryngeal and pharyngeal branches of X to supply the intrinsic muscles of the larynx and pharynx and all palatine muscles except the tensor veli palatini, which is innervated by the mandibular division of trigeminal (V3).

Preganglionic X fibres travel to the intramural ganglia in the walls of the heart, bronchi, and foregut and midgut parts of the alimentary tract (the hindgut is innervated by the sacral parasympathetic). Visceral afferents from these regions, and from the larynx and pharynx, have unipolar cell bodies in the nodose ganglion and project to the commissural nucleus of the nucleus tractus solitarii (NTS).

SUGGESTED READINGS

Andresen MC. Nucleus tractus solitarii — gateway to neural circulatory control. *Ann Rev Physiol.* 1994;56:93—117.

Eman AB, Kejner AE, Hogikyan ND, et al. Disorders IX and X. *Semin Neurol.* 2009;29:85—92.

Fitzgerald MJT, Sachithanandan SR. The structure and source of lingual proprioceptors in the monkey. *J Anat.* 1979;128:523—552.

Fitzgerald MJT, Comerford PT, Tuffery AR. Sources of innervation of the neuromuscular spindles in sternomastoid and trapezius. *J Anat.* 1982;144:184—190.

Lin HC, Barkhaus PE. Cranial nerve XII: the hypoglossal nerve. *Semin Neurol.* 2009;29:45—52.

Massey EW. Spinal accessory nerve lesions. *Semin Neurol.* 2009;29:82—84.

Mtui EP, Anwar M, Reis DJ, et al. Medullary visceral reflex circuits: local afferents to nucleus tractus solitarii synthesize catecholamines and project to thoracic spinal cord. *J Comp Neurol.* 1995;351:5—26.

Ryan S, Blyth P, Duggan N, et al. Is the cranial accessory nerve really a portion of the accessory nerve? Anatomy of the cranial nerves in the jugular foramen. *Anat Sci Int.* 2007;82:1—7.

Thompson PD, Thickbroom GW, Mastaglia FL. Corticomotor representation of the sternocleidomastoid muscle. *Brain.* 1997;120:245—255.

Vestibular Nerve

STUDY GUIDELINES

1. Describe the components of the static labyrinth and its primary role.
2. Describe the components of the dynamic labyrinth and its primary role.
3. Describe the procedure for performing a *warm water caloric test*.

INTRODUCTION

The *vestibulocochlear nerve* is primarily composed of the centrally directed axons of bipolar neurons housed in the petrous portion of the temporal bone (Fig. 19.1). The peripheral processes project to neuroepithelial cells in the vestibular labyrinth and cochlea. The nerve enters the brainstem at the junctional region of the pons and medulla oblongata.

VESTIBULAR SYSTEM

The *bony labyrinth* of the inner ear is a very dense bony shell containing **perilymph**, which resembles extracellular fluid in general. The perilymph provides a water jacket for the *membranous labyrinth*, which encloses the sense organs of balance and of hearing. The sense organs are bathed in **endolymph**. The endolymph resembles intracellular fluid, being potassium rich and sodium poor.

The vestibular labyrinth comprises the **utricle**, the **saccule**, and three *semicircular ducts* (Fig. 19.2). The utricle and saccule contain a 3×2-mm^2 *macula*. Each semicircular duct contains an *ampulla* at one end, and the ampulla houses a crista. (It should be pointed out that clinicians commonly speak of 'canals' where 'ducts' would be strictly more appropriate.)

The two maculae are the sensory organs of the *static labyrinth*, which signals head position. The three cristae are the organs of the *kinetic* or *dynamic labyrinth*, which signals head movement.

The bipolar cells of the *vestibular (Scarpa) ganglion* occupy the internal acoustic meatus. Their peripheral processes are applied to the five sensory end organs. Their central processes, which constitute the *vestibular nerve*, cross the subarachnoid space and synapse in the vestibular nuclei previously seen in Figs. 17.14 and 17.15.

Static Labyrinth: Anatomy and Actions

The position and structure of the maculae are shown in Fig. 19.3. The *utricular macula* is relatively horizontal, while the *saccular macula* is relatively vertical. The cuboidal cells lining the membranous labyrinth become columnar *supporting cells* in the maculae. Among the supporting cells are so-called *hair cells* (two morphologically different types are found that differ in their properties), to which vestibular nerve endings are applied. Some hair cells are almost completely enclosed by large nerve endings (type 1), whereas others (phylogenetically older) receive only small contacts (type 2). At the cell bases are *ribbon synapses*, the synaptic vesicles being lined up along synaptic bars. Projecting from the free surface of each hair cell are about 100 *stereocilia* and, close to the cell margin, a single, long *kinocilium*. The hair cells discharge continuously, at a resting rate of about 100 Hz.

The hair cell stereocilia of the maculae are embedded in a gelatinous matrix (*otolithic membrane*) containing protein-bound calcium carbonate crystals called *otoconia* ('ear sand'). The cilia 'move' as a unit when the otolithic membrane is displaced. (The term 'otoliths', when used, refers to the larger 'ear stones' of reptiles.) The otoconia exert 'gravitational drag' on the hair cells. Whenever the stereocilia are deflected towards the kinocilium the hair cell is depolarised; deflection in the opposite direction results in hyperpolarisation of the hair cells. Each macula has a central groove *(striola)* and the hair cell orientations have a mirror arrangement in relation to the groove. Polarisation of the hair cells, with respect to the striola, results in the hair cells on one side becoming depolarised and those on the other side becoming hyperpolarised whenever the otolithic membrane is displaced.

The arrangement of the maculae allows them to be responsive to gravitational forces and to 'communicate' head position as well as linear acceleration. In response to this signal the vestibular nuclei initiate compensatory movements, with the effect of maintaining the centre of gravity between the feet (in standing) or just in front of the feet (during locomotion), and of keeping the head horizontal. These effects are mediated by the vestibulospinal tracts.

The *lateral vestibulospinal tract*, seen earlier in sections of medulla oblongata in Chapter 17, arises from large neurons in

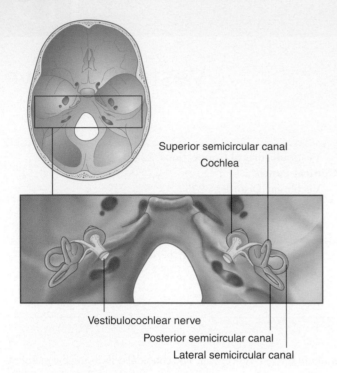

Superior semicircular canal
Cochlea

Vestibulocochlear nerve
Posterior semicircular canal
Lateral semicircular canal

Fig. 19.1 Bony labyrinth, viewed from above.

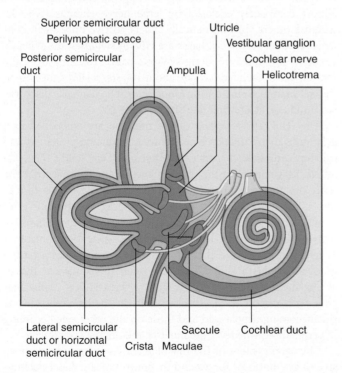

Superior semicircular duct
Perilymphatic space
Posterior semicircular duct
Ampulla
Utricle
Vestibular ganglion
Cochlear nerve
Helicotrema

Lateral semicircular duct or horizontal semicircular duct
Crista   Maculae
Saccule   Cochlear duct

Fig. 19.2 Locations of the five vestibular sense organs.

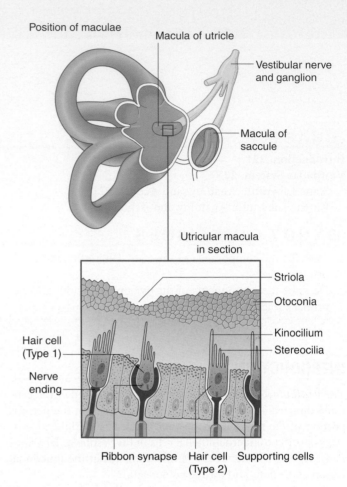

Position of maculae
Macula of utricle
Vestibular nerve and ganglion
Macula of saccule

Utricular macula in section

Striola
Otoconia
Kinocilium
Stereocilia
Hair cell (Type 1)
Nerve ending

Ribbon synapse   Hair cell (Type 2)   Supporting cells

Fig. 19.3 Static labyrinth.

loop (Chapter 16). During standing, the tract is tonically active on both sides of the spinal cord. During walking, activity is selective for the quadriceps motor neurons of the leading leg; this commences following heel strike and continues during the stance phase (when the other leg is off the ground). Deiters nucleus is somatotopically organised and the functionally appropriate neurons are selected by the flocculonodular lobe of the cerebellum. The flocculonodular lobe (Chapter 27) has two-way connections with all four vestibular nuclei.

Antigravity action is triggered mainly from the horizontal macula of the utricle. The vertical macula of the saccule, on the other hand, is maximally activated by a *free fall*. The shearing effect on the macula produces a powerful extensor thrust in anticipation of a hard landing.

A small, **medial vestibulospinal tract** arises in the medial and inferior vestibular nuclei (Fig. 17.6). It descends bilaterally in the medial longitudinal fasciculus and terminates upon excitatory and inhibitory interneurons in the cervical spinal cord. It operates *head-righting reflexes* that serve to keep the head—and the gaze—horizontal when the body is craned forward or to one side. Good examples of head-righting reflexes are to be seen around pool tables and in bowling alleys. An added twist can be provided, if required, by torsion of the eyeballs (up to 10 degrees) within the orbital sockets. This *eye-righting reflex* is

the **lateral vestibular nucleus (of Deiters)**. The fibres descend in the ventral funiculus on the same side of the spinal cord and synapse upon extensor (lower extremity antigravity) motor neurons. Both α and γ motor neurons are excited, and a significant part of the increased muscle tone is exerted by way of the γ

mediated by axons contributed to the *ascending* medial longitudinal fasciculus from the superior and medial vestibular nucleus to reach nuclei controlling the extraocular muscles. These reflex movements of the eyes will be opposite to the direction of movement perceived by the vestibular system. Evidence derived from unilateral vestibular destruction (Clinical Panel 19.1) indicates that the horizontal position of the eyes in the upright head is the result of a cancelling effect of bilateral tonic activity in these vestibuloocular pathways. The medial vestibulospinal tract is also activated by the kinetic labyrinth.

The static labyrinth contributes to the sense of position. The sense of position of the body in space is normally provided by three sensory systems: the visual system, the conscious proprioceptive system, and the vestibular system. Deprived of one of the three, the individual can stand and walk by using information provided by the other two. Following loss of vision, for example, the subject can get about, although the constraints imposed by blindness are known to all. Following loss of conscious proprioception instead, the subject uses vision as a substitute for proprioceptive sense and closure of the eyes (sensory ataxia, see Chapter 15) may lead to instability and a fall.

Kinetic Labyrinth: Anatomy and Actions

Basic features of the macular epithelium are repeated in the three cristae. Again, there are supporting cells and hair cells to which vestibular nerve endings are applied. The kinocilia of the hair cells are long, penetrating into a gelatinous projection called the **cupula** (Fig. 19.4). The cupula is bonded to the opposite wall of the ampulla.

These cristae are sensitive to angular acceleration of the labyrinths. Angular acceleration occurs during rotary 'yes' and 'no' movements of the head. The endolymph tends to lag behind because of its inertia, and the cupula balloons like a sail when thrust against it. The disposition of the kinocilia is uniform across each crista and is such that the *lateral* ampullary crista is facilitated by cupular displacement *towards* the utricle; the *superior* and *posterior* cristae are facilitated by cupular displacement *away from* the utricle. In practical terms the right lateral ampulla is stimulated by turning the head to the right and the left, while turning to the left. The superior ampullae are stimulated by flexion of the head and the posterior ampullae by extension of the head.

Efferents from the cristae terminate in the medial and superior vestibular nuclei and, as with the macula, there are also two-way connections with the flocculonodular lobe of the cerebellum. The semicircular canals are also the only peripheral sense organ directly connected to the cerebellum (uvula and nodulus).

The function of the kinetic labyrinth is to provide information for compensatory movements of the eyes in response to movement of the head. *Vestibuloocular reflexes* operate to maintain the gaze on a selected target. A simple example is our ability to gaze at the period (full stop) at the end of a sentence, while moving the head about. The two eyes move *conjugately*, that is, in parallel, in a direction that is opposite to head movement.

The horizontal vestibuloocular reflex response to a rightwards turn of the head is depicted in Figs. 19.4 and 19.5, and is

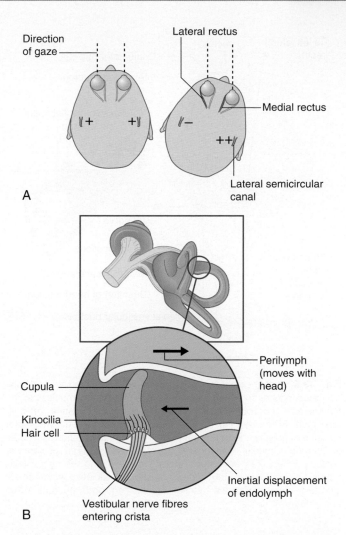

Fig. 19.4 (A) A rightwards head turn activates nerve endings in the right lateral semicircular canal, resulting in contraction of the left lateral and right medial rectus muscles. (B) The nerve endings in the cupula are excited by passive displacement of the cupula towards the ampulla. Impulse traffic increases along parent bipolar neurons whose central fibres excite the medial and superior vestibular nuclei.

described in their captions. Appropriate point-to-point connections also exist between the vestibular nuclei and gaze centres in the midbrain for similar reflexes in the vertical plane.

To control the vestibuloocular reflexes, the cerebellum is informed about the initial position of the head in relation to the trunk. This information is provided by a great wealth of muscle spindles in the deep muscles surrounding the cervical vertebral column. The spindle afferents enter the spinal cord, relay in the accessory cuneate nucleus on each side, and contribute to the cuneocerebellar tract that projects to the cerebellum via the inferior cerebellar peduncle (Fig. 17.12).

Nystagmus. A horizontal vestibuloocular reflex can be elicited artificially by warming or cooling the endolymph in the semicircular canals. In routine tests of vestibular function, advantage is taken of the proximity of the bony wall of the horizontal

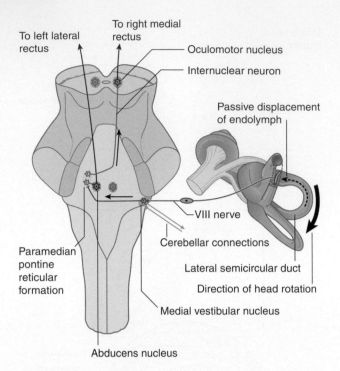

Fig. 19.5 Under cerebellar guidance, the right medial vestibular nucleus responds to a rightwards head turn by sending impulses to the contralateral horizontal gaze centre (paramedian pontine reticular formation, PPRF; see Fig. 17.15). The PPRF selects abducens motor neurons supplying the left lateral rectus and sends internuclear fibres up the right medial longitudinal fasciculus to the right oculomotor nucleus, where they seek out motor neurons serving the right medial rectus. (Not shown is the superior vestibular nucleus, which sends ipsilateral fibres having the function of inhibiting motor neurons to the two antagonist recti.)

vertigo — a sense of rotation of self in relation to the external world or vice versa.

Unilateral and bilateral vestibular syndromes are reviewed in Clinical Panel 19.1. A vascular syndrome involving the vestibular system in the medulla oblongata is described in Clinical Panel 19.2.

Caloric thermal irrigation is one test used to evaluate right versus left vestibular function, but it is also used at the bedside to determine the functional integrity of the brainstem when consciousness is depressed, such as *coma* (unarousable unresponsiveness) or in diagnosing *brain death* (permanent absence of cerebral and brainstem functions). In these clinical scenarios one canal is irrigated at a time with ice water (hence the name '*cold water caloric*') and, if the brainstem (medulla to midbrain) is intact, both eyes will slowly move towards the irrigated ear; nystagmus will be absent in this situation. Other patterns of movement or lack thereof, assuming normal prior vestibular function, are indicative of brainstem dysfunction.

Vestibulocortical Connections

Second-order sensory neurons project from the vestibular nuclei mainly to the *ipsilateral* thalamus. The fibres relay via the ventral posterior nucleus to the *parietoinsular vestibular cortex (PIVC)* and to the adjacent region of the superior temporal gyrus, as shown in Fig. 19.6. However, the PIVC cannot be named as a primary vestibular sensory area because it is in fact multisensory, receiving visual and tactile inputs as well as vestibular. (By analogy, positron emission tomography [PET] studies of tactile sensation show activity throughout most of the parietal lobe, but we know from other sources that the postcentral gyrus is the primary area, being the take-off point for analysis in the posterior parietal cortex.)

semicircular canal to the external ear canal of the middle ear. The horizontal canal is angled at 30 degrees to the horizontal plane; tilting the head back by 60 degrees brings the canal into the vertical plane, with the ampulla uppermost. In **warm water caloric thermal irrigation**, water at 44°C is then instilled into the ear. The air in the middle ear is heated, and heat transfer to the horizontal canal produces convection currents within the endolymph. Whether through displacement of the cupula or by some other mechanism, the crista of the warmer horizontal ampulla becomes more active than its opposite number. The result is a slow drift of the eyes away from the stimulated side, as if the head had been turned to the side being tested. This drift is followed by a recovery phase in which the eyes snap back to the right or their 'resting position'. These slow and fast phases are repeated several times per second. This is *vestibular nystagmus*. **Nystagmus** is a to-and-fro movement of the eyes and the direction is named in accordance with the fast phase because of the obvious 'beat'. (Trigger factors and duration also provide further diagnostic information regarding its significance.) So, a warm caloric test applied to the right ear should produce a right-beating nystagmus ('nystagmus to the right'). Instillation of cold water will result in the opposite response. Subjectively, nystagmus is accompanied by

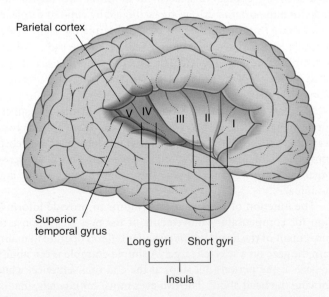

Fig. 19.6 Parietoinsular vestibular cortex (blue). *I–III*, Short insular gyri; *IV, V,* long insular gyri (IV and V are commonly fused as a single, Y-shaped long insular gyrus).

CLINICAL PANEL 19.1   Vestibular Disorders

"*Vertigo* is the sensation of self-motion when no self-motion is occurring; *dizziness* is the sensation of disturbed or impaired spatial orientation without a false or distorted sense of motion; and *imbalance* or *unsteadiness* is the feeling of being unstable while seated, standing, or walking without a particular directional preference" (Bisdorff A, et al, 2009). All of these symptoms can reflect dysfunction within the vestibular system, from the periphery to the brain, so patient and clinical features help facilitate localisation, investigation and intervention.

Unilateral Vestibular Disease

Acute dysfunction of one vestibular labyrinth may have multiple aetiologies:

- Follow a viral inflammation of the vestibular nerve *(vestibular neuronitis)*
- Migration of a portion of a calcium carbonate crystal of the utricle otoconia into a semicircular canal *(benign positional vertigo)*
- Migraine headache variant *(vestibular migraine)*
- Or represent a more serious disorder where recovery is less likely; spread of disease from the middle ear or thrombosis of the labyrinthine artery in the elderly and presenting with isolated vestibular symptoms (vertigo or dizziness).

The effects of unilateral vestibular disease are well demonstrated when the vestibular system is inactivated surgically, either during removal of an acoustic neuroma (Chapter 22) or as a last resort in treating paroxysmal attacks of vertigo. During the immediate postoperative period, the patient shows the effects of loss of tonic input from the static labyrinth:

- Loss of function in the vestibuloocular pathway on one side leads to about 10 degrees of torsion of both eyeballs towards that side. The patient's perception of the horizontal shows a corresponding tilt, so that reaching movements become inaccurate.
- The head tilts to the same side, matching the gaze with the tilted horizon.
- The patient tends to fall to the same side, because the vestibuloocular pathway no longer compensates for tilting of the head.

Because function continues in the normal lateral semicircular canal, there is a nystagmus to the normal side.

Bilateral Vestibular Disease

Following total loss of static labyrinthine function, visual guidance becomes important and the patient avoids walking in the dark. By day, any distraction causing the patient to look overhead may result in a fall. Loss of kinetic labyrinthine function makes it impossible to fix the gaze on an object while the head is moving. During walking, the scene bobs up and down *(oscillopsia)* as if it were being viewed through a handheld camera.

CLINICAL PANEL 19.2   Lateral Medullary Syndrome (Fig. 19.7)

Thrombosis of the vertebral or posterior inferior cerebellar artery may produce an *infarct* (area of necrosis) in the lateral part of the medulla. (Brainstem pathology is always suspected when a cranial nerve lesion on one side is accompanied by 'upper motor neuron signs', such as hemiplegia or increased reflexes, on the contralateral side, so-called *alternating* or *crossed hemiplegia*; seen with an infarction involving the medial medulla, *medial medullary syndrome*.)

The clinical features of a lateral medullary infarction (**lateral medullary syndrome**) depend on the extent of injury to nuclei and pathways to include:

- Damage to the vestibular nuclei leads to vertigo (often with initial vomiting or hiccups) together with the symptoms of unilateral disconnection of the labyrinth as described in Clinical Panel 19.1.
- Interruption of posterior and rostral anterior spinocerebellar fibres may produce signs of cerebellar ataxia in the ipsilateral limbs.
- Damage to the spinal tract of the trigeminal nerve interrupts fine primary afferent fibres descending the brainstem from the trigeminal ganglion (Chapter 21). These fibres are functionally equivalent to those of the Lissauer tract in the spinal cord (Chapter 15). The result of the interruption is loss of pain and thermal senses from the face on the same side.
- Interruption of the central sympathetic pathway to the spinal cord produces an ipsilateral *Horner syndrome* (ptosis, miosis, and anhidrosis).
- Damage to the nucleus ambiguus causes hoarseness and sometimes difficulty in swallowing from ipsilateral paralysis of the soft palate, larynx, and pharynx.
- Damage to the solitary nucleus can impair ipsilateral taste.
- Damage to the lateral spinothalamic tract (within the spinal lemniscus) leads to contralateral loss of pain and temperature sense in the trunk and limbs. Several months or even years later, central post stroke pain may develop within the same area (see Chapter 35).

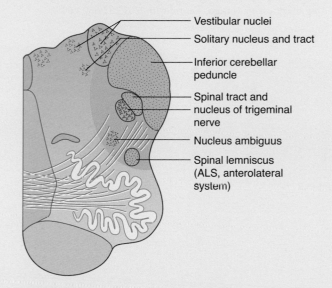

Labels:
Vestibular nuclei
Solitary nucleus and tract
Inferior cerebellar peduncle
Spinal tract and nucleus of trigeminal nerve
Nucleus ambiguus
Spinal lemniscus (ALS, anterolateral system)

Fig. 19.7 Lateral medullary infarct (shaded).

For the majority of patients presenting with isolated vertigo or dizziness, a peripheral (vestibular system or nerve) aetiology will be the explanation for their symptoms. However, in 11% of patients with an isolated episode vertigo or dizziness attack the aetiology will be vascular and most frequently involving the posterior inferior cerebellar artery area territory.

✳ Core Information

The *static labyrinth* comprises the maculae in the utricle and saccule. The *dynamic labyrinth* comprises the semicircular ducts and their cristae. Vestibular bipolar neurons supply the organs of the static and dynamic labyrinth and synapse in the vestibular nucleus, which projects to the flocculonodular lobe of the cerebellum. The static labyrinth functions to control balance, via the lateral vestibulospinal tract, by increasing antigravity tone on the side to which the head is tilted. This system is in partnership with proprioceptors and the retina in maintaining an upright posture. In the absence of good vision, or at night, a fall is likely if the system has been compromised.

The dynamic labyrinth operates *vestibuloocular reflexes* to keep the gaze on target during rotatory movements of the head. For sideways rotation, the main projection is from the medial vestibular nucleus to the contralateral paramedian pontine reticular formation (PPRF), which activates cranial nerve VI neurons supplying the lateral rectus muscle and internuclear neurons projecting via the medial longitudinal fasciculus (MLF) to the contralateral oculomotor nucleus. Together these five inner ear organs stabilise our vision and allow us to remain in the correct orientation. Clinically, the dynamic labyrinth pathway can be activated and assessed by the *caloric test*, which normally elicits nystagmus.

SUGGESTED READINGS

Balaban CD. Neurotransmitters in the vestibular system. *Handb Clin Neurol.* 2016;137:41–55.

Bisdorff A, Von Brevern M, Lempert T, Newman-Toker DE. Classification of vestibular symptoms: towards an international classification of vestibular disorders. *J Vestib Res.* 2009;19:1–13.

Brandt T, Dieterich M. The dizzy patient: don't forget disorders of the central vestibular system. *Nat Rev Neurol.* 2017;13: 352–362.

Burn JC, Stone JS. Development and regeneration of vestibular hair cells in mammals. *Semin Cell Dev Biol.* 2017;65:96–105.

Curthoys IS, MacDougall HG, Vidal PP, de Waele C. Sustained and transient vestibular systems: a physiological basis for interpreting vestibular function. *Front Neurol.* 2017;8:117.

Lee SH, Kim JO. Acute diagnosis and management of stroke presenting dizziness or vertigo. *Neurol Clin.* 2015;33:687–698.

Ó Maoiléidigh D, Ricci AJ. A bundle of mechanisms: inner-ear hair-cell mechanotransduction. *Trends Neurosci.* 2019;42: 221–236.

Ogawa K, Suzuki Y, Oishi M, Kamei S. Clinical study of 46 patients with lateral medullary infarction. *J Stroke Cerebrovasc Dis.* 2015;24: 1065–1074.

Sandhu JS, Rea PA. Clinical examination and management of the dizzy patient. *Br J Hosp Med (Lond).* 2016;77:692–698.

Seemungal BM. The cognitive neurology of the vestibular system. *Curr Opin Neurol.* 2014;27:125–132.

Shepard NT, Jacobson GP. The caloric irrigation test. *Handb Clin Neurol.* 2016;137:119–131.

Tarnutzer AA, Straumann D. Nystagmus. *Curr Opin Neurol.* 2018;31: 74–80.

van de Berg R, Rosengren S, Kingma H. Laboratory examinations for the vestibular system. *Curr Opin Neurol.* 2018;31:111–116.

Cochlear Nerve

STUDY GUIDELINES

1. Describe the mechanism of how vibrations created by sound waves result in activation of the organ of Corti.
2. Be able to identify the scala vestibuli, scala tympani, and scala media and components of the spiral organ.
3. Reproduce the central auditory pathway from the spiral ganglion to the primary auditory cortex.
4. Describe the role of the olivocochlear bundle.

AUDITORY SYSTEM

The auditory system comprises the cochlea, the cochlear nerve, and the central auditory pathway travelling from the cochlear nuclei in the brainstem to the cortex of the temporal lobe. The central auditory pathway is more elaborate (provides for more processing of the signal) than the somatosensory or visual pathways because the 'same' sounds are detected by both ears. To signal the location of a sound as well as perform further processing prior to transmission to the thalamus and cortex, a very complex neuronal network is in place. Numerous connections (mainly inhibitory) between the two central pathways exist to accomplish this task, as well as to magnify minute differences in intensity and timing of sounds that exist during normal, binaural hearing.

The Cochlea

The main features of the cochlear structure are seen in Figs 20.1 and 20.2. The cochlea is pictured as though it were upright, but in life it lies on its side, as shown earlier in Fig. 19.1. The central bony pillar of the cochlea (the **modiolus**) is in the axis of the internal acoustic meatus. Projecting from the modiolus, like the flange of a screw, is the **osseous spiral lamina**. The **basilar membrane** is attached to the tip of this lamina; it reaches across the cavity of the bony cochlea to become attached to the **spiral ligament** on the outer wall. The osseous spiral lamina and spiral ligament become progressively smaller as one ascends the two and one half turns of the cochlea, and the fibres of the basilar membrane become progressively longer.

The basilar membrane and its attachments divide the cochlear chamber into upper and lower compartments. These are the **scala vestibuli** and the **scala tympani**, respectively, and they are filled with perilymph. They communicate at the apex of the cochlea, through the **helicotrema**. A third compartment, the **scala media (cochlear duct)**, lies above the basilar membrane and is filled with endolymph. It is separated from the scala vestibuli by the delicate **vestibular membrane** (*Reissner membrane*).

Sitting on the basilar membrane is the **spiral organ** (*organ of Corti*). The principal sensory receptor epithelium consists of a single row of **inner hair cells** (sensory receptors), each one having up to 20 large afferent nerve endings applied to it. The hair cells rest upon **supporting cells**. There are also ancillary cells. The organ of Corti contains a central **tunnel**, filled with endolymph diffusing through the basilar membrane. On the outer side of the tunnel are several rows of **outer hair cells**, attended by supporting and ancillary cells (Fig. 20.2).

All the hair cells are surmounted by **stereocilia**. Unlike the vestibular hair cells, they have no kinocilium in the adult state. The stereocilia of the outer hair cells are embedded in the overlying tectorial membrane. Those of the inner hair cells lie immediately below the membrane.

Deflection of these stereocilia activates mechanically gated channels, causing the hair cell to depolarise and activate its afferent nerve endings from the *cochlea ganglion* (or *spiral ganglion*).

The outer hair cells are contractile, and they have substantial efferent nerve endings (see Fig. 20.2). It has been suggested that the oscillatory movements of outer hair cells influence the sensitivity of the inner hair cells through effects on the tectorial or basilar membrane.

Sound Transduction. Vibrations of the tympanic membrane in response to sound waves are transmitted along the ossicular chain. The footplate of the stapes fits snugly into the oval window, and vibrations of the stapes are converted to pressure waves in the scala vestibuli. The pressure waves are transmitted through the vestibular membrane to reach the basilar membrane. High-frequency pressure waves, created by high-pitched sounds, cause the short fibres of the basilar membrane in the basal turn of the cochlea to resonate and absorb their energy. Low-frequency waves produce resonance in the apical turn, where the fibres are the longest. The basilar membrane is therefore *tonotopically organized* in its fibre sequence. Not surprisingly, the inner hair cells

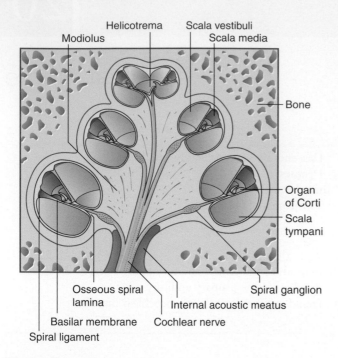

Fig. 20.1 The cochlea in section.

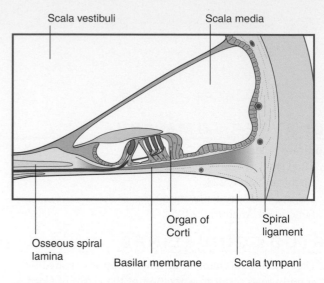

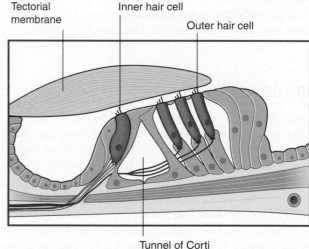

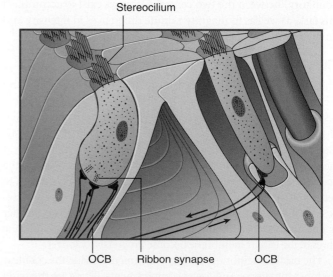

Fig. 20.2 Organ of corti at three levels of magnification. *Arrows* indicate directions of impulse traffic. *OCB*, Fibres of the olivocochlear bundle.

have a similar tonotopic sequence. In response to local resonance, the cells depolarise and liberate excitatory transmitter substance from synaptic ribbons (see Fig. 20.2).

The nerve fibres supplying the hair cells are the peripheral processes of the bipolar cochlear or spiral ganglion neurons lodged in the base of the osseous spiral lamina.

Cochlear Nerve

The bulk of the cochlear nerve consists of myelinated central processes of some 30,000 large bipolar neurons of the *cochlea (or spiral) ganglion*. Unmyelinated fibres come from small ganglion cells supplying dendrites to the outer hair cells. (Motor fibres do not travel in the cochlear nerve trunk.) The cochlear nerve traverses the subarachnoid space in company with the vestibular and facial nerves, and it enters the brainstem at the pontomedullary junction.

Central Auditory Pathways

The general plan of the central auditory pathway from the left cochlear nerve to the cerebral cortex is shown in Fig. 20.3. All entering cochlear nerve axons (first-order auditory neurons) terminate ipsilaterally on the cells of the *cochlear nuclei* located at the level of the entrance of the nerve, commonly described as the *pontomedullary junction*. From here, some second-order neurons ascend through the brainstem to reach the medial geniculate body, but most do not. Most of the second-order auditory neurons synapse along the way on one or more of several brainstem nuclei that form the 'auditory way stations' (see later). These provide further processing of the auditory information before it reaches the level of the thalamus. Students sometimes question whether these 'long neurons' should be properly referred to as 'third-order', 'fourth-order', and so on, sensory neurons in the auditory pathway because it is hard to call such long neurons 'interneurons'. It is probably best to say that second-order neurons in the auditory pathway may be comprised of two or more distinct neurons that collectively serve the 'function' of the second-order neurons in projecting (and processing) auditory information from the termination point of the peripheral nerve to the dorsal thalamus.

Almost all the neurons ascending in this pathway will synapse in the inferior colliculus, having crossed the midline as part of the trapezoid body and having contributed to the *lateral lemniscus*. After synapsing in the *inferior colliculus*, the brachium

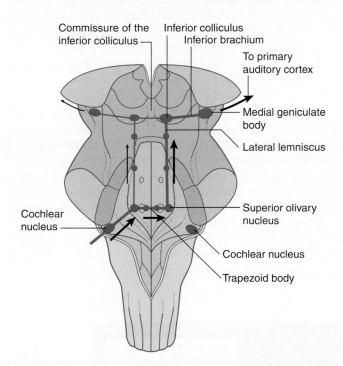

Fig. 20.3 Dorsal view of the brainstem showing the basic plan of central auditory pathways. The strand linking the two inferior colliculi is the collicular commissure.

of the inferior colliculus links the inferior colliculus with the *medial geniculate body* (the place of origin of third-order auditory neurons), which projects to *primary auditory cortex* Brodmann areas 41 and 42 in the transverse temporal gyrus. Some axons of the lateral lemniscus do bypass the inferior colliculus and go straight to the medial geniculate.

While most of the projection is bilateral, a small but important purely ipsilateral relay passes from the superior olivary nucleus to the higher auditory centres.

Functional Anatomy (Fig. 20.4)

Cochlear Nuclei. The cochlear nuclei, the *dorsal* and *ventral cochlear nucleus*, can be found encircling the lateral surface of the inferior cerebellar peduncle. Many incoming fibres of the cochlear nerve bifurcate and enter both nuclei. The cells in both are tonotopically arranged.

Responses of many cells in the ventral nucleus are called primary-like, because their frequency (firing rate) resembles that of primary afferents. Most of the output neurons from the ventral cochlear nucleus project to the nearby *superior olivary nucleus*.

The cells of the dorsal nucleus are heterogeneous. At least six different cell types have been characterised by their morphology and electrical behaviour. Most of the output neurons of the dorsal cochlear nucleus project to the contralateral inferior colliculus. Individually, they exhibit an extremely narrow range of tonal responses, being 'focused' by collateral inhibition.

Superior Olivary Nucleus. The superior olivary complex of nuclei is relatively small in the human brain. It contains *binaural neurons* affected by inputs from both ears. Ipsilateral inputs are excitatory to the binaural neurons, whereas contralateral inputs are inhibitory. The inhibitory effect is mediated by interneurons in the *nucleus of the trapezoid body* (see Fig. 20.4).

The superior olivary nucleus is responsive to differences in intensity and the short timing difference that exists between a

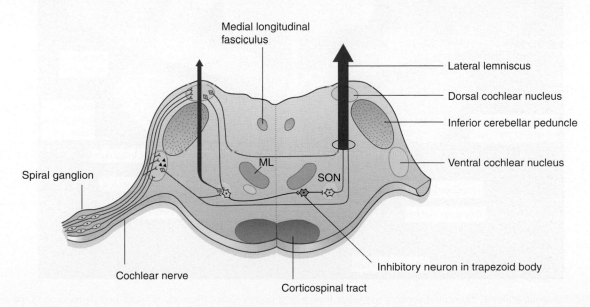

Fig. 20.4 Transverse section of the lower end of the pons showing central connections of the cochlear nerve. *ML,* Medial lemniscus; *SON,* superior olivary nucleus.

sound from a single source that enters one ear and then the same sound entering the other ear. On the side ipsilateral to the sound, stimulation of the cochlear nucleus is earlier and more intense than on the contralateral side. By exaggerating these differences through crossed inhibition, the superior olivary nucleus helps to indicate the spatial direction of incoming sounds. At the same time, the excited nucleus projects to the inferior colliculus of both sides, giving rise to binaural responses in the neurons of the inferior colliculus and beyond.

Lateral Lemniscus. Fibres of the *lateral lemniscus* arise from the dorsal and ventral cochlear nuclei, and from the superior olivary nuclei—in each case, mainly contralaterally. The tract terminates in the **central nucleus of the inferior colliculus**. Nuclei within the lateral lemniscus participate in reflex arcs (see later).

Inferior Colliculus. Spatial information from the superior olivary nucleus, intensity information from the ventral cochlear nucleus, and pitch information from the dorsal cochlear nucleus are integrated in the inferior colliculus. The main (central) part of the nucleus is laminated in a tonotopic manner. Within each tonal lamina, cells differ in their responses. Some have a characteristic 'tuning curve' (they respond only to a specific tone). Some fire spontaneously but are inhibited by sound, and some respond only to a moving source of sound.

In addition to projecting to the medial geniculate body (nucleus), the inferior colliculus exerts inhibitory effects on the opposite side through the *commissure of the inferior colliculus* (see Fig. 20.3). It also contributes to the *tectospinal tract*.

Medial Geniculate Body. The medial geniculate body is the specific thalamic nucleus for hearing. The *main (ventral) nucleus* is laminated and tonotopic, and its large (magnocellular) principal neurons project as the **auditory radiation** to the primary auditory cortex (Fig. 20.5).

Primary Auditory Cortex. The upper surface of the temporal lobe shows two or more **transverse temporal gyri**. The anterior gyrus (the *gyrus of Heschl*) contains the **primary auditory cortex** (Fig. 20.6). Tonotopic arrangement is preserved in the Heschl gyrus, its posterior part being responsive to high tones and its anterior part to low tones.

Two cortical auditory pathways exist: a dorsal pathway that serves to localise sounds and a ventral pathway that deals with identification. There is also a developmental or maturational aspect to auditory perception that, despite a certain degree of plasticity, remains an important factor in determining the prognosis and timing of an intervention when addressing hearing impairment in the young. Regarding speech, there is increasing evidence that the 'acoustic' properties of speech are matched to the physiological and response properties of the cochlea, auditory nerve, and auditory cortex. A similar relationship is seen to other 'natural' sounds and the auditory system appears to have been optimised for such relevant sounds.

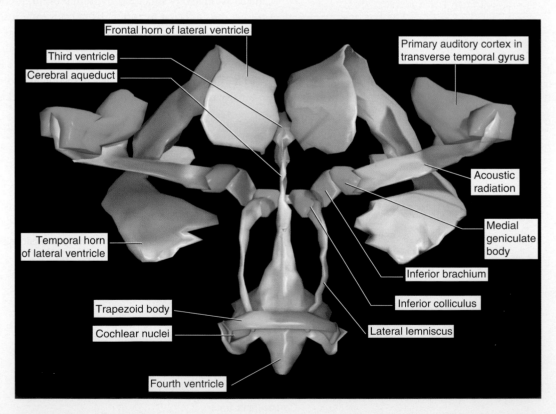

Fig. 20.5 Graphic reconstruction of the central auditory pathways from a postmortem brain. (Reproduced with kind permission of the authors and the publisher from Kretschmann H-J, Weinrich W. *Neurofunctional Systems: 3D Reconstructions with Correlated Neuroimaging: Text and CD-ROM.* New York: Thieme; 1998.)

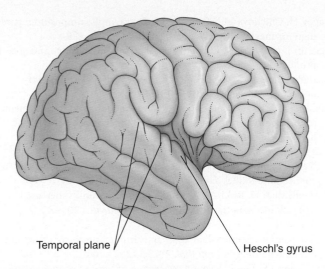

Temporal plane | | Heschl's gyrus

Fig. 20.6 Tilted view of the right cerebral hemisphere. The frontal and parietal opercula of the insula have been moved to show the anterior temporal gyrus of Heschl *(blue)*.

The auditory cortex responds to auditory stimuli within the *contralateral sound field.* In humans, ablation of the superior temporal gyrus (in the course of tumour removal) does not cause deafness, but it significantly reduces the patient's ability to judge the direction and distance of a source of sound. *Brainstem auditory evoked potentials* are described in Chapter 30. While focused on the auditory system, the shape of your ear provides further information about the vertical location of the sound (high or low) by how soundwaves reflect off the outer parts of your ear.

Brainstem Acoustic Reflexes. Collateral branches emerging from the lateral lemniscus form the interneuron linkage for certain reflex arcs:

- Fibres entering the motor nuclei of the trigeminal and facial nerves link up with motor neurons supplying the tensor tympani and stapedius, respectively. These muscles exert a damping action on the ossicles of the middle ear. The tensor tympani is activated by the subject's own voice, the stapedius by external sounds.
- Fibres entering the reticular formation have an important arousal effect, as exemplified by the alarm clock. Sudden loud sounds cause the subject to flinch; this is the '*startle response*', mediated by outputs from the reticular formation to the spinal cord and to the motor nucleus of the facial nerve.

Descending Auditory Pathways

A cascade of descending fibres flows from the primary auditory cortex to the medial geniculate nucleus and inferior colliculus, and from the inferior colliculus to the superior olivary nucleus. From the superior olivary nucleus is a projection *(olivocochlear bundle)* that emerges in the vestibular nerve and carries efferent, cholinergic fibres to the cochlea along with some for the vestibular labyrinth. The olivocochlear fibres apply large synaptic boutons to the outer hair cells and small boutons to the afferent nerve endings on the inner hair cells (see Fig. 20.2).

The primary function of the olivocochlear bundle is protective to the outer hair cells by dampening the basilar membrane response to dangerously loud noise. Activation of its supply to the inner hair cell nerve endings is thought to enhance the basilar membrane response to sounds requiring attention, such as a faint voice in a crowd.

Deafness

Deafness is a widespread problem in the general population. About 10% of adults suffer from it to some degree. The cause may lie in the outer, middle, or inner ear, or in the cochlear neural pathway. The two fundamental types of deafness are described in Clinical Panel 20.1.

CLINICAL PANEL 20.1 Two Kinds of Deafness

All forms of deafness can be grouped into two categories. **Conductive deafness** is caused by disease in the outer ear canal or in the middle ear. **Sensorineural deafness** is caused by disease in the cochlea or in the neural pathway from the cochlea to brain.

Common causes of conductive deafness include accumulation of cerumen in the outer ear and *otitis media* (inflammation in the middle ear). *Otosclerosis* is a disorder of the oval window in which the spiral ligament of the stapes is progressively replaced by bone. The stapes becomes immobilized, with severe impairment of hearing throughout the tonal range. Replacement of the stapes by a prosthesis (artificial substitute) often restores normal hearing.

Sensorineural deafness usually originates within the cochlea and is the commonest form of hearing loss of the elderly and results from deterioration of the organ of Corti; *presbycusis*, or age-related hearing loss. This typically begins by affecting high-frequency sounds (deterioration of the basal turn of the organ of Corti) and with respect to conversation, manifests as difficulty in distinguishing among high-frequency consonants (e.g., s, t, and k) while vowels, which are of low frequency, are more audible. Our hearing is most sensitive in the 2000 to 5000 Hz range, normal conversation is usually 500 to 3000 Hz, and as a result of presbycusis difficulty in understanding speech

occurs that cannot easily be overcome by just increasing loudness (measured in decibels, dB).

Occupational deafness arises from a noisy environment at work. A persistent noise, especially indoors, may eventually lead to degeneration of the organ of Corti in the region corresponding to that particular frequency.

Ototoxic deafness may follow administration of drugs, including streptomycin, neomycin, and quinine.

Infectious deafness may follow complete destruction of the cochlea by the virus mumps or congenital rubella (German measles).

An important cause of sensorineural deafness in adults is an *acoustic neuroma.* Because the trigeminal and facial nerves may be affected as well as the cochlear and vestibular, this tumour is described in Chapter 22.

Tinnitus is perception of a sound that has no external source, and further qualified as objective (generated by the person's body and measurable) or subjective. Subjective tinnitus is common, often associated with sensorineural hearing loss and frequently accompanied by a history of occupational noise exposure. In most cases it is not disruptive to lifestyle, but cases where it is or is associated with other bothersome historical features or associated symptoms may necessitate further evaluation. Guidelines exist for both interventions and patient support.

Core Information

The *bipolar cochlear neurons* occupy the osseous spiral lamina of the *modiolus*. Their peripheral processes supply hair cells in the *organ of Corti*. Their central processes terminate in the *cochlear nuclei*; from here, a polyneuronal pathway leads mainly through the *trapezoid body* and *lateral lemniscus* to the inferior colliculus, but there is a significant ipsilateral pathway too. From the *inferior colliculus*, fibres run to the *medial geniculate body* and from there to the *primary auditory cortex* on the upper surface of the temporal lobe of the brain.

Clinically, deafness is of two kinds: *conductive*, involving disease in the outer and/or middle ear, and *sensorineural*, involving disease of the cochlea (usually) or of central auditory pathways. Hearing is seldom significantly compromised by central pathway lesions because of bilateral projections to the inferior colliculus and beyond.

SUGGESTED READINGS

Basch ML, Brown RM 2nd, Rogers M, Jen HI, Groves AK. Where hearing starts: the development of the mammalian cochlea. *J Anat.* 2016;228:233–254.

Bauer CA. Tinnitus. *N Engl J Med.* 2018;378:1224–1231.

Bizley JK, Cohen YE. The what, where and how of auditory-object perception. *Nat Rev Neurosci.* 2013;14:693–707.

Chen Y, Zhang S, Chai R, Li H. Hair cell regeneration. *Adv Exp Med Biol.* 2019;1130:1–16.

Gagov H, Chichova M, Mladenov M. Endolymph composition: paradigm or inevitability? *Physiol Res.* 2018;67:175–179.

Gervain J, Geffen MN. Efficient neural coding in auditory and speech production. *Trends Neurosci.* 2019;42:56–65.

Gokhale S, Lahoti S, Caplan LR. The neglected neglect: auditory neglect. *JAMA Neurol.* 2013;70:1065–1069.

Goodyear RJ, Richardson GP. Structure, function, and development of the tectorial membrane: an extracellular matrix essential for hearing. *Curr Top Dev Biol.* 2018;130:217–244.

Kral A, Kronenberger WG, Pisoni DB, O'Donoghue GM. Neurocognitive factors in sensory restoration of early deafness: a connectome model. *Lancet Neurol.* 2016;15:610–621.

Ó Maoiléidigh D, Ricci AJ. A bundle of mechanisms: inner-ear hair-cell mechanotransduction. *Trends Neurosci.* 2019;42: 221–236.

McPherson DR. Sensory hair cells: an introduction to structure and physiology. *Integr Comp Biol.* 2018;58:282–300.

Theunissen FE, Elie JE. Neural processing of natural sounds. *Nat Rev Neurosci.* 2014;15:355–366.

Trapeau R, Schonwiesner M. The encoding of sound source elevation in the human auditory cortex. *J Neurosci.* 2018;38:3252–3264.

Wang J, Puel JL. Toward cochlear therapies. *Physiol Rev.* 2018;98: 2477–2522.

Wasserthal C, Brechmann A, Stadler J, et al. Localizing the human primary auditory cortex in vivo using structural MRI. *Neuroimage.* 2014;93:237–251.

Trigeminal Nerve

STUDY GUIDELINES

1. The motor nucleus supplies the muscles of mastication.
2. The mesencephalic unipolar neurons are proprioceptive.
3. The neurons of the principal sensory nucleus receive sensory inputs from the face and underlying mucous membranes.

4. The spinal nucleus is of special clinical importance because of its large nociceptive territory.

TRIGEMINAL NERVE

The trigeminal nerve has a very large sensory territory that includes the skin of the face, oronasal mucous membranes, teeth, dura mater, and major intracranial blood vessels. The nerve is also both motor and sensory to the muscles of mastication. The **motor root** lies medial to the large **sensory root** at the site of attachment to the pons (Fig. 17.16). The **trigeminal (Gasserian) ganglion**, near the apex of the petrous temporal bone, gives rise to the sensory root and consists of unipolar neurons.

Details of the distribution of the ophthalmic, maxillary, and mandibular divisions are available in gross anatomy textbooks. Accurate appreciation of their respective territories on the face is essential if trigeminal neuralgia is to be distinguished from other sources of facial pain (Clinical Panel 21.1).

Motor Nucleus (Figs. 17.16 and 21.1)

The motor nucleus is the special visceral efferent nucleus supplying the muscles derived from the embryonic mandibular pharyngeal arch. These comprise the masticatory muscles attached to each half of the mandible (Fig. 21.2), along with the tensor tympani, tensor veli palatini, mylohyoid, and the anterior belly of digastric muscle. The nucleus occupies the lateral pontine tegmentum. Embedded in its upper pole is a node of the reticular formation, the **supratrigeminal nucleus**, which acts as a pattern generator for masticatory rhythm.

Voluntary control is provided by corticonuclear projections from each motor cortex to both motor nuclei but mainly the contralateral one (Fig. 17.3).

Sensory Nuclei

Three sensory nuclei are associated with the trigeminal nerve: **mesencephalic, pontine (principal),** and **spinal**.

Mesencephalic Nucleus. The mesencephalic nucleus is unique in being the only nucleus in the central nervous system (CNS) that contains the cell bodies of primary unipolar sensory neurons. Their peripheral processes enter the sensory root via the mesencephalic tract of the trigeminal nerve. Some travel in the mandibular division to supply stretch receptors (neuromuscular spindles) in the masticatory muscles. Others travel in the maxillary and mandibular divisions to supply stretch receptors (Ruffini endings) in the suspensory, periodontal ligaments of the teeth.

The central processes of the mesencephalic afferent neurons descend through the pontine tegmentum in the small **tract of Probst**. Most fibres of this tract terminate in the supratrigeminal nucleus; others end in the motor nucleus or in the pontine sensory nucleus; a few travel as far as the dorsal nucleus of the vagus.

Pontine Nucleus. The pontine (principal sensory) nucleus (Fig. 17.2) is homologous with the dorsal column nuclei (gracile and cuneate). It processes discriminative tactile information from the face and oronasal cavity.

Spinal Nucleus. The spinal nucleus extends from the lower part of the pons to the third cervical segment of the spinal cord (hence the term 'spinal'). Two minor nuclei in its upper part (called **pars oralis** and **pars interpolaris**) receive afferents from the mouth. The main spinal nucleus (**pars caudalis**) receives nociceptive and thermal information from the entire trigeminal area, and even beyond.

In section, the main spinal nucleus is seen to be an expanded continuation of the outer laminae (I–III) of the dorsal horn of the cord (Fig. 21.3). The inner three laminae (IV–VI) are relatively compressed. Laminae III and IV are referred to as the magnocellular part of the nucleus. In animals, nociceptive-specific interneurons are found in lamina I. 'Polymodal' neurons are in the magnocellular nucleus and correspond to lamina V neurons lower

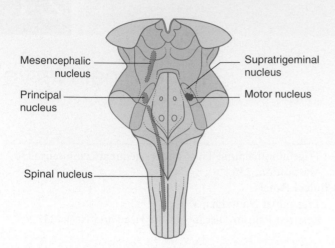

Fig. 21.1 Trigeminal nuclei. *Left,* sensory nuclei; *right,* motor nucleus, supratrigeminal nucleus.

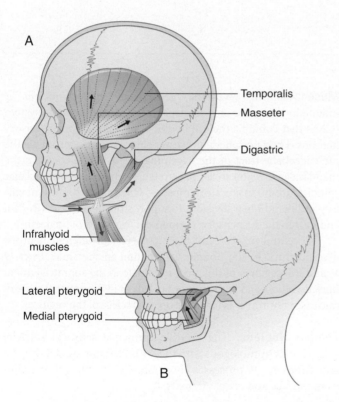

Fig. 21.2 (A) Masticatory and infrahyoid muscles viewed from the left side. (B) Lateral view of the pterygoid muscles of the left side. *Red arrows* indicate directions of pull of jaw-closing muscles. *Blue arrows* indicate directions of pull of jaw openers.

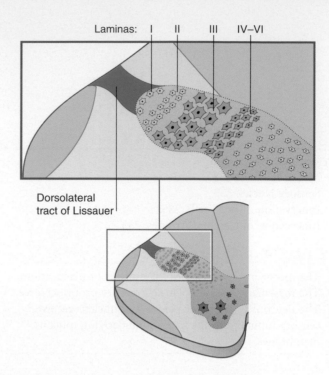

Fig. 21.3 Spinal tract and nucleus of the trigeminal nerve, at the level of the spinomedullary junction.

down. They respond to tactile stimuli applied to the trigeminal skin area and also to noxious mechanical stimuli (e.g. pinching the skin with a forceps), whereas the nociceptive-specific neurons have small receptive fields confined to one territory (a patch of skin or mucous membrane). Many of the polymodal neurons show the phenomenon of *convergence* to a marked degree. In anaesthetised animals, a single neuron may be responsive to noxious stimuli applied to a tooth, to facial skin, or to the temporomandibular joint. This finding provides a plausible basis of explanation for erroneous localisation of pain by patients. Examples are given in Clinical Panel 21.2.

Arrangements for pain modulation appear to be the same as for the spinal cord (see Chapter 24). They include the presence of enkephalinergic and γ-aminobutyric acid (GABA)ergic inter-neurons in the substantia gelatinosa and serotonergic projections from the raphe magnus nucleus.

Afferents to the spinal nucleus come from three sources (Fig. 21.4):

1. *Trigeminal afferents* are the central processes of trigeminal ganglion cells. The peripheral processes terminate in tactile and nociceptive endings in the territory of the three divisions of the nerve. Most often involved clinically are the nociceptive terminals in (1) the teeth, (2) the cornea, (3) the temporomandibular joint, and (4) the dura mater of the anterior and middle cranial fossae. In Chapter 5, it was noted that tension of the supratentorial dura gives rise to frontal or parietal headache.
2. Topographic representation of the trigeminal territory shows an onion skin-like distribution (Fig. 21.5).
3. *Facial, glossopharyngeal,* and *vagal afferents* enter from the skin of the auricle, mucous membranes of the pharyngotympanic tube, middle ear, pharynx, and larynx. These afferents are often involved in acute inflammatory processes during wintertime. Their cell bodies occupy the geniculate ganglion of the facial nerve and inferior sensory ganglia of the glossopharyngeal and vagus nerves.
4. *Cervical afferents* come from the territory of the first three cervical dorsal nerve roots. (The first dorsal nerve root is either small or absent.) Most often involved clinically are nociceptive fibres supplying (1) the intervertebral joints and spinal dura mater and (2) the dura mater of the posterior cranial fossa,

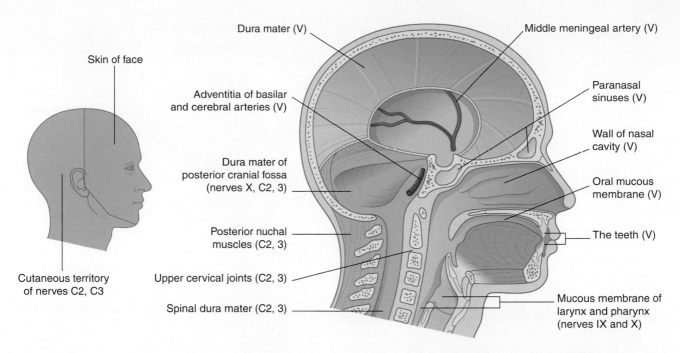

Fig. 21.4 Diagram to indicate the extensive nociceptive territory of the spinal trigeminal nucleus. Structures labelled *(V)* are supplied by the trigeminal nerve. The remainder are supplied by other nerves that have central nociceptive projections to the spinal trigeminal nucleus.

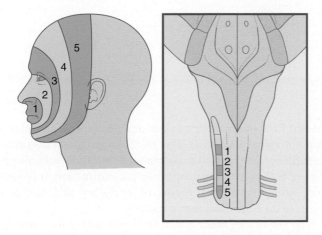

Fig. 21.5 Representation of the face in the spinal trigeminal nucleus.

reached by cervical fibres ascending through the hypoglossal canal. In Chapter 5, it was noted that infratentorial meningitis is associated with severe occipital headache and with reflex head retraction because the suboccipital muscles are supplied by the upper three cervical ventral nerve roots.

Innervation of the Teeth

From the superior and inferior alveolar nerves, Aδ and C fibres enter the root canals of the teeth and form a dense plexus within the pulp. Individual fibres terminate in the pulp, predentin, and dentinal tubules. Most dentinal tubules underlying the occlusal surfaces of the teeth contain single nerve fibres; however, the fibres are restricted to the inner ends of the tubules, whereas pain can be elicited from the outer surface of dentin after removal of enamel. Hydrodynamic and chemical factors have

been invoked to fill the gap, also with possible participation of odontoblasts as intermediaries.

The periodontal ligaments are richly innervated by the nerves supplying the oral epithelium including the gums. Some of the nerve endings are a potential source of pain during dental extraction or periodontal disease. Others function as tension receptors comparable to Ruffini endings found in joint capsules; tension receptors would be anticipated because the periodontal ligaments are arranged like hammocks around the roots of the teeth.

Innervation of Cerebral Arteries

The ophthalmic division of the trigeminal nerve comes close to the internal carotid artery in the cavernous sinus. Here it gives off afferent fibres that accompany the artery to its point of bifurcation into anterior and middle cerebral branches. The nerve fibres accompany these and also reach the posterior cerebral artery via branches accompanying the vertebral artery. Several peptide substances have been detected in these axons; they include substance P, a peptide particularly associated with nociceptive transmission.

The function of the *trigeminovascular neurons* (as they are called) is the subject of speculation. Their presence accounts well for the *frontal headache* associated with distortion of the cerebral arteries by space-occupying lesions.

Trigeminothalamic Tract and Trigeminal Lemniscus (Fig. 21.6)

The lower part of the **trigeminothalamic tract** commences in the spinal trigeminal nucleus. Nearly all of these fibres cross the midline before ascending into the pons. This component has features in common with the spinal lemniscus, which accompanies it in

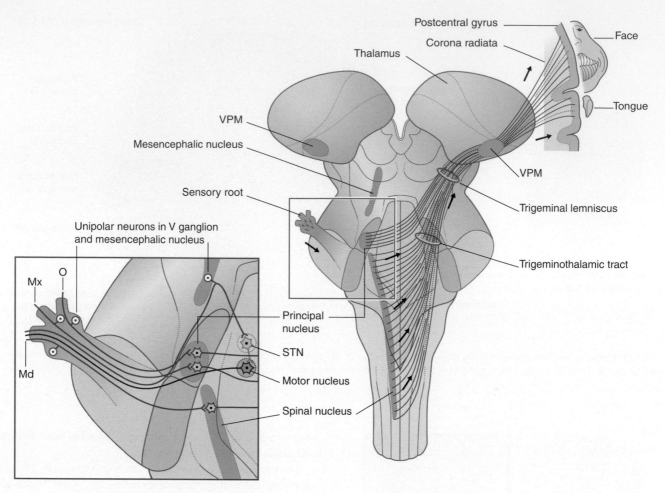

Fig. 21.6 Primary, secondary, and tertiary trigeminal *(V)* afferents. *Md*, Mandibular divisions of trigeminal nerve; *Mx*, maxillary; *O*, ophthalmic; *STN*, supratrigeminal nucleus; *VPM*, ventral posteromedial nucleus of the thalamus.

the brainstem (Figs. 17.15–17.19), mediating tactile, nociceptive, and thermal sensations. In the pons, it is joined by fibres crossing from the principal sensory nucleus, thus completing the ***trigeminal lemniscus***, which terminates in the ventral posteromedial nucleus of the thalamus (see Chapter 25). From the thalamus, third-order afferents project to the large area of facial representation in the lower half of the somatic sensory cortex.

Trigeminoreticular fibres synapse in the parvocellular reticular formation on both sides of the brainstem. They are counterparts of the spinoreticular tract, and they mediate the arousal effect of stroking or slapping the face and of old-fashioned 'smelling salts' (the ammonia irritates trigeminal afferents in the nose).

Mastication

Mastication is a complex activity requiring orchestration of the nuclear groups supplying the muscles that move the mandible, tongue, cheeks, and hyoid bone. The chief controlling centre seems to be an area of the premotor cortex directly in front of the face representation on the motor cortex. Stimulation of this area produces masticatory cycles.

The supratrigeminal nucleus receives proprioceptive information from the spindle-rich, jaw-closing muscles (masseter, temporalis, and medial pterygoid) and from the periodontal ligaments. It also receives tactile information (food in the

mouth) from the pontine nucleus, and nociceptive information from the spinal nucleus. It gives rise to an ipsilateral trigeminocerebellar projection and a contralateral trigeminothalamic projection, both containing proprioceptive information. It controls mastication directly by means of excitatory and inhibitory inputs to the trigeminal motor nucleus.

The *jaw-closing reflex* is initiated by contact of food with the oral mucous membrane. The response of the pattern generator is to activate the jaw-closing motor neurons so that the teeth are brought into occlusion.

The *jaw-opening reflex* is initiated by periodontal stretch afferents activated by dental occlusion. The pattern generator responds by inhibiting the closure motor neurons and activating the jaw openers. Muscle spindles are especially numerous in the anterior part of the masseter, and when stretch reaches a critical level the pattern generator is switched to a jaw-closing mode.

The Jaw Jerk. The jaw jerk is a tendon reflex elicited by tapping the chin with a downward stroke. The normal response is a twitch of the jaw-closing muscles, because muscle spindle afferents make some direct synaptic contacts upon trigeminal motor neurons. Supranuclear lesions of the motor nucleus (e.g. *pseudobulbar palsy*, see Chapter 18) may be accompanied by an exaggerated (abnormally brisk) jaw jerk.

The supratrigeminal nucleus is seldom dormant. In the erect posture, it activates the jaw closers to keep the mandible elevated. During sleep, it activates the lateral pterygoid so that the pharynx is not occluded by the tongue. (The root of the tongue is anchored to the mandible.) However, *the nucleus is inactivated by general anaesthesia*, in which circumstance the ramus of the mandible must be held forward constantly in order to prevent choking.

CLINICAL PANEL 21.1 Trigeminal Neuralgia

Trigeminal neuralgia is an important condition occurring in middle age or later, characterised by attacks of excruciating pain in the territory of one or more divisions of the trigeminal nerve (usually II and/or III). The patient (who is usually more than 60 years old) is able to map out the affected division(s) accurately. Because it must be distinguished from many other causes of facial pain, the clinician should be able to mark out a trigeminal sensory map (Fig. 21.7). Attacks are triggered by everyday sensory stimuli such as brushing teeth, shaving, and chewing, and the tendency of patients to wince at the onset of attacks accounts for the French term *tic douloureux*.

Episodes of paroxysmal facial pain occurring in young adults should raise a suspicion of multiple sclerosis as the cause. Postmortem histology in such cases has revealed demyelination of the sensory root of the trigeminal nerve where it enters the pons. Demyelination of large sensory fibres receiving tactile signals from skin or mucous membranes in the trigeminal territory may cause their exposed axons to come into direct contact with unmyelinated axons serving pain receptors. Animal experiments have shown that this type of contact can initiate *ephaptic transmission* of action potentials between them. It is now widely accepted that the most frequent aetiology in later years is *vascular compression*, usually by a 'sagging' posterior cerebral artery in transit around the brainstem. The trigeminal CNS/peripheral nervous system (PNS) transition zone (see Chapter 9) is several millimetres lateral to the entry zone into the pons, and postmortem histology has provided evidence of the demyelinating effect of chronic pulsatile compression.

Antiepileptic drugs that exert a blocking effect on sodium and/or calcium channels (e.g. carbamazepine) may suffice to keep relapses at bay. Surgery is indicated for those who fail to respond.

A procedure that can be performed under local anaesthesia is electrocoagulation of the affected division, through a needle electrode inserted through

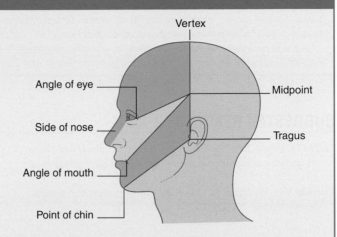

Fig. 21.7 Trigeminal nerve sensory map.

the foramen rotundum or ovale from below. The intention is to heat the nerve sufficiently to destroy only the finest fibres, in which case analgesia is produced but touch (including the corneal reflex) is preserved.

The final option is to *decompress* the afflicted nerve root through an intracranial approach whereby neighbouring vessels are lifted away from it.

A surgical procedure of historic interest is *medullary tractotomy*, whereby the spinal root was sectioned through the dorsolateral surface of the medulla. In successful cases, pain and temperature sensitivity was lost from the face but touch (mediated by the pontine nucleus) was preserved. This procedure was abandoned owing to a high mortality rate associated with compromise of underlying respiratory and cardiovascular centres.

CLINICAL PANEL 21.2 Referred Pain in Diseases of the Head and Neck

Cervicogenic Headache

Experiments on healthy volunteers have demonstrated that noxious stimulation of tissues supplied by the upper cervical nerves may induce pain referred to the head. Tissues tested include the ligaments of the upper cervical joints, the suboccipital muscles, and the sternocleidomastoid and trapezius muscles. The unilateral pain is primarily occipital, as would be expected from the cutaneous distribution of the greater occipital nerve given off by the posterior ramus of nerve C2, but it may radiate to the forehead. Diagnostic features include intensification of the pain by head movement and temporary abolition by ipsilateral local anaesthetic blockade of the greater occipital nerve. A common source of cervicogenic headache in the elderly is spondylosis, a degenerative arthritis in which bony excrescences compress the emerging spinal nerves (see Chapter 14). Another source appears to be myofascial disease of the sternocleidomastoid–trapezius continuum close to the base of the skull. *Trigger points*—tender nodules within the muscles that give rise to occipital pain when compressed—are often detected by physical therapists during palpation of these muscles.

Earache

Earache is most often the result of an acute infection of the outer ear canal or middle ear. However, pain may be referred to a perfectly healthy ear from a variety of sources. The outer ear skin receives small sensory branches from the mandibular, facial, vagus, and upper cervical nerves; the middle ear epithelium is supplied by the glossopharyngeal and vagus nerves. Earache may be a leading symptom of disease in the territory of one of these nerves. Important examples include:

• cancer of the pharynx—perhaps concealed in the piriform fossa beside the larynx or near the tonsil;
• an impacted wisdom tooth in the mandible;
• temporomandibular joint disease; and
• spondylosis of the upper cervical spine.

Pain in the Face

Important causes of pain referred to the face below the eye include:

• dental caries or an impacted maxillary wisdom tooth;
• cancer in a mucous membrane supplied by the maxillary nerve i.e. maxillary air sinus, nasal cavity, or nasopharynx;
• acute maxillary sinusitis; and
• trigeminal neuralgia affecting the maxillary nerve.

Core Information

The motor root of the V nerve enters the mandibular division to supply the four muscles of mastication and the anterior belly of digastric, the mylohyoid, tensor tympani, and tensor veli palatini. Automatic control is by the supratrigeminal nucleus, and voluntary control is from the motor cortex (mainly contralaterally).

The V ganglion (unipolar cells) sends peripheral processes into all three divisions, providing sensory endings in the face, oronasal mucous membranes, teeth, meninges, and intracranial blood vessels. Central processes synapse in the pontine (principal sensory) and spinal nuclei.

Peripheral processes proprioceptive to masticatory muscles and periodontal ligaments belong to the unipolar-celled mesencephalic nucleus. The main target of the central processes of these cells is the supratrigeminal nucleus, which is the masticatory generator.

The pontine nucleus processes tactile information from the face and oronasal mucous membranes. The spinal nucleus receives nociceptive signals from the entire trigeminal sensory field, from the oropharynx via the glossopharyngeal, from the laryngopharynx and larynx via the vagus, and from the posterior rami of upper cervical nerves.

The pontine and spinal nuclei project fibres into the reticular formation (serving arousal) and to the contralateral thalamus via the trigeminothalamic tract.

SUGGESTED READINGS

Bathla G, Hegde AN. The trigeminal nerve: an illustrated review of its imaging anatomy and pathology. *Clin Radiol.* 2013;68: 203—213.

Gonella MC, Fischbein FC. Disorders of the trigeminal system. *Semin Neurol.* 2009;29:36—44.

Joo W, Yoshioka F, Funaki T, et al. Microsurgical anatomy of the trigeminal nerve. *Clin Anat.* 2014;27:61—88.

Messlinger K, Lennerz JK, Eberhardt M, et al. CGRP and NO in the trigeminal system: mechanisms and role in headache generation. *Headache.* 2012;52:1411—1427.

Facial Nerve

CHAPTER SUMMARY

STUDY GUIDELINES

1. Cranial nerve CN VII is the most commonly paralysed of all peripheral nerves, owing to the great length of its canal in the temporal bone, where it is at risk of compression when inflamed. Since CN VII supplies the muscles of facial expression, the effects of peripheral facial nerve paralysis are obvious to all.

2. Learn the distinctions between upper and lower motor neuron lesions of CN VII.

3. Note that CN VII participates in several important reflex arcs.

FACIAL NERVE

The *facial nerve* supplies the muscles derived from the second branchial arch. These include the muscles of facial expression and four others mentioned below. It is accompanied during part of its course by the *nervus intermedius*, which is the sensory and parasympathetic component of the facial nerve. The nervus intermedius supplies secretomotor fibres to lacrimal glands in the eyes, nose, and mouth, and carries gustatory fibres from the tongue and palate.

The facial nerve arises from the branchial (special visceral) efferent cell column caudal to the motor nucleus of the trigeminal nerve (see Fig. 17.2). The *facial nucleus* occupies the lateral region of the tegmentum in the caudal part of the pons (Fig. 22.1 and see Fig. 17.15). Before emerging from the brainstem, it loops, as the *internal genu*, around the abducens nucleus, creating the *facial colliculus* in the floor of the fourth ventricle.

The nerve emerges at the lower border of the pons at the pontomedullary junction together with the nervus intermedius. Both nerves cross the subarachnoid space in company with the vestibulocochlear nerve, to the internal acoustic meatus. Above the vestibule of the labyrinth, it enters a 7-shaped bony canal having a backward bend at the *external genu* of the facial nerve. Prior to emerging from the facial canal at the stylomastoid foramen, it supplies the stapedius muscle. As the facial nerve leaves the stylomastoid foramen, it supplies the posterior belly of the occipitofrontalis, the stylohyoid, and the posterior belly of the digastric. It then turns forward within the substance of the parotid gland while dividing into the five named branches to the muscles of facial expression (Fig. 22.2).

Supranuclear/Corticobulbar Connections

All of the cell bodies of the motor nucleus receive a corticonuclear supply from the 'face' area of the contralateral motor cortex. In addition, those to the muscles of the upper face (occipitofrontalis and orbicularis oculi) receive a bilateral supply from the *ipsilateral* motor cortex as well. The bilateral supply for the upper facial muscles is reflected in their habitual paired activities in wrinkling the forehead, blinking, and squeezing the eyes closed. The muscles around the mouth, on the other hand, are often activated unilaterally for some expressive purpose. The partial bilateral supply to the facial muscles helps to distinguish a supranuclear from a nuclear or infranuclear lesion of the nerve (Clinical Panel 22.1).

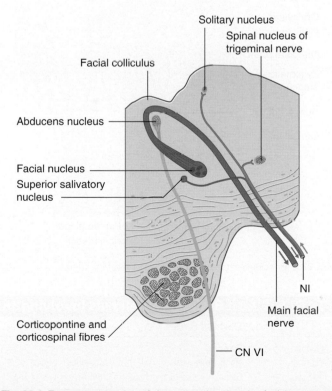

Fig. 22.1 Transverse section of the pons, showing the facial nerve and the nervus intermedius *(NI)*.

The muscles of facial expression are more responsive to emotional states than any other muscle group. A limbic contribution to the supranuclear supply is to be expected, and indeed two have been identified. One is the **nucleus accumbens** at the base of the forebrain, identified in Fig. 26.1D. The nucleus accumbens is a ventral part of the basal ganglia, which in turn influence the motor cortex. That circuit is compromised in Parkinson disease, which is often characterised by mask-like facies (see Chapter 26). The other occupies the *affective area* of the cingulate gyrus (illustrated in Fig. 33.3), an emotionally responsive region in the territory of the anterior cerebral artery. It is active during production of a spontaneous smile, and this is of clinical interest, as explained in Clinical Panel 22.1.

Nuclear Connections

Five reflex arcs engaging the facial nucleus are listed in Table 22.1. Most important clinically is the corneal reflex.

Corneal Reflex

The usual test is to touch the cornea with a cotton wisp. This should elicit a bilateral blink response. The afferent limb of the reflex is the ophthalmic division of the trigeminal nerve (nasociliary branch). The efferent limb is the facial nerve (branch to the palpebral element of orbicularis oculi). The reflex can still be elicited following a transection of the spinal tract of the trigeminal nerve (tractotomy, see Chapter 21), because the ophthalmic afferents evidently synapse in the principal (pontine) nucleus of the trigeminal. Interneurons projecting from each principal nucleus to both facial nuclei complete the reflex arc.

The corneal reflex may be lost following a lesion of either the ophthalmic or facial nerve. A gradual compression of ophthalmic fibres in the sensory root of the trigeminal nerve may damage corneal fibres selectively. For this reason, the corneal reflex must be tested in patients under suspicion of an acoustic neuroma (Clinical Panel 22.2).

NERVUS INTERMEDIUS

Nervus intermedius aligns with the facial nerve distal to the internal genu. It comprises two sets of parasympathetic and two sets of special sense fibres (Fig. 22.3).

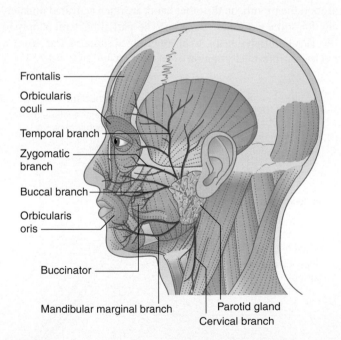

Fig. 22.2 Principal extracranial branches of the facial nerve.

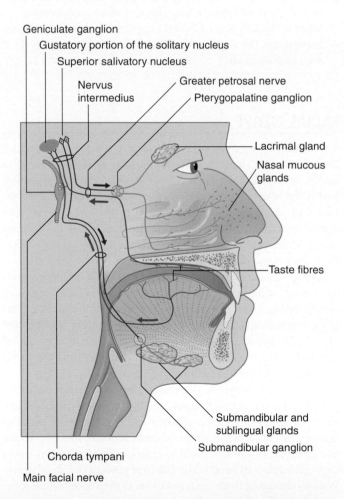

Fig. 22.3 The nervus intermedius and its branches. *Arrows* indicate the direction of the impulse.

TABLE 22.1	Brainstem Reflexes Involving the Facial Nerve.				
	Corneal Reflex	**Sucking Reflex**	**Blinking to Light**	**Blinking to Noise**	**Sound Attenuation**
Receptor	Cornea	Lips	Retina	Cochlea	Cochlea
Afferent	Ophthalmic nerve	Mandibular nerve	Optic nerve	Cochlear nucleus	Cochlear nucleus
First synapse	Spinal nucleus of trigeminal	Pontine nucleus of trigeminal	Superior colliculus	Inferior colliculus	Superior olivary nucleus
Second synapse	Facial nucleus	Facial nucleus	Facial nucleus	Facial nucleus	Facial nucleus
Muscle	Orbicularis oculi	Orbicularis oris	Orbicularis oculi	Orbicularis oculi	Stapedius

The *parasympathetic root* of the nerve arises from the **superior salivatory nucleus** in the pons. This is the motor component of the **greater petrosal** and **chorda tympani** nerves. The greater petrosal nerve synapses in the **pterygopalatine ganglion** ('the ganglion of hay fever'), whose postganglionic fibres stimulate the lacrimal and nasal glands as well as palatine and nasopharyngeal glands. The motor component of the chorda tympani synapses in the **submandibular ganglion**, whose postganglionic fibres stimulate the submandibular and sublingual glands.

The *special viscera afferent (SVA) root* of the facial nerve has unipolar cell bodies in the **geniculate ganglion**. The peripheral processes of these ganglion cells supply taste buds in the palate via the greater petrosal nerve and taste buds in the anterior two-thirds of the tongue via the chorda tympani. The central processes enter the *gustatory part* of the **solitary nucleus**, which also receives fibres from the glossopharyngeal nerve (see Chapter 18), as well as the vagus nerve (which carries taste fibres from the epiglottis). From here, second-order neurons project to the thalamus on the *same* side, through the *central tegmental tract (CTT)* for relay to anterior parts of the insula and cingulate cortex.

A few cells of the geniculate ganglion supply skin in and around the external acoustic meatus (Clinical Panel 22.1).

CLINICAL PANEL 22.1 Lesions of the Facial Nerve

Supranuclear Lesions

The commonest cause of a supranuclear lesion of the seventh nerve is a vascular stroke, in which corticobulbar and corticospinal fibres are interrupted at or above the level of the internal capsule. The usual effect of a stroke is to produce a contralateral motor weakness of the lower part of the face and of the limbs. (The lower part of the face may appear to recover momentarily when participating in a spontaneous smile, as mentioned earlier.) The upper face escapes because of the bilateral supranuclear supply to the upper part of the facial nucleus.

Nuclear Lesions

The main motor nucleus may be involved in thrombosis of one of the pontine branches of the basilar artery. As might be anticipated from the relationships depicted in Fig. 22.1, the usual result of such a lesion is an *alternating (crossed) hemiplegia*: complete paralysis of the facial and/or abducens nerve on the side of the lesion combined with motor weakness of the limbs on the opposite side owing to concomitant involvement of the corticospinal tract.

Infranuclear Lesions

Bell palsy is a common disorder caused by a neuritis (possibly viral in origin) of the facial nerve. The inflammation causes the nerve to swell and conduction is compromised by the close fit of the nerve in its bony canal in the interval between the geniculate ganglion and stylomastoid foramen. There may be some initial pain in the ear, but the condition is otherwise painless.

Facial paralysis is usually complete. On the affected side, the patient is unable to raise the eyebrow, close the eye, or retract the lip (Fig. 22.4). The patient may experience *hyperacusis*: ordinary sounds may be unpleasantly loud because of loss of the damping action of the stapedius muscle.

Tests may reveal dysfunction of nervus intermedius fibres, with ipsilateral reduced lacrimal and salivary secretions and loss of taste from the anterior part of the tongue.

Four out of five patients recover completely within a few weeks because the nerve has only suffered a conduction block *(neuropraxia)*. In the remainder of patients, the nerve undergoes Wallerian degeneration (see Chapter 9); recovery takes about 3 months and is often incomplete. During regeneration, some preganglionic fibres of the nervus intermedius may enter the greater petrosal nerve instead of the chorda tympani, with the result that the lacrimal gland becomes active at mealtimes (so-called 'crocodile tears').

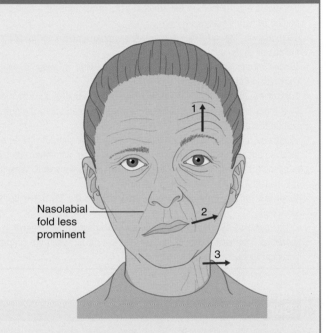

Nasolabial fold less prominent

Fig. 22.4 Complete facial nerve paralysis, patient's right side. The patient has been asked to smile and to look upward. To compare the two sides, cover the left and right halves of the photograph alternately with a card. On the normal (left) side, *(1)* the frontalis muscle has raised the eyebrow, *(2)* the buccinator has retracted the lips, and *(3)* the platysma is in moderate contraction. On the right side, the lower eyelid is drooping because of paralysis of orbicularis oculi.

Other causes of infranuclear palsy include a patch of demyelination within the pons in the course of multiple sclerosis, tumours in the cerebellopontine angle (Clinical Panel 22.2), middle ear disease, and tumours of the parotid gland. *Herpes zoster oticus* is a rare but well-recognised viral infection of the geniculate ganglion. Severe pain in one ear precedes a vesicular rash in and around the external acoustic meatus. Swelling of the geniculate ganglion may result in a complete facial palsy *(Ramsay Hunt syndrome)*.

CLINICAL PANEL 22.2   Syndromes of the Cerebellopontine Angle

The **cerebellopontine angle** is the recess between the hemisphere of the cerebellum and the lower border of the pons. The petrous temporal bone, laterally, completes a triangle having the CN V nerve at its upper corner and CN IX and CN X at its lower corner, and bisected by CN VII and CN VIII.

Several kinds of space-occupying lesions may compromise one or more of the nerves. The most frequent is an **acoustic neuroma** (Fig. 22.5), a slow-growing, benign tumour of Schwann cells (*neurolemmoma*). The tumour originates on the vestibular nerve within the internal acoustic meatus, but the initial symptoms are more often cochlear than vestibular. *An acoustic neuroma must be suspected in every middle-aged or elderly patient presenting with unilateral auditory or vestibular symptoms.* Early diagnosis is important because of the difficulty of removing a large neuroma extending into the posterior cranial fossa; also, because the cumulative motor and sensory disturbances may not show significant improvement after surgery.

The following is a fairly typical sequence of symptoms and signs in a case escaping early detection:

* *Tinnitus* is experienced on the affected side, in the form of a high-pitched ringing or fizzing sound.
* *Deafness* on the affected side is slowly progressive over a period of months or years.
* *Vertigo* occurs episodically. Severe vertigo with nystagmus signifies compression of the brainstem.
* *Loss of the corneal reflex* is an early sign of distortion of the CN V nerve by a tumour emerging from the internal acoustic meatus into the posterior cranial fossa.
* *Weakness of the masticatory muscles* is a later sign of CN V nerve involvement. The jaw deviates towards the affected side when the mouth is opened, because the normal lateral pterygoid is unopposed. Wasting of the masseter may be detected by palpation.
* *Weakness of the facial musculature* develops as the VII nerve becomes stretched.
* *Anaesthesia of the oropharynx* signifies involvement of the IX nerve.
* *Ipsilateral 'cerebellar signs'* in the arm and leg appear when the cerebellum is compressed.

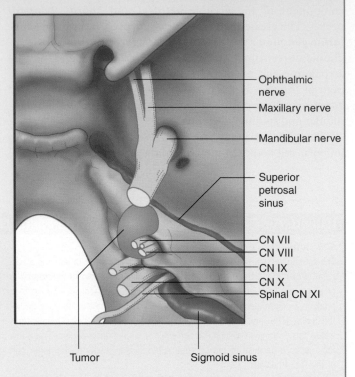

Fig. 22.5 An acoustic neuroma invading the right posterior cranial fossa.

* *'Upper motor neuron signs'* in the limbs signify compression of the brainstem.
* *Signs of raised intracranial pressure* (headache, drowsiness, papilledema) signify obstruction of cerebrospinal fluid circulation either inside or around the brainstem.

✳ Core Information

Upon leaving its nucleus, the facial nerve winds around the abducent nerve nucleus, producing the facial colliculus. It emerges at the lower border of the pons, and at the internal auditory meatus, enters a long bony canal opening at the stylomastoid foramen at the base of the skull. It supplies the muscles of facial expression, the occipital portion of occipitofrontalis, the stapedius, the stylohyoid, and the posterior belly of the digastric. The upper half of the facial nucleus receives a bilateral corticobulbar innervation from the motor cortex; the lower half receives only a contralateral innervation.

The nervus intermedius travels in part with CN VII. The superior salivatory nucleus provides the motor components of the greater petrosal nerve (for lacrimal and nasal glands by the pterygopalatine ganglion) and the chorda tympani (for submandibular and sublingual glands via the submandibular ganglion). The geniculate ganglion of CN VII has pseudounipolar neurons receiving taste from the palate via the greater petrosal nerve and tongue via the chorda tympani. A few pseudounipolar neurons supply the skin in and around the external acoustic meatus.

SUGGESTED READINGS

Cattaneo L, Pavesi G. The facial motor system. *Neurosci Biobehav Rev.* 2014;38:135–159.

Chaudhari N, Roper SD. The cell biology of taste. *J Cell Biol.* 2010; 190:285–296.

Gilchrist JM. Seventh cranial neuropathy. *Semin Neurol.* 2009;29:5–13.

Gordin E, Lee TS, Ducic Y, Arnaoutakis D. Facial nerve trauma: evaluation and considerations in management. *Craniomaxillofac Trauma Reconstr.* 2015;8(1):1–13.

Morales D, Donnan P, Daly F. Impact of clinical trial findings on Bell's palsy management in general practice in the UK 2001-2012: interrupted time series regression analysis. *BMJ Open.* 2013;3: e003121.

Shoja MM, Oesiku NM, Griessenauer CI, et al. Anastomoses between lower cranial and upper cervical nerves. *Clin Anat.* 2014; 27:118–130.

Takezawa K, Townsend G, Ghabriel M. The facial nerve: anatomy and associated disorders for oral health professionals. *Odontology.* 2018;106(2):103–116.

Toulgoat F, Sarrazin JL, Benoudiba F, et al. Facial nerve: from anatomy to pathology. *Diagn Interv Radiol.* 2013;94:1033-1042.

Weiss MS, Hajnal A, Czaja K, Di Lorenzo PM. Taste responses in the nucleus of the solitary tract of awake obese rats are blunted compared with those in lean rats. *Front Integr Neurosci.* 2019;13:35.

You YP, Zhang JX, Lu AL, et al. Vestibular schwannoma surgical treatment. *CNS Neurosci Ther.* 2013;19:289–293.

Ocular Motor Nerves

STUDY GUIDELINES

General

Because of the immense diagnostic and therapeutic importance of ocular muscle innervation, and because of its inherent complexity, neuro-ophthalmology has become its own branch of medicine.

It is especially important to describe the way in which premotor centres can operate bilaterally to keep the gaze on target, even when the head is moving.

Specific

1. Describe the function of cranial nerves (CN) III, IV, and VI on eye movements; identify which extraocular muscles are 'yoked' and work together to keep both eyes in their cardinal position of gaze.
2. Indicate the nerve supply to the six muscles that move the eyeball and describe how the CN III elevates the upper eyelid.
3. Contrast the effects of the sympathetic and parasympathetic autonomic nerve supply to the eye; explain the changes and anatomic pathways that are responsible for the pupillary changes noted in a dark room, in a well-lit room, and when focusing on an object held close to one's nose.

THE NERVES

The ocular motor nerves comprise the **oculomotor** (CN III), **trochlear** (CN IV), and **abducens** (CN VI) **nerves**. They provide the motor nerve supply to the four recti and two oblique muscles controlling movements of the eyeball on each side (Fig. 23.1). The oculomotor nerve contains two additional sets of neurons: one to supply the levator of the upper eyelid and the other to control the sphincter muscle of the pupil and the ciliary muscle.

The nuclei serving the extraocular muscles (extrinsic muscles of the eye) belong to the somatic efferent cell column of the brainstem, in line with the nucleus of the hypoglossal nerve. The oculomotor nucleus has an additional, parasympathetic nucleus that belongs to the general visceral efferent cell column.

Oculomotor Nerve

The nucleus of the third nerve is at the level of the superior colliculus of the midbrain. It is partly embedded in the periaqueductal grey matter (Fig. 23.2A). It is composed of five individual subnuclei, which supply striated muscles (ipsilateral subnuclei innervate the inferior rectus, inferior oblique, and medial rectus, and the contralateral superior rectus muscle; the levator palpebrae superioris is innervated by a single midline nucleus) and one parasympathetic nucleus.

The nerve passes through the tegmentum of the midbrain and emerges into the interpeduncular fossa. It crosses the apex of the petrous temporal bone, pierces the dural roof of the

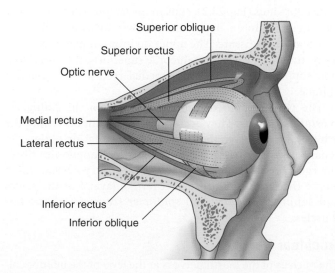

Fig. 23.1 Extrinsic ocular muscles.

Labels: Superior oblique; Superior rectus; Optic nerve; Medial rectus; Lateral rectus; Inferior rectus; Inferior oblique

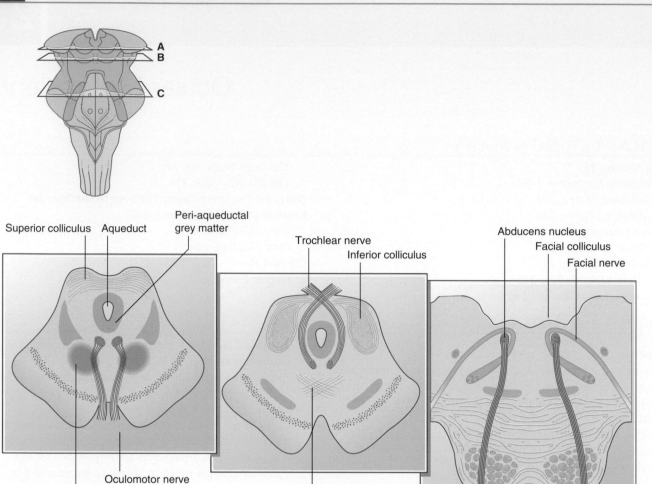

Superior colliculus   Aqueduct   Peri-aqueductal grey matter

Trochlear nerve   Inferior colliculus

Abducens nucleus   Facial colliculus   Facial nerve

Oculomotor nerve

Red nucleus

A Upper midbrain

Decussation of superior cerebellar peduncles

B Lower midbrain

Abducens nerve

C Lower pons

Fig. 23.2 (A–C) Transverse sections of the brainstem showing the origins of the ocular motor nerves.

cavernous sinus (Fig. 23.3), runs in the lateral wall of the sinus, and divides into an upper and a lower division within the superior orbital fissure. The upper division supplies the superior rectus and the levator palpebrae superioris; the lower division supplies the inferior and medial recti and the inferior oblique.

The parasympathetic fibres originate in the **Edinger–Westphal nucleus**. They accompany the main nerve into the orbit and then leave the branch to the inferior oblique to synapse in the **ciliary ganglion**. Postganglionic fibres emerge from the ganglion in the **short ciliary nerves**, which pierce the lamina cribrosa ('sieve-like layer') of the sclera and supply the *ciliary* and *sphincter (constrictor) pupillae* muscles.

Trochlear Nerve

The nucleus of the fourth nerve is at the level of the inferior colliculus of the midbrain. The nerve itself is unique in two respects

(Fig. 23.2B): it is the only nerve to emerge from the dorsum of the brainstem and the only nerve to fully decussate.

The CN IV winds around the crus of the midbrain and travels in the wall of the cavernous sinus accompanied by CN III (Fig. 23.3). It passes through the superior orbital fissure and supplies the *superior oblique* muscle.

Abducens Nerve

The nucleus of the sixth nerve is in the floor of the fourth ventricle, at the level of the facial colliculus in the lower pons (Fig. 23.2C). The nerve descends to emerge at the lower border of the pons (pontomedullary junction) and runs up the pontine subarachnoid cistern beside the basilar artery. It angles over the apex of the petrous part of the temporal bone and passes through the cavernous sinus inferolateral to the internal carotid artery (Fig. 23.3). It enters the orbit through the superior orbital fissure and supplies the *lateral rectus* muscle, which abducts the eye.

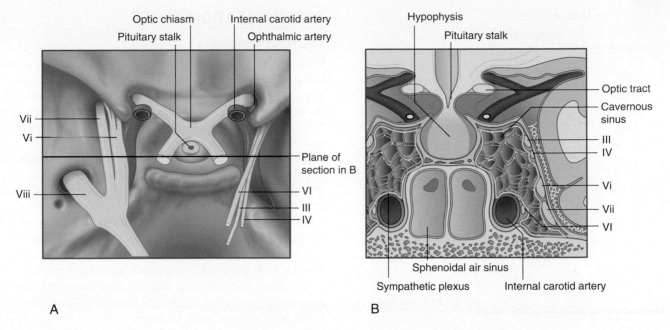

Fig. 23.3 (A) Middle cranial fossa with cavernous sinuses removed. (B) Coronal section in the plane of the hypophysis with the cavernous sinuses in place. *III*, Oculomotor nerve; *IV*, trochlear nerve; *VI*, abducens nerve; *Vi, Vii, Viii*, ophthalmic, maxillary, mandibular divisions of trigeminal nerve.

NERVE ENDINGS

Motor Endings

All the ocular motor units are small, containing 5 to 10 muscle fibres (compared with 1000 or more in the tibialis anterior muscle). These motor units can be divided into three groups, of which two are most relevant: motor neurons that form single 'en plaque' endings that innervate muscle fibres and respond with a fast twitch and those that form multiple small 'en grappe' endings on muscle fibres that respond with a slow tonic contraction. The fast twitch muscle fibres are likely involved with saccadic or rapid eye movements, while the slow twitch fibres are involved in gaze holding (e.g. fixation, smooth pursuit). As extraocular muscles execute multiple functions it is likely to occur through unique groupings of motor units that allow independent activation to produce a repertoire of actions.

Sensory Endings

Neuromuscular spindles and Golgi tendon organs are not prominent in the extraocular muscles of humans. However, other assumed sensory axons approach the central portion of slow twitch muscle fibres, but then turn back towards the distal muscle zone forming a spiral of nerve endings around their tips. This unique nerve ending type, the ***palisade ending***, is believed to provide such proprioceptive information and contribute to the monitoring of eye position.

The cell bodies of these ***palisade ending*** nerves and the cell bodies of the motor neurons that innervate the slow twitch muscle fibres are most likely found around the periphery of the cranial motor nuclei. If these motor neurons function in the same role as γ motor neurons, then the palisade ending neurons would function in a similar manner to a muscle spindle and provide proprioceptive information rather than contribute to eye movement.

There are other sensory afferents from extraocular muscles (some may provide proprioceptive information, others nociception or vasodilatation), which travel through the ophthalmic nerve to the trigeminal ganglion. The trigeminal ganglion also receives proprioceptive terminals from the neck muscles and projects both to the ipsilateral cerebellum and to the contralateral superior colliculus. The conjunction of ocular and cervical proprioceptive information presumably assists in the coordination of simultaneous movements of the eyes and head.

PUPILLARY LIGHT REFLEX (FIG. 23.4)

Constriction of the pupils in response to light optimises visual acuity and protects the retina from overexposure to bright light. It involves four sets of neurons:

1. The afferent limb commences in melanopsin-containing retinal ganglion cells (small subset of ganglion cells that provide luminance information; *intrinsically photosensitive retinal ganglion cells, ipRGC*) that generate an electrical signal, independent of rod or cone synaptic input, and travels within the optic nerve.
2. Fibres leaving the optic chiasm enter both optic tracts and terminate in the ***pretectal nuclei***, situated just rostral to the superior colliculus on each side (Fig. 17.19).
3. Each pretectal nucleus is linked by interneurons to both Edinger–Westphal (parasympathetic) nuclei; the two nuclei are connected by the ***posterior commissure (PC)***.
4. Preganglionic parasympathetic fibres enter the oculomotor nerve, exit through the inferior division of the oculomotor nerve, and synapse in the ciliary ganglion.

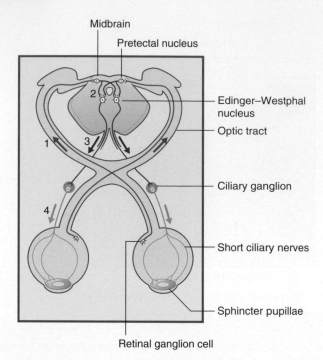

Fig. 23.4 Pupillary light reflex. For numbers, see text.

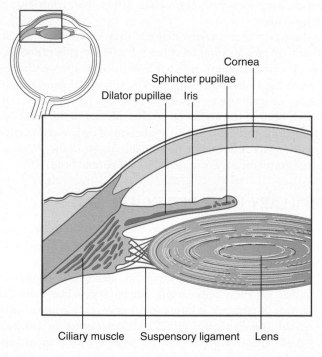

Fig. 23.5 Intrinsic muscles of the eye.

5. Postganglionic fibres run in the short ciliary nerves and enter the iris to supply the sphincter (constrictor) pupillae (Fig. 23.5). The normal response is consensual; that is, both pupils constrict equally when the light is applied to one eye only.

ACCOMMODATION REFLEX

The Near Response

When the eyes view a near object, the ciliary muscles contract reflexively, thereby relaxing the suspensory ligament of the lens (Fig. 23.5). Because the lens at rest is somewhat flattened or stretched by tension exerted on the lens capsule by the suspensory ligaments, the lens bulges passively when the ciliary muscle contracts. The thicker lens has the greater refractive power required to bring near objects into focus on the retina. This response of the lens is termed *accommodation*.

This **accommodation reflex**, as understood clinically, involves two additional features. The sphincter pupillae contracts to eliminate passage of light through the peripheral, thinner part of the lens. At the same time, the visual axes of the two eyes converge, as a result of increased tone in the medial rectus muscles. The convergence is clinically known as *vergence*.

The three features described are also known as the *near response*:

- The lens becomes more biconvex.
- The pupil constricts.
- The eyes converge.

Pathway for the Accommodation Reflex. To execute the near response, a stereoscopic analysis of the object is carried out at the level of the visual association cortex. The afferent limb of the reflex passes from the retina to the occipital lobe via the lateral geniculate body. The efferent limb passes from the occipital lobe to the midbrain, where some fibres activate the Edinger–Westphal nucleus and others activate *vergence* (convergence) cells in the reticular formation. The convergence cells activate the nuclear groups serving the medial recti, with the effect of *fixating* the object onto the fovea centralis of each eye. The (con)vergence response is called the *fixation reflex*.

Pupillary constriction can be caused by light and by accommodation. A bright light stimulus usually produces greater pupillary constriction than accommodation. When the light reflex pathway is damaged, but the near reflex pathway remains intact, a condition known as **light-near dissociation** results. The near reflex results in a (greater) pupillary constriction compared to light. The most common cause of light-near dissociation is blindness from optic neuropathy. The condition may also result from lesions in the dorsal midbrain that interrupt the afferent optic nerve fibres where they travel to the Edinger–Westphal nucleus but not those of the near reflex that reach this nucleus via a more ventral route. While other causes for light-near dissociation exist, two need to be specifically mentioned: *Argyll Robertson pupil* that classically results from the inflammatory response of neurosyphilis disrupting the light pathway in the midbrain and *Adie tonic pupil* from an idiopathic (unknown) injury to the parasympathetic ciliary ganglion.

The Far Response

Just as the state of the pupil depends upon the balance of sympathetic and parasympathetic activity, so does the state of the lens. At rest both are in midposition. The resting focal length of the lens averages 1 metre (with considerable variation between individuals). This is because the ciliary muscle is tonically active. To bring a distant object into focus, the ciliary muscle must be inhibited, so that the suspensory ligament becomes taut and the lens flat. The sphincter of the pupil is inhibited as well.

The sympathetic system innervates all the intrinsic muscles. It has a dual mode of action. It causes contraction of the dilator pupillae via α receptors on the muscle fibres, and it causes *relaxation* of the ciliary muscle and pupillary sphincter via β receptors. This dual effect constitutes the *far response*, and it is used to focus the eyes upon objects at a distance. (**Note**: The unqualified use of α and β receptors signifies α_1 and β_2, respectively.)

In stressed individuals, heightened sympathetic activity may interfere with the normal process of accommodation. For example, nervous students taking an important written test may have difficulty in bringing the questions into proper focus.

NOTES ON THE SYMPATHETIC PATHWAY TO THE EYE

The great length of the sympathetic pathway to the eye is indicated in Fig. 23.6.

1. *Central fibres* descending from the hypothalamus cross to the other side in the midbrain. In the pons and medulla, they are joined by ipsilateral fibres descending from the reticular formation.

2. *Preganglionic fibres* emerge in the first thoracic ventral nerve root and run up in the sympathetic chain to the superior cervical ganglion.

3. *Postganglionic fibres* from the superior cervical ganglion run along the external and internal carotid arteries and their branches.

Interruption of this 'three-neuron' oculosympathetic pathway anywhere along its course can result in **Horner syndrome** (small pupil *(miosis)*, ipsilateral ptosis, and variable anhidrosis depending on the site of the lesion; Chapter 13). The external carotid sympathetic fibres accompany all the branches of the external carotid artery. Those accompanying the facial artery supply the arterioles of the cheek and lips and are particularly responsive to emotional states. Those accompanying the maxillary artery supply the cavernous tissue covering the nasal conchae (turbinate bones).

Two sets of sympathetic fibres accompany the *internal carotid artery*. One set leaves it to join the ophthalmic division of the CN V in the cavernous sinus, then leaves this in the *long and short ciliary nerves* to supply the vessels and smooth muscles of the eyeball (ptosis results from paralysis of the smooth muscle fibres within the aponeurosis of the levator palpebrae superioris, the *superior tarsal muscle of Muller*). The second set forms a plexus around the internal carotid artery and its branches, including the ophthalmic artery. The ophthalmic artery gives off supratrochlear and supraorbital branches, which carry sympathetic fibres to the skin of the forehead and scalp.

Interruption of the postganglionic (sympathetic internal carotid plexus) fibres near the jugular foramen (see *jugular foramen syndrome*, Chapter 18), or in the cavernous sinus, produces anhidrosis (loss of sweating) on the forehead and scalp.

CONTROL OF EYE MOVEMENTS

The eyes normally move as a pair. This *conjugate* movement is of two fundamentally different kinds, as follows:

1. *Gaze shifting*. Cortical and subcortical areas are responsible for these volitional eye movements.
   a. **Saccadic** are conjugate, high velocity, ballistic eye movements under the control of the cerebral cortex, particularly the frontal and parietal eye fields, that redirect fixation to a new object of interest and onto the fovea of the eye. During this rapid eye movement, visual acuity is diminished, reestablishing itself once the target is again on the fovea, but this change in acuity goes unnoticed as this discontinuity is 'filled in' by the visual system.
   b. **Vergence** are dysconjugate eye movements that shift the gaze from far to near targets (e.g. fixation reflex).
2. *Gaze holding*. The visual system (retina to visual cortex) provides feedback with respect to the position of the target of gaze and the eye position that keeps the target on the retina (fovea) when the target or we move. (While the eyes may appear stationary, there are involuntary, fast, but small fixational eye movements that continue to occur, shifting the projection of an object over different retinal receptors, and facilitating feature extraction. If the retina

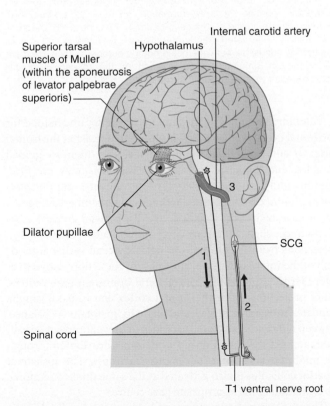

Fig. 23.6 Sympathetic innervation of the eye; three neuron pathways from the hypothalamus to the eye. *Arrows* indicate directions of impulse conduction. *SCG*, Superior cervical ganglion. For numbers, see text.

were truly immobile, the visual system would function poorly as it is relatively insensitive to unchanging input.)

a. *Tracking*, or *smooth pursuit*, occurs as the eyes follow an object of interest that is moving slowly across the visual field; eye velocity matches that of the visual target and maintains visual acuity by keeping the image on the fovea. (Without an object to track, it is not possible for an individual to volitionally move his or her eyes at such a slow speed. Attempts to do so result in small saccadic eye movements.)

b. *Vestibuloocular reflex* occurs when the gaze is held on an object of interest during movements of the head and is dependent upon displacement of endolymph in the kinetic labyrinth (Chapter 19).

Gaze Shifting

Four separate *gaze* centres in the brainstem pick out motor neurons appropriate to the direction of movement—leftwards, rightwards, upwards, or downwards—and are involved in both shifting and gaze-holding eye movements. The centres are small nodes in the reticular formation. They contain *burst cells*, which discharge at 1000 Hz (impulses/s) and entrain the appropriate motor neurons momentarily at this rate because it is necessary to overcome the elastic properties of the orbit to initiate eye movements.

The paired centres (left and right) for horizontal eye movements are in the **paramedian pontine reticular formation** (**PPRF**; Fig. 17.15). When each is activated, it will result in a conjugate (both eyes) movement to its own side (Fig. 23.7); for example, activation of the left PPRF moves both eyes so that they gaze to the left. The midbrain contains a bilateral centre for vertical eye movements located at the rostral end of the *medial longitudinal fasciculus (MLF)*, at the level of the pretectal nucleus, called the *rostral interstitial nucleus of the MLF (riMLF)*; perhaps its neurons for upgaze are more dorsal, for downgaze more ventral (Fig. 17.19). (Other nuclei that are often mentioned for vertical eye movements include the *interstitial nucleus of Cajal (INC)*, which is at the same level but a little ventral and plays a role in integrating information from the medulla and pons. The *nucleus of the posterior commissure (PCom)* contributes to upward gaze generation and coordination with eyelid movements.)

Automatic scanning movements are activated through the superior colliculus on receipt of visual information from the retina through the optic tract. Examples of automatic scanning include the quick sideward glance towards an object attracting attention in the peripheral visual field. The tectoreticular projections concerned cross the midline before engaging the gaze centres. Saccadic accuracy is controlled by the midregion (vermis) of the cerebellum, which receives afferents from the superior colliculi and projects to the vestibular nucleus. The posterior parietal cortex is likely involved in shifting gaze to such novel targets, and the *parietal eye field* (Brodmann area 7a) is involved when exploring visual scenes via visually guided saccades; both areas have significant interaction with the *frontal eye fields*.

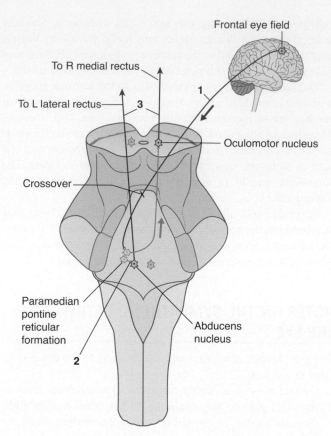

Fig. 23.7 Pathways involved in a voluntary ocular saccade to the left. *(1)* A projection from the right frontal eye field activates the left paramedian pontine reticular formation (PPRF). *(2)* Some PPRF neurons activate adjacent abducens neurons. *(3)* Other PPRF neurons send heavily myelinated (fast) internuclear fibres along the medial longitudinal bundle to activate oculomotor neurons serving the right medial rectus. Simultaneous contraction of the respective medial rectus muscles yields a saccade to the left.

Voluntary saccadic eye movements are better understood for horizontal eye movements and multiple areas exist in the frontal cortex (*frontal eye field*: voluntary saccades, memory-guided saccades, and vergence movements; *supplementary eye field*: planning and learning saccadic eye movements; and *dorsolateral prefrontal cortex*: planned saccades to remembered targets), which have reciprocal interactions with parietal cortical areas to produce such voluntary eye movements (Chapter 28). Projections from the frontal eye fields descend in the anterior limb of the internal capsule, and most of these fibres cross over before terminating in the contralateral brainstem gaze centres. Other projections from the frontal cortex end in basal ganglia (caudate, substantia nigra) and help to maintain a 'balance' between reflex and volitional saccades to prevent unwanted saccades and act through a group of neurons distributed through the midbrain and pons (*omnipause neurons*). The ipsilateral superior colliculus is also activated at the same time, to reinforce the excitation of the appropriate gaze centre.

There is hemispheric control of horizontal saccades, but the left hemisphere is responsible for saccadic eye movements to the right side and vice versa. Some patients who experience an acute frontal lobe lesion (usually an ischemic stroke) may temporally exhibit an inability to volitionally look to the side opposite the lesion (*gaze paralysis* or *acquired oculomotor apraxia*) while their vestibuloocular reflex remains intact. This gaze paralysis usually vanishes within a week, even if the hemiplegia remains profound. Unilateral parietal lobe lesions, especially of the right side, may cause delayed or hypometric (short of the planned target) saccades to the side contralateral (opposite) to the lesion (Chapter 32).

Gaze Holding

The neural mechanisms for tracking are complex because of the following basic requirements: (1) intact visual pathways to monitor the position of the object throughout the movement; (2) neurons to signal the rate of movement of the object (velocity detectors); (3) neurons to coordinate movements of the eyes and head (neural integrator); and (4) a system to monitor smooth execution of the tracking movement. An example of this system for horizontal smooth pursuit would include the following:

- Object movement detection begins in the retina and through the optic nerve projects to the lateral geniculate nucleus and from there to the primary visual cortex. With further cortical input from the frontal, parietal, and temporal cortex, it converges on the *temporoparietooccipital junction (TPO)* that projects ipsilaterally to the pons.
- The ipsilateral *dorsolateral pontine nucleus (DLPN)* receives that input and projects to the contralateral cerebellar flocculus, which projects to the vestibular nucleus.

- The vestibular nuclei project back (same side of origin of the cortical response) to the pons and the PPRF so the result is a conjugate horizontal movement of the eyes. It is important to remember that smooth pursuit movements are ipsilateral; the right hemisphere is responsible for rightward smooth pursuit movements and vice versa.

Vertical eye movements are generated bihemispherically with projections to the riMLF, which then projects to the respective motor neurons of cranial nerves III and IV. The INC integrates additional information from vestibular, pons, and medulla neurons, and the PCom further contributes with respect to upgaze and eyelid movement.

The vestibuloocular reflex is signalled by the dynamic labyrinth and is integrated with spatial and velocity information in the *nucleus prepositus hypoglossi*, a node of the reticular formation that helps to position and hold the eyes steady in an eccentric position of gaze. The nucleus prepositus hypoglossi projects to the PPRF or, for vertical eye movements, the riMLF, which integrates conjugate eye movements. Cortical input (frontal, parietal, and insular) further modulates these responses. As a reflex, it also needs to be suppressed when a target and the head (and eyes) are moving synchronously in the same direction; otherwise the reflex would move the eyes in a direction opposite to the head movement!

The dynamic labyrinth and cerebellum cooperate to keep the eyes on target during movement of the head, as described in Chapter 19.

CLINICAL PANEL 23.1 Ocular Palsies

One or more of the three ocular motor nerves may be paralysed by disease within the brainstem (e.g. multiple sclerosis, vascular occlusion), in the subarachnoid space (e.g. meningitis, aneurysm in the circle of Willis, distortion by an expanding intracranial lesion), in the cavernous sinus (e.g. thrombosis of the sinus, aneurysm of the internal carotid artery there), or by microvascular ischemia to the nerve in the setting of atherosclerotic risk factors. There is a significant prevalence of structural lesions, and it may be prudent to consider contrast-enhanced MRI for all patients presenting with acute, isolated ocular motor mononeuropathies irrespective of age.

Oculomotor Nerve
Complete III Nerve Palsy
Characteristic signs of complete third nerve paralysis (left eye) are shown in Fig. 23.8A. They are:
1. Complete ptosis of the upper eyelid (held open by the examiner in this figure so the position of the left eye can be seen).
2. A fully dilated, non-reactive pupil (unopposed dilator pupillae).
3. A fully abducted eye (unopposed lateral rectus), which is also depressed (unopposed superior oblique).

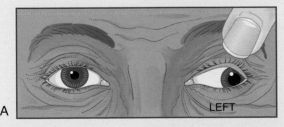
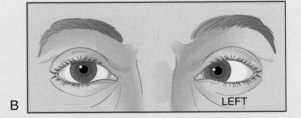

Fig. 23.8 (A) Complete left III nerve paralysis. The closed eyelid has been raised by the examiner's finger. (B) Complete left VI nerve paralysis.

Partial III nerve palsy

The pupils are always monitored when cases of head injury come to medical attention. Rapidly increasing intracranial pressure, resulting from an acute extradural or subdural hematoma (Chapter 5), often compresses the third nerve against the crest of the petrous temporal bone. The parasympathetic fibres are superficially placed and are the first to suffer, and the pupil dilates progressively on the affected side. Pupillary dilatation is an urgent indication for surgical decompression of the brain.

Trochlear Nerve

The IV nerve is rarely paralysed alone. The cardinal symptom is diplopia (double vision) on looking down, such as when going downstairs. This happens because the superior oblique normally assists the inferior rectus in pulling the eye downwards, especially when the eye is in an adducted position.

Abducens Nerve

The effect of a complete VI nerve paralysis is shown in Fig. 23.8B (right eye is affected and in this diagram the individual is attempting to look towards their right). The eye is fully adducted by the unopposed pull of the medial rectus. The abducens nerve has the longest course in the subarachnoid space of any cranial nerve. It also bends sharply over the crest of the petrous temporal bone. A space-occupying lesion affecting either cerebral hemisphere may cause compression and paralysis of one abducens nerve.

'Spontaneous' paralysis of the VI nerve may be caused by an arterial aneurysm at the base of the brain, atherosclerosis of the internal carotid artery in the cavernous sinus, or microvascular ischemia to the nerve in the setting of atherosclerotic risk factors.

Internuclear Ophthalmoplegia (INO)

Interruption of the linkage between the abducens nucleus and the contralateral oculomotor nucleus, via the MLF, gives rise to a disorder of conjugate gaze referred to as ***internuclear ophthalmoplegia***.

As an example, a lesion of the right MLF is shown in Fig. 23.9 and would leave the gaze to the right unaffected, whereas attempting to gaze to the left, the right eye adducts minimally and the contralateral left eye abducts, but nystagmus (towards the left) is seen. On looking to the left the left abducens nucleus is

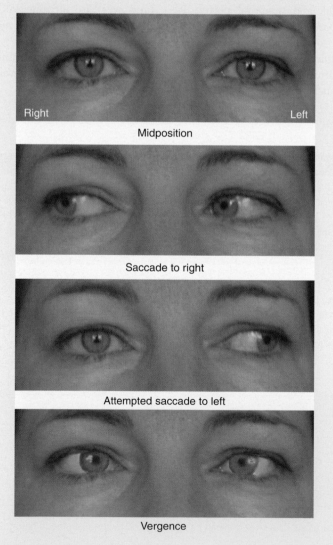

Right   Left

Midposition

Saccade to right

Attempted saccade to left

Vergence

Fig. 23.9 Right internuclear ophthalmoplegia.

activated (causing contraction of the left lateral rectus muscle and abduction of the left eye) and the PPRF also projects into the right MLF that would normally activate the right oculomotor nucleus and result in contraction of the right medial rectus (and adduction of the right eye), but this pathway is blocked so, the right medial rectus does not contract. The individual experiences diplopia when looking to the left (two images side-by-side). Integrity of the III nucleus and the right medial rectus is shown by its normal behaviour during the vergence component of the near response (this involves a different and unaffected pathway).

Below the age of 40, the chief cause of internuclear ophthalmoplegia is a demyelinating plaque from multiple sclerosis disrupting the MLF. Above the age of 60, the chief cause is a stroke from an occlusion of a pontine branch of the basilar artery causing an ischemic injury to the MLF.

Ocular Sympathetic Supply

Any one of the three sequential sets of neurons depicted in Fig. 23.6 may be interrupted by local pathology.

1. The central set may be interrupted by a vascular lesion of the pons or medulla oblongata or by demyelinating disease (multiple sclerosis). The usual picture is one of Horner syndrome (ptosis and miosis, as described in Chapter 13) with cranial nerve involvement on one side, together with motor weakness and/or sensory loss in the limbs on the contralateral side. *Horner syndrome* is associated with anhidrosis—absence of sweating—in the face and scalp on the same side, together with congestion of the nose (engorged turbinates).
2. The *preganglionic* set is most often interrupted by infection/tumour of the lung, by trauma, or cervical spine disease. Horner syndrome is again associated with anhidrosis of the face and scalp (and nasal congestion) on the same side.
3. The *postganglionic* set accompanying the external carotid artery can be injured by disease of the carotid artery *(dissection of the carotid artery)* or by a tumour of the base of the skull. The set accompanying the internal carotid artery may be interrupted as part of a *jugular foramen syndrome* (Chapter 18) or by pathology in the cavernous sinus. Horner syndrome is now accompanied by anhidrosis of the forehead and anterior scalp (territory of the supraorbital and supratrochlear arteries).

✳ Core Information

Oculomotor Nerve

Somatic efferent fibres of cranial nerve (CN) III arise from the main nucleus at the level of the superior colliculus. The nerve passes in the wall of the cavernous sinus and its two divisions exit the cranium through the superior orbital fissure. The upper division supplies the superior rectus and levator palpebrae superioris muscles; the lower division supplies the inferior oblique as well as the inferior and medial recti muscles.

Parasympathetic fibres emerge from the *Edinger–Westphal nucleus*, travel in the main nerve, and synapse in the ciliary ganglion to supply the sphincter pupillae and ciliary muscles. Paralysis of CN III causes dilation of the pupil, ptosis, and divergent squint.

Trochlear Nerve

The nucleus of the CN IV is at the level of the inferior colliculus. The nerve crosses the midline before emerging below the inferior colliculus. It passes in the lateral wall of the cavernous sinus to supply the superior oblique muscle. Paralysis is characterised by diplopia on looking down.

Abducens Nerve

The nucleus is at the level of the facial colliculus in the pons. The CN VI runs in the subarachnoid space from lower border of the pons to the apex of the petrous part of the temporal bone and passes through the cavernous sinus and the superior orbital fissure to supply the lateral rectus muscle. Paralysis is characterised by convergent squint with inability to abduct the affected eye.

(A simple memory device useful to remember which nerve innervates which eye muscle is: LR6(SO4)3. This fictitious chemical formula reminds us that the lateral rectus (LR) is innervated by the VI nerve, the superior oblique (SO) is innervated by the IV nerve, and the rest of the eye muscles are innervated by the III nerve.)

Sympathetic

Muscles stimulated (via α_1 receptors) are the dilator pupillae, a smooth muscle in the anterior deeper part of the levator palpebrae superioris (known as the *tarsal muscle of Muller*). Paralysis is characterised by ptosis with a constricted pupil *(Horner syndrome)*. Muscles inhibited (via β_2 receptors) are the sphincter pupillae and the ciliary muscles.

Parasympathetic

Muscles stimulated are the sphincter (constrictor) pupillae and the ciliary muscles.

Reflex Pathways

For the *pupillary light reflex*: from the retina to the pretectal nucleus, to both Edinger–Westphal nuclei, to the ciliary ganglion, and finally, the sphincter pupillae muscle.

For the *accommodation reflex*: from the retina to the lateral geniculate body, to the occipital cortex, to the Edinger–Westphal nucleus, to the ciliary ganglion, and then to the ciliary muscles.

Oculomotor controls

Gaze shifting (*saccadic*) eye movements are locally activated by six gaze centres. Most important clinically is the *paramedian pontine reticular formation (PPRF)*, which operates to pull the ipsilateral lateral rectus and contralateral medial rectus conjugately to its own side. Automatic scanning is controlled by the superior colliculi and voluntary scanning by the frontal eye fields. Gaze holding is complex and involves the occipital cortex, dynamic labyrinth, cerebellum, superior colliculus, and reticular formation.

SUGGESTED READINGS

Bac YJ, Kim JH, Choi BS, et al. Brainstem pathways for horizontal eye movement: pathologic correlation with MR imaging. *RadioGraphics.* 2013;33:47–59.

Baird-Gunning JJD, Lueck CJ. Central control of eye movements. *Curr Opin Neurol.* 2018;31:90–95.

Binda P, Morrone MC. Vision during saccadic eye movements. *Annu Rev Vis Sci.* 2018;4:193–213.

Detwiler PB. Phototransduction in retinal ganglion cells. *Yale J Biol Med.* 2018;91:49–52.

Kim SH, Zee DS, du Lac S, et al. Nucleus prepositus hypoglossi lesions produce a unique ocular motor syndrome. *Neurology.* 2016;87:2026–2033.

Larsen RS, Waters J. Neuromodulatory correlates of pupil dilation. *Front Neural Circuit.* 2018;12:21.

Martin TJ. Horner Syndrome: a clinical review. *ACS Chem Neurosci.* 2018;9:177−186.

Paduca A, Bruenech JR. Neuroanatomical structures in human extraocular muscles and their potential implication in the development of oculomotor disorders. *J Pediatr Ophthalmol Strabismus.* 2018;55:14−22.

Pretegiani E, Optican LM. Eye movements in Parkinson's disease and inherited Parkinsonian syndromes. *Front Neurol.* 2017;8:592.

Rucci M, Victor JD. The unsteady eye: an information-processing stage, not a bug. *Trends Neurosci.* 2015;38:195−206.

Spering M, Carrasco M. Acting without seeing: eye movements reveal visual processing without awareness. *Trends Neurosci.* 2015; 38:247−258.

Takahashi M, Shinoda Y. Brain stem neural circuits of horizontal and vertical saccade systems and their frame of reference. *Neuroscience.* 2018;392:281−328.

Tamhankar MA, Volpe NJ. Management of acute cranial nerve 3, 4 and 6 palsies: role of neuroimaging. *Curr Opin Ophthalmol.* 2015;26:464−468.

Tarnutzer AA, Straumann D. Nystagmus. *Curr Opin Neurol.* 2018; 31:74−80.

Reticular Formation and the Neuromodulatory System

STUDY GUIDELINES

1. Outline the subdivisions and functions of the reticular formation.
2. Describe the location, type, and role of aminergic brainstem neurons of the neuromodulatory system.
3. Define a chemoreceptor and its role in respiratory control.
4. Summarise how the central nervous system monitors and controls respiration.
5. Define a baroreceptor and its role in cardiovascular control.
6. Summarise how the central nervous system monitors and controls blood pressure.
7. Define nociception and pain, and outline the pathway of nociceptive transmission within the spinothalamic and spinobulbar pathways.
8. Describe the role of the periaqueductal grey (PAG) substance and the magnus raphe nucleus in pain modulation.
9. Define the gate control of nociceptive transmission and its clinical importance.
10. Explain how a 'flip-flop' mechanism can explain the relationship between wake versus sleep and nonrapid eye movement (NREM) versus rapid eye movement (REM) sleep.
11. Define the ascending reticular activating system (ARAS) and how our understanding of its origin has changed.

RETICULAR FORMATION

The term **reticular formation** refers only to the polysynaptic network in the brainstem, although the network continues rostrally into the thalamus and hypothalamus, and caudally into the propriospinal network of the spinal cord. The ground plan is shown in Fig. 24.1A. The **medial reticular (tegmental) field** contains large-celled neurons and the **lateral reticular (tegmental) field** small-celled neurons.

The medial field is a predominantly *efferent system*. The axons are relatively long, and some ascend to synapse in the midbrain reticular formation or in the thalamus. Others have both ascending and descending branches contributing to a polysynaptic network. Projections from the premotor cortex, *corticoreticular fibres*, project here and give rise to the **pontine** and **medullary reticulospinal tracts**.

Neurons within the lateral field have long dendrites that branch at regular intervals. They have a predominantly transverse orientation, and their interstices are penetrated by long pathways running to the thalamus. The lateral network is mainly afferent in nature and receives fibres from all sensory pathways, including the special senses:

- Olfactory fibres are received through the medial forebrain bundle, which passes alongside the hypothalamus.
- Visual pathway fibres arise from the superior colliculus.
- Auditory pathway fibres originate from the superior olivary nucleus and vestibular fibres from the medial vestibular nucleus.
- Somatic sensory fibres are received from the *spinoreticular tracts* and from the spinal cord and principal (chief or main pontine) nucleus of the trigeminal nerve.

Axons from these neurons ramify extensively among the dendrites of the medial field and some synapse within the nuclei of cranial nerves and act as pattern generators.

Functional Anatomy

The range of functions served by different parts of the reticular formation is indicated in Table 24.1.

Pattern Generators

Central pattern generators (CPG) are integrated neuronal circuits that generate repetitive or stereotyped patterns of motor behaviour that can be independent of any sensory input or feedback. However, CPGs are subject to significant modulation that

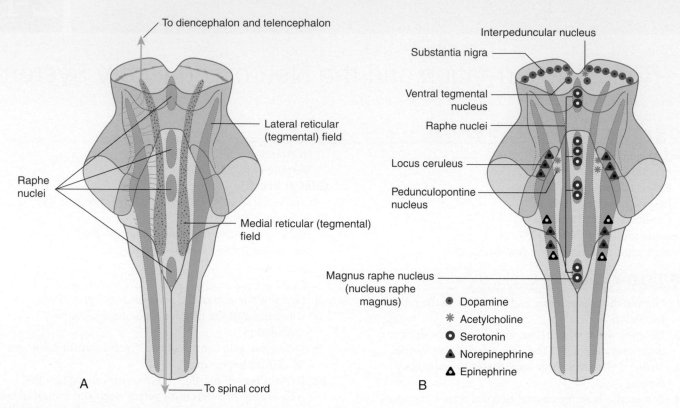

Fig. 24.1 (A) Reticular formation and subdivisions. (B) Aminergic and cholinergic cell groups of the neuromodulatory system.

TABLE 24.1 **Components of the Reticular Formation and their Perceived Functions.**

Function	Component
Bladder control	Pontine micturition centre
Cardiovascular control	Caudal ventrolateral medulla (CVLM)
	Posterior ventrolateral medulla (PVLM)
	Parabrachial nuclear complex
Locomotion	Mesencephalic locomotor region (pedunculopontine and cuneiform nucleus)
	Pontomedullary reticular formation
Patterned cranial nerve activities (chewing, coughing, conjugate eye movements, sneezing, swallowing, vomiting, yawning)	Premotor cranial nerve nuclei (central pattern generators)
Respiratory control	Dorsal respiratory group (DRG)
	Ventral respiratory group (VRG)
	Parabrachial nuclear complex
	Retrotrapezoid nucleus
Salivary secretion, lacrimation	Salivatory nuclei
Wake and sleep	Parabrachial nuclear complex
	Parafacial zone
	Pedunculopontine nucleus
	Subcoeruleus region

allows flexibility of response and integration with other systems. Patterned activities involving cranial nerves include:

- Conjugate (parallel) movements of the eyes locally controlled by premotor nodal points (*gaze centres*) in the midbrain and pons linked to the nuclei of the ocular motor nerves (see Chapter 23).
- Rhythmic chewing movements are controlled by the supratrigeminal premotor nucleus in the pons (see Chapter 21).
- Swallowing, vomiting, coughing, yawning, and sneezing are controlled by separate premotor nodal points in the medulla and linked to specific cranial nerves and the respiratory centres.
- Higher-level bladder controls are described in Basic Science Panel 24.1.
- Locomotor pattern generators are described in Basic Science Panel 24.2.
- An overview of gait controls is shown in Fig. 24.2.
- The salivatory nuclei belong to the parvocellular reticular formation of the pons and medulla and they contribute preganglionic parasympathetic fibres to the facial and glossopharyngeal nerves.

Respiratory Control

Groups of neurons located along either side of the upper medulla oblongata and organised into a *dorsal respiratory nucleus (DRN)* and *ventral respiratory nucleus (VRN)* regulate the respiratory cycle (Fig. 24.3). Neurons of the DRN lie around and ventrolateral to the nucleus tractus solitarius and integrate sensory information (e.g. from cranial nerves IX and X via peripheral chemoreceptors) related to respiration, while other neurons project to related inspiratory motor neurons within the spinal cord.

The VRN lies ventral to the DRN. This column of neurons extends from the pons to the spinal cord and consists of three

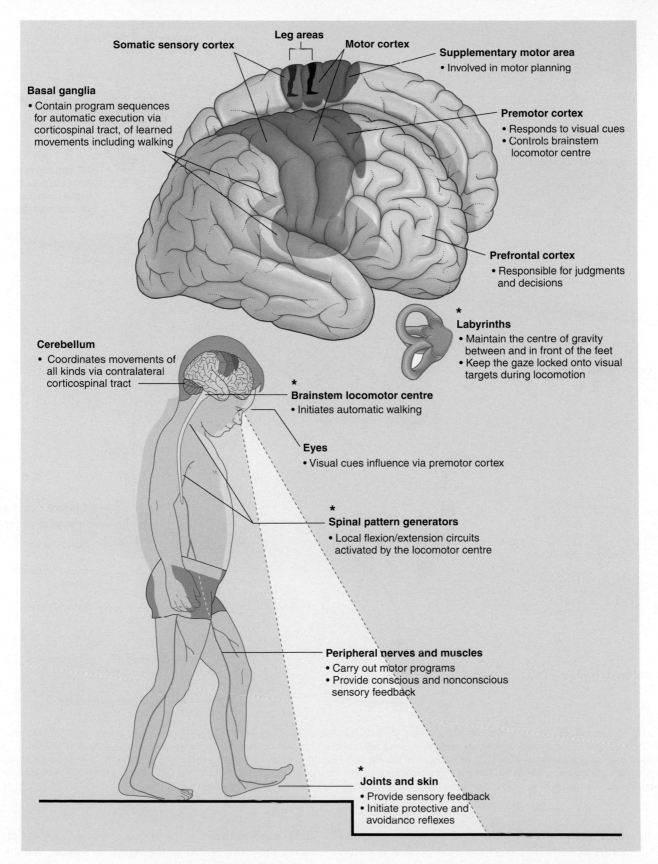

Somatic sensory cortex

Leg areas

Motor cortex

Supplementary motor area
• Involved in motor planning

Basal ganglia
• Contain program sequences for automatic execution via corticospinal tract, of learned movements including walking

Premotor cortex
• Responds to visual cues
• Controls brainstem locomotor centre

Prefrontal cortex
• Responsible for judgments and decisions

*
Labyrinths
• Maintain the centre of gravity between and in front of the feet
• Keep the gaze locked onto visual targets during locomotion

Cerebellum
• Coordinates movements of all kinds via contralateral corticospinal tract

*
Brainstem locomotor centre
• Initiates automatic walking

Eyes
• Visual cues influence via premotor cortex

*
Spinal pattern generators
• Local flexion/extension circuits activated by the locomotor centre

Peripheral nerves and muscles
• Carry out motor programs
• Provide conscious and nonconscious sensory feedback

*
Joints and skin
• Provide sensory feedback
• Initiate protective and avoidance reflexes

Fig. 24.2 Overview of gait controls. Key nodes are indicated by an *asterisk*. (The assistance of Professor Tim O'Brien, Director, Gait Laboratory, Central Remedial Clinic, Dublin, is gratefully acknowledged.)

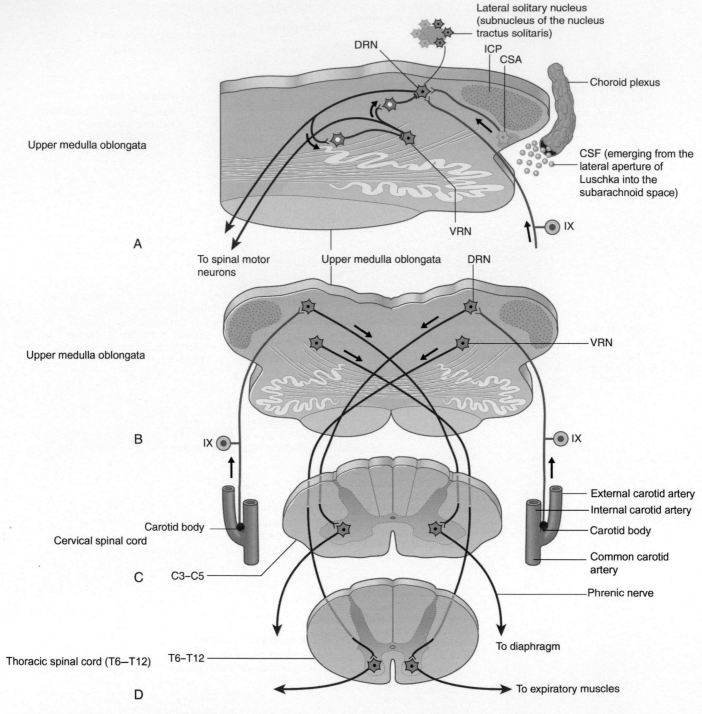

Fig. 24.3 Respiratory control systems. All sections are viewed from below and behind. (A) is an enlargement taken from (B). (A) Inhibitory interaction between dorsal and ventral respiratory nuclei *(DRN, VRN)*. Choroidal capillaries discharge cerebrospinal fluid *(CSF)* close to the medullary chemosensitive area *(CSA)*, whence neurons project to DRN. (B) The glossopharyngeal nerve *(IX)* contains chemoreceptive neurons reaching from the carotid body to the DRN. (C) Phrenic motor neurons are activated by the contralateral DRN. (D) Muscles of the abdominal wall are activated by the contralateral VRN to produce forced expiration. *ICP,* Inferior cerebellar peduncle.

regions which receive sensory (afferent) information from the DRN. The ***rostral VRN*** (*Bötzinger complex*) portion is within the *parafacial respiratory group* of neurons and contains expiratory interneurons that project to other respiratory nuclei and the caudal VRN. In the ***intermediate VRN***, the most rostral portion consists of inspiratory neurons *(pre-Bötzinger complex)* and possibly functions as the CPG of inspiration and for coordinating the other phases of the respiratory cycle. Within and near the intermediate VRN is the *nucleus ambiguus* (motor neurons of CN IX and X that when activated prevent collapse of upper airway during inspiration) and the *nucleus paraambigualis* that projects to inspiratory motor neurons in the spinal cord and inspiratory accessory muscles. The **caudal VRN** contains the *nucleus retroambigualis* (dorsal to the nucleus ambiguus; see Fig. 17.13) and is comprised of expiratory premotor neurons which project to spinal cord motor neurons that innervate accessory muscles of expiration (e.g. internal intercostals). As expiration is normally a passive process, these neurons are relatively inactive during normal breathing but become active during exercise.

The *parabrachial nuclear complex* surrounds the superior cerebellar peduncle and is in the dorsolateral pons. It participates in the regulation of cardiovascular and respiratory function. Stimulation of this nucleus by the amygdala in anxiety states results in characteristic hyperventilation (see Chapter 33).

Through numerous complementary and regulatory interactions between these brainstem structures and higher CNS centres, respiratory control is seamlessly integrated with speaking, swallowing, sleep—wake cycles, and emotions.

Medullary Chemosensitive Area. The choroid plexus of the fourth ventricle produces cerebrospinal fluid (CSF) that passes through the lateral aperture (of Luschka) of the fourth ventricle (Fig. 24.3). At this location, cells of the lateral reticular formation at the medullary surface are exquisitely sensitive to the hydrogen (H^+) ion concentration in the neighbouring CSF. In effect, this medullary chemosensitive area (*CSA; retrotrapezoid nucleus*) samples the partial pressure of carbon dioxide (P_{CO2}) level in the CSF, which is a direct reflection of the P_{CO2} in the blood supplying the brain (CSA also receives input from the peripheral chemoreceptors). Any increase in H^+ ions stimulates the dorsal respiratory nucleus through a direct synaptic linkage. (Several other nuclei within the medulla are also chemosensitive.)

Carotid Chemoreceptors. The **carotid body** is close to the bifurcation of the carotid artery (Fig. 24.3) and receives a small branch from the external carotid artery that ramifies within the carotid body. Blood flow through the carotid body is so intense that the arteriovenous partial pressure of oxygen (P_{O2}) changes by less than 1% during passage. The glomus cells chemoreceptors are neuroectodermal in origin, and release of their neurotransmitters triggers an action potential in the sensory endings of branches of the sinus nerve (branch of IX). The carotid chemoreceptors respond primarily to a fall in P_{O2} or rise in P_{CO2} and cause reflex adjustment of blood gas levels by altering the rate of breathing. Chemoreceptors in the **aortic bodies** (beneath the aortic arch) are relatively insignificant in humans but play a similar role and their afferents arise from the X cranial nerve.

Cardiovascular Control

Through **baroreceptors**, which facilitate cardiopulmonary reflexes, the cardiovascular, endocrine, and central and peripheral nervous systems confine blood pressure fluctuations to physiological normal ranges (Fig. 24.4). The baroreceptor system begins with receptors; afferent nerve endings within the adventitia of the carotid sinus and aortic arch that serve as mechanoreceptors and increase their firing pattern with increased arterial blood pressure. Within the carotid sinus are afferent fibres of CN IX and in the aortic arch, afferent fibres of

CN X. Both terminate in the caudal portion of the nucleus of the solitary tract from which two projections arise.

One projection is to neurons of the reticular formation within the *caudal ventrolateral medulla* (*CVLM*) and from there, through an inhibitory projection, to the *posterior ventrolateral medulla* (*PVLM*). Those neurons project to preganglionic sympathetic neurons of the intermediolateral cell column within the spinal cord, inhibit sympathetic activity, and decrease blood pressure (through vasodilation) and heart rate. The other projection is to the ventral lateral portion of the nucleus ambiguus and vagal preganglionic parasympathetic neurons. These neurons will then project to the *cardiac ganglia*, increasing their inhibition and lowering the heart rate.

The balance of parasympathetic and sympathetic activity reflects the continuous monitoring by these baroreceptors. Similarly, cardiorespiratory mechanoreceptors within the walls of the cardiopulmonary veins, atria, and left ventricle serve as low-pressure receptors and play a complementary role in maintaining blood pressure.

NEUROMODULATORY SYSTEM

Aminergic Neurons of the Brainstem

Interspersed among the reticular formation are sets of *aminergic (or monoaminergic)* neurons that share several cellular properties (Fig. 24.1B), and whose neurotransmitters are synthesised from an aromatic amino acid. One set produces the neurotransmitter *serotonin*, three sets produce **catecholamines** (*dopamine, norepinephrine, and epinephrine*), and one set produces *histamine* (Table 24.2).

- The **serotonergic neurons** have the largest territorial distribution of any set of central nervous system (CNS) neurons. In general terms, those of the midbrain project rostrally into the cerebral hemispheres; those of the pons ramify in the brainstem and cerebellum; and those of the medulla supply the spinal cord (Fig. 24.5). All parts of the CNS grey matter are permeated by serotonin-secreting axonal varicosities. Clinically, enhancement of serotonin activity is part of the treatment for a prevalent condition known as major depression.
- The **dopaminergic neurons** of the midbrain fall into two groups. At the junction of tegmentum and crus are those of the **substantia nigra** (see Chapter 26). Medial to these are those of the **ventral tegmental nuclei** (Fig. 24.6) that project *mesocortical fibres* to the frontal lobe and *mesolimbic fibres* to the nucleus accumbens (see Chapter 33).
- The **noradrenergic (norepinephrine) neurons** are only marginally less prodigious than the serotonergic ones. About 90% of the somas are pooled in the **locus coeruleus** (*coeruleus nucleus*), a 'violet spot' in the floor of the fourth ventricle at the upper part of the pons (Fig. 24.7). Neurons of the locus coeruleus project in *all* directions, as indicated in Fig. 24.8.
- *Epinephrine-secreting neurons* are relatively scarce and are confined to the medulla oblongata. Some project rostrally to the hypothalamus, others project caudally to synapse upon preganglionic sympathetic neurons in the spinal cord.

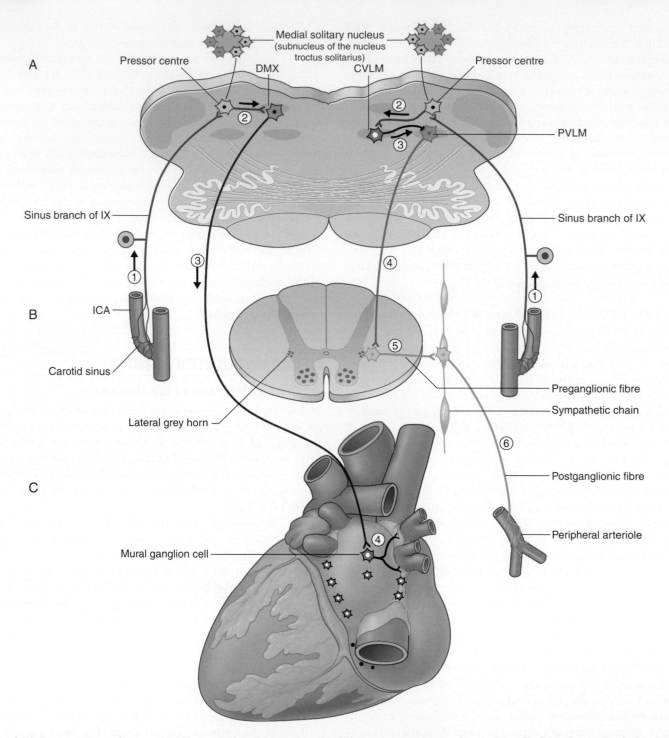

Fig. 24.4 Baroreceptor reflexes. (A) Upper medulla oblongata. (B) Spinal cord segments T1 to L3. (C) Posterior wall of the heart. Baroreceptor–parasympathetic reflex *(left)*. *1,* Mechanoreceptors in the carotid sinus (and the aortic arch) excite fibres in the sinus branch of the glossopharyngeal nerve (and vagus nerve). *ICA,* internal carotid artery. *2,* Baroreceptor neurons of nucleus of the solitary tract respond by stimulating cardioinhibitory neurons in the dorsal (motor) nucleus of the vagus *(DMX)*. *3,* Preganglionic, cholinergic parasympathetic vagal fibres synapse upon mural ganglion cells on the posterior wall of the heart. *4,* Postganglionic, cholinergic parasympathetic fibres reduce sinoatrial node pacemaker activity, thus reducing the heart rate. Baroreceptor–sympathetic reflex *(right)*. *1,* Carotid sinus (and aortic arch) mechanoreceptor afferents excite baroreceptor neurons of the nucleus of the solitary tract. *2,* Baroreceptor neurons respond by exciting the inhibitory neurons of the reticular formation in the caudal ventrolateral medulla *CVLM)*. *3,* The CVLM projects to the adrenergic and noradrenergic neurons of the posterior ventrolateral medulla *(PVLM)*, inhibiting them. *4,* Tonic excitations of the lateral grey horn are reduced. *5* and *6,* Preganglionic and postganglionic sympathetic tone to peripheral arterioles is reduced, thus lowering peripheral arterial resistance. *IX,* Glossopharyngeal nerve.

TABLE 24.2 Aminergic Neurons of the Neuromodulatory System.

Neurotransmitter	Location
Acetylcholine	Basal forebrain (nucleus basalis of Meynert), pons (pedunculopontine nucleus and laterodorsal tegmental nuclei)
Dopamine	Midbrain (ventral tegmental area and substantia nigra pars compacta)
Epinephrine	Medulla
Histamine	Diencephalon (tuberomammillary nucleus)
Norepinephrine	Midbrain, pons (locus coeruleus), medulla
Serotonin	Midbrain (raphe nuclei), pons (raphe nuclei), medulla (magnus raphe nucleus)

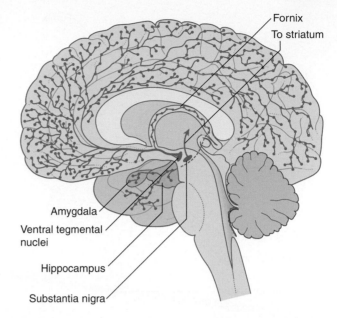

Fig. 24.6 Dopaminergic projections from the midbrain nuclei.

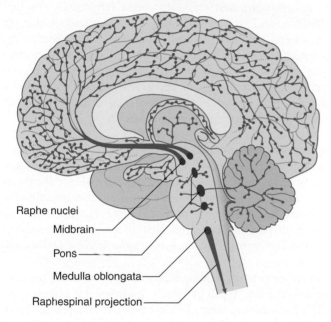

Fig. 24.5 Serotonergic projections from the brainstem midline (raphe) nuclei.

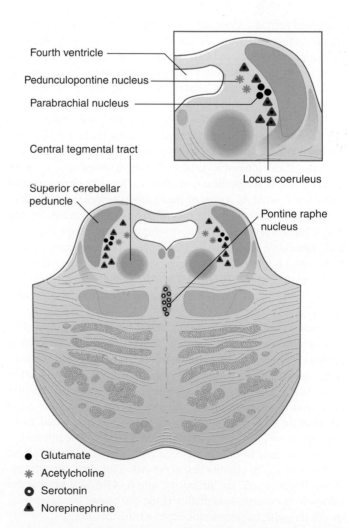

Fig. 24.7 Part of a transverse section through the upper part of the pons, showing elements of the neuromodulatory system.

In the cerebral cortex, the ionic and electrical effects of aminergic neuronal activity are quite variable. First, more than one kind of postsynaptic receptor exists for each of the amines. Second, some aminergic neurons also liberate a peptide substance capable of modulating the transmitter action, usually by prolonging it. Third, the larger cortical neurons receive many thousands of excitatory and inhibitory synapses from local circuit neurons, and have numerous different receptors. Activation of a single kind of aminergic receptor may have a large or small effect, depending on the existing excitatory state.

Although our understanding of the physiology and pharmacology of the aminergic neurons is far from complete, their relevance to a wide range of behavioural functions is unquestioned.

Nociception and Pain

Nociception is detection of potential or actual stimuli that can cause tissue injury. While *pain* involves nociception in that it encompasses the negative affective or emotional aspects,

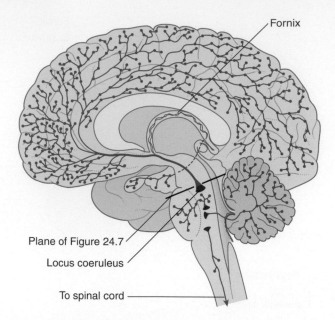

Fornix

Plane of Figure 24.7

Locus coeruleus

To spinal cord

Fig. 24.8 Noradrenergic projections from the pons and medulla oblongata nuclei.

perceived pain is dependent upon environmental context, emotional factors, attentional mechanism, and prior experience. Pain and our associated behaviours are dynamic, causing our attention to shift from other relevant environmental and intrinsic stimuli. Those same stimuli may shift our attention and change our response and behaviour to pain.

Nociceptive transmission from the trunk and limbs enters the dorsal horn of the spinal cord, whereas transmission from the head and upper part of the neck enters the spinal trigeminal nucleus. These afferents consist of *unmyelinated type C axons* that respond to temperature, mechanical force or chemicals and finely *myelinated Aδ axons* or mechanoreceptors from the skin. Within the spinal cord, the type C axons will terminate in the dorsal horn layers I and II *(substantia gelatinosa)* (see Fig. 15.5) and signal dull or poorly localised pain. Their primary neurotransmitter is glutamate, but many use *substance P* or *calcitonin gene–related peptide (CGRP)*. The Aδ axons terminate in layers II and V and signal sharp well-localised pain; their neurotransmitter is glutamate.

These afferents terminate on dorsal horn interneurons predominantly found within lamina I, II, IV, V and the trigeminal nucleus where some will give rise to the trigeminothalamic tract. Other interneurons within the spinal cord are also projection neurons that give rise to the spinothalamic tract, spinoreticular tract, and other spinobulbar sensory pathways that will cross the midline and are collectively called the *anterolateral pathway*, based on location within the spinal cord. Other interneurons are intrinsic to the spinal cord and trigeminal nucleus and form various local circuits that serve either an excitatory (transmitter is glutamate) or inhibitory role (GABA and glycine for some interneurons; enkephalin (Enk; an opiate pentapeptide) for others) with respect to nociceptive transmission.

There are also non-nociceptive afferents (e.g. touch, vibration) that project to inhibitory interneurons and this 'crosstalk'

can impact nociceptive sensory information transmission. This is referred to as the **gate control of nociceptive transmission** and believed to account for the relief afforded by 'rubbing the sore spot'. It is also the rationale for the use of *transcutaneous electrical nerve stimulation (TENS)* where a stimulating electrode applied to the skin within the area of discomfort activates non-nociceptive afferents, and by inhibitory interneuron activation, blocks nociceptive transmission in the spinal cord.

Ascending fibres that predominantly constitute the spinothalamic tract will terminate in different nuclei of the thalamus (e.g. the ventral posterolateral nucleus for those afferents representing the trunk and limb and the ventral posteromedial nucleus for those originating from the trigeminal nucleus). Thalamocortical projections include those to the somatosensory cortex (where, how much), insular cortex (what type of nociceptive information), and cingulate cortex (emotional, affective, autonomic, and aversive response). The other tracts within the anterolateral pathway (e.g. spinoreticular) will project to the brainstem (nucleus of the solitary tract, locus coeruleus, nucleus raphe magnus, *periaqueductal grey substance (PAG)*, and parabrachial nucleus) and from there reach the hypothalamus, thalamus, and amygdala (emotional and aversive responses with PAG as a 'centre' for pain modulation).

Supraspinal Antinociception. This network of connections is responsible for the processing of nociceptive information, subsequent behavioural responses, and the rationale for the therapeutic targeting of analgesic medications or other modalities of intervention. Modulation of nociceptive transmission and subsequent pain involves areas that all have opioid receptors (i.e. *cingulate cortex*, **PAG**, **magnus raphe nucleus (MRn)**, and *locus coeruleus*).

In response to descending forebrain and ascending nociceptive information, PAG (normally inhibited by interneurons within PAG that are themselves inhibited by enkephalin (Enk)-containing interneurons, opioid peptides, cannabinoids, and β-endorphins released from a small set of hypothalamic neurons projecting to the Enk-containing interneurons) projects to the MRn and locus coeruleus. Their projections to the dorsal horn and trigeminal nucleus inhibit nociceptive afferents and projection neurons or act through inhibitory interneurons (Fig. 24.9). The result is analgesia, but other sensory modalities remain intact.

Sleeping and Wakefulness

Electroencephalography (EEG) reveals characteristic patterns in the electrical activity of cerebral cortical neurons that accompany various states of consciousness. The normal waking state is characterised by high frequency, low amplitude waves. The onset of sleep is accompanied by slow frequency, high amplitude waves, with the higher amplitude being a result of the synchronised activity of a larger number of neurons. This type of sleep is called *slow wave* (synchronised) or **nonrapid eye movement (NREM) sleep**. At the initiation of sleep, this first NREM stage lasts for about 60 minutes and transitions into the next stage where the EEG pattern resembles the waking state. Dreams occur during this stage of sleep as do rapid eye

A

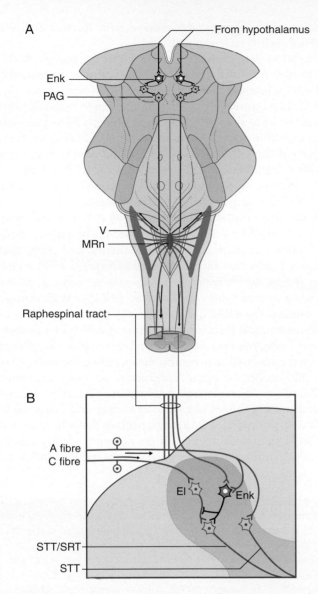

Enk

PAG

V
MRn

Raphespinal tract

B

A fibre
C fibre

EI   Enk

STT/SRT

STT

Fig. 24.9 Antinociceptive pathways. (A) Posterior view of the brainstem. (B) Right dorsal grey horn of the spinal cord viewed from above. The periaqueductal grey matter *(PAG)* contains an excitatory projection to the magnus raphe nucleus *(MRn)* and locus coeruleus (not shown), and enkephalinergic interneurons *(Enk)* that inhibit interneurons that tonically inhibit those projection cells. Inhibitory fibres from the hypothalamus release (disinhibit) the excitatory MRn projection neurons. The effects within the trigeminal spinal nucleus and dorsal grey horn are the same: serotonin liberated by MRn neurons excites Enk interneurons, which inhibit nociceptive projection cells. The nociceptive pathway at cord level is represented by the C-fibre input to an excitatory interneuron *(EI)*, which in turn excites the spinothalamic or spinoreticular projection cell *(STT/SRT)* unless inhibited by an Enk interneuron. Rubbing the sore spot sends impulse trains along A afferent axons inducing the Enk cell to exert presynaptic inhibition on the EI terminal, and postsynaptic inhibition on the STT/SRT projection cell. Passage of purely tactile information into the spinothalamic tract *(STT)* is not impeded.

movements, hence the more usual term, **rapid eye movement (REM) sleep**. Several alternating cycles of NREM and REM sleep occur throughout a normal night's sleep, as described in Chapter 29.

The cycling between sleep and wakefulness reflects two networks in the brain, one for the waking state and the other for sleep. These networks are antagonistic to one another in a relationship referred to as a 'flip—flop' or sleep—wake switch (which enables transitions between them to be rapid and complete). A similar type of circuitry exists between NREM and REM sleep.

Sleep follows a cyclical pattern or a *circadian rhythm* that originates from the **suprachiasmatic nucleus**, the primary biological clock. Its neurons are synchronised by light input from the retina, melatonin from the pineal gland, and environmental signals that all allow it to inform the sleep—wake cycle, set cellular clocks of other CNS nuclei, and synchronise the physiologic systems of tissues and organs (homeostatic input from changing cellular metabolic states) and allostatic activities (feeding and locomotor activity) or behaviour. These rhythms change slowly and, without the rapid transitions of a flip—flop mechanism, transitions from sleep to wake would occur in a slow and undesirable (or unsafe) way.

Wake Promoting or Arousal System (Caudal Midbrain and Rostral Pons). Nuclei that serve to modulate activity of the cerebral cortex include:

- Cholinergic neurons of the *pedunculopontine* and *laterodorsal tegmental nuclei.*
- Monoaminergic neurons of the locus coeruleus (noradrenergic), dorsal and median raphe nuclei (serotonergic), and the tuberomammillary nucleus (histaminergic).

These cholinergic and monoaminergic neurons innervate the thalamus, facilitating transfer of information to the cerebral cortex and influencing two additional areas:

- peptidergic *(orexin/hypocretin)* neurons within the lateral hypothalamus (promotes active wakefulness and the consolidation of both wake and sleep states; degeneration of these neurons results in the condition called *Narcolepsy*, see Chapter 29); and
- cholinergic neurons within the *basal forebrain* (area in front of the hypothalamus and below the striatum; *nucleus basalis of Meynert* and *substantia innominata*) project to the cerebral cortex.

Despite their roles in promoting wakefulness, the destruction of these neurons (separately or in groups) often results in little effect on the total amount of wake or sleep, suggesting a role for other wake—sleep regulatory systems. Those other systems employ glutamate or GABA and their innervation serves not a neuromodulator but a typical neurotransmitter ('fast') role or action.

Arousal neurons are found in the *basal forebrain* (GABAergic) that project to wide areas of the cerebral cortex. The *parabrachial nucleus* (glutaminergic) and *pedunculopontine nucleus* (glutaminergic) respond to specific activating conditions (e.g. noxious stimuli) and project to the hypothalamus and amygdala or become active during specific states (wake or REM sleep). Other neurons within the hypothalamus (glutamatergic or GABAergic) also promote wakefulness directly or inhibit those systems that promote sleep. What these arousal systems have in common is that their activation promotes wakefulness and their destruction results in behavioural unresponsiveness.

Sleep-Inducing System (Hypothalamus and Brainstem)

- *Ventrolateral preoptic nucleus* neurons (producing GABA and galanin, an inhibitory neuropeptide) and *median preoptic nucleus* (GABAergic; believed to respond to homeostatic signals to indicate an accumulated need to sleep) inhibit most of the components of the arousal system and are mainly active during sleep.
- *Parafacial zone* (ventrolateral to the genu of the facial nerve, GABAergic and believed to respond to homeostatic signals or 'indicate' an accumulated need to sleep) inhibits the parabrachial nucleus and therefore inhibits the wake or arousal state.
- *Lateral hypothalamus* (*melanin-concentrating hormone neurons,* GABAergic and glutamatergic) innervates neurons in the brainstem that control REM sleep.

The 'flip–flop' switch for waking and sleep. During sleep, the GABAergic neurons of the sleep-inducing system actively inhibit, via GABAergic input, the wake-promoting neurons. The reverse occurs when this arousal system inhibits these sleep-inducing circuits to maintain the waking state.

REM and NREM Sleep Centres (Pons).

Neurons in the upper pons (*subcoeruleus region*, glutamatergic neurons located ventral to the locus coeruleus) generate REM sleep and constitute the *REM sleep centre*. Different subgroups of these neurons send ascending projections to the hypothalamus and the basal forebrain nuclei (believed to generate the REM EEG pattern and dreaming) and descending projections to the brainstem and spinal cord (responsible for rapid eye movements and loss of muscle tone by suppression of motor activity through inputs to inhibitory spinal interneurons).

The REM sleep centre is normally under GABAergic inhibition from nearby interneurons (rostrally located in the *ventrolateral PAG substance*) that represent an *NREM sleep centre*. The NREM sleep centre receives input from multiple areas and helps to regulate REM sleep. When active, it prevents REM sleep, but when the REM sleep centre is active, the NREM sleep centre is suppressed (flip–flop switch for REM and NREM sleep) and this allows rapid transitions between REM and NREM sleep.

A variety of sleep disorders can be explained by disturbance of these wake–sleep and NREM–REM systems.

Ascending arousal system (ascending reticular activating system or ARAS). Earlier studies proposed the brainstem reticular formation as playing a role in wakefulness and sleep. That anatomic localisation and its observed widespread effect on the brain led to the designation of this arousal network as the *ascending reticular activating system (ARAS)*. With further investigation, the ARAS did not appear to arise from the reticular formation, and the neuromodulatory system (monoaminergic and cholinergic neurons) was discovered to play a significant role so, the preferred term became the *ascending arousal system*, but this model is again undergoing revision. Currently, GABAergic and glutamatergic neurons have a role in promoting arousal and REM sleep, whereas NREM sleep and inhibition of REM sleep incorporates GABAergic neurons that inhibit arousal and REM sleep, and neurons of the neuromodulatory system serve a role in adjusting wake–sleep states to specific conditions.

CLINICAL PANEL 24.1 Congenital Central Hypoventilation Syndrome

The integration of peripheral and central chemoreceptors with brainstem and CNS centres allows the seamless regulation of respiration with other activities (e.g. speaking, swallowing, and sleep–wake cycles) by adjusting the rate and depth of respiration to maintain P_{O2} and P_{CO2} levels within appropriate limits. This balance is disrupted as hypoventilation can occur with pulmonary, cardiac, neurologic, neuromuscular, or metabolic disorders.

Congenital central hypoventilation syndrome (*CCHS*, or *Ondine curse*) occurs in the absence of any of these medical conditions and is a rare disorder of autosomal inheritance that shows variable penetrance. It typically presents in the neonatal period when a newborn presents with central apnoeas (temporary cessation of breathing) and cyanosis resulting in the need for assisted ventilation. This hypoventilation is significantly worse during sleep, particularly NREM sleep, where breathing is dependent on the automatic control of breathing. These infants do not exhibit signs of respiratory distress, despite hypercapnia and hypoxemia from significant hypoventilation. Affected individuals may have associated conditions due to autonomic nervous system dysfunction including tumours of neural crest origin, gastrointestinal manifestations, ophthalmologic and endocrinological regulation abnormalities. The onset of CCHS may occur later, so children or adults can present with unexplained apnoeas or hypoventilation without significant changes in their breathing pattern to both hypercapnia and hypoxemia.

CCHS is caused by a mutation in the PHOX2B gene, located in chromosome 4p12 that plays an essential role in the development of respiratory control neurons and the autonomic nervous system. PHOX2B protein contains polyalanine repeats (9 to 20) and the majority (90%) of CCHS patients are heterozygous for an increased number of these repeats. Those individuals with a smaller number of excess repeats will have milder symptoms, later onset, and may not need ventilatory assistance. Those with more repeats typically present in the newborn period and require full-time ventilatory support.

The PHOX2B mutation affects neurons within the brainstem (i.e. the retrotrapezoid nucleus (RTN) and other brainstem nuclei (Fig. 24.9)) and their ability to integrate both central and peripheral chemoreceptor inputs that mediate sympathetic and parasympathetic control of the respiratory system. Clinical suspicion of CCHS requires confirmation by PHOX2B gene mutation analyses and if abnormal, genetic counselling for those diagnosed and their families. As lung disease is typically minimal, ventilators provide the necessary support to ensure adequate ventilation. Diaphragm pacing represents a recent intervention that uses surgically implanted electrodes to activate the phrenic nerve and cause diaphragm contraction. Rate is controlled through an implanted phrenic nerve pacemaker and allows the individual mobility by separation from an immobile ventilator.

BASIC SCIENCE PANEL 24.1 Higher-Level Urinary Bladder Control

The lower urinary tract comprises two functional systems that act as a coordinated system for storage and elimination of urine. The sacral parasympathetic system at the S2–S4 spinal cord level (reaches the bladder through the pelvic splanchnic nerve) causes contraction of the urinary bladder (detrusor muscle) and relaxes the urethral smooth muscle facilitating micturition, whereas the lumbar sympathetic system (T10–L2 preganglionic neurons synapse in the inferior mesenteric ganglia and those post-ganglionic fibres travel in the hypogastric nerve to reach the bladder) relaxes the detrusor muscle, but contracts the urethral smooth muscle allowing the bladder to fill. Spinal cord neurons at S2–S4 (*Onuf nucleus*) innervate the external urethral

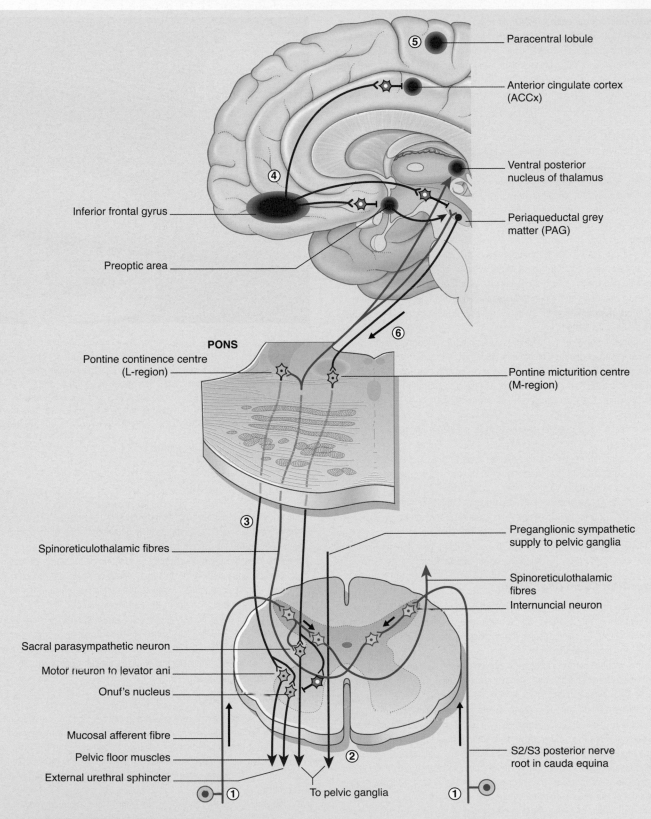

Fig. 24.10 Higher-level bladder controls.

sphincter (through the pudendal nerve), contributing to the function of both autonomic systems; when active, it facilitates storage by contracting the sphincter, and when inhibited, micturition.

Several CNS circuits integrate these systems, but a *voiding reflex*, through a spinobulbospinal neural circuit, results in a switch between storage and micturition. Afferents in the bladder wall, activated as it fills, transmit their signal through the pelvic splanchnic nerve to lumbosacral spinal interneurons circuits, and to a projection into the lateral funiculus that reaches the midbrain *periaqueductal grey (PAG) substance*. As this afferent signal increases, a 'set point' (bladder volume) is reached when PAG activates neurons within the *pontine micturition centre* (*PMC, M-region* or *Barrington nucleus*; this may have a role beyond micturition and be time for a name change, e.g. *pelvic organ stimulating centre*), a paramedian reticular nucleus, with interconnections across the midline. PMC neurons project to micturition-related, parasympathetic preganglionic neurons in segments S2 to S4 of the spinal cord (Fig. 24.10) that initiate micturition by a rise in intravesical pressure (contraction of the smooth muscle of the urinary bladder wall). PMC neurons also project to GABAergic interneurons inhibiting Onuf's nucleus (see Chapter 13) whose projections travel in the pudendal nerve and their inhibition results in relaxation of the *external urethral striated sphincter* facilitating the expulsion of urine. The PMC is responsible for this coordinated reflex activity and receives essentially all its input from PAG, which also plays a role in the storage of urine through the sympathetic nervous system. (Another brainstem nucleus may facilitate storage of urine by increasing contraction of the urethral sphincter; ventral and lateral to the PMC in the reticular formation is the *pontine continence centre* (or *L-region*).)

The voiding reflex is under multiple levels of central nervous system control that ensure micturition occurs when appropriate or socially acceptable and these cortical areas may be lateralised to the right side. This complexity also helps to explain the multiple ways that loss of voluntary control *(incontinence)* can occur by injury, medical disease, or medications that affect the nervous system.

Functional brain imaging (fMRI) is beginning to identify various brain regions involved in bladder control and delineate their pathways (Fig. 24.11). The focal point of influence is PAG that receives afferent information from the bladder, but this sensory information is also transmitted to the thalamus. fMRI suggests the following cortical areas play a role in control of micturition:

- The insular cortex generates conscious sensation of normal bladder filling.
- The medial prefrontal cortex affects decision-making in emotional or social contexts and by inhibiting PAG, it can raise the set point or threshold to initiate a voiding reflex.
- The dorsal anterior cingulate cortex and supplementary motor area generate a sensation of urgency and reinforce the ability to postpone micturition by bladder relaxation and sphincter contraction.
- The parahippocampal area of the temporal lobe, with the inclusion of PAG, allows an unconscious monitoring of bladder filling.

Micturition Cycle (Fig. 24.10)

1. When the bladder is half full, vesical afferents from stretch receptors in the detrusor and in the mucous membrane of the trigone relay this information along spinoreticular fibres reaching the pons (PMC), midbrain (PAG), and insula via the thalamus

   The insular cortex projects to the decision centre in the medial prefrontal cortex and parahippocampal area, keeping them informed about the level of bladder filling.
2. As indicated in Chapter 13, activity in the sympathetic system is stepped up so that bladder compliance can be increased by detrusor muscle ceptors) and urethral and bladder neck smooth muscle contraction (via α_1 adrenergic receptors). Parasympathetic neurons are silenced.
3. Spinoreticular fibres synapsing in the *pontine continence centre (L-centre)* of the pons activate the Onuf nucleus in the sacral cord, thereby raising the tone of the external urethral sphincter.
4. With completion of filling, there is perception of urgency. If time or place is not suitable, part of the medial prefrontal gyrus comes alive. This area puts the *dorsal anterior cingulate cortex (ACCx)* 'on hold' by reducing its

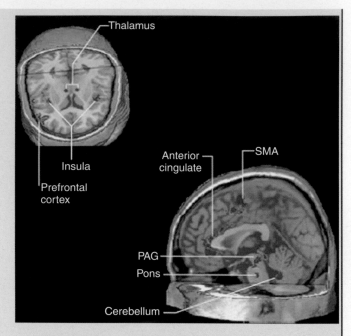

Fig. 24.11 Depiction of areas showing increased functional magnetic resonance imaging (fmri) activity at some time during the storage phase of the micturition cycle. Pons is the assumed pontine micturition control centre. *PAG,* Periaqueductal grey matter; *SMA,* supplementary motor area. (From De Wachter SG, Heeringa R, van Koeveringe GA, Gillespie JI. On the nature of bladder sensation: the concept of sensory modulation. *Neurourol Urodyn.* 2011;30:1220–1226.)

activity via association fibre projections to the local inhibitory interneurons. Likewise, projections to hypothalamus and midbrain inhibit the PAG by activating appropriate interneurons.

5. As a final measure there is voluntary contraction of the entire pelvic floor to further enhance continence, but this cannot be sustained for long. The command for this contraction is sent to the perineal representation on the medial side of the motor cortex in the paracentral lobule.
6. When time and place permit, the medial prefrontal cortex releases its inhibition on the PAG, which switches from storage to micturition by activating the PMC (and inactivating the pontine continence centre via inhibitory interneurons), thus resulting in detrusor muscle contraction and sphincter muscle relaxation.

Role of Monoamines

The motor and sensory spinal cord nuclei serving the bladder are abundantly supplied with serotonergic neurons descending from the MRn in the medulla oblongata. Distension of the bladder is known to stimulate the MRn (via spinoreticular activation of the PAG). A quick review of the lower-level bladder controls (Fig. 13.12) suggests that the MRn sets the general tone in favour of bladder filling.

Noradrenergic fibres descending to the ventral grey horn from the locus coeruleus potentiate the effect of local glutamate release onto Onuf nucleus, thereby enhancing external sphincter tone during the filling phase.

BASIC SCIENCE PANEL 24.2 Locomotor Pattern Generator

During the initiation of a behaviour, and as the brain sends a signal to the motor system, it simultaneously sends an internal neural model or 'copy' of the sensory consequences of that activity to other sensory processing and monitoring areas (e.g. basal ganglia and cerebellum) or a feed-forward prediction of the effects of that behaviour. This *efference copy* is compared to the actual sensory information that will later result from the behaviour *(reafferent)* as well as other environmental sensory information *(afferent)* and any mismatch can be addressed to ensure the desired behaviour is the one that occurs. Efference copies enable the brain to predict the effects of a behaviour, playing a critical role in producing the complicated motor activities mediated through locomotor regions located in the brainstem, and ultimately affect the CPGs.

Locomotor CPGs exist in vertebrates (and other animals) within their spinal cord grey matter and are responsible for the oscillating circuits that deliver rhythmically entrained signals to extremity flexor and extensor muscle groups that enable balance, posture, and locomotion. However, locomotor CPGs are subject to supraspinal commands from a **mesencephalic locomotor region (MLR),** which itself follows directions from motor areas of the cerebral cortex. The MLR is also reciprocally connected to the basal ganglia and cerebellum and with their efference copy will both modulate and integrate sensory information to allow appropriate 'adjustments' to the MLR to effectively implement its intended action. The MLR consists of nuclei of the reticular formation (**pedunculopontine nucleus,** close to the superior cerebellar peduncle where it passes along the upper corner of the fourth ventricle to enter the midbrain (Fig. 17.16) and the *cuneiform nucleus* that lies dorsal to it) and its projections are predominantly sent to the next, and critical, locomotor control centre, the **pontomedullary reticular formation**. This formation is a collection of separate reticular nuclei located in the pons and medulla and is the origin of the *reticulospinal tracts*. Influenced by cortical motor and premotor areas, the cerebellum, vestibular nuclei, and spinoreticular proprioceptive input allows the pontomedullary reticular formation to make the final determinants of muscle tone and postural adjustments that facilitate adaptive posture and locomotion.

Output from the medullary reticular nuclei will form the **lateral reticulospinal tract** and descend bilaterally while the pontine nuclei contribute to the ipsilateral *medial reticulospinal tract.* The reticulospinal tracts descend into the spinal cord, and most fibres will synapse on premotor interneurons influencing the activity of alpha and gamma motoneurons and spinal CPGs, which together generate and modulate locomotion and associated postural support. The CPGs also receive direct somatosensory input from the limbs, allowing further refinement of their activity.

This fundamental CNS organisation that allows ambulation also informs the major focus of spinal cord injury rehabilitation: activation of spinal locomotor reflexes to enable ambulation. Research has investigated how to support regenerating axons both physically and chemically to improve the possibility that supraspinal ambulatory motor fibres will 'bridge the gap' in a cervical or thoracic cord injury. However, other technologies to restore ambulation for those who suffered spinal cord injuries are also under development and one, *epidural electrical stimulation (ESS),* deserves further comment.

A series of electrodes are surgically implanted over the dorsal roots of the cauda equina (which convey proprioceptive information), and when activated by ESS, electrical pulses transmit responses into the spinal cord, activating existing locomotor CPGs and other intrinsic neural circuits. Combined with extensive physical therapy, empirically determining the proper temporal and spatial activation of dorsal roots allows ESS to sequentially activate lower extremity extensor or flexor muscles that result in standing and walking. An unexpected outcome is that after a period, some level of locomotion persists without the need of ESS.

The explanation for this persistence is that despite the severity of a spinal cord injury (SCI) there are often areas of white matter that are spared and contain descending fibres from supraspinal centres, but alone are unable to elicit volitional movements. However, the spatiotemporal sequencing of ESS not only activates proprioceptive dorsal root afferents but promotes extensive reorganisation of these residual descending neural pathways, corticoreticular in origin, and this task-specific sensory information also improves the responsiveness and functionality of intrinsic spinal cord circuits. This secondary reorganisation and neuroplasticity restore some level of locomotion that persists without the need of ESS.

✳ Core Information

Reticular Formation

The reticular formation is phylogenetically a very old neural network that originated as a slowly conducting, polysynaptic pathway intimately connected with olfactory and limbic regions. In the human brain, the reticular formation continues to be of importance in automatic and reflex activities and has retained its linkages to the limbic system.

The reticular formation extends as columns of neurons along the entire length of the brainstem and continues into the intermediate zone of the spinal cord. Within the brainstem, it is divided into two functional zones. A **medial reticular (tegmental) field** consists of large-celled neurons and gives rise to a descending tract (reticulospinal) and participates in the control of posture and coordination of the related head and eye movements. A **lateral reticular (tegmental) field** contains smaller neurons that help to coordinate automatic or limbic functions. These neurons receive specific afferents that help to coordinate the output of brainstem sensory or motor nuclei that are nearby.

The reticular formation can be further divided into about ten subnuclei that are more easily defined by their cytoarchitecture, functionality, and neurochemical characteristic, but are less conspicuous on routine stained sections of the brainstem. Their roles in coordinating brainstem sensory and motor nuclei endows them with a **central pattern generator (CPG)** function. Gaze centres in the midbrain and pons control conjugate eye movements; a midbrain locomotor area regulates walking; a pontine supratrigeminal nucleus regulates chewing rhythm; and a pontine micturition centre controls the bladder. In the medulla oblongata are respiratory, emetic, coughing, and sneezing centres, as well as pressor and depressor centres for cardiovascular control. In addition, the medullary chemosensitive area contains reticular formation neurons sensitive to H^+ ion levels in the CSF.

Neuromodulatory System

The neuromodulatory system is interspersed around the reticular formation and forms discrete nuclei with extensive projections to the CNS. Responsible for facilitating the different states of arousal, attention, sleep, and wakefulness, it is also a major part of the anatomical-physiological correlate of the ascending reticular activating system through effects on the thalamus and cortex.

Neuronal cytoarchitecture of the nuclei in this system displays, specific neurochemical characteristics and, through their extensive projections, unique connectivity with diffuse areas of the brain, brainstem, or spinal cord. Using their specific neurochemical characteristics, they can be classified into several groups. Those neurons that synthesise acetylcholine are located within the basal forebrain and tegmentum of the midbrain and pons and contribute to memory and attention. Monoaminergic neurons are found in nuclei within the midbrain and those that are dopaminergic play a role in motor activity and related behaviour. Serotonergic neurons are in nuclei along the midline of the brainstem *(raphe nuclei)* and through their extensive connections play a role in mood, sleep, and nociception. Norepinephrine neurons are almost exclusively found in the locus coeruleus nucleus located in the tegmentum of the upper pons where they participate in arousal or attention. Epinephrine-secreting neurons of the medulla project to the hypothalamus and spinal cord. Within the tuberomammillary nucleus of the hypothalamus are neurons that synthesise histamine and contribute to wakefulness.

The sleep—wake state requires a complex interplay between the nuclei within the reticular and neuromodulatory systems, as they participate through cyclical activation or reciprocal inhibition of their nuclei. Sleep is an active phenomenon and characterised by the temporary impairment of consciousness.

Supraspinal antinociception occurs through neurons within the brainstem midline *(raphe nuclei)* and specifically at the level of the medulla from the ***magnus raphe nucleus (MRn*** or ***nucleus raphe magnus)***, which is activated by the hypothalamus and midbrain. Efferents from the MRn descend the entire length of the spinal cord, releasing serotonin from their terminals onto the substantia gelatinosa of the spinal dorsal horn (and trigeminal nucleus), and activating enkephalinergic interneurons that inhibit transmission in spinothalamic/trigeminothalamic neurons.

SUGGESTED READINGS

Albrecht U, Ripperger JA. Circadian clocks and sleep: impact of rhythmic metabolism and waste clearance on the brain. *Trends Neurosci.* 2018;41:677—688.

Asboth L, Friedli L, Beauparlant J, et al. Cortico-reticulo-spinal circuit reorganization enables functional recovery after severe spinal cord contusion. *Nat Neurosci.* 2018;21:576—588.

Benarroch EE. Brainstem integration of arousal, sleep, cardiovascular, and respiratory control. *Neurology.* 2018;91:958—966.

Bishara J, Keens TG, Perez I. The genetics of congenital central hypoventilation syndrome: clinical implications. *Appl Clin Genet.* 2018;11:135—144.

Dampney R. Emotion and the cardiovascular system: postulated role of inputs from the medial prefrontal cortex to the dorsolateral periaqueductal gray. *Front Neurosci.* 2018;12:343.

Del Negro CA, Funk GD, Feldman JL. Breathing matters. *Nat Rev Neurosci.* 2018;19:351—367.

Duan B, Cheng L, Ma Q. Spinal circuits transmitting mechanical pin and itch. *Neurosci Bull.* 2018;34:186—193.

Ferreira-Pinto MJ, Ruder L, Capelli P, Arber S. Connecting circuits for supraspinal control of locomotion. *Neuron.* 2018;100: 361—374.

Griffiths D. Functional imaging of structures involved in neural control of the lower urinary tract. In: Vodušek BD, Boller F, eds. *Neurology of Sexual and Bladder Disorders. Handbook of Clinical Neurology.* Vol 130. 3rd series. Philadelphia, PA: Elsevier; 2015: 121—133.

Groh A, Krieger P, Mease RA, Henderson L. Acute and chronic pain processing in the thalamocortical system of humans and animal models. *Neuroscience.* 2018;387:58—71.

Holst SC, Landolt HP. Sleep-wake chemistry. *Sleep Med Clin.* 2018;13: 137—146.

Joiner WJ. The neurobiological basis of sleep and sleep disorders. *Physiology.* 2018;33:317—327.

Keller JA, Chen J, Simpson S, et al. Voluntary urination control by brainstem neurons that relax the urethral sphincter. *Nat Neurosci.* 2018;21:1229—1238.

MacKinnon CD. Sensorimotor anatomy of gait, balance, and falls. In: Day BL, Lord SR, eds. *Balance, Gait and Falls. Handbook of Clinical Neurology.* Vol 159. 3rd series. Philadelphia, PA: Elsevier; 2018:3—26.

Mena-Segovia J, Bolam JP. Rethinking the pedunculopontine nucleus: from cellular organization to function. *Neuron.* 2017;94: 7—18.

Miyazato M, Kadekawa K, Kitta T, et al. New frontiers of basic science research in neurogenic lower urinary tract dysfunction. *Urol Clin N Am.* 2017;44:491—505.

Paxinos G, Furlong T, Watson C. *Human Brainstem: Cytoarchitecture, Chemoarchitecture, Myeloarchitecture.* New York, NY: Academic Press; 2019.

Straka H, Simmers J, Chagnaud BP. A new perspective on predictive motor signaling. *Curr Biol.* 2018;28:R232—R243.

Wagner FB, Mignardot JB, Le Goff-Mignardot CG, et al. Targeted neurotechnology restores walking in humans with spinal cord injury. *Nature.* 2018;563:65—71.

Thalamus, Epithalamus

CHAPTER SUMMARY

STUDY GUIDELINES

1. Describe the characteristics of the thalamic nuclei within the relay, association, and 'non-specific' nuclei groups.
2. List the afferent and efferent projections for the following relay nuclei: anterior, ventral lateral, ventral posterior, medial, and lateral geniculate bodies.
3. List the afferent and efferent projections for the dorsomedial nucleus.
4. Describe how the thalamic reticular nucleus differs from the other thalamic nuclei.
5. Discuss the thalamocortical and corticothalamic projections that pass through the thalamic peduncles.

THALAMUS

The thalamus is a prominent feature in *magnetic resonance imaging (MRI)* scans in each of the three planes in which views are taken. The primary afferent and efferent connections of the main nuclear groups are listed in Table 25.1. The connections are diverse but in general serve to provide sensorimotor integration through conscious perception of sensation (either external or internal to the body) to guide the motor system and facilitate corticocortical communication for higher cortical functions.

As noted in Chapter 2, the two thalami lie at the centre of the brain. Their medial surfaces may be 'linked' (*massa intermedia* or *interthalamic adhesion*) across the third ventricle, and their lateral surfaces are in contact with the posterior limb of the internal capsule. The upper surface of each occupies the floor of a lateral ventricle. The inferior aspect receives sensory, cerebellar, and basal ganglia inputs as well as an upward continuum of the reticular formation and neuromodulatory system.

Thalamic Nuclei

All thalamic nuclei except one (*reticular nucleus*) have reciprocal excitatory connections with the cerebral cortex. The Y-shaped **internal medullary lamina** of white matter divides the thalamus into three large cell groups: anterior, medial dorsal (MD), and lateral nuclear groups (Fig. 25.1). The lateral group consists of dorsal and ventral nuclear tiers. At the back of the thalamus are the **medial** and **lateral geniculate bodies**. The *external medullary lamina* separates the thalamus from the shell-like **reticular nucleus**. The thalamic nuclei are categorised into three functional groups: *relay (specific) nuclei, association nuclei,* and *'non-specific' nuclei.*

Within each thalamic nucleus, most neurons are glutamatergic excitatory projection neurons (e.g. thalamocortical, thalamostriatal) and the remainder are inhibitory GABAergic interneurons. The projection neurons are further organised into *core* (driver) and *matrix* (modulatory) cells, but the number of each cell type again differs among the nuclei. Core cells receive modality-specific inputs and project in a topographically organised manner; those projecting to the cerebral cortex predominantly transmit to layer 4. Matrix cells receive less precise inputs, project more diffusely, and those projecting to the cerebral cortex predominantly transmit to layer 1 and have the potential to synchronise activity across broad areas of the cortex.

Input to the thalamic nuclei is predominantly glutaminergic and excitatory and can be divided into two main types. Some are specific (driver) and represented by the medial lemniscus input to the ventral posterior lateral (VPL) or cortical (layer 5) for the medial dorsal (MD). However, the majority is regulatory (modulatory) and serves as a feedback system.

The result of this excitatory and inhibitory input on thalamic projection neurons causes them to assume two different states and firing patterns. **Tonic firing** is the 'typical' state of neurons where firing frequency reflects input and the magnitude of that input. The other state is **burst firing** where activation of a thalamic neuron produces a burst of action potentials followed by a period of inactivation. Discreteness of response does not occur, but a burst firing pattern functions as an 'alerting' response to a novel or unexpected stimulus or event.

Relay Nuclei. Table 25.1 and Fig. 25.1 provide details for each of these nuclei and define the reciprocal connection to their corresponding area of cerebral cortex.

TABLE 25.1   Thalamic Nuclei and Their Connections.

Functional Group	Nucleus	Afferents	Efferents
Relay nuclei	Anterior	Mammillothalamic tract, cingulate cortex, hippocampus	Prefrontal and cingulate cortex
	Ventral anterior (VA)	Substantia nigra (pars reticulata)/Globus pallidus internum (GPi)	Prefrontal cortex, frontal eye field
	Ventral lateral (VL), anterior part	Globus pallidus (internal segment)	Supplementary motor area
	Ventral lateral (VL), posterior part	Deep cerebellar nuclei	Motor and premotor association cortex
	Ventral posterolateral (VPL)	Medial lemniscus and spinothalamic tract (body)	SI and SII somatosensory cortex
	Ventral posteromedial (VPM)	Medial lemniscus and spinothalamic tract (head)	SI, SII, and parietal association cortex Brodmann areas 5 and 7
	Medial geniculate	Inferior colliculus	Primary auditory cortex
	Lateral geniculate	Optic tract	Primary visual cortex
Association nuclei	Lateral dorsal (LD)	Pretectum, cingulate cortex, hippocampus	Cingulate cortex
	Mediodorsal (MD)	Prefrontal cortex (olfactory), amygdala, striatum, superior colliculus	Prefrontal and cingulate cortex, frontal eye fields
	Lateral posterior (LP)/ Pulvinar complex	Superior colliculus, primary visual cortex, somatosensory cortex, auditory cortex, cingulate cortex, prefrontal (motor related), amygdala	Posterior parietal, temporal and visual association cortex; somatosensory cortex, cingulate and prefrontal (motor related) cortex; amygdala
'Non-specific' nuclei	Intralaminar (centromedian, parafascicular and others)	Reticular formation, neuromodulatory system, spinothalamic tract, basal ganglia, cerebellum, cingulate cortex	Corpus striatum, cerebral cortex
	Midline nuclei	Reticular formation, neuromodulatory system, amygdala	Cingulate cortex, hippocampus, corpus striatum
Reticular	Reticular	Thalamic nuclei, reticular formation, cortex	Thalamic nuclei

The ***anterior nucleus*** is involved in cognition (memory), emotion, and executive (behavioural) control and is a component of the Papez circuit (see Chapter 33).

The ***ventral posterior nucleus (VP)*** (Fig. 25.2) receives fibres of the medial, spinal, and trigeminal lemnisci. It projects to the somatosensory cortex (SI), and a smaller projection is sent to the second somatic sensory area (SII) at the foot of the postcentral gyrus. The VP is somatotopically organised (Fig. 25.3). The portion of the nucleus devoted to the face and head is called the ***ventral posteromedial nucleus (VPM)*** and that for the trunk and limbs is called the ***ventral posterolateral nucleus (VPL)***.

Modality segregation is a feature of both VP nuclei, with proprioceptive neurons most anterior and tactile neurons posterior. Most spinothalamic nociceptive input does not project to the VP nucleus, but further posteriorly to other nuclei (*ventromedial posterior, ventral posterior inferior nucleus,* and *anterior nucleus of the thalamus*). In addition, there is no evidence in the VP of an antinociceptive mechanism comparable to that found in the substantia gelatinosa region of the spinal cord and spinal trigeminal nucleus. However, an unexplained disorder, the *thalamic pain syndrome*, may follow a vascular lesion that interferes with the spinothalamic system and these other posterior thalamic nuclei. In this condition, a period of complete sensory loss may occur on the contralateral side of the body and later bouts of severe pain occurring either spontaneously or in response to tactile stimuli. (See also Chapter 35, *central post-stroke pain.*)

The ***medial geniculate nucleus*** is the thalamic nucleus of the auditory pathway. It receives the inferior brachium from the inferior colliculus (which carries auditory signals from both ears, see Chapter 20), and it projects to the primary auditory cortex in the superior temporal gyrus.

The ***lateral geniculate nucleus*** is the principal thalamic nucleus for vision. It receives retinal inputs from both eyes via the optic tract, and it projects to the primary visual cortex in the occipital lobe. The visual pathways are described in Chapter 31.

Association Nuclei. The association nuclei are reciprocally connected to association areas of the cerebral cortex and subcortical areas. These nuclei play a critical role in regulating the 'connectivity' between different cortical (and other) areas that is based on behavioural goals. Goal-directed control needs to be rapid and occurs both through selectivity in transmission of information to cortical areas, modifying the activity within those areas and the connectivity between different cortical areas or networks.

The roles of these nuclei include:

• ***Lateral dorsal nucleus*** has a role similar to the anterior nucleus. (see Chapter 33).

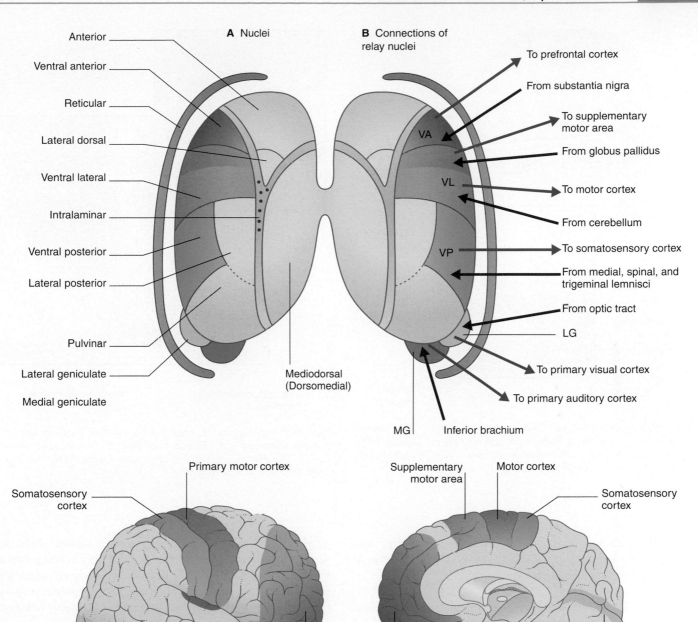

Fig. 25.1 (A) Thalamic nuclei viewed from above. (B) Connections of the relay nuclei. (C) Lateral and (D) medial surface of the hemisphere showing cortical areas receiving projections from the relay nuclei. *LG,* Lateral geniculate nucleus; *MG,* medial geniculate nucleus; *VA,* ventral anterior nucleus; *VL,* ventral lateral nucleus; *VP,* ventral posterior nucleus.

- **Mediodorsal nucleus** (or dorsomedial) function includes cognition (memory), direction and shifting of attention, mood (emotional processing), and olfaction.
- **Lateral posterior nucleus** and **pulvinar** belong to a single nuclear complex. An 'extrageniculate visual pathway' that functions to draw attention to objects of interest in the peripheral field of vision and limits distraction to play a critical role in spatial attention.

'Non-specific' Nuclei. While the name is a misnomer, these nuclei play the following roles:
- **Intralaminar nuclei** are contained within the internal medullary lamina of white matter. Through their input and projections, they play critical roles in arousal, cognitive function, regulation of the basal ganglia, and cortical synchronisation.

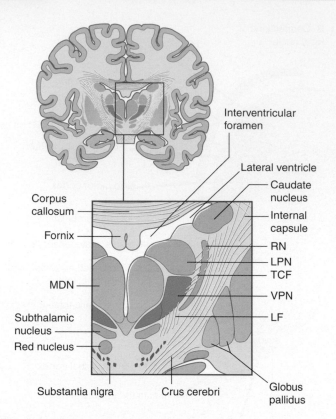

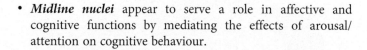

Fig. 25.2 Coronal Section Through the Thalamus and Related Structures. *LF,* Lemniscal fibres; *LPN,* lateral posterior nucleus; *MDN,* mediodorsal nucleus; *RN,* reticular nucleus; *TCF,* thalamocortical fibres; *VPN,* ventral posterior nucleus.

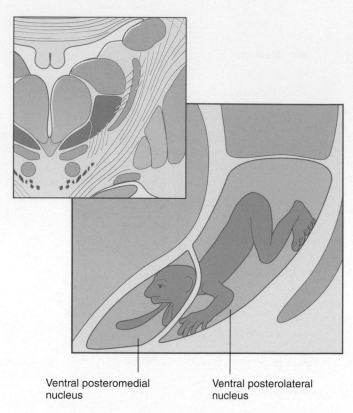

Fig. 25.3 Somatosensory map in the ventral posterior thalamic nucleus. (Redrawn and modified from Ohye C. Thalamus. In: Paxinos G, ed. *The Human Nervous System.* San Diego: Academic Press; 1990;439–468, with permission.)

- *Midline nuclei* appear to serve a role in affective and cognitive functions by mediating the effects of arousal/attention on cognitive behaviour.

Thalamic Reticular Nucleus. The thalamic reticular nucleus (TRN) is shaped like a shield around the front and lateral side of the thalamus and separated from the main thalamus by the *external medullary lamina.* All thalamocortical and corticothalamic projections pass through the TRN and provide collateral excitatory branches to it (Fig. 25.4); the TRN projects back to the corresponding thalamic nuclei, and controls (modulates) the rate of discharge of those thalamic projection neurons by their inhibition. The TRN is exclusively made up of inhibitory GABAergic neurons.

The specificity of modulation reflects the topographical organisation of the TRN with respect to relay nuclei (a distinct sector of the TRN projects to a specific portion of the nucleus), but a more diffuse projection for the other thalamic nuclei. Other inputs to the TRN (e.g. reticular formation, brainstem nuclei) are typically diffuse.

An organisational outcome of the TRN results in both specificity and generalisability of activation that allows functional diversity as groups (networks) of TRN neurons which are differentially modulated or engaged, based on sensory, motor, or cognitive circumstances. A novel auditory, visual, or tactile experience can be isolated (*saliency*) from the normal background 'noise' of cortical

activity in the awake state. This process is known as 'centre-surround' and occurs when feedback from the cerebral cortex or other input decreases TRN activity of a stimulated patch of the sensory nucleus (the centre), and simultaneously suppresses ongoing, random activity in the surrounding neurons not directly involved.

Oscillation

A histologic feature of TRN neurons is the possibility of electrical coupling of those neurons and their synchronisation of thalamocortical activity. This arrangement may form the anatomic basis of the phenomenon of *oscillation* if thalamic neurons change from tonic to a burst firing state at a rate of 5 to 15 Hz, usually for a few seconds at a time. These oscillations can produce bursts of cortical activity known as *sleep spindles,* so called because they are detectable by means of electroencephalography at specific stages of sleep. Sleep—wake cycles are further described in Chapter 29.

Thalamic Peduncles

The reciprocal connections between the thalamus and the cerebral cortex travel in four thalamic peduncles (Fig. 25.5). The **anterior thalamic peduncle** passes through the anterior limb of the internal capsule to reach the prefrontal cortex and cingulate gyrus. The **superior thalamic peduncle** passes through the posterior limb of the internal capsule to reach the premotor, motor, and somatosensory cortex. The **posterior thalamic peduncle** passes through the

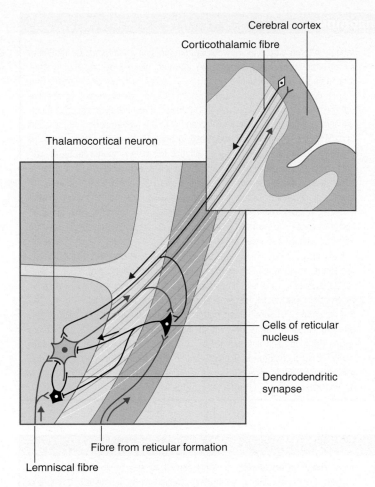

Fig. 25.4 Basic synaptic relationships of the thalamic reticular nucleus. (Modified from Pinault D. The thalamic reticular nucleus: structure, function and concept. *Brain Res Rev.* 2004;46:1–31.)

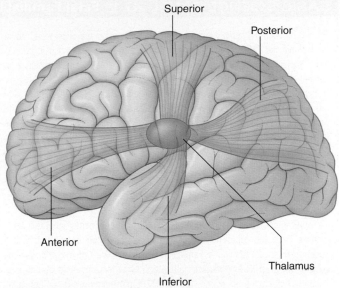

Fig. 25.5 The thalamic peduncles (left hemisphere).

posterior limb of the internal capsule to reach the occipital lobe and the posterior parts of the parietal and temporal lobes. The **inferior thalamic peduncle** passes below the lentiform nucleus to reach the anterior temporal and orbital cortex. Each of the four peduncles are incorporated into the corona radiata.

EPITHALAMUS

The epithalamus includes the pineal gland (considered in Chapter 34) and the habenula and stria medullaris, which are included with the limbic system in Chapter 33.

CLINICAL PANEL 25.1 **Thalamic Territory Strokes**

Blood supply to the thalamus typically arises from small perforating branches of the posterior cerebral artery and posterior communicating artery (Fig. 4.1). Vessel occlusion causes thalamic infarction and is encountered in approximately 11% of strokes within the vertebrobasilar system, based on large stroke registries.

Divided into four groups that reflect arterial territories, specific groupings of nuclei are affected that result in different clinical features that can mimic those associated with strokes involving the cerebral cortex and exemplify the prominent role of the thalamus in cortical function.

These four groups include:

• Anterior territory — *tuberothalamic arteries* that arise from the posterior communicating artery supply the anterior nucleus, ventral anterior, and part of the ventral lateral (12% of thalamic strokes). Infarction results in cognitive (anterograde amnesia, perhaps in part secondary to disruption of the mammillothalamic tract and superimposition of unrelated information when speaking) and behavioural changes (apathy and perseveration or repeating the same comment or action) and impaired visuospatial processing.

• Paramedian territory — *thalamoperforating arteries* that arise from the posterior cerebral artery (P1 segment or the portion between the top of the

basilar artery and the origin of the posterior communicating artery) supply the intralaminar group and most of the dorsomedial nucleus (35% of thalamic strokes). After infarction there can be a period of loss of consciousness or somnolence that with resolution is followed by behavioural (disinhibited behaviour or speech, apathy, or motivation) and cognitive impairment (amnesia, confusion, aphasia) accompanied by vertical gaze impairment.

• Inferolateral territory — *thalamogeniculate arteries* whose origin is the posterior cerebral artery (P2 segment or the portion after the posterior communicating artery) provide circulation to the ventral lateral nuclear groups (45% of thalamic strokes). Infarction results in some degree of *hypoesthesia* (diminished sensory loss, but possible sparing of proprioception) and ataxia accompanied by difficulties with planning, initiating, and regulating goals and behaviour (*executive functions*).

• Posterior territory — *posterior choroidal artery* that originates from the P2 segment supplies the lateral geniculate and the pulvinar (8% of thalamic strokes). After infarction there can be hypoesthesia, visual field deficit (because of involvement of the lateral geniculate and producing a contralateral *homonymous horizontal sectoranopia*), and deficits in attentional processes related to visual stimuli.

BASIC SCIENCE PANEL 25.1   Fatal Familial Insomnia

Prion proteins (PrP^c or PrP) are a normal cellular membrane constituent, abundant within the CNS (pre- and postsynaptic localisation), but whose function is not completely understood. Consisting of 253 amino acids and a structure of several flexible alpha helices, it can be easily degraded by cellular proteases. Structural alterations in PrP^c cause abnormal folding that result in their assuming a transmissible pathogenic role, referred to as 'prions,' that are resistant to proteases. They accumulate within and destroy neurons. These prions can also induce a conformational change within normal cellular PrP, converting them into a 'similar' pathogenic agent without requiring nucleic acid, and these abnormal prion proteins multiply, a process referred to as the *Prion theory*. Prion diseases are described in humans and animals and remain unique as an infectious disorder since they do not require nucleic acids and exist in hereditary, sporadic, and infectious forms.

Fatal familial insomnia (FFI) is a rare, autosomal dominantly inherited, prion disease (sporadic cases can occur but are rare). A point mutation within codon 178 (substitution of asparagine for aspartic acid) of the *prion protein gene (PRNP)* results in a mutated allele and when accompanied by the presence of methionine at codon 129 (met129) polymorphic site in the same allele, causes FFI. This leads to the accumulation of this abnormal prion protein *(FI-PrP129)* within neurons and its metabolism by proteases is disrupted.

FFI case-based descriptions provide an age of onset that extends from the third to eighth decade, but with an average age of 51. Initial symptoms lack specificity but include lack of concentration and insomnia resistant to accepted modalities of treatment and despite increasing symptoms of fatigue. Altered autonomic nervous system function *(dysautonomia)* manifests as elevated heart rate *(tachycardia)*, elevated blood pressure, temperature regulation *(hyperthermia)*, and weight loss. Motor manifestations appear that reflect dysfunction of the basal ganglia *(tremor, bradykinesia)*, cerebellum *(ataxia)*, and pyramidal tract (increased reflexes). Relentlessly progressive memory and language impairment develop and with the progression of motor manifestations the individual is soon bed bound. On average, from onset of symptoms, death occurs within one year, and this time is shorter for those who have two alleles homozygous for the met129 polymorphism. Pathological changes are most marked within the thalamus (mediodorsal and anterior nucleus predominantly) where neuron loss and astrocyte proliferation are found. Similar changes occur within the hippocampus and temporal and cingulate cerebral cortex. To variable degrees, this abnormal prion protein can be detected within these same areas.

Early diagnosis of FFI is hindered by its rarity and non-specificity of early symptoms, so initial clinical suspicion of FFI occurs when there is rapid clinical deterioration, constellation of symptoms and findings, and lack of another explanation. Diagnostic testing includes electroencephalography (to identify the disruption of normal sleep patterns) and neuroimaging (e.g. MRI of the brain to detect abnormalities within the thalami). There are no biomarkers within the blood and unlike other prion disorders, cerebrospinal fluid examination is not as helpful. Molecular genetic testing can identify this abnormal variant in the PRPN gene but is not yet widely available. There are currently no treatment protocols for affected individuals.

✳ Core Information

Thalamus

The thalamus is the largest component of the diencephalon, and the largest nuclear mass in the entire nervous system. The two thalami lie at the centre of the brain. Their medial surfaces contribute to the walls of the third ventricle and are often 'linked' across the third ventricle. Their lateral surfaces are in contact with the posterior limb of the internal capsule. The upper surface of each occupies the floor of a lateral ventricle. The ependyma lining the ventricular surface of the two thalami stretches across its superior part to form the roof of the third ventricle. The tela choroidea (vascular pia mater opposed to the ependymal lining and giving rise to the choroid plexus) lies exterior to the ependyma in this region.

Thalamic nuclei are identified by their cytoarchitecture and myeloarchitecture. An internal medullary lamina (band of white matter) subdivides the thalamus anatomically into an anterior, dorsomedial and lateral nuclear groups, the lateral being separable into a dorsal and a ventral tier. Except for olfaction, each sensory system projects to the thalamus, but it is not just a passive relay station, as local processing occurs within its nuclei and its activity is modulated by inputs from the brainstem and feedback from the *reticular nucleus* of the thalamus and from the cortex.

Each thalamic nucleus has a reciprocal connection to a specific area of the cerebral cortex and the pattern of input and output defines three functional groups. **Relay nuclei** receive specific sensory and motor inputs and project to specific sensorimotor areas of the cerebral cortex or serve as a first-order relay. **Association nuclei** are aptly named as they receive and project to cortical association areas, facilitating 'communication' between them, and serve as a higher order relay capable of shifting functional cortical connectivity that allows focusing on one aspect of the environment while decreasing another. The last group is classified by the location of its nuclei, **intralaminar** and **midline**; each nucleus receives specific inputs that arise from the reticular formation, cortex, striatum, cerebellum, and spinothalamic pathway, and project to the striatum and cerebral cortex. This group was once considered 'nonspecific' but plays a role in modulating and synchronising cortical arousal, motor function, cognition, and responsiveness to sensory stimuli. The one exception to this organisational grouping is the **thalamic reticular nucleus** which receives input from the reticular formation (all thalamic nuclei may also be influenced by the neuromodulatory system), other thalamic nuclei, and the cerebral cortex, but only projects to those thalamic nuclei from which it received input.

Epithalamus

The epithalamus lies posterior to the thalamus and forms the posterior part of the roof of the third ventricle. It includes the *pineal gland* (which secretes melatonin and plays a role in the circadian cycle), *habenula* (which receives afferents from the forebrain and projects to midbrain reticular nuclei) and the *stria terminalis* (which contains afferents that originate in the amygdala and project to the hypothalamus).

SUGGESTED READINGS

Benarroch EE. Pulvinar: associative role in cortical function and clinical correlations. *Neurology*. 2015;84:738–747.

Carrera E, Bogousslavsky J. The thalamus and behavior: effects of anatomically distinct strokes. *Neurology*. 2006;66:1817–1823.

Crabtree JW. Functional diversity of thalamic reticular subnetworks. *Front Syst Neurosci*. 2018;12:41.

Danet L, Barbeau EJ, Eustache M, et al. Thalamic amnesia after infarct: the role of the mammillothalamic tract and mediodorsal nucleus. *Neurology*. 2015;85:2107–2115.

Golden EC, Graff-Radford J, Jones DT, Benarroch EE. Mediodorsal nucleus and its multiple cognitive functions. *Neurology*. 2016;87: 2161–2168.

Halassa MM, Kastner S. Thalamic functions in distributed cognitive control. *Nat Neurosci*. 2015;20:1669–1679.

Hintzen A, Pelzer EA, Tittgemeyer M. Thalamic interactions of cerebellum and basal ganglia. *Brain Struct Func*. 2018;223: 569–687.

Llorens F, Zarranz JJ, Fischer A, et al. Fatal familial insomnia: clinical aspects and molecular alterations. *Curr Neurol Neurosci Rep*. 2017;17:30.

Moustafa AA, McMullan RD, Roston B, et al. The thalamus as a relay station and gatekeeper: relevance to brain disorders. *Rev Neurosci*. 2017;28:203–218.

Nakajima M, Halassa MM. Thalamic control of functional cortical connectivity. *Curr Opin Neurobiol*. 2017;44:127–131.

Noseda R, Borsook D, Burstein R. Neuropeptides and neurotransmitters that modulate thalamo-cortical pathways relevant to migraine headache. *Headache*. 2017;57:97–111.

Patel N, Jankovic J, Hallet M. Sensory aspects of movement disorders. *Lancet Neurol*. 2014;13:100–112.

Powell R, Hughes T. A chamber of secrets: the neurology of the thalamus: lessons from acute stroke. *Pract Neurol*. 2014;14:440–445.

Sherman SM. Functioning of circuits connecting thalamus and cortex. *Compr Physiol*. 2017;7:713–739.

Vartiainen N, Perchet C, Magnin M, et al. Thalamic pain: anatomical and physiological indices of prediction. *Brain*. 2016;139:708–722.

Basal Ganglia

STUDY GUIDELINES

1. Identify basal ganglia nuclei in brain sections.
2. List the four different basal ganglia circuits (or loops) and describe their function.
3. Summarise the major neurotransmitters involved in the basal ganglia circuits and their function (excitatory or inhibitory): cortical input, globus pallidus, striatum, substantia nigra, subthalamic nucleus, and thalamus.
4. Draw the direct and indirect basal ganglia pathways and predict the outcome of dysfunction of each.
5. Explain the origin of the clinical features of Parkinson disease with respect to its known pathogenesis: bradykinesia, rigidity, postural instability, and tremor.
6. Contrast the clinical features of Huntington chorea, hemiballism, and cerebral palsy with potential sites of basal ganglia dysfunction.

OVERVIEW

The term **basal ganglia** designates the areas of the basal forebrain and midbrain known to be involved in the control of movement and motor learning (Fig. 26.1). The basal ganglia comprise the following:

- The **striatum** (caudate nucleus, putamen, and nucleus accumbens; the nucleus accumbens and the olfactory tubercle are known as the *ventral striatum*)
- The **globus pallidus**, which is comprised of an **external (lateral) segment** (GPe) and an **internal (medial) segment** (GPi); together they are known as the *dorsal pallidum*. The internal segment extends into the midbrain as the **pars reticulata** (or reticular part) of the **substantia nigra (SNpr)**.

    Anteriorly and inferiorly at the level of the anterior commissure the lentiform nucleus is indented by the commissure, and that portion of the globus pallidus below the commissure is called the *ventral pallidum*.
- The **subthalamic nucleus (STN)**
- The pigmented **pars compacta** (or compact part) of the substantia nigra (SNc)
- The putamen and pallidum together are also called the **lentiform nucleus**.

Most neurons (90%) within the striatum are GABAergic inhibitory projection neurons *(medium-sized spiny neurons)* that form two functional subgroups expressing different receptors. One subgroup projects to the GPi and the SNpr; this constitutes what is called the **direct pathway** that promotes activity ('go'). The other subgroup projects to the GPe, which then projects to the STN; this is the **indirect pathway** that elicits inhibition ('no go').

Both groups of projection neurons receive excitatory glutaminergic cortical inputs as well as modulatory dopaminergic inputs from the SNc. While different receptors exist on striatal projection neurons, dopaminergic receptors appear 'unique' and receive their input from nigrostriatal (SNc) afferents. Dopamine receptors on direct pathway projection neurons are referred to as D_1-type and neurons of the indirect pathway are called D_2-type; however, dopaminergic input is excitatory for D_1 neurons, promoting the direct pathway, and inhibitory for the D_2 neurons of the indirect pathway.

The striatum can be subdivided into multiple topographic areas that receive their input from different cortical areas and project to different thalamic nuclei or SNc and functional areas called the **matrix** and **striosome**. The striatal neurons of the direct and indirect pathways are within the matrix and receive input from the cortex, thalamus, and portions of the SNc. Those neurons within the striosome receive their input from the limbic cortex, amygdala, and different areas of the SNc, and a mechanism by which the basal ganglia influence and are influenced by the limbic system.

The GPi and SNpr represent the output nuclei of the basal ganglia; these are tonically active inhibitory GABAergic neurons that project to the thalamus and brainstem nuclei, and whose activity is modified by the direct and indirect pathway (Fig. 26.2). (There is one other projection from the cerebral cortex directly to the subthalamic nucleus, the **hyperdirect pathway**, which allows the cerebral cortex to 'bypass' the striatum and directly activate this nucleus to inhibit motor activity.) While shown as separate pathways, the direct and indirect pathways' main role is to reinforce a chosen motor act, inhibit

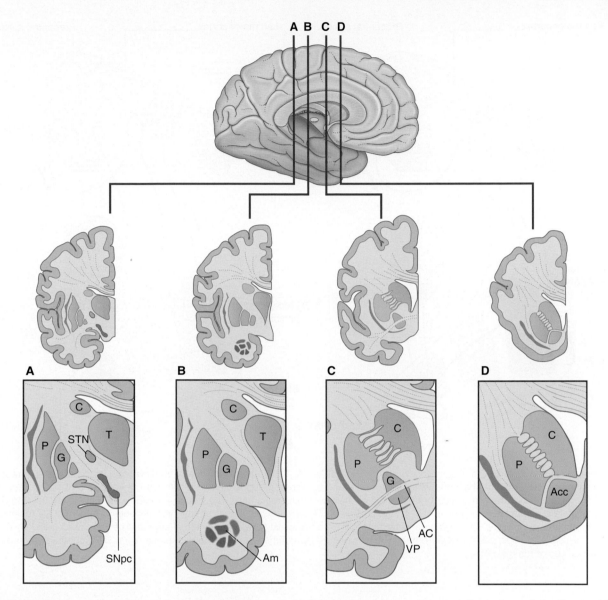

Fig. 26.1 (A–D) Four coronal sections of the brain, viewed from behind. Ventral parts are enlarged at the bottom of the figure. *AC,* Anterior commissure; *Acc,* nucleus accumbens; *Am,* amygdala; *C,* caudate nucleus; *G,* globus pallidus; *P,* putamen; *SNpc,* substantia nigra pars compacta; *STN,* subthalamic nucleus; *T,* thalamus; *VP,* ventral pallidum.

those that are unchosen and thereby ensure the activation of the specific motor program that is required.

The remaining striatal neurons (10%) are interneurons. Most use acetylcholine as their neurotransmitter *(giant aspiny cholinergic interneurons)* and the remainder are GABAergic. These interneurons have a direct modulating effect on both subgroups of striatal projection neurons through their presynaptic effects on glutamate release from corticostriatal pathways and dopamine release from nigrostriatal terminals. Some of these interneurons receive dopaminergic input from the SNc, while others modulate the activity of striatal interneurons.

BASIC CIRCUITS

It is possible to demonstrate at least four circuits that predominantly begin in the cerebral cortex, traverse the basal ganglia, and return to the cortex:

1. A *motor loop,* concerned with voluntary and learned movements.
2. A *cognitive loop,* concerned with planning and motor intentions.
3. A *limbic loop,* concerned with emotional aspects of movement.
4. An *oculomotor loop,* concerned with voluntary eye movements, *saccades.*

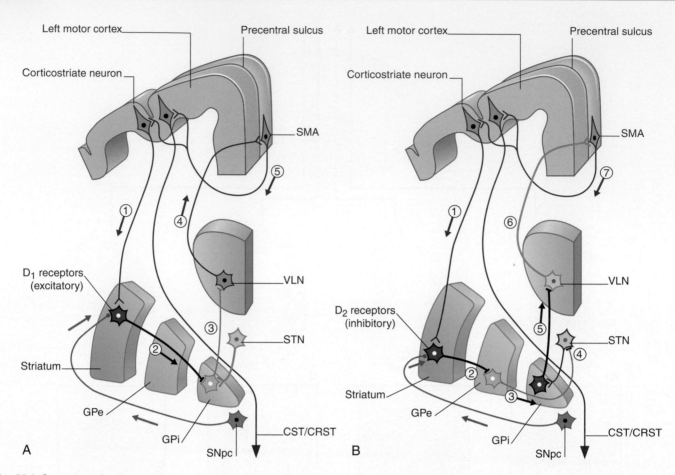

Fig. 26.2 Coronal section through the motor loop, based on Fig. 26.1A. (A) The sequence of five sets of neurons involved in the 'direct' pathway from the sensorimotor cortex to the thalamus with final return to the sensorimotor cortex via the SMA. (B) The sequence of seven sets of neurons involved in the 'indirect' pathway. The *red/pink* neurons are excitatory utilising glutamate. The *black/grey* neurons are inhibitory utilising GABA. The *brown*, nigrostriatal neuron utilises dopamine, which is excitatory via D_1 receptors on target striatal neurons and inhibitory via D_2 receptors on the same and other striatal neurons. *CRST*, Corticoreticular fibre; *CST*, corticospinal fibre; *GPe*, external segment of the globus pallidus; *GPi*, internal segment of the globus pallidus; *SMA*, supplementary motor area; *SNpc*, compact part of the substantia nigra; *STN*, subthalamic nucleus; *VLN*, ventral lateral nucleus of the thalamus.

Motor Loop

The motor loop commences in the sensorimotor cortex and returns there via the striatum (predominantly the putamen), thalamus, and the supplementary motor area (SMA).

Fig. 26.2 is a schematic wiring diagram depicting the component parts of this motor loop. Two pathways are known. The **direct pathway** involves five consecutive sets of neurons (see Fig. 26.2A). The **indirect pathway** adds the STN to the circuitry and involves seven sets of neurons (see Fig. 26.2B). Two pathways comprise the output from the GPi (***ansa lenticularis*** and ***lenticular fasciculus***) and project to the thalamus, as shown in Fig. 26.3.

All projections from the cerebral cortex arise from pyramidal cells and are excitatory (glutaminergic). So too is the projection from the thalamus to the SMA. Those from the striatum and from both segments of the *globus pallidus* (GPi, GPe, and the ventral pallidum) arise from medium-sized spiny neurons and are inhibitory. They are GABAergic and also contain neuropeptides of an uncertain role.

The **nigrostrial pathway** projects from the SNc to the striatum, where it forms two types of synapses upon those projection neurons (see Fig. 26.2): those synapsing upon direct pathway neurons are facilitatory, by way of *dopaminergic type 1 (D_1)* receptors on their dendritic spines; and those synapsing upon indirect pathway neurons are inhibitory, by way of *dopaminergic type 2 (D_2) receptors*. Cholinergic interneurons within the striatum are excitatory to projection neurons and are inhibited by dopamine.

A healthy substantia nigra is tonically active, favouring activity in the direct pathway. Facilitation of this pathway is necessary for the SMA to become active before and during movement. SMA activity immediately prior to movement can be detected by means of recording electrodes attached to the scalp. This activity is known as the (electrical) *readiness potential*, and its manner of production is described in the caption to Fig. 26.4. Impulses pass from the SMA to the motor cortex, where a cerebello–thalamo–cortical projection selectively enhances pyramidal and corticoreticular neurons within milliseconds prior to discharge.

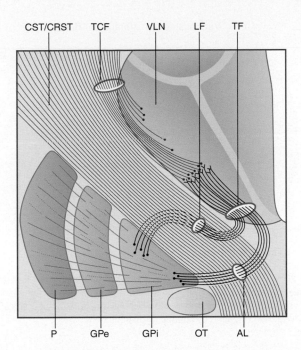

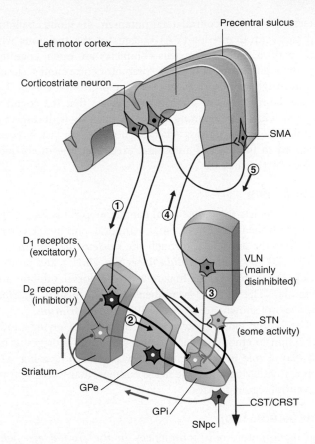

Fig. 26.3 Part of the projection from the internal segment of globus pallidus *(GPi)* to the ventral lateral nucleus *(VLN)* and ventral anterior nucleus of the thalamus sweeps around the base of the internal capsule as the **ansa lenticularis** *(AL)*; the remainder traverses this region as the **lenticular fasciculus** *(LF)*. The two parts come together as the **thalamic fasciculus** *(TF)* before entering the thalamus. *CRST,* Corticoreticular fibre; *CST,* corticospinal fibre; *GPe,* external segment of globus pallidus; *OT,* optic tract; *P,* putamen; *TCF,* thalamocortical fibres.

Fig. 26.4 Activities in the striatal motor loops, prior to movement. The supplementary motor area *(SMA)* is activated through the direct pathway as follows: *(1)* Corticostriate fibres from the sensorimotor cortex activate those GABAergic spiny neurons in the striatum having D₁ receptors tonically facilitated by nigrostriatal inputs (SNpc). *(2)* The activated striatal neurons inhibit internal pallidal *(GPi)* neurons *(3)* with consequent *disinhibition* of the ventral lateral nucleus *(VLN)* thalamocortical neurons *(4)* and activation of the SMA *(5)*, which both modifies ongoing corticostriate activity and initiates impulse trains along corticospinal *(CST)* and corticoreticular *(CRST)* fibres. Activity along the indirect pathway is relatively slight because of tonic dopaminergic inhibition of the relevant striatal neurons via D₂ receptors that releases GPe inhibitory neurons and results in further inhibition of the subthalamic nucleus *(STN)*. Activity of the STN is further modulated by corticosubthalamic fibres *(hyperdirect pathway)*. *GPe,* External segment of globus pallidus; *SNpc,* compact part of the substantia nigra.

The putamen and globus pallidus are somatotopically organised, permitting selective facilitation of neurons relevant to (say) arm movements via the direct route, with simultaneous inhibition of unwanted (say) leg movements via the indirect route. For suppression of unwanted movements, the STN, acting upon that segment of the body map in the GPi, is especially important. Progressive failure of dopamine production by the SNpc is the precipitating cause of *Parkinson disease* (PD) (Clinical Panel 26.1).

What are the Normal Functions of the Motor Loop? Although movements can be produced on the opposite side of the body by direct electrical stimulation of the healthy putamen, the basal ganglia do not normally initiate movements. Nevertheless, they are active during all movements, whether fast or slow. They seem to be involved in scaling the strength of muscle contractions and, in collaboration with the SMA, in organising the requisite sequences of cell columns in the motor cortex. They come into action after the corticospinal tract has already been activated by 'premotor' areas (including the cerebellum). Because patients with PD have so much difficulty in performing internally generated movement sequences, it is believed that the basal ganglia have a 'reservoir' of learned

motor programs, which they are able to assemble in the appropriate sequence for the movements decided upon and to transmit the coded information to the SMA.

Cognitive Loop

The head of the caudate nucleus receives a large projection from the prefrontal cortex and it participates in goal-based motor learning. *Positron emission tomography (PET)* scan studies have demonstrated increased contralateral blood flow through the head of the caudate nucleus when novel motor actions are performed with one hand. There is also increased activity in the anterior part of the contralateral putamen, the globus pallidus, and the ventral anterior (VA) nucleus of the thalamus with hand actions. The VA nucleus completes an 'open' cognitive loop through its projection to the premotor cortex and a 'closed' loop through a return projection to the prefrontal cortex. The cortical connections of the caudate suggest that the cognitive loop participates in planning ahead, particularly with respect to complex motor intentions. When the novel motor task has been practiced to the level of automatic execution, the motor loop becomes active instead.

Limbic Loop

Fig. 26.5 depicts the *limbic* basal ganglia loop. This loop originates from the inferior prefrontal, temporal, and limbic cortex, as well as the amygdala, through the **nucleus accumbens** (see Fig. 26.1D) and **ventral pallidum** (see Fig. 26.1C), and projects back to those areas via the thalamus (mediodorsal, midline, and habenula). The nucleus accumbens and the nearby *olfactory tubercle* (not shown) are known as the **ventral striatum**.

The limbic loop is likely to be involved in giving motor expression to emotions, such as through smiling or gesturing, and play a role in reinforcing or reward-based learning. The loop is rich in dopaminergic nerve endings, many arising from the ventral tegmental area.

Oculomotor Loop

The oculomotor loop commences in the *frontal eye fields* (area 8) and *posterior parietal cortex* (area 7). It passes through the caudate nucleus and the SNpr. It returns to the frontal eye field and prefrontal cortex via the VA nucleus of the thalamus. The SNpr sends an inhibitory GABAergic projection to the superior colliculus, where it synapses upon cells controlling automatic saccades (Chapter 23). These cells are also supplied directly from the frontal eye field. *Saccades* are the fast eye movements made when looking towards an object

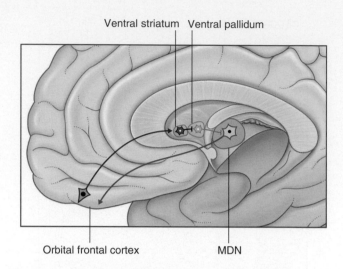

Fig. 26.5 The limbic basal ganglia loop, right hemisphere. Excitatory cortical projections to the ventral striatum result in further inhibition of the ventral pallidum and the mediodorsal nucleus of the thalamus (MDN) is then released by means of disinhibition.

that is already present, going to be present, or was present but no longer visible.

While the eyes are fixated, the SNpr is tonically active, maintaining their position. Whenever a deliberate saccade is about to be made towards another object, the oculomotor loop is activated and the superior colliculus is *disinhibited (inhibition is released)*. Without the normal inhibition from the basal ganglia, the superior colliculus then discharges to reinforce the activity of the direct pathway. Maximum speed (22 m/s) is rapidly achieved, the eyeballs are moved to the target, and the SNpr resumes its vigilance once the object is again fixated.

CLINICAL PANEL 26.1 Hypokinetic-Rigid Syndromes

Parkinson disease (PD) is a progressive neurodegenerative disorder, uncommon before the age of 50 years and increasing in frequency with age to affect 1% to 3% of those over the age of 65 years. The following motor manifestations, initially asymmetric, impact volitional activities and characterise the disorder, and while their presence is used to support the diagnosis, vary in prominence and may not all be present in an individual patient, suggesting clinical subtypes:

- **Bradykinesia**

  Bradykinesia means slowness of movement. Patients report that routine activities, such as opening a door, require deliberate planning and consciously guided execution. Normally, the basal ganglia contribution to movement is initiated some milliseconds after the premotor cortex and cerebellum have raised the firing rate of motor cortex neurons to threshold at a spinal lower motor neuron level. In PD the boost to lower motor neuron activation is weak because of the weakened contribution from the supplementary motor area (SMA).

- **Muscular Rigidity**

  A resistance to passive flexion and extension of the joint of a limb through its range of motion (most easily elicited at the elbow or wrist),

rigidity, is found when checking muscle tone, affecting all somatic musculature, but a predilection for flexors imposes a stooped posture. This steady and uniform resistance is also termed *'lead pipe rigidity'* to distinguish it from the *'clasp knife phenomenon'* or an initial resistance to movement that yields as the limb is moved and characteristic of the spasticity that accompanies upper motor neuron lesions. The clinician may detect a subtle underlying tremor in the form of a ratchety *'cogwheel'* sensation (tremor superimposed on rigidity) when checking motor tone. Difficulty in writing is another common early feature of PD. The individual written letters become small and irregular. Loss of writing skill is attributable to cocontraction of wrist flexors and extensors.

Because muscle spindle stretch reflexes are not exaggerated in PD, attention has focused on the Golgi tendon organ afferents responsible for *autogenic inhibition* as an explanation for rigidity. As illustrated in Chapter 10, these afferents synapse upon inhibitory, Ib premotor interneurons, which, when activated by muscle contraction, dampen the activity of motor neurons supplying the same muscle and any homonymous contributors to the same movement (e.g., impulses generated in biceps brachii tendon organs will depress both brachialis and biceps motor neurons). In PD patients, autogenic inhibition is reduced and it may contribute to rigidity, because in PD there is some degree of cocontraction of prime movers and antagonists. The function of the Ib inhibitory reflex pathway may be modulated by the basal ganglia in a context- and task-dependent manner.

- **Impairment of Postural Reflexes**

Patients go off balance easily and tend to fall stiffly ('like a telegraph pole') in response to a mild accidental push that compromises their maintenance of balance. The underlying fault is an impairment of anticipatory postural adjustments; normally, a push to the upper part of the body elicits immediate contraction of lower limb muscles appropriate for the maintenance of equilibrium.

- **Tremor**

Tremor, at 3 to 6 Hz in a limb, is the initial feature in two-thirds of patients with PD. Typically, the tremor only involves muscle groups that are at rest and diminishes during voluntary movement, hence a **resting tremor**. The term resting tremor is used to distinguish it from the *intention tremor* of cerebellar disease that is absent at rest and elicited by voluntary movement. It is also different from *essential tremor*, discussed later. Resting tremor is characterised as a rhythmic tremor of the lips and tongue, pronation—supination of the forearm, and flexion—extension of the fingers. A *'pill-rolling'* movement of the index and middle fingers against the thumb pad is also characteristic. While resting tremor characterises PD, other types of tremor may coexist.

The pathophysiology of resting tremor is unclear and does not correlate with the other motor symptoms of PD, progress at the same rate as bradykinesia, rigidity, or gait problems, and may not demonstrate the same response to treatment as these other motor findings. These observations all support a different pathophysiology. While the aetiology is unknown, evidence suggests dysfunction within two circuits, basal ganglia and the cerebello—thalamo—cortical pathway ('dimmer-switch model', where basal ganglia dysfunction acts as the trigger and the cerebello—thalamo—cortical circuit produces the tremor).

Listed below are **non-motor symptoms** in PD that reflect its neuropathology extending beyond the sole loss of dopaminergic neurons within the SNpc:

- Cognitive impairments and dementia (after 15—20 years of progression of PD, dementia is identified in 80% of patients and coexists with other non-motor symptoms)
- Neuropsychiatric symptoms (depression is reported in up to 50% of PD patients)
- Sleep disorders in 25% of PD patients
- Autonomic symptoms (e.g., bladder dysfunction, orthostatic hypotension, dysphagia).

'The' neuropathological feature of PD is dopaminergic neuron loss in the SNpc and intraneuronal cytoplasmic inclusions of α-synuclein aggregations termed **'Lewy bodies'** in remaining SNpc neurons that induces their death. The main site of projection of these neurons is to the putamen; adjacent dopaminergic neurons projecting to the caudate are not as significantly affected, but symptom onset in PD does not occur until approximately 60% of the SNpc neurons have been lost. The consequence of this neuronal loss is a 'shift' from the direct to the indirect motor pathway (Fig. 26.6). However, the presentation of PD with its nonmotor findings reflects neurodegeneration that extends beyond dopaminergic neurons to include noradrenergic, serotonergic and cholinergic neurons, the cerebral cortex, and the autonomic nervous system.

Visualisation of changes in dopaminergic systems can be achieved by *[18 F]DOPA (fluorodopa F-18) position emission scanning* (PET) that uses a mildly radioactive compound which, when injected intravenously, binds with dopamine receptors in the striatum. In symptomatic PD a significant reduction in binding (and therefore of receptors) is revealed (Fig. 26.7). Similarly, single-photon emission computed tomography (SPECT) imaging of the

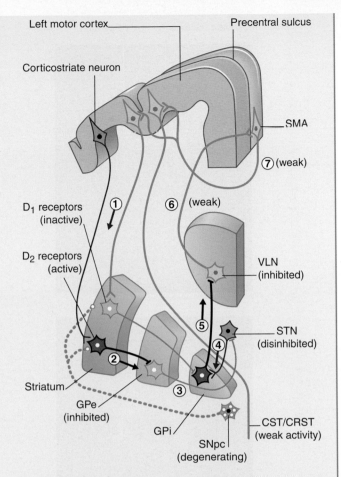

Fig. 26.6 Consequences of degeneration of the pathway from the compact part of the substantia nigra *(SNpc)* to the striatum (S) in parkinson disease. The effects arise from loss of tonic facilitation of spiny striatal neurons bearing D1 receptors, together with loss of tonic inhibition of those bearing D_2 receptors. The direct pathway is disengaged, and the indirect pathway is activated by default. *(1)* Corticostriate neurons from the sensorimotor cortex now strongly activate those D2 receptor GABAergic neurons *(2)* in the striatum that synapse upon and inhibit those *(3)* in the external pallidal segment *(GPe)* and result in disinhibition of the subthalamic nucleus *(STN)*. The STN discharges strongly *(4)* onto the GABAergic neurons of the internal pallidal segment *(GPi)*; these in turn discharge strongly *(5)* into the ventral lateral nucleus *(VLN)* of the thalamus, resulting in reduced output along thalamocortical fibres *(6)* travelling to the supplementary motor area *(SMA)*. Inputs *(7)* from the SMA to the corticospinal and corticoreticular fibres *(CST/CRST)* become progressively weaker, with consequences for initiation and execution of movements.

uptake of *ioflupane I123 (DaTscan)* by the presynaptic dopamine transporter serves as a marker of integrity of the dopaminergic nigrostriatal pathway and detects its degeneration. While these imaging studies support a clinical diagnosis of PD, they are more frequently used to exclude it, and the gold standard for diagnosis of PD is the presence of neuronal loss of the SNpc and Lewy bodies at postmortem pathological examination.

The onset of PD is sporadic and likely a combination of environmental and genetic factors; however, 10% to 15% of patients have a positive family history and a monogenetic cause (e.g., *Pink1* or *Parkin*). The initiation of sporadic PD is hypothesised to occur when a pathogen enters the body, initiating α-synuclein aggregation and spread in the central nervous system, perhaps by a prion-like mechanism.

Head of caudate nucleus   Putamen

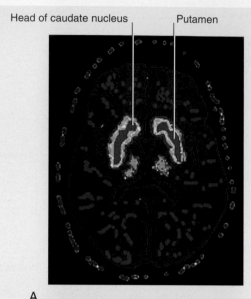

A

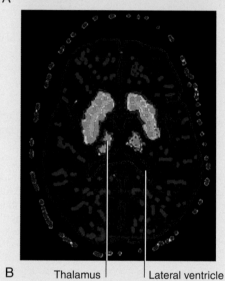

B   Thalamus   Lateral ventricle

Fig. 26.7 Diagram showing typical results of brain scans following intravenous injection of [^{18}F]fluorodopa. Intensity of uptake is indicated as *red* (greatest), *yellow*, *green*, and *blue* (least). (A) Control. (B) Parkinson disease.

Misdiagnosis

The diagnosis of PD is 'reconsidered' at each clinic visit, since one in five people initially diagnosed and treated for PD are eventually found to have another diagnosis. These other hypokinetic-rigid syndromes are also referred to as *parkinsonism* as the clinical features resemble PD, but their pathophysiology, prognosis (worse), and responsiveness to treatment (little or none,

while a clear and beneficial response is typically seen with therapy in PD) differ. The most common neurogenerative disorders that 'mimic' PD and distinguishing features follow:

- *Multiple system atrophy* is an α-synucleinopathy like PD, but its major pathology is in oligodendroglia rather than neurons, and while neuronal inclusions occur, they do not resemble Lewy bodies.
  - Prominence of autonomic dysfunction (e.g., orthostatic hypotension, bladder/bowel dysfunction) accompanied by either parkinsonism (unresponsive to levodopa) or cerebellar ataxia
- *Lewy body disease* is also an α-synucleinopathy and the deposition of α-synuclein is within neurons, but most prominent within axons.
  - Dementia, either preceding or appearing with parkinsonism, fluctuations in mental status, visual hallucinations, sleep disorder, and sensitivity to dopamine receptor blocking agents
- *Progressive supranuclear palsy* is a neurodegenerative disorder characterised by the accumulation of abnormally phosphorylated tau (proteins that normally stabilise microtubules within cells) in specific brain regions.
  - Characterised by early falls, hypokinesia/rigidity with little or no tremor, and slow vertical saccades (eventually leading to restricted vertical eye movements; *supranuclear vertical ophthalmoplegia*).
- *Nondegenerative parkinsonism* refers to those disorders that have an aetiology attributed to a toxin, drug (antipsychotic medications with dopamine receptor blocking effects), infection, and, less frequently, cerebrovascular (result of multiple cerebral infarctions).

Essential tremor is more than twice as prevalent as PD, and is often mistaken for it since it commonly becomes manifest during the fifth decade and is sometimes called familial tremor because of autosomal dominant inheritance. It is characterised initially by a faint trembling, tremulous handwriting, and is most noticeable when the arms are fully outstretched. Head bobbing or vocal tremor can also occur. The aetiology is felt to be Purkinje cell dysfunction and reduced cerebellar cortical dysfunction. Levodopa (L-dopa) is ineffective, but pharmacotherapeutic agents that serve to enhance GABAergic neurotransmission are beneficial.

Treatment of Parkinson Disease
Medications
The most effective form of treatment that improves quality of life for PD remains L-dopa, which can cross the blood—brain barrier and is metabolised to dopamine by surviving nigral neurons. Some 75% of patients benefit, with a reduction of symptoms, but effectiveness of L-dopa declines as there is a progressive loss of nigral neurons, and dopamine agonist drugs may be used to stimulate striatal postsynaptic dopamine receptors. Administration of dopamine agonists can result in *impulse control disorders*, when a person fails to resist the drive to behave in ways that result in impaired social behaviour. In PD this can include pathological gambling, excessive spending, hypersexuality, and overeating. After several years of L-dopa therapy, many patients develop medication-related dyskinesias (hyperkinetic), also known as spontaneous movements.

Other less efficacious medications include monoamine oxidase B inhibitors, *N*-methyl-D-aspartate receptor blockers, and anticholinergic drugs. *Anticholinergic drugs* reduce activity of the cholinergic interneurons in the striatum and can ameliorate tremor, but the required dosage is liable to produce one or more of the autonomic side effects listed in Fig. 13.13.

CLINICAL PANEL 26.2   Other Movement Disorders

Cerebral Palsy

Cerebral palsy (CP) is an umbrella term covering a variety of motor disorders arising from damage to the brain during fetal life or in the perinatal period. CP manifests as a disorder of movement or posture. The incidence is about 2 to 3.5 per 1000 live births in all countries. About 10% of cases develop in the postnatal period, and these are usually attributed to infection or head injury.

Various classifications of CP exist, based on the anatomic site of injury, clinical symptoms and signs, pattern of involvement of the limbs, timing of the presumed injury, and muscle tone but, increasingly, clinical descriptive criteria are used to define the disorder but pathophysiology is less clear or attributable to specific brain lesions.

- A frequent type of presentation is *spastic diplegia*. During the early postnatal months most affected children are usually described as being 'floppy' (atonic), changing to a spastic state (of the lower limbs in particular) by the end of the first year. Some children will appear clinically normal by the age of 5 years, but if the condition is progressive (evident on reexamination at the age of 4 or 5 years) then other disorders (e.g., genetic, metabolic) need to be excluded and the diagnosis of CP is in doubt. Most children will have abnormal neuroimaging, but this is not required for the diagnosis. The ventricular system in spastic diplegia can appear dilated owing to maldevelopment of periventricular oligodendrocytes in the sixth to eighth month of gestation. Notably, those myelinating corticospinal fibres destined for lumbosacral segments of the spinal cord are affected. Intrauterine infection (Fig. 26.8), ischemia, and metabolic disorders are etiological suspects.
- *Extrapyramidal* or *dyskinetic CP* can result from perinatal asphyxia. In this condition the striatum is particularly affected, perhaps because it is normally highly active metabolically in establishing synaptic connections with the pallidum.
- *Choreoathetosis* is characteristic. *Chorea* refers to momentary spontaneous writhing of muscle groups in a random manner, interfering with voluntary movements and *athetosis* describes similar, slower movements that are continuous. The similarity of chorea and athetosis and their 'blending' together make the term *choreoathetosis* more appropriate.

Huntington Disease

Huntington disease is an autosomal (chromosome 4) dominant, inherited disease that is caused by a CAG repeat expansion in exon 1 of the *huntingtin (HTT)* gene. The pathogenesis is assumed to be a gain of function that results in striatal neuron death. Prevalence is estimated at 4 to 10 per 100,000 people, and the mean age of symptom onset is 40 years, but younger and older ages of onset are described. The clinical history is one of a primary neurodegenerative disorder (other organ systems are involved as *huntingtin* is expressed in other tissues) manifested by progressive chorea, behavioural changes, and eventually a progressive dementia. Death results from the resulting motor impairment, dysphagia, and inanition.

Hemiballism

Hemiballism (or *hemiballismus*) tends to occur in the elderly and is initially described as (and typically results from) thrombosis of a small branch of the posterior cerebral artery supplying the subthalamic nucleus (STN). It is marked by the abrupt onset of wild, flailing movements of the contralateral arm, sometimes of the leg as well. The appearances suggest that the thalamocortical pathway from the ventral lateral nucleus (VLN) of the thalamus to the supplementary motor area (SMA) has become intensely overactive. It is assumed that the STN, and other basal ganglia nuclei, influence the firing pattern of the internal segment of the globus pallidus (GPi), and when 'eliminated' result in random fluctuations of inhibition and disinhibition within these motor circuits.

(This question may well be asked: If vascular destruction of the STN results in hemiballism, why does STN paralysis by high-frequency stimulation not have the same effect? The explanation is not completely clear, but the STN is not just a relay nucleus for the indirect pathway, but is functionally subdivided and plays a role within all of the functional loops (motor, cognitive, oculomotor, and limbic) of the basal ganglia through its reciprocal connections with the GPe (and GPi as well as the SNpr). It also receives direct excitatory glutamatergic inputs from the cortex ('hyperdirect pathway' that could allow the cortex to use contextual information to determine what motor programs are transmitted though the basal ganglia) and excitatory glutamatergic input from the thalamus (centromedian and parafascicular nucleus). The observed effects of deep brain stimulation of the STN in PD could occur by activation of adjacent pathways, more likely not through the STN's role in the indirect pathway, but through another circuit(s) in which it serves a functional role.)

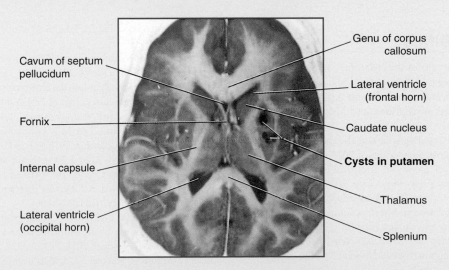

Fig. 26.8 Horizontal magnetic resonance imaging (MRI) slice at the level of the corpus striatum from a 2-year-old girl suffering from severe choreoathetosis as a result of intrauterine damage to her basal ganglia by toxoplasmosis. The putamen on both sides has been partly replaced by cysts. (MRI kindly provided by Professor J. Paul Finn, Director, Magnetic Resonance Research, Department of Radiology, David Geffen School of Medicine, UCLA, CA, USA.)

BASIC SCIENCE PANEL 26.1   Deep Brain Stimulation for Parkinson Disease

First identified within animal models and later humans with Parkinson disease (PD), functional changes of basal ganglia 'behaviour', predicted by the loss of dopaminergic innervation, ... were identified as tonic firing of neurons in the subthalamic nucleus (STN) and internal segment of the globus pallidus (GPi) was recorded, representing increased transmission within the indirect pathway. Modifying techniques of stereotaxic surgery and electrical stimulation developed to map areas of the cerebral cortex prior to resection, the STN or GPi could be identified and ablated, resulting in amelioration of PD motor symptoms. As constant stimulation of these same structures produced similar clinical effects assumed to arise from the modulation of their abnormal signalling, stimulation replaced ablation and the current approach used in functional neurosurgery or *deep brain stimulation (DBS)*. Under stereotaxic guidance electrodes are now placed within the GPi or STN, and using high-frequency stimulation the optimum site of stimulation is guided by observation of the patient as they perform different motor tasks. DBS can be performed either unilaterally or bilaterally and is effective in lessening the tremor, bradykinesia, and rigidity in PD, improving the patient's quality of life.

The choice of target, GPi or STN, is guided by patient-related features and goals as well as technical that are related to the programming strategies or requirements for effective stimulation. The larger size of the GPi lessens the chance of inadvertent spread of the stimulating current to the internal capsule or to association or limbic GPi projection areas. Less functional segregation with overlapping of motor, cognitive, and association areas within the STN, as well as its smaller size, may make it a less favourable target for DBS when there is an increased risk of cognitive or behavioural decline, but improvement of motor symptoms may be better. Regardless of choice, DBS has a significant impact and role in PD patient care.

✳ Core Information

The basal ganglia are nuclear groups involved in movement control and motor learning. They comprise the *striatum* (*putamen, caudate nucleus*, and the *nucleus accumbens, globus pallidus, subthalamic nucleus (STN)*), and *substantia nigra*. The globus pallidus has an *external (GPe)* and an *internal segment (GPi)*, the latter tapering into the midbrain as the *substantia nigra reticular part (SNpr)*. The GPi provides the 'output' from the basal ganglia that exert control over the thalamus. Four circuits (loops) commence in the cerebral cortex, pass through the basal ganglia, and return to the cortex, ultimately modulating cortical activity: the *cortico-basal ganglia-thalamo-cortical circuits*. The *substantia nigra pars compacta (SNc)* stands separately to these circuits but influences them by way of nigrostriatal pathways.

Cortical inputs to the striatum and STN are excitatory. Striatal outputs are inhibitory to the globus pallidus; so, too are the pallidal outputs to the STN and the thalamus. The STN is excitatory to the GPi.

The **direct pathway**, striatum → GPi, is facilitated by the normal tonic activity of SNc dopaminergic neurons. The **indirect pathway**, striatum → GPe → STN → GPi, is inhibited by the SNc.

The striatum and globus pallidus are somatotopically organised, permitting selective activation of body parts; the STN is especially important for inhibition of unwanted movements.

In the *motor loop*, facilitation of the direct pathway is necessary for the supplementary motor area (SMA) to become active before and during movement. SMA activity immediately prior to movement is detectable as the *readiness potential* and is produced by silencing of GPi neurons with consequent liberation (disinhibition) of thalamocortical neurons to the SMA, with follow-through to the motor cortex for initiation of movement. The main function of the motor loop seems to be the appropriate sequencing of serial order actions for the execution of learned motor programs. In PD, the loss of SNc dopaminergic neurons causes the indirect pathway to become dominant, with follow-through suppression of the ventral lateral nucleus (VLN) of the thalamus and reduced SMA activity thus accounting for the characteristic bradykinesia. PD symptomatology also includes rigidity, impairment of postural reflexes, and tremor.

The *cognitive loop* begins in the association cortex and returns via the VA nucleus of the thalamus to the premotor and prefrontal cortex. It is actively engaged during motor learning and appears concerned with planning ahead for later movements.

The *limbic loop* begins in the cingulate cortex and amygdala, passes through the nucleus accumbens, and returns to the SMA; it is probably involved in giving physical expression to the current emotional state.

The *oculomotor loop* disinhibits the SNpr, thereby liberating the superior colliculus to execute a saccade.

SUGGESTED READINGS

Benarroch EE. Intrinsic circuits of the striatum: complexity and clinical correlation. *Neurology.* 2016;86:1531–1542.

Borghammer P. How does Parkinson's disease begin? Perspectives on neuroanatomical pathways, prions, and histology. *Mov Disord.* 2018;33:48–57.

Bostan AC, Strick PL. The basal ganglia and the cerebellum: nodes in an integrated network. *Nat Rev Neurosci.* 2018;19:338–350.

Brandenburg JE, Fogarty MJ, Sieck GC. A critical evaluation of current concepts in cerebral palsy. *Physiology.* 2019;34:216–229.

Conte A, Defazio G, Hallett M, et al. The role of sensory information in the pathophysiology of focal dystonias. *Nat Rev Neurol.* 2019;15:224–233.

Fazl A, Fleischer J. Anatomy, physiology and clinical syndromes of the basal ganglia: a brief review. *Semin Pediatr Neurol.* 2018;25:2–9.

Ghosh R, Tabrizi SJ. Huntington disease. *Handb Clin Neurol.* 2018;147:255–278.

Grillner S. The enigmatic "indirect pathway" of the basal ganglia: a new role. *Neuron.* 2018;99:1105–1107.

Hassan A, Benarroch EE. Heterogeneity of the midbrain dopamine system. Implications for Parkinson disease. *Neurology.* 2015;85:1795–1805.

Haubenberger D, Hallet M. Essential tremor. *N Engl J Med.* 2018;378:1802–1810.

Helmich RC. The cerebral basis of Parkinsonian tremor: a network perspective. *Mov Disord.* 2018;33:219–231.

Jamwal S, Kumar P. Insight into the emerging role of striatal neurotransmitters in the pathophysiology of Parkinson's disease and Huntington's disease: a review. *Curr Neuropharmacol.* 2019;17:165–175.

Joutsa J, Horn A, Hsu J, Fox MD. Localizing parkinsonism based on focal brain lesions. *Brain.* 2018;141:2445–2456.

Kogan M, McGure M, Riley J. Deep brain stimulation for Parkinson disease. *Neurosurg Clin N Am.* 2019;30:137–146.

McGregor MM, Nelson AB. Circuit mechanisms of Parkinson's disease. *Neuron.* 2019;101:1042–1056.

Ramirez-Zamora A, Ostrem JL. Globus pallidus interna or subthalamic nucleus deep brain stimulation for Parkinson disease: a review. *JAMA Neurol.* 2018;75:367–372.

Raza C, Anjum R, Shakeel NUA. Parkinson's disease: mechanisms, translational models and management strategies. *Life Sci.* 2019;226:77–90.

Wessel JR, Aron AR. On the globality of motor suppression: unexpected events and their influence on behavior and cognition. *Neuron.* 2018;93:259–280.

Cerebellum

STUDY GUIDELINES

1. Describe the functional organisation of the cerebellum and the relationship to the deep cerebellar nuclei.
2. Classify the microscopic organisation of the cerebellar cortex and the cell types found in each layer.
3. Contrast the two types of afferents to the cerebellar cortex with respect to origin, termination, and neurotransmitters.

4. Characterise the origin of output from the cerebellum, the neurotransmitter released, and the effect on the deep cerebellar nuclei.
5. List the cerebellar efferent pathways from the deep cerebellar nuclei to their eventual point of 'termination'.
6. Provide examples of the expected clinical manifestations of dysfunction of the *vestibulocerebellum*, *spinocerebellum*, and *pontocerebellum* or *neocerebellum*.

OVERVIEW

Phylogenetically, the initial development of the cerebellum (in fish) took place in relation to the vestibular labyrinth. With the development of quadrupedal locomotion, the anterior lobes of the cerebellum (in particular) became richly connected to the spinal cord. Assumption of the erect posture and achievement of a whole new range of physical and cognitive skills have been accompanied by the appearance of massive linkages between the anterior and posterior lobes of the cerebellum and the cerebral cortex. In general, cerebellar connections with the vestibular system, spinal cord, and cerebral cortex are arranged such that each cerebellar hemisphere is primarily concerned with the coordination of movements ipsilaterally.

The gross anatomy of the cerebellum is described briefly in Chapter 3, where it may be reviewed at this time.

FUNCTIONAL NEUROANATOMY

Phylogenetic and functional aspects can be combined (to an approximation) by dividing the cerebellum into functional regions (Figs. 27.1 and 27.2). The *flocculonodular lobe* is also known as the *vestibulocerebellum* because it receives input and directs its output to the vestibular nuclei; it controls eye movements through the vestibular system. (Other contributions from the brainstem and through the pons from the parietal and occipital cortex provide further input and contribute to eye movement control.) Portions of the vermis receive input from the reticular formation, frontal eye fields, and superior colliculus and then project to the deep cerebellar

nuclei (the *fastigial nuclei*) in the white matter (Fig. 27.2). The fastigial nuclei project to the gaze centres of the brainstem and vestibular nuclei to control saccadic eye movements (Chapter 23).

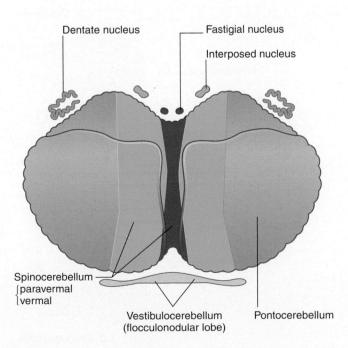

Fig. 27.1 Zonation of the cerebellum. The deep (intra) cerebellar nuclei are represented separately.

The *spinocerebellum* includes the vermis and paravermal (next to the vermis) cerebellar cortex, and receives input from the spinocerebellar tracts (and through the pons cortical input and input from the vestibular nuclei and reticular formation).

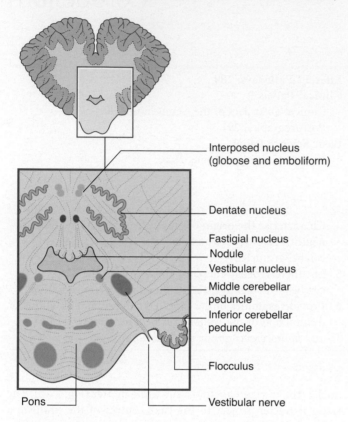

Fig. 27.2 Transverse section of the lower pons and cerebellum showing the position of the deep cerebellar and vestibular nuclei.

Labels in Fig. 27.2:
- Interposed nucleus (globose and emboliform)
- Dentate nucleus
- Fastigial nucleus
- Nodule
- Vestibular nucleus
- Middle cerebellar peduncle
- Inferior cerebellar peduncle
- Flocculus
- Vestibular nerve
- Pons

The vermis projects to the *fastigial nuclei* and, through projections to the reticular formation and vestibular nuclei where the *reticulospinal* and *vestibulospinal tracts* arise, influences postural reflexes of the head and trunk. The paravermal area receives cortical input via the pons and spinal cord input via the spinocerebellar tracts, and projects to the **globose** and **emboliform nuclei**; the two nuclei together are called the **interposed nucleus** (Fig. 27.2). The interposed nucleus projects to the parvocellular part of the red nucleus and ventrolateral thalamus. The parvocellular nucleus projects to the Inferior olivary nucleus through the rubro-olivary tract and with the cerebral cortex, involved in motor learning and correcting motor activity of the limbs.

The remaining lateral strip is the largest and projects to the **dentate nucleus** (Fig. 27.2). This area is called the *pontocerebellum* because of its numerous inputs from the contralateral nuclei pontis. It is also called the **neocerebellum** because the pontine nuclei convey information from large areas of the cerebral neocortex (phylogenetically the most recent). It is uniquely large in the human brain and plays a significant role in the planning, initiation, control, and correction of voluntary movements as well as cognitive, speech, behaviour, affect, and executive functions.

MICROSCOPIC ANATOMY

The structure of the cerebellar cortex appears uniform throughout. It is made up of three principal layers: the innermost *granular layer* (directly adjacent to the white matter), the *Purkinje cell layer* composed primarily of Purkinje cells, and the outermost *molecular layer* (Fig. 27.3).

The **granular layer** contains billions of **granule cells**, whose somas are only 6 to 8 μm in diameter. Their short dendrites receive so-called **mossy fibres** from all sources except the

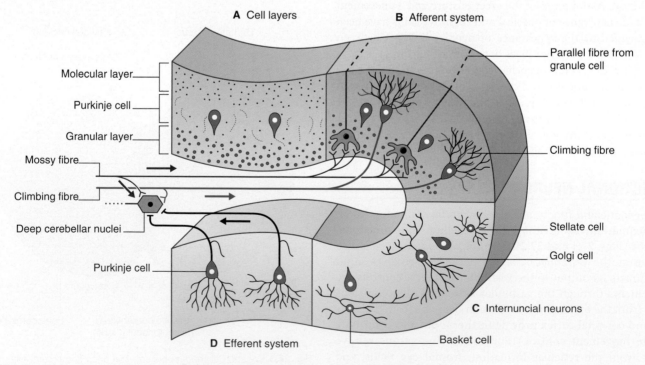

A Cell layers

B Afferent system

Labels:
- Molecular layer
- Purkinje cell
- Granular layer
- Mossy fibre
- Climbing fibre
- Deep cerebellar nuclei
- Purkinje cell
- Parallel fibre from granule cell
- Climbing fibre
- Stellate cell
- Golgi cell
- Basket cell

D Efferent system

C Internuncial neurons

Fig. 27.3 Cerebellar cortex. (A) Cell layers. (B) Afferent systems. (C) Interneurons. (D) Efferent system.

inferior olivary nucleus. Before reaching the cerebellar cortex, the mossy fibres, which are excitatory in nature, give off collateral branches to the deep cerebellar nuclei.

The axons of the granule cells extend into the molecular layer where they divide in a T-shaped manner to form *parallel fibres* (they run parallel to the transverse fissures of the cerebellum) that are parallel to other parallel fibres, but perpendicular to the axes of the Purkinje cell dendritic tree. They make excitatory (glutamatergic) contacts with the distal dendrites of Purkinje cells. The granular layer also contains *Golgi cells* (see later) whose dendrites are stimulated by the parallel fibres of the granule cells. The *Purkinje cell layer* consists of very large *Purkinje cells*. The fan-shaped dendritic trees of the Purkinje cells are the largest dendritic trees in the entire nervous system and at right angles to the parallel fibres (Fig. 27.4).

The dendritic tree of Purkinje cells receives synapses from a huge number of parallel fibre axons (as many as 100,000, but only a small number are active at any one time) of granule cells, each one making successive synapses (one or two per Purkinje

cell) on the dendritic spines of about 400 (possibly more) Purkinje cells. Not surprisingly, stimulation of only a small number of granule cells by mossy fibres has a small facilitatory effect upon many Purkinje cells. Many thousands of parallel fibres must act simultaneously to bring the membrane potential of the Purkinje cell to threshold.

Each Purkinje neuron also receives a single *climbing fibre* from the contralateral inferior olivary nucleus. In stark contrast to the one-per-cell synapses of parallel fibres, the olivocerebellar fibre divides at the Purkinje dendritic branch points and makes numerous synaptic contacts (thousands) with those dendritic spines (Fig. 27.4). A single action potential applied to one climbing fibre is enough to elicit a short burst of action potentials from its Purkinje cell, known as a *complex spike* (see later). The complex spike is so powerful that, for some time after it ceases firing, the synaptic effectiveness of these parallel fibres undergoes a *long-term depression (LTD)*. In this sense, the Purkinje cells *remember* that they have been excited by olivocerebellar fibres.

The axons of the Purkinje cells are the *only* axons to emerge from the cerebellar cortex. Remarkably, they are entirely inhibitory (the neurotransmitter is GABA) in their effects. Their principal targets are their corresponding deep cerebellar nuclei. They also give off collateral branches, mainly to *Golgi cells*.

The *molecular layer* is almost entirely taken up with Purkinje dendrites, parallel fibres, supporting neuroglial cells, and blood vessels. However, two sets of inhibitory interneurons are also found there, lying in the same plane as the Purkinje cell dendritic trees, but perpendicular to the granule cell axons or parallel fibres (Fig. 27.3). Near the cortical surface are small *stellate cells*; close to the Purkinje cell layer are larger *basket cells*. Both sets are contacted by parallel fibres, and they both inhibit Purkinje cells. The stellate cells synapse upon dendritic shafts, whereas the basket cells form a 'basket' of synaptic contacts around the soma, as well as forming axoaxonic synapses upon the initial segment of the axon. A single basket cell synapses upon some 250 Purkinje cells. As one group, or row, of Purkinje cells becomes active, the rows on either side will be inhibited by these interneurons.

The final cell type in the cortex is the *Golgi cell*, whose dendrites are contacted by parallel fibres and whose axons divide extensively before synapsing upon the short dendrites of granule cells. The synaptic ensemble that includes a mossy fibre terminal, granule cell dendrites, and Golgi cell boutons is known as a *glomerulus* (Fig. 27.5). Golgi cells function to limit the output of the mossy fibre inputs onto the granule cells.

Spatial Effects of Mossy Fibre Activity (Fig. 27.6)

As already noted, cerebellar afferents (except for olivocerebellar ones) form mossy fibre terminals after giving off excitatory collaterals to one of the deep cerebellar nuclei. The afferents excite groups of granule cells, which in turn facilitate many hundreds of Purkinje cells arranged in rows beneath the parallel fibres of the granule cells. Along the row of excitation, known as a *microzone* (smallest efferent unit of the cerebellar cortex), the Purkinje cells begin to fire and to inhibit neurons in one of the deep nuclei. At the same time, weakly facilitated Purkinje cells along the edges of the microzone are inhibited by stellate and basket cells. As a result, a row of Purkinje cells is sharply focused, while those rows on

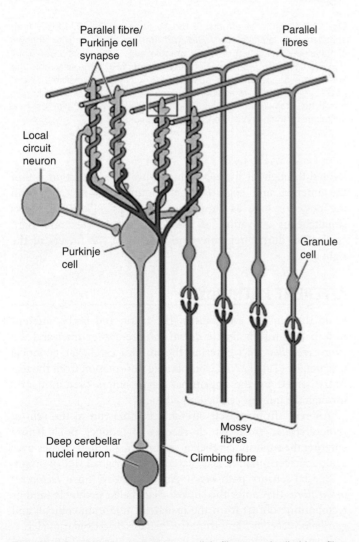

Fig. 27.4 Relationship between parallel fibres and climbing fibre synapses upon the dendritic spines of a purkinje cell. (Modified from Purves D, Augustine GJ, Fitzpatrick D, et al., eds. *Neuroscience*, 5th ed. Sunderland, MA: Sinauer Associates; 2012.)

Granule cell dendrite   Golgi cell axon

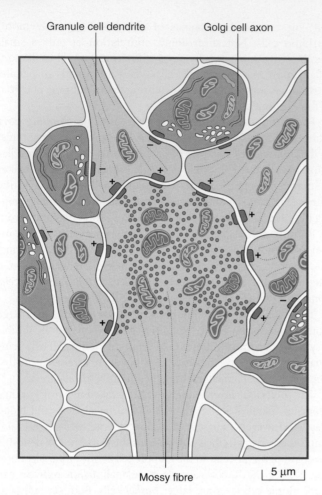

Mossy fibre | 5 µm |

Fig. 27.5 A synaptic glomerulus. + or − indicate excitation/inhibition.

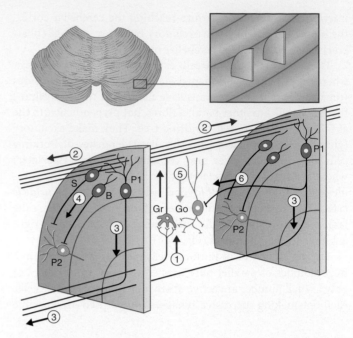

Fig. 27.6 Scheme of effects of mossy fibre activity. *(1)* Mossy fibre stimulating a granule cell *(Gr)*. *(2)* Parallel fibre activity follows simultaneous activation of many granule cells. *(3)* Activation of distal Purkinje cells *(P1)* results in selective inhibition of neurons within the appropriate deep cerebellar nucleus. *(4)* Activation of stellate *(S)* and basket cells *(B)* inhibits adjacent Purkinje cells *(P2)*. *(5)* Golgi cells *(Go)* terminate granule cell activity. *(6)* Intense online activity can be sustained by inhibition of Golgi cells by Purkinje cells.

either side will be inhibited. The excitation is terminated by Golgi cell inhibition via the granule cells that stimulated them (self-limiting). Powerful excitation will last longer because highly active Purkinje cells inhibit underlying Golgi cells, thereby allowing the granule cells to continue to fire.

REPRESENTATION OF BODY PARTS

Representation of body parts in the human cerebellar cortex can be investigated by means of *functional magnetic resonance imaging (fMRI)*. These investigations, along with evidence from clinical cases, indicate the presence of somatotopic maps in the anterior and posterior lobes (Fig. 27.7).

The body is represented on the cerebellar cortex more than once and the axial musculature is represented in a medial position, whereas the distal musculature is represented more laterally. The expression *'fractionated somatotopy'* refers to the patchy nature of the representation of body parts. Simple representations as shown in Fig. 27.7A are inaccurate, and it is likely that multiple homunculi exist, as shown in Fig. 27.7B. The cumulative results of fMRI studies, clinical manifestations of individuals with cerebellar lesions, and cerebellar stimulation performed as an adjunctive procedure during brain surgery all suggest that motor and cognitive functions are both integrated and 'discretely'

located throughout the cerebellum with motor function within the anterior, and cognitive, behavioural, and speech within the posterior lobe as shown in Fig. 27.7C. Fig. 27.8 shows simultaneous activation of the left motor cortex and right cerebellum during repetitive movements of the fingers of the right hand.

AFFERENT PATHWAYS

From the muscles and skin of the trunk and limbs, afferent information travels in the *dorsal spinocerebellar tract* and the *cuneocerebellar tract* entering the inferior cerebellar peduncle ipsilaterally (Table 27.1). Comparable information from the territory served by the trigeminal nerve enters predominantly through the inferior cerebellar peduncle.

Afferents from muscle stretch receptors run in the *ventral spinocerebellar tract*, which reaches the upper pons before entering the superior cerebellar peduncle, and then crosses over again so its termination is ipsilateral to its original side of origin.

Special sensory pathways (visual, auditory) form *tectocerebellar fibres* that enter the superior cerebellar peduncle (and as tectopontine fibres) from the ipsilateral midbrain colliculi and *vestibulocerebellar fibres* from the ipsilateral vestibular nuclei.

Two large pathways enter from the contralateral brainstem. The *pontocerebellar tract* enters through the middle peduncle, and the *olivocerebellar tract* enters through the inferior cerebellar peduncle.

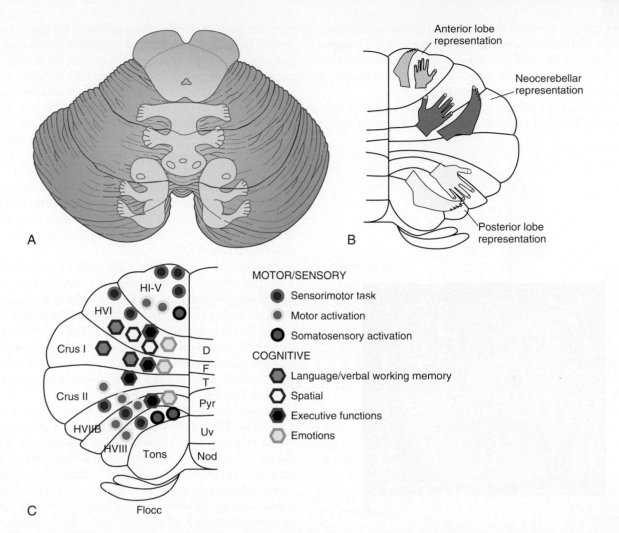

Fig. 27.7 (A) Dorsal surface of cerebellum showing orientation of somatotopic maps (Modified from Snider RS. Interrelations of cerebellum and brainstem. *Assoc Res Nerv Men Dis*. 1952;30:267–281). (B) Illustration of our current understanding that multiple cerebellar somatotopic homunculi maps exist in the cerebellum and those in the neocerebellum respond to more complex movements. (C) Based on functional imaging studies, this illustration shows the localisation of cerebellar structures controlling motor/sensory (more anterior) versus cognitive (more posterior) tasks. While shown as separated from one another, it is unlikely that this is the actual case and greater connectivity (between the cerebellar as well as the cerebral cortex) probably exists. The abbreviations used refer to specific anatomic names. (B and C are reproduced with the kind permission of Grimaldi G, Manto M. Topography of cerebellar deficits in humans. *Cerebellum* 2012;11:336–351.)

Reticulocerebellar fibres enter the inferior cerebellar peduncle from reticular nuclei (paramedian and lateral) of the medulla oblongata.

Finally, aminergic fibres enter all three peduncles from noradrenergic and serotonergic cell groups in the brainstem. Under experimental conditions, both kinds of neurons appear to facilitate excitatory transmission in mossy and climbing fibre terminals.

Olivocerebellar Tract

The sensorimotor cortex projects, via corticospinal collaterals, in an orderly, somatotopic manner onto the ipsilateral inferior and accessory olivary nuclei. The order is preserved in the *olivocerebellar tract* projections onto the 'body maps' in the contralateral cerebellar cortex (from principal nucleus to the cerebellar hemisphere, from the accessory nuclei mainly to the vermis and flocculus). Under resting conditions in animal experiments, groups of olivary neurons discharge synchronously at 5 to 10 Hz

(impulses/s). The synchrony is likely due to the presence of electrical synapses (gap junctions) between dendrites of neighbouring neurons. In the cerebellar cortex, the response of Purkinje cells takes the form of *complex spikes* (multiple action potentials in response to single pulses), because of the spatiotemporal effects of climbing fibre activity along the proximal branches of the dendritic tree.

It is believed that motor learning is by means of a phenomenon called *long-term depression (LTD)*. This refers to depression of ongoing parallel fibre activity for up to several hours, following a burst of complex spikes (Fig. 27.9). Both neurons concerned are glutamatergic and Purkinje dendrites possess both α-amino-3-hydroxy-5-methyl-4-isoxazolepropionic acid (AMPA) and metabotropic receptors. The key molecule in the interaction is the second messenger protein kinase C (PKC), which is activated by parallel fibre activity and mediates protein phosphorylation in ion channels. The molecular sequence is as illustrated in Fig. 8.8.

Complex spikes are associated with a large increase in intracellular calcium and this interacts with PKC to diminish the postsynaptic response of the AMPA receptors to glutamate stimulation, thereby producing long-term depression until the intracellular calcium is returned to normal concentrations.

When a monkey has been trained to perform a motor task, increased discharge of Purkinje cells during task performance takes the form of simple spikes produced by bundles of active parallel fibres. If an unexpected obstacle is introduced into the task (e.g. momentary braking of a lever that the monkey is operating), bursts of complex spikes occur each time the obstacle is encountered. As the animal learns to overcome the obstacle so that the task is completed in the set time, the complex spikes dwindle in number and finally disappear. This is just one of several experimental indicators that the inferior olivary nucleus has a significant *learning function* in the acquisition of new motor skills.

The olivary nucleus receives direct ipsilateral projections from the premotor and motor areas of the cerebral cortex and from the visual association cortices, providing a suitable substrate for its activities. It also receives sensory information through the *spinoolivary tract* (Chapter 15).

In theory, the red nucleus of the midbrain could function as a 'novelty detector' because it receives collaterals both from cortical fibres descending to the olive and from cerebellar output fibres ascending to the thalamus. Most of the output from the red nucleus is to the ipsilateral olivary nucleus, which it appears to inhibit. Upon detection of a mismatch between an intended movement and an actual movement performed, the red nucleus (parvocellular part) inhibits the appropriate cell groups in the olive until the two are harmonised.

As mentioned in Chapter 15, *motor adaptation* is primarily a function of the cerebellum. The cerebellum oversees modification of routine motor programs in response to changes in the environment (e.g. walking uphill versus walking on a flat surface). Experimental evidence indicates that prolonged motor adaptation, such as walking over a period of weeks while wearing an ankle cast, is accompanied by long-term potentiation (LTP) of cerebellothalamic synapses, thereby facilitating the influence of the cerebellum on the motor cortex.

Motor sequence learning, for example learning to walk during infancy, is primarily a function of the basal ganglia (Chapter 26).

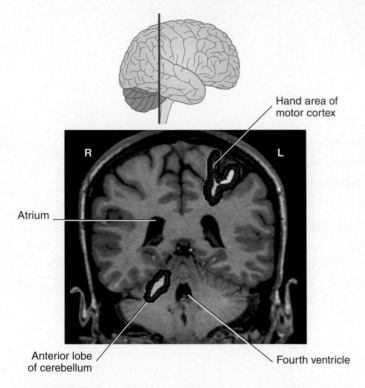

Hand area of motor cortex

Atrium

Anterior lobe of cerebellum

Fourth ventricle

Fig. 27.8 Representation of fMRI activity in a volunteer executing repetitive movement of the fingers of the right hand. (From a series kindly provided by Professor J. Paul Finn, Director, Magnetic Resonance Research, Department of Radiology, David Geffen School of Medicine at UCLA, California, USA.)

TABLE 27.1 Primary Afferents to the Cerebellum.

Tract	Origin	Termination	Peduncle
Vestibulocerebellar	Vestibular ganglia	Nodulus and uvula (ipsilateral)	Inferior
Vestibulocerebellar	Vestibular nuclei	Flocculus, nodulus, and vermis (bilateral)	Inferior
Ventral spinocerebellar	Ascends in contralateral spinal cord (T12–L5)	Vermis and intermediate zone (ipsilateral)	Superior
Dorsal spinocerebellar	Clarke nucleus /Nucleus dorsalis (T1–L2/3)	Vermis and intermediate zone (ipsilateral)	Inferior
Cuneocerebellar	Accessory cuneate nucleus (medulla)	Vermis and intermediate zone (ipsilateral)	Inferior
Rostral spinocerebellar	Ipsilateral spinal cord (cervical)	Vermis and intermediate zone? (ipsilateral)	Inferior and superior
Reticulocerebellar	Lateral, paramedian and reticulotegmental reticular nuclei	Vermis and intermediate zone (ipsilateral)	Inferior (middle—reticular tegmental nucleus)
Trigeminocerebellar	Spinal and main sensory nucleus of V	Vermis and intermediate zone (ipsilateral)	Inferior
Tectocerebellar	Inferior (and superior) midbrain colliculi	Anterior and posterior lobes (bilateral)	Superior
Olivocerebellar	Inferior olivary, accessory olivary nuclei	All contralateral areas	Inferior
Pontocerebellar	Pontine nuclei	Anterior and posterior lobes (contralateral) Vermis (ipsilateral)	Middle

EFFERENT PATHWAYS (FIG. 27.10)

From the *vestibulocerebellum* (flocculonodular lobe), axons project to the vestibular nuclei bilaterally through the inferior cerebellar peduncle. The contralateral projection crosses over within the cerebellar white matter. Portions of the vermis project to the fastigial nucleus, which projects to the gaze centres of the brainstem and vestibular nuclei. Cerebellovestibular outputs to the medial and superior vestibular nuclei control movements of the eyes through the medial longitudinal fasciculus (Chapters 17 and 23). A separate output to the ipsilateral lateral vestibular nucleus (of Deiters) contributes to balance control. Some Purkinje axons bypass the fastigial nucleus and exert direct tonic inhibition on the nucleus of Deiters.

From the *spinocerebellum* the vermis projects to the contralateral reticular formation *(reticulospinal)* and to the vestibular nuclei *(vestibulospinal)*; axons travel in the inferior cerebellar peduncle. They assist in relation to posture and locomotion. The paravermal area projects to the *interposed nucleus*. The interposed nucleus projects to the red nucleus and thalamus that, through their connections to the spinal cord *(rubrospinal tract)* and cortex, monitor and correct motor activity of the limbs.

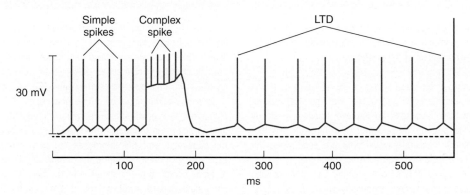

Fig. 27.9 Recording from a purkinje cell. The complex spike elicited by activation of a climbing fibre results in a depression of the frequency of the simple spikes elicited by a parallel fibre. *LTD*, Long-term depression.

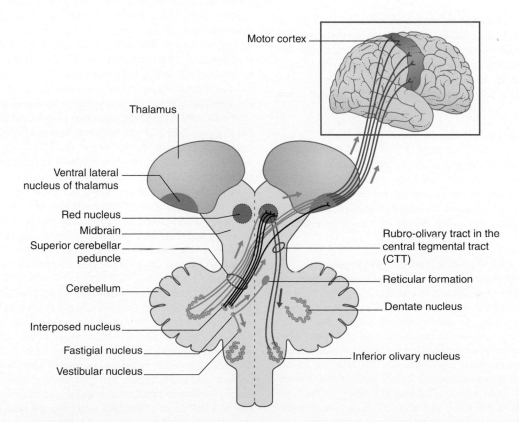

Fig. 27.10 Principal cerebellar efferents. *Arrows* indicate directions of impulse conduction. The central tegmental tract contains the rubro-olivary tract, spinoreticular tract, and fibres conveying taste.

From the *neocerebellum*, the massive **dentatorubrothalamic tract** forms the bulk of the superior cerebellar peduncle. It decussates in the lower midbrain and gives collaterals to the red nucleus before synapsing in the ventrolateral nucleus of the thalamus (a few fibres synapse in the ventroanterior nucleus of the thalamus) that project to the motor cortex. In addition to the sensorimotor cortex, the neocerebellum receives input from all cortical areas (except for the primary visual cortex) and corticopontine fibres that originate from cortical association areas of the prefrontal and temporal area may contribute the majority. This cerebrocerebellar loop is completed by projections from the dentate nucleus to the midline and intralaminar thalamic nuclei (which also receive input from the basal ganglia, reticular formation, and spinal cord) that project to those corresponding cortical areas that contributed those corticopontine fibres.

CLINICAL PANEL 27.1   Clinical Disorders of the Cerebellum

Diseases involving the cerebellum usually involve more than one lobe and/or more than one of the three sagittal strips. However, characteristic clinical pictures occur in association with lesions of the cerebellum.

Midline Cerebellar Lesion: Rostral Vermis Syndrome
Rostral vermis syndrome presents with gait ataxia that manifests as an increased base (spreading their legs apart to improve stability), unsteady walking, and an inability to perform *tandem gait* (walking with one foot placed in front of the other). Inaccurate movements are seen when the patient attempts heel-to-shin testing and referred to as *dysmetria*.

Clinical presentations of lesions of the rostral vermis and anterior lobe often occur in children because of a tumour, *medulloblastoma*, in the roof of the fourth ventricle. These tumours expand rapidly and soon produce signs of raised intracranial pressure (headache, vomiting, drowsiness, and papilledema) by blocking the pathway of cerebrospinal fluid drainage from the ventricular system.

Another aetiology is disease of the anterior lobe observed in chronic alcoholics. In postmortem studies of individuals with *alcoholic cerebellar degeneration*, pronounced atrophy of the cerebellar cortex of the anterior lobe and vermis, with loss of granule and Purkinje cells, and reduction in the thickness of the molecular layer are found. The lower limbs are most affected, and a staggering, broad-based gait is evident even when the individual is not intoxicated.

Midline Cerebellar Lesion: Caudal Vermis Syndrome
Lesions of the flocculonodular and posterior lobe of the cerebellum are associated with *truncal ataxia* that results in the patient swaying when sitting still, unsupported by their hands, and being unable to stand with their feet together. Eye movements can be involved and are slow, inaccurate, and often accompanied by *nystagmus* (a to-and-fro rhythmic and involuntary movement of the eyes usually elicited by looking in a specific direction).

Cerebellar Hemispheric Lesion: Hemispheric syndrome
The cerebellar hemispheres are largely concerned with motor planning and coordination of complex tasks. Damage to one hemisphere leads to symptoms that are most notable in the ipsilateral limbs. Disease of the neocerebellar cortex, dentate nucleus, or superior cerebellar peduncle leads to this incoordination of voluntary movements, particularly in the upper limbs. When fine, purposeful movements are attempted (e.g. grasping a glass, using a key), an *intention tremor (action tremor)* develops: the hand and forearm quiver as the target is approached owing to faulty agonist/antagonist muscle synergies around the elbow and wrist. The hand may travel past the target ('overshoot'). Because cerebellar guidance is lost, the normal smooth trajectory of reaching movements may be replaced by stepped flexions, abductions, and so forth ('*decomposition of movement*').

Rapid alternating movements performed under command, such as pronation/supination, become quite irregular *(dysdiadochokinesia)*. The 'finger-to-nose' and 'heel-to-knee' tests are performed with equal clumsiness whether the eyes are open or closed—in contrast to dorsal column disease where performance is adequate when the eyes are open (Chapter 15).

Speech may be impaired *(dysarthria, scanning speech)* regarding both phonation and articulation. Phonation (production of vowel sounds) is uneven and often tremulous owing to loss of smoothness of contraction of the diaphragm and the intercostal muscles. The terms slurred, jerky, or explosive have been applied to this feature. Articulation is affected because of faulty coordination of impulses in the nerves supplying the lips, mandible, tongue, palate, infrahyoid muscles, and all the muscles that assist with phonation.

The Cerebellum and Higher Brain Functions
The cellular circuitry of the cerebellum results in a modular organisation that facilitates its function as a forward controller and allows it to independently learn, process, and properly sequence fragments of what will become a more complex motor activity. This modular organisation is reflected anatomically and physiologically by fractionated somatotopy (Fig. 27.7B,C) and different cerebellar cortical areas, representing simple movements, can be dynamically 'recombined' into a more complex motor activity. These complex sensorimotor functions are segregated, and fMRI supports their location in the anterior lobe.

Similarly, fMRI supports the localisation of emotional and cognitive function to the posterior lobe with pontine input originating from the prefrontal and temporal associative cerebral cortex.

Further subdivision of cognitive activity is demonstrated when cortical areas associated with specific tasks activate specific cerebellar areas. This is exemplified by lateral cerebellar activity that is greatest during speech, with a one-sided predominance consistent with a possible linkage (via the thalamus) with the motor speech area of the dominant frontal cortex (Chapter 32). Something more than mere motor control may be involved, because lateral cerebellar activity is greater during functional naming of an object, for example 'dig' or 'fly', than during simple object identification, for example 'shovel' or 'airplane'.

Cerebellar cognitive affective syndrome (CCAS) is an inclusive term introduced to indicate cerebral functional deficits that follow sudden, severe damage to the cerebellum, such as thrombosis of one of the three pairs of cerebellar arteries, or the unavoidable damage inflicted during removal of a cerebellar tumour. Such patients show *cognitive* defects in the form of diminished reasoning power, inattention, grammatical errors in speech, poor spatial sense, and patchy memory loss. If the vermis is included in the damage, *affective* (emotional) symptoms also appear, sometimes in the form of *flatness of affect* (dulling of emotional responses), and other times in the form of aberrant emotional behaviour. These functions appear to be segregated to the posterior lobe of the cerebellum.

CLINICAL PANEL 27.2   Posturography

Posturography is the instrumental recording of the erect posture. The subject stands on a platform and spontaneous body sway is detected by strain gauges beneath the corners of the platform. Linkage of the strain-gauge data to a computer can yield a graphic record of anteroposterior and side-to-side sway.

Recordings are done first with the eyes open and then with the eyes closed. This is *static posturography* and it helps to distinguish between different causes of ataxia. *Dynamic posturography* provides information on the effects of an abrupt 4° backward tilt of the supporting platform. For this phase of the examination, surface electromyographic (EMG) electrodes are applied over the gastrocnemius (ankle plantar flexor) and over the tibialis anterior (ankle dorsiflexor). The normal response to the backward tilt is threefold:

a. A monosynaptic, spinal, stretch reflex contraction of the calf muscles after 45 ms
b. A polysynaptic stretch reflex contraction of the calf muscles after 95 ms
c. A long-loop contraction of the ankle dorsiflexors after 120 ms. The ascending limb of the long loop is via the tibial–sciatic nerve and the dorsal column–medial lemniscal pathway to the somatosensory cortex; the descending limb is via the corticospinal tract and the sciatic–peroneal/fibular nerve.

Dynamic posturography helps to distinguish among a wide variety of disorders affecting different levels of the central nervous system and peripheral nervous system.

Anticipatory Function of the Cerebellum

The cerebellum has a sophisticated function in relation to *postural stabilisation* and *postural fixation*, as indicated by the following examples.

Postural stabilisation. Fig. 27.11 illustrates the anticipatory contraction of the gastrocnemius muscle to stabilise the body prior to a voluntary contraction of the biceps brachii. In more general terms, displacement of the upper trunk away from the centre of gravity by a voluntary movement of the head or upper limb is anticipated by the cerebellum. Having received instructions from premotor areas of the frontal lobe (Chapter 28) concerning the *intended* movement, the cerebellum ensures proportionate contractions of postural muscles in a distal to proximal sequence, from lower leg to thigh to trunk, to keep the centre of gravity balanced over the base of support (the feet). Damage to the cerebellar vermis affects normal anticipatory activation (via the lateral vestibulospinal tract) of slow-twitch, postural control muscles, resulting in loss of balance as a result of failure to counter the effect of gravity displacement produced by movement of any body part (see Clinical Panel 27.1).

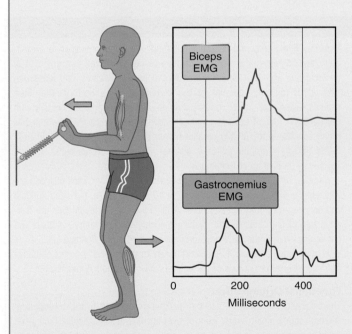

Fig. 27.11 Postural Stabilisation. The subject is pulling a stiff spring attached to the wall. Flexion of the elbow during contraction of biceps brachii tends to pull the trunk forward *(arrow)*. This movement is prevented by equivalent contraction of the gastrocnemius, exerting downward pressure on the forefoot, which tends to thrust the trunk backward *(arrow)*. Simultaneous electromyographic *(EMG)* recordings show that onset of (automatic) gastrocnemius contraction precedes voluntary biceps contraction by 80 ms. (Modified from Nashner LM. Reflex control of posture and movement. *Progr Brain Res.* 1979;50:177–184.)

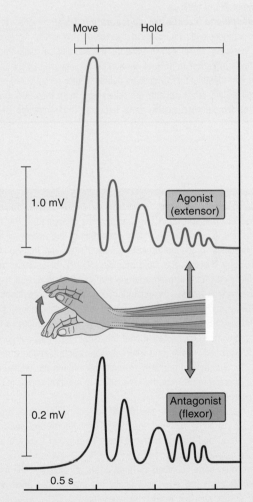

Fig. 27.12 Postural Fixation. The subject was instructed to perform sudden wrist extension and to briefly hold the extended posture. Electromyographic (EMG) recordings show that wrist flexors come into action before completion of the movement. In the 'hold' position note alternation of electrical activity between agonist and antagonist. Antagonist EMG activity is much weaker, as indicated by the scale bars on the left. (Modified from Topka H, Mescheriakov S, Boose A, et al. A cerebellar-like terminal and postural tremor induced in normal man by transcranial magnetic stimulation. *Brain* 1999;122:1551–1562.)

Damage to the anterior lobe is associated with failure of the reticulospinal tracts to anticipate the gravitational effects produced by locomotion, resulting in gait disturbances (see Clinical Panel 27.1).

Postural fixation. Fig. 27.12 illustrates an experiment where the subject was instructed to execute sudden wrist extension and to maintain the extended wrist posture for 2 seconds, while electromyographic records were being taken from the primary wrist extensors (extensors carpi radialis longus and brevis) and a primary antagonist (flexor carpi radialis). The data revealed that the *antagonist* began to contract prior to completion of the movement, resulting in oscillations with the agonist muscles during the fixation period. The contribution of the antagonist is to prevent spontaneous oscillatory torques (tremors) caused by viscoelastic properties of the muscles.

BASIC SCIENCE PANEL 27.1 **Paraneoplastic syndrome**

Paraneoplastic syndromes are clinical syndromes secondary to tumour secretion of functional peptides/hormones or related to immune cross-reactivity with normal host tissue and not attributed to direct tumour invasion. They may develop prior to the presentation of the original tumour, herald its recurrence, or the clinical presentation suggests the underlying malignancy. Paraneoplastic syndromes may present with neurological, endocrine, dermatological, or rheumatological symptoms or findings.

Paraneoplastic cerebellar degeneration (PCD) is one of the most common paraneoplastic neurological syndromes and while these syndromes occur in less than 1% of cancer patients, the neurological syndrome predates the diagnosis of cancer in 65% of cases. PCD is diagnosed by the clinical presentation and identification of specific autoantibodies (onconeural) in serum or cerebrospinal fluid. Most patients are female and more than 90% have breast, ovarian, or female reproductive tract tumours. The symptoms of PCD can include dysfunction of any area of the cerebellum and can include disorders of ocular motility (diplopia or nystagmus), limb, and gait ataxia. Onset is often abrupt and progression can be very rapid, occurring over days or weeks.

While over 30 autoantibodies are described in PCD, *anti-Yo antibody* (anti-Purkinje cell cytoplasmic antibody-type 1, PCA1) is the most common antibody detected. The onconeural antibodies can involve intracellular antigens (anti-Yo) or cell-surface antigens, but those that involve intracellular antigens tend to demonstrate relentless progression; most patients will become wheelchair-bound or bedridden, and have a poor response to treatment (against the tumour itself or in attempts to modify the immune attack with immunosuppressive therapy).

Anti-Yo antibodies are an epiphenomenon of cellular immunity and the actual aetiology of PCD are antigen-specific CD8+ T lymphocytes that result in cytotoxic activity and Purkinje cell death.

✴ **Core Information**

The cerebellum is made up of two *hemispheres* connected in the midline by the *vermis* and a *flocculonodular lobe* consisting of the nodule of the vermis and the flocculus in the hemisphere on each side. The hemispheres show numerous deep fissures, the most prominent being the *primary fissure* that divides the hemisphere into an anterior and posterior lobe, and the *posterolateral fissure* that divides the posterior lobe from the flocculonodular lobe. The cerebellar surface is extensively folded into *folia* and about 80% of the cortex (surface grey matter) is hidden from view on the surfaces of the folia.

The cerebellum is connected to the brainstem via three paired cerebellar peduncles (*superior, middle,* and *inferior*). Fibre tracts carrying afferent information to the cerebellum primarily traverse the inferior and middle cerebellar peduncles; the efferents from the cerebellum to cerebral cortex leave via the superior cerebellar peduncle.

Within the cerebellar white matter are several paired nuclei; from medial to lateral they are the *fastigial, interposed (emboliform and globose nuclei)*, and most lateral and largest is the *dentate*; as a group they are referred to as the *deep cerebellar nuclei*.

The cerebellar cortex consists of three layers; *molecular* is the most superficial, then *Purkinje cell layer*, and finally the *granule cell layer*. Within the cerebellar cortex are five major cell types (*basket, Golgi, granule, Purkinje,* and *stellate* cells). Only the granule cells are excitatory (using the neurotransmitter glutamate) and the remainder are inhibitory (GABA is their neurotransmitter). The only output cells of the cerebellar cortex are the Purkinje cells, which are inhibitory to the deep cerebellar and vestibular nuclei. Projections from the deep cerebellar and vestibular nuclei are excitatory and represent the final output from the cerebellum.

There are two main types of excitatory inputs to the cerebellum: *mossy fibres* that have multiple origins (pontine nuclei, spinal cord, and other brainstem nuclei) and *climbing fibres* that arise from the inferior olivary nucleus within the medulla, which receives input from the cerebral cortex, red nucleus, and spinal cord.

Mossy fibres enter the cerebellum through its three peduncles, are excitatory, and contact granule cells (and deep cerebellar nuclei) that give rise to an ascending axon that enters the molecular layer, bifurcates, and forms *parallel fibres* (that run parallel to the cerebellar folia). Each parallel fibre extends several millimetres, passes through, and makes synaptic contact with the dendritic tree of several hundred Purkinje cells; each Purkinje cell has synapses with up to 100,000 parallel fibres. The basic input–output circuit is mossy fibres → granule cells → parallel fibres → Purkinje cells → deep nucleus → brainstem or thalamus.

Climbing fibres arise from the contralateral inferior olive. Each of these olivocerebellar axons will contact only 7 to 10 Purkinje cells, but each Purkinje cell only receives one climbing fibre. A climbing fibre extends over the dendritic tree of one Purkinje cell, making thousands of excitatory synapses and powerfully exciting the cell body and dendritic tree of the Purkinje cell.

Another group of afferents project diffusely to the cerebellar cortex and arise from monoaminergic neurons of the neuromodulatory system (Chapter 24).

Functional Organisation

The cerebellum is connected to the ipsilateral body and to the contralateral cerebral cortex, so it exerts control over ipsilateral movement. Through its modular organisation it plays a major role in motor control through circuits or loops (cerebrocerebellar and cerebellospinal) that allows it to modulate activity of motor neurons without directly contacting them. This occurs as the cerebral cortex sends a copy of its motor commands to the cerebellum *(efference copy)* and the cerebellum makes a prediction of the sensory consequences of the activity (serves as a *forward controller*). Comparing predicted versus actual sensory feedback allows the cerebellum to affect the motor activity through the brainstem if 'errors' are detected, or through the loop to the cerebral cortex, change the motor command itself. Through this forward controller role, the cerebellum matches the intended action to what occurs in real time or through learning, modifies its own internal forward model.

As prominent as its role in motor control, the cerebellum plays an integrative role in cognition, behaviour, speech, affect, and executive functioning (e.g. modifying behaviour to the meet the context of the environment). This is facilitated through cerebrocerebellar connections with the prefrontal, parietal, and temporal cerebral cortex.

A terminology persists that is useful, although not entirely accurate, but attempts to align cerebellar phylogeny, macroanatomy, and function. This separates the cerebellum based on afferents into a *vestibulocerebellum* (archicerebellum) or flocculonodular lobe, *spinocerebellum* or vermis and medial hemisphere, and *pontocerebellum* (cerebrocerebellum or *neocerebellum*) or lateral hemisphere. However, the spinocerebellum receives afferents from the cerebral cortex and the pontocerebellum from the brainstem and spinal cord.

The vestibulocerebellum (flocculonodular lobe) primarily receives afferents from and projects to the vestibular system and assists with vestibuloocular processing. Dysfunction results in impaired control of eye movements and imbalance or disequilibrium.

The spinocerebellum (vermis and medial hemisphere or paravermian region) receives input from sensory systems via the spinal cord and brainstem, projects to the fastigial (connects to the vestibular and reticular formation) and interposed cerebellar nuclei (connects to the red nucleus), and functions in postural reflexes of the head and trunk. Dysfunction impairs posture and gait.

The pontocerebellum or neocerebellum (lateral cerebellar hemispheres) receives its input via the pontine nuclei that are connected to the cerebral cortex, projects to the dentate nucleus, which connects to the contralateral thalamus and functions in sensorimotor coordination and cognitive functions. Dysfunction of the anterior lobe is associated with difficulty in carrying out complex planned voluntary movement. Posterior lobe injury is associated with cognitive, behaviour, speech, affect, and executive dysfunction.

SUGGESTED READINGS

Apps R, Hawkes R, Aoki S, et al. Cerebellar modules and their role as operational cerebellar processing units: a consensus paper. *Cerebellum*. 2018;17:654–682.

Ashida R, Cerminara NL, Brooks J, Apps R. Principles of organization of the human cerebellum: macro- and microanatomy. *Handb Clin Neurol*. 2018;154:45–58.

Berzero G, Psimaras D. Neurological paraneoplastic syndromes: an update. *Curr Opin Oncol*. 2018;30:359–367.

Bodranghien F, Bastian A, Casali C, et al. Consensus paper: revisiting the symptoms and signs of cerebellar syndrome. *Cerebellum*. 2016;15:369–391.

Bostan AC, Strick PL. The basal ganglia and the cerebellum: nodes in an integrated network. *Nat Rev Neurosci*. 2018;19:338–350.

Canto CB, Onuki Y, Bruinsma B, van der Werf YD, De Zeeuw CI. The sleeping cerebellum. *Trends Neurosci*. 2017;40:309–323.

D'Angelo E. Physiology of the cerebellum. *Handb Clin Neurol*. 2018;154:85–108.

Grimaldi G, Manto M. Topography of cerebellar deficits in humans. *Cerebellum*. 2012;11:336–351.

Kansal K, Yang Z, Fishman AM, et al. Structural cerebellar correlates of cognitive and motor dysfunctions in cerebellar degeneration. *Brain*. 2017;140:707–720.

Kratochwil CF, Maheshwari U, Rijli FM. The long journey of pontine nuclei neurons: from rhombic lip to cortico-ponto-cerebellar circuitry. *Front Neural Circuits*. 2017;11:33.

Kuo SH. Ataxia. *Continuum*. 2019;25:1036–1054.

Noorani I, Carpenter RH. Not moving: the fundamental but neglected motor function. *Philos Trans R Soc Lond B Biol Sci*. 2017;19(372):1718.

Sathyanesan A, Zhou J, Scafidi J, et al. Emerging connections between cerebellar development, behaviour and complex brain disorders. *Nat Rev Neurosci*. 2019;20:298–313.

Schmahmann JD. The cerebellum and cognition. *Neurosci Lett*. 2019;688:62–75.

Cerebral Cortex

STUDY GUIDELINES

1. The cerebral cortex is the part of the body that makes us truly human. Its structure is enormously complex, and assignment of functions to different parts is made difficult, and often unrealistic, by the multiplicity of interconnections.
2. Sensory, motor, and cognitive areas of the cortex are taken in turn.
3. Although damage often leads to permanent disability, the *plasticity* of the cortex is of special interest to all concerned with neurorehabilitation. Examples are taken from sensory and motor areas.

STRUCTURE

The cerebral cortex (*pallium; Gr.* 'shell') varies in thickness from 2 to 4 mm, being thinnest in the primary visual cortex and thickest in the primary motor area. More than half of the total cortical surface is hidden from view in the walls of the sulci. The brain contains approximately 86 billion neurons (the cerebral cortex contains only 19% of this total but represents 81% of the brain's mass), a similar number of neuroglial cells, and a dense capillary bed.

Microscopy reveals the cortex to have a layered or laminar appearance reflecting the arrangement of its cells and nerve fibres as well as a radial organisation of these cellular elements. The general *cytoarchitectonic* structure (patterns based on the appearance of cells; patterns based on the arrangement of myelinated fibres are referred to as the *myleoarchitectonic* structure) varies in detail from one region to another, permitting the cortex to be mapped into dozens of histologically different 'areas'. Considerable progress has been achieved in relating these areas to 'specific' functions, but while conceptually useful, the relationships represent a simplification because they often represent only nodal points of more widespread functional systems with connectivity to other parts of the brain.

Laminar Organisation

A laminar arrangement of neurons is apparent in sections taken from any part of the cortex. Phylogenetically 'old elements', including the *paleocortex* (olfactory cortex) and the *archicortex* (hippocampal formation and dentate gyrus; concerned with memory) are made up of three cellular laminae, but transition into six laminae is seen in the **neocortex** (*neopallium;* or *isocortex,* which refers to its uniform cortical neurogenesis that results in these six laminae) representing the remaining 90% or the majority of the cerebral cortex.

Cellular Laminae of the Neocortex (Fig. 28.1)

 I. The **molecular layer** contains the tips of the apical dendrites of pyramidal cells (see later), and the most distal branches of axons projecting to the cortex from the intralaminar nuclei of the thalamus.
 II. The **outer granular layer** contains small pyramidal and stellate cells (see later).
III. The **outer pyramidal layer** contains medium-sized pyramidal cells and stellate cells.
IV. The **inner granular layer** contains stellate cells receiving afferents from the thalamic relay nuclei. (*Stellate (granule) cells* are especially numerous in the primary somatic sensory cortex, primary visual cortex, and primary auditory cortex, which all receive afferent sensory information. The term *granular cortex* is applied to these areas. In contrast, the primary motor cortex that gives rise to corticospinal and corticobulbar projections contains relatively few stellate cells in lamina IV and prominent pyramidal cells in laminae III

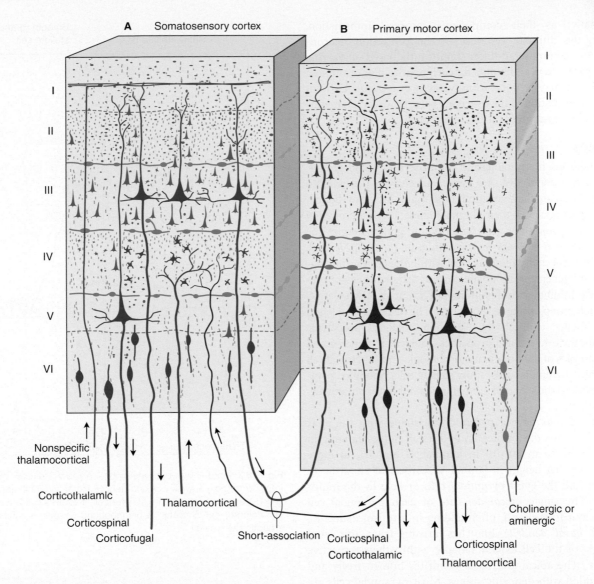

A Somatosensory cortex

B Primary motor cortex

Nonspecific
thalamocortical

Corticothalamic

Corticospinal

Corticofugal

Thalamocortical

Short-association

Corticospinal

Corticothalamic

Corticospinal

Thalamocortical

Cholinergic or
aminergic

Fig. 28.1 Cerebral (Six-Layered) isocortex. (A) Somatosensory cortex and (B) primary motor cortex; cortical laminae I to VI are numbered.

and V, which further obscure individual layers. This area is called the *agranular cortex*.)

V. The ***inner pyramidal layer*** contains large pyramidal cells projecting to the striatum, brainstem, and spinal cord.

VI. The ***fusiform layer*** contains modified pyramidal cells projecting to the thalamus.

Columnar Organisation (Fig. 28.1)

While the laminar organisation of the cerebral cortex is often emphasised, there is also a radial or 'columnar' organisation of these cellular components. This columnar organisation of the neocortex provided the initial conceptual framework to investigate the functionality of its neuronal components in the somatic sensory cortex of animals. This radial grouping of cellular components was felt to represent discrete units with similar physiologic findings and to form the building block for more complex functions. Groups of columns could form modules, characterised by dealing with different aspects of a specific sensory modality or function. It is now clear that columns are not homogeneous across the cortex because multiple characteristics can vary, including their actual cellular constituents and their numbers, ontogeny, synaptic connectivity, and molecular markers, which all contribute to variable functional and stimulus response properties. As an organising principle, the concept of a column is helpful, but it is equally useful to consider the cortex as being organised in both horizontal (laminar) and vertical (radial) dimensions. While not resulting in an analogous structure (column) with visibly discrete edges, this concept is more faithful to the underlying anatomy, observed experimental functionality, and the 'economy' and plasticity that exist within the cortex. Interconnectivity between groups of columns allows more complicated activities, behaviour or cognitive, to emerge.

This underlying 'circuitry' of cortical organisation can result in the cells of each column becoming modality-specific (functionally) as their components 'process' information. However, the ultimate response of the projection neurons within those columns can differ significantly based on varying stimulus parameters and inputs for each neuron. For example, a given column may respond to movement of a particular joint but not to stimulation of the overlying skin; however, if circumstances differ, so may their ultimate response.

Cell Types

Cortical neurons morphologically comprise two broad groups. The majority, 60% to 85%, are *pyramidal neurons* (referring to their shape) that are the sole output (and major input) of the cortex and the rationale for their alternate name, *cortical projection neurons;* their projections are excitatory and glutamatergic. The remaining 15% to 40% are *nonpyramidal* or *interneurons* and, while their connectivity remains local within the cortex, they significantly influence and modulate cortical activity; they are predominantly inhibitory and γ-aminobutyric acid (GABA)ergic. Within each group, multiple subtypes can be distinguished based on morphology, connectivity, electrophysiological properties, cellular lineage, physiologic properties, molecular markers, and so on. Examples of the principal morphologic and functional cell types include pyramidal cells, spiny stellate cells (modified pyramidal cells), and the group of nonpyramidal inhibitory interneurons (Fig. 28.2).

- *Pyramidal cells* have a pyramid-like shape with the apex pointed toward the surface and with cell bodies ranging in height from 20 to 30 μm in laminae II and III, to more than twice that height in lamina V. Largest of all, at 80 to 100 μm, are the *giant pyramidal cells of Betz* in the motor cortex. The single *apical dendrite* of each pyramidal cell reaches out to lamina I, often ending in a tuft of dendrites. Several *basal dendrite* branches arising from the basal 'corners' of the cell extend radially within their respective laminae. The apical and basal dendrites branch freely and are studded with dendritic spines. Most pyramidal cells are found in cortical layers II to III and V to VI. The axons of pyramidal cells arise from their base and give off recurrent branches, capable of exciting neighbouring pyramidal cells, before entering the underlying white matter.
- *Spiny stellate cells* are one type of atypical pyramidal cell, located in lamina IV and abundant in the primary sensory cortex. Their spiny dendrites are limited to lamina IV, but their axons may ascend or descend, making excitatory glutamatergic synaptic contacts with pyramidal cells. They receive most of the thalamic afferent input to lamina IV and likely have a major role in its radial propagation.
- *The nonpyramidal, inhibitory interneurons* share GABA as their neurotransmitter, but otherwise are morphologically heterogeneous and classified in various ways. (Neocortical neurons are represented by a complicated and evolving nomenclature. *Smooth stellate (or granule) cells* are found in all cortical layers; their dendrites radiate in all directions, and their axons form an arborisation locally within that same territory, often referred to as *local plexus neurons.* However, *neurogliaform, chandelier,* and *basket cells* are all considered special classes of stellate cells despite their unique morphologic

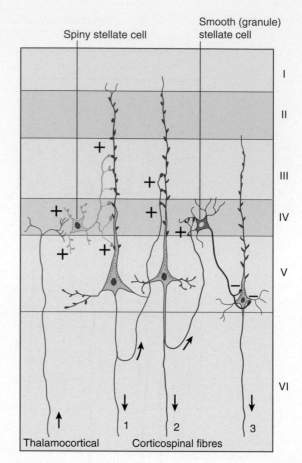

Fig. 28.2 Input–output connections. *Arrows* indicate directions of impulse traffic. *+ and –* signs denote excitation/inhibition. Pyramidal cell 1 is excited by the spiny stellate cell; it excites cell 2 within its own cell column; cell 3 within a neighbouring column is inhibited by the smooth stellate cell.

characteristics. Our only advice is when encountering the term granule or smooth stellate cell, conceptually substitute the word interneuron to guide your reading and comprehension.) For our organisational purposes these cells can be subdivided into three large families based on markers their interneurons express: parvalbumin, somatostatin, and the serotonin (5-hydroxytryptamine; 5HT) 3a receptor (5HT3aR).

- *Parvalbumin-expressing interneurons* have nonspiny dendrites and receive excitatory inputs from the thalamus and cortex but inhibitory inputs from other similar interneurons. They are believed to play a role in stabilising the activity of cortical networks of cells. As is the case in the cerebellar cortex (Chapter 27), these neurons exert a focusing action in the cerebral cortex by silencing weakly active cell columns. *Chandelier cells* (so named because of the candle-shaped clusters of axoaxonic boutons) are most common in lamina II, synapse on the initial axon segment of pyramidal cells, and principally affect cortico–cortical connections. *Basket cells* are predominantly found in laminae II and V, and as their name implies, their axons form pericellular baskets around pyramidal cell bodies, their distal dendrites and axons, and other basket cells (Fig. 28.3).

- **Somatostatin-expressing interneurons** are exemplified by the *Martinotti cells*, located in laminae V and VI, which send their axons into lamina I. Receiving input from pyramidal cells, they can cause lateral restriction of activation and may serve to integrate nonsensory input that results in behaviour-dependent control of dendritic integration of stimuli by their pyramidal cells.

- **5HT3a-expressing interneurons** are a heterogeneous group but represent the most numerous interneurons in superficial cortical laminae. They may have a role in learning through their effects on cortical circuits via their cortical and thalamic inputs. Dendrites of *neurogliaform cells (spiderweb cells)*, one prominent type of interneuron in laminae II and III, spread radially but are unique because they establish synapses with each other and other interneuron types; this suggests a prominent role in synchronising cortical circuits. Another morphologically diverse group of interneurons releases vasoactive intestinal polypeptide (VIP) in addition to GABA; other interneurons in this group coexpress cholecystokinin (CCK) and other peptide receptors.

Afferents

Afferents to a given region of the cortex can be derived from four sources (primarily from the cortex) and have distinctive patterns of termination:

1. Long and short **association fibres** from small- and medium-sized pyramidal cells in laminae II and III in other parts of the ipsilateral cortex.
2. **Commissural fibres** from medium-sized pyramidal cells in laminae II and III project through the corpus callosum from matching or modality-related (homotopic) areas of the opposite hemisphere.
3. **Thalamocortical fibres** from the appropriate specific or association nucleus, for example fibres from the ventral posterior thalamic nucleus to the somatic sensory cortex and from the dorsomedial thalamic nucleus to the *prefrontal* cortex (defined below) terminate in lamina IV. *Nonspecific thalamocortical fibres* from the intralaminar nuclei terminate in all laminae.
4. **Cholinergic and aminergic fibres** from the basal forebrain, hypothalamus, and brainstem. These fibres are represented in *green* in Fig. 28.1, and while they innervate the entire cortex, this does not result in a generalised or nonspecific response. Their anatomic specificity (cortical, laminar, and cell) results in activation or inhibition of limited collections of neurons. The relevant nuclei of origin, and the transmitters/modulators involved, are:
   - nucleus basalis of Meynert (basal forebrain nuclei), acetylcholine;
   - tuberomammillary nucleus (posterior hypothalamus), histamine;
   - substantia nigra pars compacta (ventral midbrain tegmentum), dopamine;

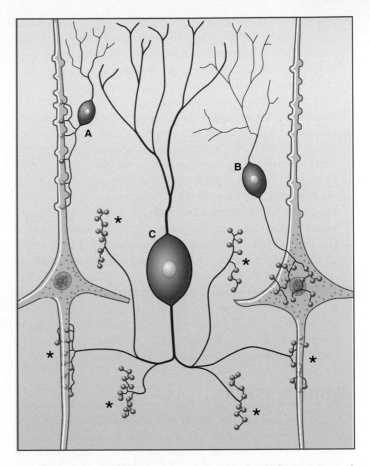

Fig. 28.3 Three morphologic types of gabaergic inhibitory neuron. *A*, Axodendritic cell, synapsing upon the shaft of the apical dendrite of a pyramidal cell; *B*, basket cell, forming axosomatic synapses on a pyramidal cell; *C*, chandelier cell, forming axoaxonic synapses *(*)* upon the initial segments of the two pyramidal cell axons shown, and upon four other initial segments not shown. (Based on DeFelipe J. Chandelier cells and epilepsy. *Brain*. 1999;122:1807–1822, with permission.)

- raphe nuclei (midbrain and rostral pons), serotonin;
- locus coeruleus (rostral pons), norepinephrine.

These five sets of neurons are of particular relevance to psychiatry and are considered in Chapter 33.

Efferents

All efferents from the cerebral cortex are axons of pyramidal cells, and all are excitatory in nature. Axons of some pyramidal cells contribute to short or long association fibres; others form commissural or projection fibres; association and commissural fibres make up the bulk of white matter of the cerebral hemisphere.

- Examples of short association fibre pathways (which pass between adjacent cortical areas through the superficial white matter as *U fibres*) are those entering the motor cortex from the sensory cortex and vice versa (Fig. 28.1). Examples of long association fibre pathways are projections between the *prefrontal cortex* (cortex anterior to the motor areas) and sensory association areas. Pyramidal cells that primarily reside in laminae II and III are the source of these fibres.

- The commissural fibres of the brain are *entirely* composed of pyramidal cell axons running through the corpus callosum and posterior and anterior commissures (and in other, minor commissures) to corresponding cortical areas in the opposite hemisphere (e.g. the primary cortical area projecting to its equivalent contralateral association area) and noncorresponding areas. (These commissural connections are lacking between the primary visual cortex (area 17) and the primary somatosensory and motor cortex representing the distal part of the upper limb.) Pyramidal cells that primarily reside in laminae II and III are the source of these fibres.

- Projection fibres from the primary sensory and motor cortex form the largest input to the basal ganglia (Chapter 26). The thalamus receives projection fibres from all parts of the cortex. Other major projection systems are corticopontine (to the ipsilateral pontine nuclei), corticonuclear (to contralateral motor and somatic sensory cranial nerve nuclei in the pons and medulla), and corticospinal. Pyramidal cells that primarily reside in laminae V and VI (preferentially projecting to specific thalamic relay nuclei) are the source of these fibres.

CORTICAL AREAS

The most widely used reference map is that of Brodmann, who divided the cortex into 44 areas (his numbering scheme extended to 52, but not all numbers were used) based on cytoarchitectonic characteristics. Most of these areas are shown in Fig. 28.4, but 'sharp' borders between areas do not exist. (These numbers are often used to refer to functional areas, although Brodmann rejected any such correlation.) Coloured in Fig. 28.4 are the three principal primary sensory areas (somatic, visual, and auditory) and the single primary motor area. The adjacent cortex to each primary sensory or motor cortical area is the association cortex referred to as the *unimodal association area* (same modality). The rest of the neocortex consists of *multimodal (polymodal) association areas* receiving fibres from more than one unimodal association area (e.g. receiving tactile and visual inputs, or visual and auditory) and other multimodal or paralimbic areas.

Investigating Functional Anatomy

The term *connectome* was coined to represent a 'comprehensive map of neural connections whose purpose is to illuminate brain function'. However, the desire to develop a complete functional map of the human brain necessitates collection of empirically derived data on that structural connectivity, but much remains unknown. Contemporary approaches are providing unique opportunities to achieve this goal through advances in computing capabilities and data storage, neuropsychologic testing, and magnetic resonance imaging (MRI) capabilities that allow imaging of the living human brain.

These new advances in understanding the brain are accompanied by a shift from looking at individual areas of the cortex to considering all areas and their interactions at once. New methodical or theoretical frameworks have been deployed to

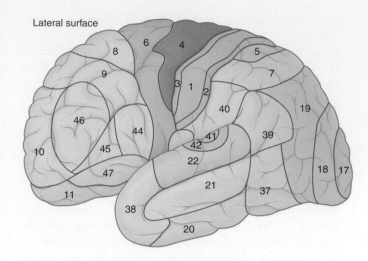

Lateral surface

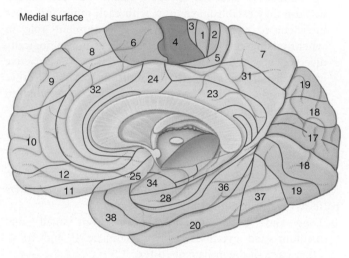

Medial surface

Fig. 28.4 Cytoarchitectural areas of brodmann. Coloured areas indicate motor *(red)*, *4*, primary motor cortex; *6 on medial surface*, supplementary motor area; *6 on lateral surface*, premotor cortex, and Sensory *(blue)*, *3/1/2*, primary somatic sensory cortex; *40*, secondary somatic sensory cortex; *17*, primary visual cortex; *18, 19*, visual association cortex; *41, 42*, primary auditory cortex*; *22*, auditory association cortex. (*The primary auditory cortex is not in fact visible from the side, being entirely on the *upper* surface of the superior temporal gyrus.)

describe and predict these complex system dynamics using *network analysis* and a mathematical approach based on *graph theory*. Network models use collections of 'elementary' cortical units and their connections to demonstrate how functions can emerge dynamically or 'capture the brain in action'. These models remain limited by the known connections between areas, but some connections are inferred to exist based on primate studies. However, models may also predict functional relationships unsupported by a known structural basis or pathways predicted to exist based on a performed behaviour. While imaging of living brain pathways and connectivity will advance through the use of these neuroradiologic techniques and mathematical modelling, the development of new and continued use of 'old' techniques of neuroanatomy are required to provide the structural evidence for these emerging pathways and systems of cortical activation.

Two dominant methods are in use for 'identification and localisation' of functions in the human brain. Both techniques depend upon the local increases in blood flow that meet the additional oxygen demand imposed by localised neural activity.

Positron Emission Tomography. *Positron emission tomography (PET)* measures oxygen consumption following injection of water labelled with oxygen-15 (^{15}O) into a forearm vein. ^{15}O is a positron-emitting isotope of oxygen; the positrons react with nearby electrons in the blood to create γ rays, which are counted by γ-ray detectors. Alternatively, fluorine-18-labelled deoxyglucose (^{18}F-deoxyglucose) may be used to measure glucose consumption. ^{18}F-deoxyglucose is taken up by neurons as readily as glucose.

Image subtraction and *image averaging* are required for meaningful interpretation of PET studies, as explained in the caption to Fig. 28.5, and a similar signal extraction process is deployed in functional MRI (fMRI).

For specialised investigations, radiolabelled drugs are used to quantify receptor function, for example, radiolabelled dopamine in the corpus striatum in relation to Parkinson disease (Chapter 26); radiolabelled serotonin in the brainstem and cortex in relation to depression (Chapter 34); and radiolabelled acetylcholinesterase in relation to Alzheimer disease (Chapter 34).

Functional Magnetic Resonance Imaging (fMRI). Does not require introduction of any extraneous material. It depends upon the different magnetic properties of oxygenated versus deoxygenated blood. As it happens, the local increases in blood flow are more than sufficient to meet oxygen demands, and it is the increase in the ratio of oxyhaemoglobin to deoxyhaemoglobin that is exploited to generate the MRI signal. Functional and structural connectivity can be demonstrated as the fMRI signal changes covary or fluctuate together in various cortical areas, even in the absence of 'direct' cortical links. The discussion that follows is based on the findings of such functional imaging, clinical observations, and insights from nonhuman studies.

SENSORY AREAS

Somatic Sensory Cortex (Areas 3, 1, 2)

Components. The somatic sensory or *somaesthetic* cortex occupies the entire postcentral gyrus (Fig. 28.6). Representation of contralateral body parts is inverted (except for the face) and the hand, lips, and tongue have disproportionately large representations. The familiar homunculus diagrams shown in Fig. 28.6A and B are only intended to serve as schematic representations of different parts of the body and ignore the extensive overlap of those representations.

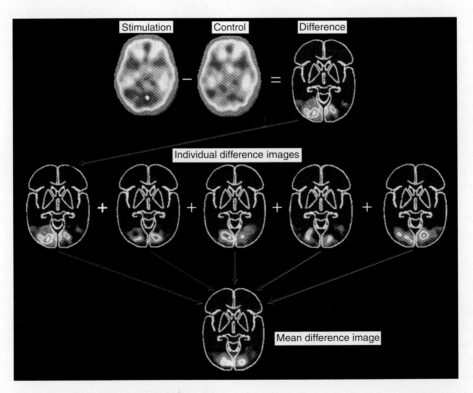

Fig. 28.5 Image subtraction and image averaging in positron emission tomography (pet) scans. *Top:* The middle image is from a control mode, where the subject lies at rest. Uptake of ^{15}O is active throughout the cortex and subcortical grey matter. The left image is from the same subject staring at dots moving on a screen. The high level of background activity obscures the effect. The right image is produced by subtracting the control value to reveal the additional activity in the visual cortex produced by the staring task. *Middle:* Four other subjects have performed the same task. Subtraction of background 'noise' reveals varying differences among the five. Because brains vary in size between individuals, activities in all five brains have been projected onto a common, 'average' brain (hence the identical brain profiles in this row). *Bottom:* A mean value for the five brains produces a 'mean difference image' representative of the five as a group. (Modified from Posner and Raichle: Images of the mind, New York, 1994, Sci. Amer. Library, p. 65.)

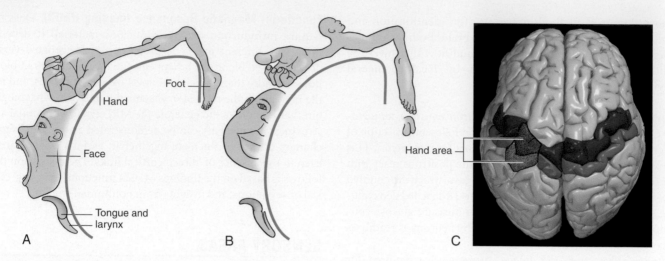

Foot

Hand

Face

Tongue and larynx

A

B

Hand area

C

Fig. 28.6 (A) Figure (modified from Penfield and Rasmussen, 1950) depicting the inverted disposition of the motor homunculus in the left precentral gyrus excepting the face. Overlap among body part representations is not shown. (B) Figure (modified from Penfield and Rasmussen, 1950) depicting the inverted disposition of the sensory homunculus in the left postcentral gyrus excepting the face. Overlap among body part representations is not shown. (C) The primary motor cortex *(red)* and primary somatosensory cortex *(blue)* viewed from above. The relatively larger representation of the motor and sensory areas in the left hemisphere is typical of right-handed individuals. (Modified from Kretschmann HJ, Weinrich W. Neurofunctional Systems: 3D Reconstructions with Correlated Neuroimaging: Text and CD-ROM, New York, 1998, Thieme.)

In a vertical section (Fig. 28.7C) the somesthetic cortex is divisible into areas 3, 1, and 2. Area 3 (divided into smaller area 3a and larger area 3b) receives thalamocortical projections (from the ventroposterior medial and lateral nuclei), and to a lesser extent, areas 1 and 2 share similar projections. Cutaneous receptor input is segregated, and rapidly adapting projections dominate area 1; area 2 is more complex having both cutaneous and noncutaneous receptors. Receptor field size and organisation becomes more complex on moving from area 3b to 1. Areas 3 (3a is usually included in the motor cortex), 1, and 2 are considered as *primary somatosensory cortex (S1)*, but area 3b alone more clearly 'deserves' the distinction as primary. Functional properties of sensory cortex neurons are neither fixed (especially in the associative cortex) nor just extracting relevant sensory information but organising that information with respect to the current context or situation. This contextual processing allows flexible, goal-oriented behaviour to emerge; repeated processing leads to learning.

Afferents. In addition to thalamic afferents from the ventral posterior nucleus (Fig. 28.7B), the somesthetic cortex receives commissural fibres from the opposite somatic sensory cortex through the corpus callosum and short association fibres from the adjacent primary motor cortex. Many of the fibres from the motor cortex are collaterals of corticospinal fibres travelling to the ventral horn of the spinal cord, and they may contribute to the sense of weight (*baragnosia* is a loss of this sensation) when an object is lifted.

It is not unusual for the somesthetic cortex to be compromised by occlusion of a branch of the middle cerebral artery supplying the sensory cortex. *Cortical-type sensory loss* in such cases is shown by a reduction in sensory acuity on the opposite side of the body, especially in the forearm and hand (evidenced by a raised sensory threshold, poor two-point discrimination,

and impaired vibration and position sense), but also in the recognition of more complex stimuli despite touch, pain, temperature, and even vibration sense remaining intact. This can manifest as inability to recognise common objects placed in the hand (*astereognosis*), inability to identify numbers traced onto the palm (*agraphesthesia*), or inability to recognise two tactile stimuli applied simultaneously to bilateral, opposite parts of the body (*extinction*). Loss of ability to recognise the size and shape of objects because of deficits between sensory receptors and up to the cortex is referred to as *stereoanaesthesia*. Complex clinical deficits are observed with parietal injuries usually of the nondominant hemisphere (more often right), which together are called *agnosias* (*tactile agnosia*, inability to recognise shape by tactile stimuli alone; *anosognosia*, denial of illness or deficit; and *autopagnosia*, inability to identify, orient, or recognise body parts). Parietal injuries (more often left) may also result in an *apraxia*, or the inability to carry out a purposeful skilled act or to use an object appropriately despite otherwise normal motility and comprehension.

Efferents. Efferents from the somesthetic cortex comprise association, commissural, and projection fibres. *Association fibres* pass to the ipsilateral motor cortex, to area 5 and to area 40 (the supramarginal gyrus). *Commissural fibres* pass to the contralateral somesthetic cortex. *Projection fibres* descend within the posterior part of the pyramidal tract (PT) and terminate upon interneurons in sensory relay nuclei, namely the ventral posterior nucleus of the thalamus of the same side, and the dorsal column and spinal dorsal grey horn of the opposite side. As explained in Chapter 15, sensory transmission in the spinothalamic pathway may be suppressed (via inhibitory interneurons) during vigorous activities such as running, whereas in the dorsal column—medial lemniscal pathway (DCML), transmission may be enhanced (via excitatory interneurons) during exploratory activities such as palpation of textured surfaces.

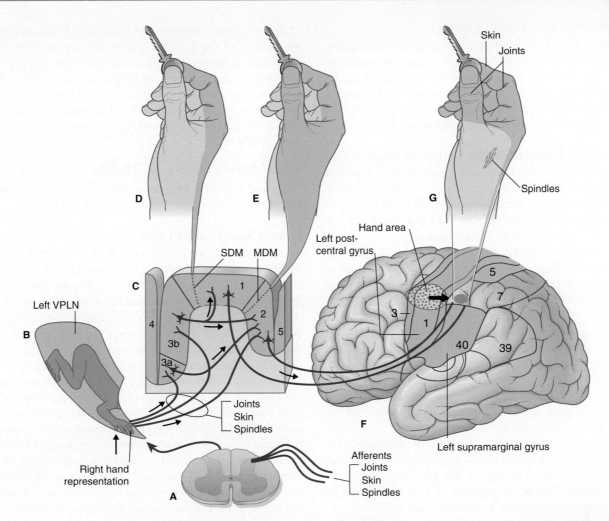

Fig. 28.7 Sensory sequence enabling identification of a key by touch alone. (A) Coded sensory information from the right hand enters the spinal cord through the medial part of the dorsal root entry zone and ascends in the fasciculus cuneatus of the dorsal column pathway in the cervical spinal cord to synapse in the nucleus cuneatus in the medulla oblongata on the same side. Second-order axons from the nucleus cuneatus cross in the sensory decussation (internal arcuate fibres) and ascend as the medial lemniscus to reach the thalamus. (B) The hand area of the ventral posterior lateral nucleus *(VPLN)* of the thalamus contains somas of third-order sensory neurons. (C) The third-order neurons project to areas 3, 1 (indirectly), and 2 of the somatic sensory cortex. (D) *SDM*, 'single' digit cortical module. (E) *MDM*, 'multi' digit cortical module. (F) Surface view of the left parietal lobe (hatched area indicates the hand area). Area 7 receives short association fibres from areas 1, 2, and 5 and integrates information from (G) skin, muscle spindles, and joint capsules. Connections with tactile memory stores in area 7 and in area 5 enable an image of the key to be perceived without the aid of vision.

Somatic Sensory Association Area (Area 5)

This term is used with respect to area 5, directly behind the somatic sensory cortex. Most of the area is active during reaching movements of the contralateral arm taking place under visual guidance (the *dorsal visual pathway* is discussed later).

Superior Parietal Lobule (Area 7)

Clinically, the term *superior parietal lobule* is equated with area 7. The *lower* part of area 7 receives inputs from areas 1, 2, and 5. Receipt of tactile and proprioceptive information from skin, muscles, and joints causes area 7 to tap into its own 'memory' stores concerning the recognition of objects held in the (opposite) hand, whereby an unseen object can be identified (Fig. 28.7).

The *upper* part of area 7 contains a cell station in the 'Where?' visual pathway (see later).

Inferior Parietal Lobule (Areas 39 and 40)

The inferior parietal lobule comprises areas 39 (angular gyrus) and 40 (supramarginal gyrus). Both are concerned with language, a mainly left hemisphere function described in Chapter 32; disturbance of language caused by a brain lesion is *aphasia*. (Lesions in the right hemisphere may result in the inability to understand or use emotions in oral language, *aprosodia*.)

Intraparietal Cortex

The cortex in the walls of the intraparietal sulcus is especially active during tasks involving visuomotor coordination, such as reaching for and grasping objects identified in the contralateral visual field and subjecting them to simultaneous visual and tactile three-dimensional analysis. This area includes the parietal eye field (see later).

Secondary Somatic Sensory Area

On the medial surface of the parietal operculum of the insula is a small *secondary somatic sensory area (SII)*. It receives a nociceptive projection from the thalamus, and it is highlighted during PET scans of the brain during peripheral painful stimulation (Chapter 25). SII also appears to collaborate with SI in aspects of tactile discrimination or localisation of painful stimuli.

Plasticity of the Somatic Sensory Cortex. In monkeys, cortical sensory representations of the individual digits of the hand can be defined very exactly by recording the electrical response of cortical cell columns to tactile stimulation of each digit in turn. These digital maps can be altered by peripheral sensory experience, as the following experiments indicate:

- The median nerve supplies the ventral surface of the outer three and a half digits of the hand, whereas the radial nerve supplies their dorsal surfaces. If the median nerve is crushed, the representation of the dorsal surface on the digital map increases at the expense of the ventral representation. The increase begins within hours and progresses slowly over a period of weeks. With regeneration of the median nerve, the cortical map reverts to normal.
- If the middle digit is denervated, the corresponding cortical area is unresponsive for a few hours then becomes progressively (over weeks) taken over by expansion of the representations of the second and fourth digits.
- If the pad skin of a digit is chronically stimulated, for example by having to press a rotating sanded disc to release pellets of food, representation of the pad may increase to twice its original size over a period of weeks, reverting to normal after the experiment is discontinued.

These experiments show that somatic sensory maps are *plastic*, being modified by peripheral events. A purely anatomic explanation (e.g. sprouting of nerve branches within the central nervous system, or peripherally) is not appropriate for the earliest changes, which begin within hours. Instead they can be accounted for based on sensory competition.

Sensory Competition. Sensory maps made at the level of the dorsal grey horn, dorsal column nuclei, thalamus, and somesthetic cortex all show evidence of anatomic overlap. For example, the thalamocortical somesthetic projection for the third digit overlaps the projections for the second and fourth digits. Within the zone of overlap, cortical columns are shared by afferents from two adjacent digits. Cortical interneurons can exert lateral inhibition upon weakly stimulated columns. Under experimental conditions (e.g. in cats), the number of columns responding to a particular thalamocortical input can be increased by local infusion of a GABA antagonist drug (bicuculline), which suppresses lateral inhibition. The effect of removal of a peripheral sensory field may be comparable; if one set of thalamocortical neurons falls silent owing to loss of sensory input, it no longer exerts lateral inhibition and cortical columns within its territory are 'taken over' by neighbouring, active sets. These synaptic connections between cells are subject to both long-term and short-term modifications during development and are also a reflection of learning.

In the human somatosensory body map, the digits are represented next to the face. In several well-documented cases of upper limb amputation, patients had later experiences of 'phantom finger' sensations on touching their face on that side with an implement such as a comb held in the other hand. This illusion may occur within 2 weeks of amputation. This can be explained based on the unmasking of preexisting overlap of thalamocortical neurons.

Visual Cortex (Areas 17, 18, 19)

The visual cortex comprises the *primary visual cortex* (area 17) and the *visual association cortex* (areas 18 and 19).

Primary Visual Cortex (Area 17). As noted in Chapter 31, the primary visual cortex is the target of the geniculocalcarine tract, which relays information from the ipsilateral halves of both retinas, and therefore from the contralateral visual field. This myelinated tract creates a pale *visual stria* *(line of Gennari)* within the primary visual cortex before synapsing upon spiny stellate cells of the highly granular lamina IV. The visual stria (first noted by medical student Francesco Gennari circa 1775) has provided the alternative name, *striate cortex*, for area 17.

The spiny stellate cells belong to *ocular dominance columns*, so named because alternating columns are dominated by inputs from the left and right eyes (Chapter 31). If the input of each eye could be separately marked and the visual cortex viewed from the surface, this alternating columnar arrangement would form bands in the form of whorls (resembling fingerprints), and each alternating band would respond to the input of one or the other eye. The geniculocalcarine projection is so ordered that matching points from the two retinas are registered side by side in contiguous columns. This arrangement is ideal for binocular vision because collections of these columns form modules, and the edge responds to inputs from both eyes.

The nondiscriminative inputs from the lateral geniculate nucleus are 'transformed' into a range of properties within the primary visual cortex, lamina VI. This occurs through the arrangement of neurons within lamina VI into functional columns. The wiring of these neurons results in the appearance of specific sensitivity to contour, direction of motion, size, and orientation of visual stimuli; distinctly demonstrated in Fig. 28.8. Complex interpretations emerge through further cortical connectivity.

Plasticity of the Primary Visual Cortex. The basic pattern and balance of ocular dominance columns are established before birth and preserved in animals reared in complete darkness. If one eye is deprived of sensory experience in childhood, the corresponding cortical columns remain small and those from the visually experienced eye become larger than normal.

Visual Association Cortex (Areas 18 and 19). The visual association cortex comprises areas 18 and 19, which are also conjointly called the *peristriate* or *extrastriate* cortex (Fig. 28.4). Afferents are received mainly from area 17 but they include some direct thalamic projections from the pulvinar. The cell columns are concerned with *feature extraction*. Some columns

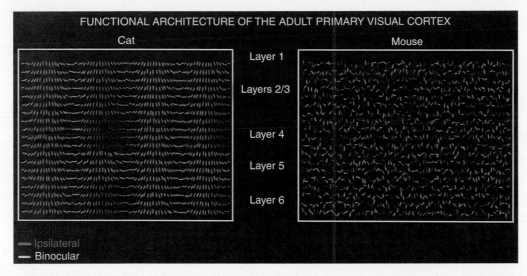

Fig. 28.8 Representation of the selectivity of neurons in the primary visual cortex (v1) that receive inputs from the lateral geniculate nucleus. Recordings from neurons in the adult cat *(left)* consist of neurons highly selective for specific orientations (denoted by the angle of the lines) and dominated to varying degrees by the contralateral *(red)* or ipsilateral *(green)* eye, with many cells driven by both eyes *(yellow)*. Both orientation and ocular dominance (neurons responding better to stimulation of one eye or the other) properties are organised into columns. Preferred orientation columns span all cortical layers, while ocular dominance is most pronounced in layer 4, where many cells are driven monocularly. The mouse V1 *(right)* does not have columnar organisation of orientation or ocular dominance. However, neurons are still highly orientation-selective and display a range of ocular dominance, but with a bias toward the contralateral eye. (Legend is modified from and the figure is reproduced from Espinosa JG, Stryker MP. Development and plasticity of the primary visual cortex, *Neuron.* 2012;75:230–249, with the kind permission of the authors and publishers.)

respond to geometric shapes, some respond to colour, some to stereopsis (depth perception), and some to more complex representations such as facial recognition.

Many of the peristriate columns have large receptive fields. Some of these straddle the physiologic 'blind spot' (optic nerve head) and may be responsible for 'covering up' the blind spot during monocular vision.

The projection from the pulvinar to the visual association cortex is considered part of the pathway involved in 'blindsight' (residual visual processing after destruction of the primary visual cortex). This remarkable condition has been observed in patients following thrombosis of the calcarine branch of the posterior cerebral artery. Although blindness in the contralateral field appears complete, these patients are nonetheless able to point to a moving spot of light—without any perception of it—merely a 'feeling' that it is there. The actual anatomic pathway concerned remains unclear, but visual input via the medial root of the optic tract or superior colliculus, and from the pulvinar to the association visual cortex or from the lateral geniculate nucleus to the cortex are possibilities.

The most functionally advanced visual association modules occupy the lateral and medial parts of area 19. The lateral set of modules is colloquially described as belonging to a dorsal, 'Where?' visual pathway. The medial set belongs to a ventrally placed, 'What?' pathway; both pathways operate in parallel and should not be considered dichotomous.

The 'Where?' Visual Pathway (Fig. 28.9). Consistent with electrical recordings taken from alert monkeys, PET scans of human volunteers reveal the lateral part of area 19 to be especially responsive to *movement* taking place in the contralateral

visual hemifield. The main projection from this area is to area 7, known to clinicians as the *posterior parietal cortex.* In addition to movement perception, area 7 is involved in *stereopsis* (three-dimensional vision), which with *spatial sense* is defined as perception of the position of objects in relation to one another.

Area 7 receives 'blindsight' fibres from the pulvinar, and it projects via the superior longitudinal fasciculus to the ipsilateral frontal eye field and premotor cortex (PMC).

In monkeys, cell columns in area 7 are activated when a significant object (e.g. fruit) appears in the contralateral visual hemifield. Through association fibres, the active cell columns increase the resting firing rate of columns in the frontal eye field and PMC, but without producing movement. The effect is called *covert attention,* or *covert orientation.* It becomes *overt* when the animal responds with a saccade (high velocity conjugate eye movement) with or without a reaching movement directed toward the object. Following a lesion to area 7, the motor responses to significant targets occur late, and reaching movements of the contralateral arm are inaccurate.

In human volunteers, PET scans show increased cortical metabolism in area 7 in response to object movement in the contralateral visual hemifield. During reaching of the opposite arm toward an object, areas 5 and 7 are both active. In humans (as in monkeys), a lesion that includes area 7 is associated with clumsy, inaccurate reaching into the contralateral visual hemifield. The 'Where?' system is also a 'How?' system because visuospatial information is used by the motor system to guide movement.

In volunteers, two additional areas of cortex become active when items of special interest appear. Shown in Fig. 28.9, and mentioned again later, is the *dorsolateral prefrontal cortex*

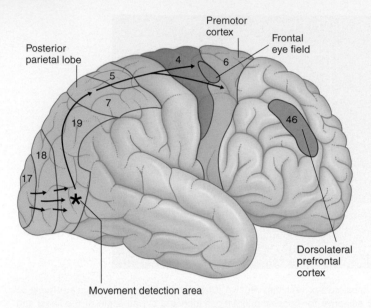

Fig. 28.9 Lateral surface of right hemisphere, showing the 'where?' visual pathway from the visual cortex to the parietal and frontal lobes. The *asterisk* marks the area for detection of movement in the left visual field. Activity of the right frontal eye field facilitates a saccade toward the left visual field.

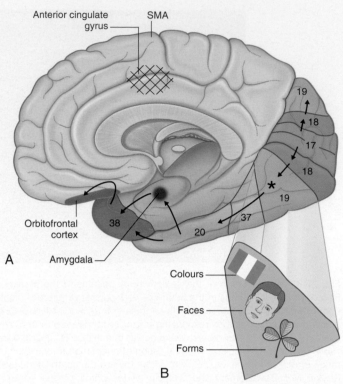

Fig. 28.10 (A) Medial view of right hemisphere, showing the 'what?' pathway. The *asterisk* marks the visual identification area within the fusiform gyrus on the inferior surface. Ventral area 19 is enlarged in (B). *SMA*, Supplementary motor area.

(DLPFC; roughly corresponding to Brodmann area 46), a significant decision-making area, notably in relation to an *approach* or *withdraw* decision. Shown in Fig. 28.10 is a patch in the cortex of the anterior cingulate gyrus. This area is considered in Chapter 33, but it may be mentioned here that it is activated by the dorsolateral cortex when subjects are *paying attention* to a visual task.

The 'What?' Visual Pathway (Fig. 28.10).

The ventral visual pathway converges onto the anteromedial part of area 19, mainly within the fusiform gyrus part of the occipitotemporal gyrus (Fig. 2.5). This region is concerned with three kinds of visual identification (neurons within these areas further integrate these visual features with nonsensory cognitive and behavioural variables), indicated in Fig. 28.10B:

- Relatively lateral are modules activated by the *forms* (shapes) of objects of all kinds, including the shapes of letters. It is regarded as a centre for generic (categorical/canonical) object identification (e.g. a dog *as such*, without connotation).
- In the mid-region are modules specifically devoted to the generic identification of human faces.
- Relatively medial is the *colour recognition area*, essential for recognition of all colours except black and white. A state of *achromatopsia* (colour blindness can result from dysfunction of any part of the visual pathway) may occur following a sustained fall in blood pressure within both posterior cerebral arteries, for example, caused by an embolus blocking the top of the parent basilar artery, resulting in cerebral infarction. Such patients see everything only in black and white (grey scale).

Recognition of individual objects and faces is a function of the anterior part of the 'What?' pathway in the *inferotemporal cortex* (area 20) and in the cortex of the temporal pole (area 38). These two areas are engaged during identification of, for example, *Mary's* face or *my* dog. Failure of facial recognition (a type of agnosia called *prosopagnosia*) is a frequent and distressing feature of Alzheimer disease (Chapter 33), where the patient may cease to recognise family members despite retaining the sense of familiarity of common objects.

Threatening sights or faces cause areas 20 and 38 to activate the *amygdala*, especially in the right hemisphere; the right amygdala in turn activates the fear-associated *right orbitofrontal cortex*, the purple area in Fig. 28.10A (Chapter 33).

How might visual association areas become activated, such as in execution of a decision to look for an apple in a bowl of mixed fruit, or for a particular word in a page of text? In PET studies the frontal lobe is active whenever attention is being paid to a task at hand. The DLPFC is particularly active during visual tasks involving form and colour. During visual searching, the role of the frontal lobe seems to be to activate memory stores within the visual association areas, so that the relevant memories are held online during the search. The anterior part of the cingulate cortex is also active. Just as information is 'passed' from the primary to the visual associative cortex of the dorsal and ventral pathways, there is also a 'top-down' process that allows cognition and behavioural states (e.g. attention and expectation) to interact with earlier steps of visual processing.

This allows the visual scene to become stable despite continuous eye movements (an internal model of the external world that is kept in alignment by vestibular, somatosensory, and visual input) and facilitates interpretation of the visual scene and attributes different meanings depending on the behavioural context.

The V1 to V5 Nomenclature. Specialists in vision research use the following designations in relation to cortical visual processing:

V1 equates with Brodmann area 17.

V2 and V3 equate with Brodmann areas 18 and 19, respectively.

V4 includes the three sets of identification modules in the fusiform gyrus (anteromedial Brodmann area 19), the 'What?' visual pathway.

V5 equates with the movement detection modules in the lateral occipital cortex (anterolateral Brodmann area 19), the 'Where?' visual pathway.

Auditory Cortex (Areas 41, 42, 22)

The *primary auditory cortex* occupies the anterior transverse temporal gyrus of Heschl, described in Chapter 20. The Heschl gyrus corresponds to areas 41 and 42 on the upper surface of the superior temporal gyrus; most of the input from the medial geniculate body projects to area 41. Columnar organisation in the primary auditory cortex has been suggested to take the form of *isofrequency stripes*, each stripe responding to a particular tonal frequency. Higher frequencies activate lateral stripes in the Heschl gyrus, and lower frequencies activate medial stripes. Because of incomplete crossover of the central auditory pathway in the brainstem (Chapter 20), *each ear is represented bilaterally*. In experimental recordings the primary cortex responds equally well from both ears in response to monaural stimulation, but the contralateral cortex is more responsive during simultaneous binaural stimulation.

The auditory association cortex corresponds to area 22, for speech perception (considered in Chapter 32). Visual and auditory data are brought together in the polymodal cortex bordering the superior temporal sulcus (junction of areas 21 and 22).

Excision of the entire auditory cortex on one side (in the course of removal of a tumour) has no obvious effect on auditory perception. The only significant defect is loss of *stereoacusis*; on testing, the patient has difficulty in appreciating the direction and the distance of a source of sound.

MOTOR AREAS

Primary Motor Cortex

The primary motor cortex (area 4) is a strip of agranular cortex within the precentral gyrus. It gives rise to 60% to 80% (estimates vary) of the corticospinal tract (CST). The remaining fibres originate in the premotor, cingulate, supplementary motor areas, and parietal cortex, as illustrated in Chapter 16. The densest terminations of the CST within the spinal cord are in those areas that will innervate distal muscles of the extremities.

There is an inverted somatotopic representation of contralateral body parts except the face, with relatively large areas devoted to the hand (important for control of fine finger movements), circumoral region, and tongue (Fig. 28.6A). The hand area can usually be identified as a backward projecting knob 6 to 7 cm from the upper margin of the hemisphere.

Ipsilateral body parts are also represented in the somatotopic map, ipsilateral motor neurons being supplied by the 10% of PT fibres that remain uncrossed but are unlikely to innervate distal limb muscles.

Direct stimulation of the human motor cortex indicates that the cell columns control *movement direction*. The primary motor cortex 'synthesises' movement commands but is not where the commands originate. The primary motor cortex's projections are transmitted to the spinal cord through CST fibres, which branch extensively as they approach their targets. The act of picking up a pen, for example, requires a moderate contraction of opponens pollicis as prime mover, a matching level of contraction of the portion of flexor digitorum profundus providing the tendon to the terminal phalanx of the index finger, and lesser levels of contraction of adductor and flexor brevis pollicis. Steadying the upper limb as a whole during any kind of manipulative activity is a function of the PMC (see later) and reflects the importance of unconscious postural adjustments associated with voluntary movements. Larger cortical motor areas are also formed where adjoining columns of neurons are 'grouped' with respect to function and the production of complex movement sequences (Fig. 28.11).

Plasticity in the Motor Cortex. In monkeys and in lower mammals, small lesions of the motor cortex produce an initial paralysis of the corresponding body part, followed within a few days (sometimes within hours) by progressive recovery. The recovery is attributable to a change of allegiance of cell columns close to the lesion, which take on the missing motor function. Instead of inflicting a lesion, it is possible to enlarge the motor territory of a patch of cortex merely by injecting a GABA antagonist drug locally into the cortex. Expansion of motor territories at spinal cord level is already provided for by extensive overlap of projections from area 4 to the motor cell columns in the ventral grey horn, but the degree of plasticity is less than in the cortex. Connections between the CST (and other descending tracts) and motor neurons in the spinal cord occur through interneurons. These interneurons integrate sensory and cortical information that results in a specific and orderly activation of motor neuron pools and the muscles that they innervate.

Sources of Afferents to the Primary Motor Cortex

1. *The opposite motor cortex,* through the corpus callosum. The strongest commissural linkages are between matching cell columns that control the vertebral and abdominal musculature. This is to be expected since these muscle groups routinely act bilaterally in maintaining the upright position of the trunk and head. The weakest commissural linkages are between cell columns controlling the distal limb muscles, where the two sides tend to act independently.

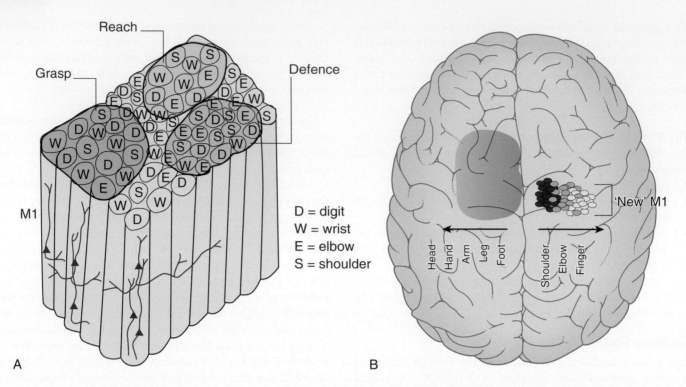

Fig. 28.11 (A) Proposed functional organisation of the hand—forearm segment of the primary motor cortex *(M1)* in monkeys and other primates. Although the M1 has an overall somatotopy, the local somatotopy is fractured to form a mosaic of radial rows of neurons that evoke small, specific movements. Minicolumns for digit movement may adjoin those for wrist, elbow, or shoulder movements, and subsets of these minicolumns are grouped to function in the production of more complex movement sequences, such as grasping, reaching, or defending the head against a blow. (Legend is modified from and the figure is reproduced from Levine AJ, et al. Spatial organization of cortical and spinal neurons controlling motor behaviour. *Curr Opin Neurobiol.* 2012;22:812—821, with the kind permission of the authors and publishers.) (B) Spatial organisation of primate motor cortical cells that control movement of muscle groups. Cells are located in a medial-to-lateral progression of foot, leg, arm, hand, and head *(blue)*. Within the caudal portion of M1 are corticomotoneurons that directly reach motor neurons and are suited to control highly precise movements that subserve fine motor skills. These neurons are organised in a medial-to-lateral progression of proximal *(red)* to distal *(yellow)* muscle targets. The authors referred to this region as a 'new M1', subdivision of the 'old M1' region *(blue)*, to reflect the recent appearance of this refined form of motor activity and an evolutionally 'new' region of motor cortex. (Legend is modified from and the figure is reproduced from Kaas JH. Evolution of columns, modules, and domains in the neocortex of primates, *Proc Natl Acad Sci USA.* 2012;109(Suppl 1):10655—10660, with the kind permission of the authors and publishers.)

2. ***Somatosensory cortex.*** *Cutaneous* cell columns in areas 1, 2, and 3 feed forward via short association fibres. (Linkages for the hand are especially numerous; the distance is short because the hand areas of the motor and somatic sensory cortex mainly occupy the corresponding walls of the central sulcus.) *Proprioceptive* cell columns receive afferent relays from the annulospiral endings of muscle spindles; they send short association fibres to the corresponding motor columns for execution of the long-loop stretch reflex (Chapter 16).

3. ***Contralateral dentate nucleus.*** The cerebellum assists in the selection of appropriate muscles for synergic activities, and in the timing and strength of their contractions.

4. ***Supplementary motor area (SMA).***

Premotor Cortex

The PMC (area 6 on the lateral surface of the hemisphere) is about six times larger than the primary motor cortex. It receives cognitive inputs from the frontal lobe in the context of motor intentions, and a rich sensory input from the parietal lobe (area 7) incorporating tactile and visuospatial signals. It is especially active when motor routines are run in response to visual or somatic sensory cues, such as reaching for an object in full view or identifying an object out of sight by manipulation. The PMC is usually active bilaterally if at all. One explanation is the need for interhemispheric transfer of motor plans through the corpus callosum. It is also the case that the PMC has a major projection to the brainstem nuclei that give origin to the reticulospinal tracts (and a minor one to the CST). Lesions confined to the human PMC are rare, but they are characterised by postural instability of the contralateral shoulder and hip. A significant function of the PMC therefore seems to be that of bilateral postural fixation, for example, to fixate the shoulders during bimanual tasks and to stabilise the hips during walking. The PMC may contribute to recovery of function in cases of pure motor hemiplegia (Chapter 35) following a vascular lesion confined to the CST within the corona radiata. The PMC shows increased activity on PET scans following such a lesion; the cortico—reticulospinal pathway descends anterior to the CST.

Supplementary Motor Area

In contrast to the PMC's responsiveness to external cues, the SMA (area 6 on the medial surface of the hemisphere) responds to *internal cues*. In particular, it is involved in *motor planning*, as exemplified by the fact that the SMA is activated by the frontal lobe (DLPFC) the moment we *intend* to make a movement, even if the movement is not performed. The principal function of the SMA seems to be that of preprogramming movement sequences that have already been built into motor memory. It functions in collaboration with a motor loop passing through the basal ganglia (Chapter 26) and projects to area 4 as well as contributing directly to the CST. Unilateral lesions of the SMA can be associated with *akinesia* (inability to initiate movement) of the contralateral arm and leg. Bilateral lesions are accompanied by total akinesia, including akinesia for speech initiation.

Cortical Eye Fields

Fig. 28.12 illustrates the *cortical eye fields* involved in scanning movements (saccades). Their connections and functions are summarised in Table 28.1.

Dorsolateral Prefrontal Cortex. This is a higher-level cognitive centre engaged in assessment of the visual scene, in decisions about making voluntary saccades, and in voluntary repression of reflexive saccades. (*Voluntary* saccades result from internally generated decisions. *Reflexive* saccades are automatic responses to objects appearing in the peripheral visual

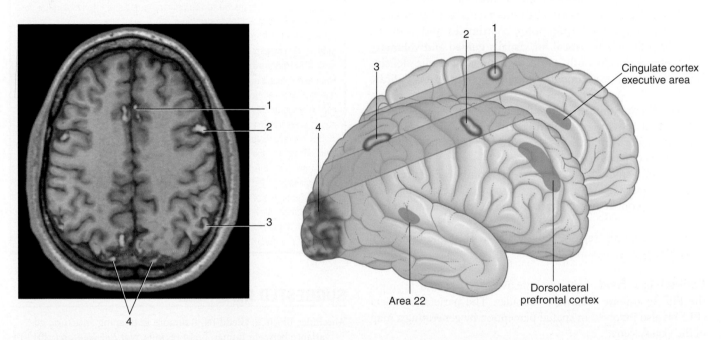

Fig. 28.12 Areas of cerebral cortex involved in saccadic movements. *1*, Supplementary eye field; *2*, frontal eye field; *3*, parietal eye field; *4*, visual association cortex.

TABLE 28.1 Cortical Eye Fields.[a]

Eye Field	Primary Afferents From	Primary Efferents to	Function
Dorsolateral prefrontal cortex (DLPFC)	Visual association areas	Ipsilateral FEF, SEF, SC, and CCx	Advanced planning for voluntary saccades
Cingulate cortex (CCx)	DLPFC, FEF, SEF	Ipsilateral FEF and SC	Assessment of emotional significance
Supplementary eye field (SEF)	DLPFC, PEF, area 22	Ipsilateral FEF and SC	Learning, planning, and triggering of saccades
Frontal eye field (FEF)	DLPFC, FEF, PEF	Contralateral PPRF, ipsilateral CCx, and SC	Voluntary and visually guided saccades
Parietal eye field (PEF)	'Where' visual pathway, pulvinar, and DLPFC	Ipsilateral FEF and SC	Reflexive saccades
Area 22	Auditory association cortex, PEF	Ipsilateral SC	Saccades to source of sound

Note: The left paramedian pontine reticular formation (PPRF) moves the eyes to the left. The right superior colliculus (SC) also moves the eyes to the left, because of a crossed projection from it to the left PPRF.
[a]At times SC is also included in this group, despite its brainstem location, because of its critical role in generating saccades.

field. Strictly speaking, reflexive saccades should be called *responsive*; they are not true reflexes, being amenable to voluntary suppression.)

Cingulate Cortex. Participates with the DLPFC in decision-making and in assessing the emotional significance, or *valence*, of visual targets.

Supplementary Eye Field. Occupies the anterior part of the SMA and is engaged in motor planning, especially when multiple saccades are required.

Frontal Eye Field. Initiates voluntary saccades that shift attention towards stimuli or suppresses the tendency to direct gaze to a new stimulus in response to one or more of the three inputs listed. The frontal eye field (FEF) 'maintains' a map of visual space with respect to oculomotor coordinates and with the superior colliculus is critical for visually guided and voluntary saccades; lesions to both cause permanent saccadic deficits. Both clinical and experimental (monkey) observations indicate that:

- The FEFs are tonically active, bilaterally.
- Increased activity in the mid-region of the FEF on one side causes a horizontal saccade toward the contralateral visual hemispace (a *contraversive saccade*).
- Increased activity in the upper region on one side produces an obliquely downward contraversive saccade; bilateral upper region activation causes both eyes to look straight down.
- Increased lower region activity has corresponding effects with respect to upward gaze.

Parietal Eye Field. Initiates reflexive saccades and prompts the FEF to initiate voluntary saccades. The parietal eye field (PEF) is also involved in spatial perception by generating a map of the visual scene.

For prefrontal cortex and frontal lobe dysfunction, see Chapter 32.

CLINICAL PANEL 28.1 Stiff Person Syndrome

An unusual but well-recognised condition known as *stiff person syndrome (SPS)* is an autoimmune central nervous system disorder associated with the presence of circulating antibodies to glutamic acid decarboxylase (GAD65), a key enzyme that converts glutamate to GABA. SPS is manifested as a state of muscle rigidity, with episodic muscle spasms (produced by co-contraction of prime movers and antagonists predominantly of the proximal limb and axial muscles) and task-specific phobias. Normally the upper motor neurons are held in check by tonic activity of nearby GABAergic inhibitory interneurons. Some areas of the cortex are affected more than others, and the clinical effects relate to impaired function of these GABAergic neurons resulting in motor cortex hyperexcitability. The actual relationship of these circulating antibodies to the pathogenesis of SPS is currently being explored.

Core Information

The cerebral cortex has both a laminar and juxtaposed interconnected columnar organisation. The two basic cell types are pyramidal and nonpyramidal (interneurons). Pyramidal cells occupy laminae II, III, and V and (as fusiform cells) lamina VI. Lamina IV is rich in spiny stellate cells (modified pyramidal neurons). Small pyramidal cells link the gyri within the hemisphere, medium-sized pyramidal cells link matching areas of the two hemispheres, and the largest pyramidal cells project to the thalamus, brainstem, and spinal cord. All pyramidal cell projections are excitatory; spiny stellate cells are also excitatory to pyramidal cells. Cortical interneurons are inhibitory. Columnar organisation takes the form of cell columns, which are considered the basic functional unit of cortical processing. Each cell column consists of a characteristic 'microcircuit' of neurons.

The somatic sensory cortex contains an inverted representation of body parts. Important inputs come from the ventral posterior nucleus of the thalamus; important outputs go to the primary motor and inferior parietal cortex. The primary visual cortex receives the geniculocalcarine tract. Cellular responses of differing complexity depend upon convergence of simpler onto more complex cell types. The visual association areas are characterised by feature extraction, for example, of motion, colour, and shape. Form and colour extraction continue into the cortex on the underside of the temporal lobe, motion into the posterior parietal lobe. The primary auditory cortex occupies the upper surface of the superior temporal gyrus and the auditory association cortex is lateral to it.

The primary motor cortex occupies the precentral gyrus. It gives rise to most of the PT, the body parts being represented upside down. Its main inputs are from the somatosensory cortex, cerebellum (via the ventral posterior nucleus of the thalamus), and the premotor and supplementary motor areas. The premotor area operates mainly in response to external cues, the supplementary motor area in response to internally generated cues. Under control of the dorsolateral prefrontal cortex, four distinct cortical areas are involved, in different contexts, in producing contraversive saccades.

SUGGESTED READINGS

Alexander-Bloch A, Giedd JN, Bullmore E. Imaging structural covariance between human brain regions. *Nat Rev Neurosci.* 2013;14:322–336.
Allen Brain Atlas. <http://www.brain-map.org/>. Accessed 12.06.14.
Amunts K, Zilles K. Architectonic mapping of the human brain beyond Brodmann. *Neuron.* 2015;88(6):1086–1107.
Arslan S, Ktena SI, Makropoulos A, Robinson EC, Rueckert D, Parisot S. Human brain mapping: a systematic comparison of parcellation methods for the human cerebral cortex. *NeuroImage.* 2018;170:5–30.
Blumberg J, Kreiman G. How cortical neurons help us see: visual recognition in the human brain. *J Clin Invest.* 2010;120:3054–3063.
Bonini L, Ferrari PF, Fogassi L. Neurophysiological basis underlying the organization of intentional actions and the understanding of others' intention. *Conscious Cogn.* 2013;22:1095–1104.
Borst G, Thompson WL, Kosslyn SM. Understanding the dorsal and ventral systems of the human cerebral cortex: beyond dichotomies. *Amer Psych.* 2011;66:624–632.
Bullmore E, Sporns O. The economy of brain network organization. *Nat Rev Neurosci.* 2012;13:336–349.
Burr DC, Morrone MC. Constructing stable spatial maps of the world. *Perception.* 2012;41:1355–1372.

Catani M, de Schotten MT, Slater D, et al. Connectomic approaches before the connectome. *Neuroimage*. 2013;80:2—13.

Child ND, Benarroch EE. Differential distribution of voltage-gated ion channels in cortical neurons: implications for epilepsy. *Neurology*. 2014;82:989—998.

Cowey A. The blindsight saga. *Exp Brain Res*. 2010;200:3—24.

da Costa NM, Martin KAC. Whose cortical column would that be? *Front Neuroanat*. 2010;4:16.

DeFelipe J. Chandelier cells and epilepsy. *Brain*. 1999;122: 1807—1822.

Espinosa JS, Stryker MP. Development and plasticity of the primary visual cortex. *Neuron*. 2012;75:230—249.

Fedurco M. Long-term memory search across the visual brain. *Neural Plast*. 2012; Article ID 392695.

Gilaie-Dotan S, Saygin AP, Lorenzi LJ, et al. The role of the human ventral visual cortex in motion perception. *Brain*. 2013;136: 2784—2798.

Gilbert C, Li W. Top-down influences on visual processing. *Nat Rev Neurosci*. 2013;14:350—363.

Greig LC, Woodworth MB, Galazo MJ, et al. Molecular logic of neocortical projection neuron specification, development and diversity. *Nat Rev Neurosci*. 2013;14:755—769.

Grill-Spector K, Malach R. The human visual cortex. *Annu Rev Neurosci*. 2004;27:649—677.

Han W, Sestan N. Cortical projection neurons sprung from the same root. *Neuron*. 2013;80:1103—1105.

Harris KD, Mrsic-Flogel TD. Cortical connectivity and sensory coding. *Nature*. 2013;503:51—58.

Human Brain Project. <http://humanbrainproject.eu>. Accessed 12.06.14.

Innocenti GM, Vercelli A. Dendritic bundles, minicolumns, columns, and cortical output units. *Front Neuroanat*. 2010;4:11.

Joukal M. Anatomy of the human visual pathway. In: Skorkovská K, ed. *Homonymous Visual Field Defects*. Cham, Switzerland: Springer; 2017:1—16.

Kaas JH. Evolution of columns, modules, and domains in the neocortex of primates. *Proc Natl Acad Sci USA*. 2012;109(suppl 1): 10655—10660.

Kretschmann H-J, Weinrich W. *Neurofunctional systems: 3D reconstructions with correlated neuroimaging: text and CD-ROM*. New York: Thieme; 1998.

Larkum M. A cellular mechanism for cortical associations: an organizing principle for the cerebral cortex. *Trends Neurosci*. 2013;36:141—151.

Le Magueresse C, Monyer H. GABAergic interneurons shape the functional maturation of the cortex. *Neuron*. 2013;77:388—405.

Lein E, Hawrylycz M. The genetic geography of the brain. *Sci Am*. 2014;310:71—77.

Lent R, Azevedo FAC, Andrade-Moraes CH, et al. How many neurons do you have? Some dogmas of quantitative neuroscience under revision. *Eur J Neurosci*. 2012;35:1—9.

Loukas M, Pennell C, Groat C, et al. Korbinian Brodmann (1868—1918) and his contributions to mapping the cerebral cortex. *Neurosurgery*. 2011;68:6—11.

Mesulam M. The evolving landscape of human connectivity: facts and inferences. *Neuroimage*. 2012;62:2182—2189.

Miller EK, Buschman TJ. Cortical circuits for the control of attention. *Curr Opin Neurobiol*. 2013;23:216—222.

NIH Blueprint: The Human Connectome Project. <http://human-connectome.org>. Accessed 12.06.14.

Penfield W, Rasmussen T. *The Cerebral Cortex of Man: A Clinical Study of Localization and Function*. New York: The Macmillan Company; 1950.

Posner MI, Raichle ME. Images of the brain. In: Posner MI, Raichle ME, eds. *Images of the Mind*. New York: Scientific American Library; 1994:57—82.

Prasad S, Galetta SL. Anatomy and physiology of the afferent visual system. *Handb Clin Neurol*. 2011;102:3—19.

Sporns O. The human connectome: origins and challenges. *Neuroimage*. 2013;80:53—61.

Tiberi L, Vanderhaeghan P, van den Ameele J. Cortical neurogenesis and morphogens: diversity of cues, sources and functions. *Curr Opin Cell Biol*. 2012;24:269—276.

Van Essen DC, Glasser MF. Parcellating cerebral cortex: how invasive animal studies inform noninvasive mapmaking in humans. *Neuron*. 2018;99(4):640—663.

Wedeen VJ, Rosene DL, Wang R, et al. The geometric structure of the brain fiber pathways. *Science*. 2012;335:1628—1634.

Weiner KS, Grill-Spector K. Neural representations of faces and limbs neighbor in human high-level visual cortex: evidence for a new organization principle. *Psych Res*. 2013;77:74—97.

Zhang X, Kedar S, Lynn MJ, Newman NJ, Biousse V. Homonymous hemianopias: clinical-anatomic correlations in 904 cases. *Neurology*. 2006;66(6):906—910.

Electroencephalography

STUDY GUIDELINES

1. Be able to describe the origin of the recorded EEG, underlying rationale for the 10–20 recording system, and the significance of the letter/number combinations used to define electrode placements.
2. Contrast the patterns that typify the waking EEG from that associated with sleep, both REM and NREM sleep.
3. Discuss why the phenomenon of *phase reversal* is useful in the interpretation of an EEG abnormality.

4. Describe the classification of epileptic seizures and how an epileptic seizure is different from epilepsy.
5. List the characteristics of narcolepsy and its pathogenesis.
6. We suggest you review the concepts expressed regarding transmitters and receptors in Chapter 8 before reading about drug therapy in the Clinical Panels.

NEUROPHYSIOLOGIC BASIS OF THE ELECTROENCEPHALOGRAM

Since its initial development, electroencephalography has remained a unique tool for the study of cortical function and a valuable supplement to history, physical examination, and information gained by radiologic studies.

When small metallic disc electrodes are placed on the surface of the scalp, oscillating currents of 20 to 100 µV can be detected and are referred to as an *electroencephalogram (EEG)*. Their origin is a direct consequence of the additive effect of groups of cortical pyramidal neurons being arranged in radial (outward-directed) columns. The columns relevant here are those beneath the surface of the cortical gyri. As the membrane potentials of these columns fluctuate, an *electrical dipole* (adjacent areas of opposite charge) develops. The dipole results in an electrical field potential as current flows through the adjacent extracellular space as well as intracellularly through the neurons (Fig. 29.1). It is the extracellular component of this current that is recorded in the EEG, and variations in both the strength and density of the current loops result in its characteristic sinusoidal waveform.

The oscillations of the EEG, measured in microvolts (µV), are thought to be generated by reciprocal excitatory and inhibitory interactions of neighbouring cortical cell columns.

TECHNIQUE

After careful preparation of the skin of the scalp to ensure good contact, electrodes are affixed in a placement that is in conformity with the 10–20 international system of electrode placement (with the modified combinatorial nomenclature), in which the scalp is divided into a grid in accordance with Fig. 29.2.

By defining a consistent placement of electrodes, direct comparison in follow-up studies is feasible, as is a method to compensate for differences in head size. Each electrode placement allows it to preferentially record over a cortical surface area of approximately 6 cm^2. The nomenclature employed to define each electrode position combines a letter with a number, as shown in Fig. 29.2.

Actual EEG recordings are made from all sites simultaneously. The potential difference between electrode pairs is recorded (as a rule), and this is displayed as a separate individual graph or channel. Often other physiologic recordings are performed at the same time (e.g. an electrocardiograph (ECG) and/or a surface electromyograph (EMG)).

If varying pairs of electrodes are used, the montage (output) is termed *bipolar* (Fig. 29.3A). If they have one recording site in common (auricle, or mastoid area), it is called *referential* (Fig. 29.3B). Fig. 29.4 provides a complete set of normal tracings.

TYPES OF PATTERNS

Normal EEG Rhythms

Awake State EEG. The EEG demonstrates prominent changes both with the level of alertness and during the various stages of sleep. Each of these patterns is specific and is considered during EEG interpretation. A routine EEG study will usually take 30 minutes and will include recordings made during wakefulness and during early stages of sleep, because specific abnormalities (especially epileptiform ones) may only be detected during the sleep portion of the recording.

In the alert awake state (Fig. 29.5A) the pattern is described as desynchronised because the waveforms are quite irregular.

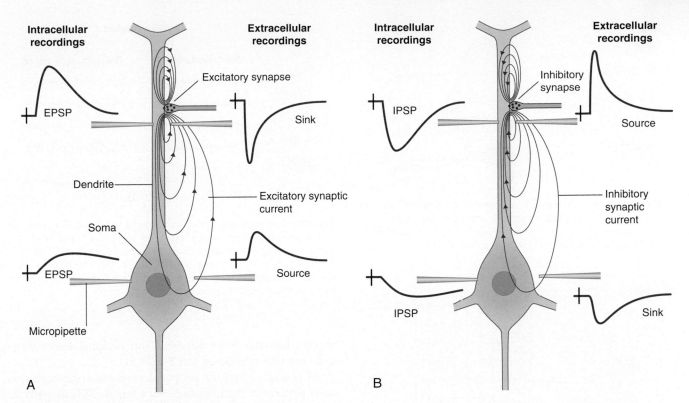

Fig. 29.1 Diagram illustrating the contribution of individual excitatory and inhibitory synaptic currents to the extracellular field potentials. Micropipettes are being used to sample intracellular and extracellular events. (A) Intracellular recordings show that the excitatory synapse generates a rapid excitatory postsynaptic potential *(EPSP)* at the synaptic site on the dendrite and a slower and smaller EPSP at the soma. Extracellular recordings show that the source *(+)* of excitatory synaptic current flows outward through the membrane of the proximal dendrite and soma and inward (the sink) at the synaptic site. (B) An inhibitory synapse is seen to have the opposite effect. The inhibitory postsynaptic potential *(IPSP)* is associated with a current source at the synaptic site and a sink along the proximal dendrite and soma.

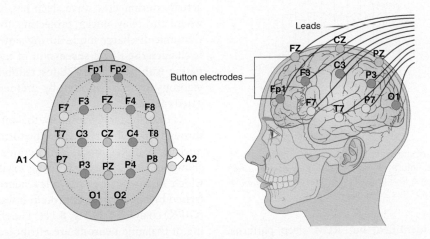

Fig. 29.2 Deployment of surface electrodes on the scalp. *Letters: C,* coronal; *F,* frontal; *FP,* frontopolar; *O,* occipital; *P,* parietal; *T,* temporal; *Z,* midline. *Numbers: Odd numbers,* left side; *even numbers,* right side. *A1, A2* are reference electrode positions (see text).

The background frequency is usually around 9.5 Hz. A beta frequency of more than 14 Hz may be superimposed over anterior head regions.

In a relaxed state with the eyes closed, rhythmic waveforms called the **alpha rhythm** appear in the alpha frequency (8 to 14 Hz), notably over the parietooccipital area (Fig. 29.5B).

Normal Sleep EEG

- **Rapid eye movement (REM)** sleep. Dreamy light sleep accompanied by REMs; also called paradoxical sleep because the EEG resembles that for the awake state.
- **Non-REM (NREM)** sleep. NREM sleep (stages 1–3); stage 3 is also called slow wave sleep. In a routine EEG, NREM

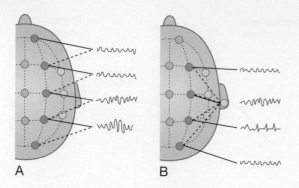

Fig. 29.3 (A) Bipolar recording. A succession of adjacent pairs of electrodes is used. Only four sample tracings are shown. (B) Referential recording. The reference electrode is attached to the ear in this example. Again, only four sample tracings are shown.

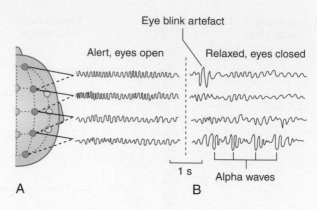

Fig. 29.5 Electroencephalogram in the awake state. (A) Subject is alert with eyes open. Beta waves are seen in Fp2–F4 and F4–C4. (B) Subject is relaxed with eyes closed. An eye-blink artefact is seen in the Fp2–F4 tracing. Alpha waves are seen in P4–O2. The beta waves are characterised by low amplitude and high frequency; the alpha waves, by a sinusoidal rhythmic waxing and waning.

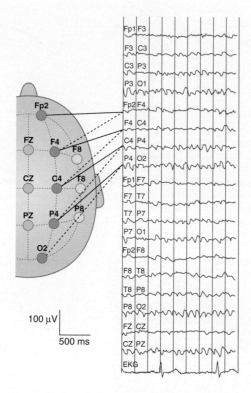

Fig. 29.4 A complete set of normal tracings. Figure is tagged in accordance with the nomenclature in Fig. 29.2. (An ECG has been taken simultaneously.) Note the low amplitude of the waves (20 μV or less) and their high frequency in this 2-second sample.

rhythm becomes more apparent (on occipital leads) during quiet rest with eyes closed (see Fig. 29.5).

By general agreement, proper sleep is associated with slow-wave patterns in the EEG and characteristic EEG patterns that allow sleep stages to be recognised. This begins with a rapid descent through stage 1, characterised by a steady theta rhythm, into stage 2, characterised by delta waves interrupted by fast sinusoidal waveforms called *sleep spindles*, and occasional *K complexes*; stage 3 is characterised by the slow delta waves—hence the term *slow wave sleep* for that stage (see Fig. 29.6).

It is generally agreed that the waxing and waning of cortical activity during slow wave sleep has its origin in the thalamus, where the relay nuclei projecting to the cortex also enter a rhythmic discharge mode during slow wave sleep. This rhythm is characterised by a succession of hyperpolarised states alternating with depolarised states, exhibiting bursts of firing. The vigorous firing is triggered by momentary opening of voltage-gated calcium channels.

As described in Chapter 25, thalamocortical projections pass through an inhibitory shell in the form of the thalamic reticular nucleus, with reciprocal connections to parent relay cells as shown in Fig. 25.4. Burst firing excites the reticular nucleus, which in turn causes the relay neurons to become hyperpolarised by opening the G protein inwardly rectifying potassium (GIRK) channels (see Fig. 8.11). The rhythmic waxing and waning of thalamic neurons are attributed to a pulsatile discharge pattern inherent to the cells of the reticular nucleus.

After about an hour's sleep, the stage 2 wave pattern is repeated and is succeeded by a longer period of slow wave sleep. Then time is spent in REM sleep, a 'dream' state accompanied by:
- visual imagery,
- REMs generated by extraocular muscle contractions,
- EMG silence in the musculature of trunk and limbs, and
- EEG beta rhythm characteristic of the waking state—hence the term *paradoxical sleep*.

REM sleep is the dominant state during the final two cycles in the 8 hours spent in bed. Although the significance of dreams is a matter of endless debate, activation of the visual cortex is

sleep will usually be identified, but REM sleep patterns, because of the briefness of the EEG, would be unusual.

Sleep can be defined at both a behavioural level (e.g. immobility) and by patterns of neuronal activity of the brain (e.g. cortical neuronal firing patterns). There are various purported reasons for sleep, but its universal occurrence among animals implies its primary nature. In terms of NREM sleep, two functions appear to be fundamental. One allows time for neurons to perform their own cellular maintenance, not possible during the high activity states of wakefulness. The other supports learning and memory.

People normally pass through three to five sleep cycles per night, the first within the initial 90 minutes of sleep. The sequence of events is summarised in Fig. 29.6. Alpha

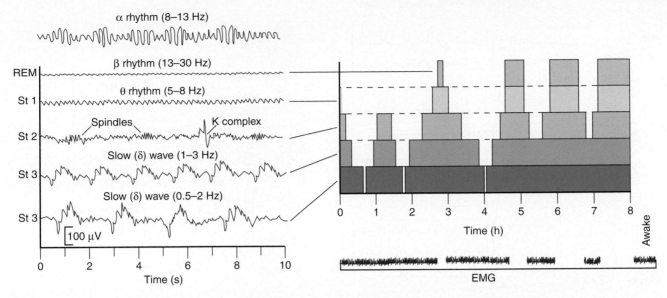

Fig. 29.6 Typical 8-hour sleep and electroencephalogram patterns. Note that the rapid eye movement *(REM)* period *(in pink)* is not one of the official three sleep stages despite being routinely referred to as REM sleep. The electromyogram *(EMG)* trace shows that skeletal muscles are 'paralysed' during REM sleep.

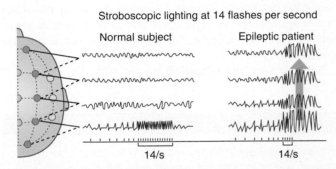

Fig. 29.7 Effects of stroboscopic lighting. In normal subjects, stroboscopic lighting induces matching spikes in occipital recording sites (referred to as *driving*). This represents one of the activation procedures performed during an electroencephalogram in the hopes of eliciting an abnormality; some patients with epilepsy are at risk of experiencing an epileptic seizure precipitated by this procedure.

brought about by the ponto-geniculo-occipital (PGO) pathway, from pontine reticular formation to lateral geniculate body to occipital cortex. (In individuals blind from birth, dreams have a purely auditory content, perhaps associated with activation of the lateral geniculate body.)

Because of the brief time that an EEG is recorded, a patient does not often cycle through REM sleep patterns. It should be noted that in normal circumstances, REM sleep almost never occurs during the first descent into sleep. Should it do so, the strange sleep disorder called narcolepsy should come to mind (Clinical Panel 29.1). It should also be mentioned that volunteers awakened during REM sleep do not invariably report a dream, and that dreaming occasionally happens during NREM sleep.

EEG Activation Procedures. To increase the diagnostic yield of an EEG, certain procedures are performed, usually at the end of the recording, in the hope that an abnormality will appear. In addition to sleep, two common procedures are a brief period of

hyperventilation and another of photic stimulation using strobe (flickering) light at varying frequencies (Fig. 29.7).

Maturation of Wave Format. Accurate interpretation of an EEG necessitates familiarity on the part of the electroencephalographer with those patterns that are age-specific and hence represent normal maturational stages of development. Earliest recordings, from premature babies, show only intermittent electrical activity, which is asynchronous between the hemispheres. Continuous symmetric activity emerges during childhood, with increasingly distinctive wakeful and sleeping patterns. During early teenage years, the adult EEG pattern is established.

Abnormal EEG Rhythms

Focal Abnormalities Without Seizures. *Focal slowing* in the form of delta waves (Fig. 29.8) indicates presence of a mass or lesion of some kind.

Phase reversal of focal spike or sharp wave discharges are occasionally seen over localised areas of the cortex. Both appear as abrupt events distinguishable from the background; individual spikes last 20 to 70 ms and sharp waves 70 to 200 ms; both are usually followed by a slow wave(s). Such discharges project to the surface with a negative polarity, and their electrical field is seen at more than two adjacent electrodes, but with a point of *phase reversal* between adjacent electrodes that 'defines' their EEG localisation (Fig. 29.9). In anterior temporal and frontal areas, they may be indicative of an *ictal focus*, a term denoting a locus of origin of seizures. In the occipital region any correlation is usually with visual impairment.

Generalised Abnormalities Without Seizures. Disorders that cause generalised dysfunction within cortical or subcortical structures result in a diffuse pattern of abnormalities on EEG. Such disorders include hypoglycaemia, hypoxia, and dementia. This can be manifested by replacement of normal background

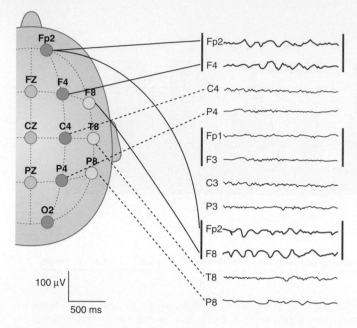

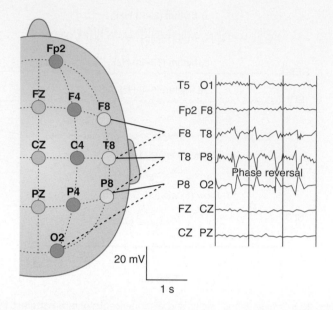

Fig. 29.8 Bipolar montage illustrating focal slowing. Printouts from right lateral frontal areas display delta waves in this 60-year-old female suffering from headache and drowsiness for several months without overt physical signs. Coronal magnetic resonance imaging slices showed compression of the right lateral ventricle. Surgery revealed the cause to have been an astrocytoma. (Analogous tracings from the left frontal area are normal.)

Fig. 29.9 Phase reversal. This patient suffered from primary focal seizures. Phase reversal between the T8 and P8 electrodes suggests an ictal focus located in the right posterior temporal lobe.

frequency by diffuse slowing. Disorders involving the white matter of the brain are more often associated with delta waves and are often polymorphic (of variable appearance and less sinusoidal).

Seizures, See Clinical Panel 29.2

CLINICAL PANEL 29.1   Narcolepsy

Narcolepsy is a chronic sleep disorder characterised by **excessive daytime sleepiness (EDS),** which is necessary for the diagnosis. Additional features can be present:

- EDS manifests as an irresistible desire to sleep for periods of minutes to an hour and occurs several times during the day; these 'naps' are refreshing. These are often associated with REM sleep.
- **Cataplexy** is brief episodes of sudden muscle paralysis that occur during the wake state and is often triggered by emotion, notably by surprise of any kind. These episodes represent the atonia associated with REM sleep that occurs during the wake state. Cataplexy may range from mild (e.g. dropping the head or jaw, dropping something held in the hand) to severe, with collapse due to flaccid paralysis of the trunk and limbs with consciousness fully preserved. Occasionally, it may be the only presenting symptom, but typically, EDS is the first symptom to appear. When EDS and cataplexy occur together, the patient has *Narcolepsy type 1*.
- Sleep paralysis and hallucinations occur in the general population and can accompany narcolepsy; both reflect an intrusion of normal REM-associated events into the wake state. *Sleep paralysis* occurs most often upon awakening, manifests as a state of complete awareness but an inability to speak or move the limbs, lasts from seconds to minutes, and is accompanied by the sensation of fear or suffocation. *Hypnopompic hallucinations* occur at the transition from sleep to wakefulness to sleep and are characterised by striking visual imagery.

The diagnosis of narcolepsy is based on a through sleep history that looks for other causes of EDS and begins with the performance of a diagnostic sleep study or *polysomnogram* (*PSG*). A PSG is an extended recording of sleep that includes an EEG (allows the staging or time spent in the different stages of sleep to be determined), records motor activity, respiratory effort, and oxygen saturation, and serves to detect other sleep disorders. Lacking another explanation for EDS, the next study is a *multiple sleep latency test* that consists of multiple short naps for timing the onset to REM, which is short in those with narcolepsy, and supports the diagnosis.

Narcolepsy can be very distressing as the patient may be accused of laziness or incompetence at work and is at risk of accidents when driving a car or merely crossing the street. The underlying aetiology of Narcolepsy type 1 is a loss of neurons located in the lateral walls of the hypothalamus that results in impaired production of the excitatory peptide *orexin* (*hypocretin*) whose role is stabilising the state of wakefulness. Orexin receptors are normally present on the histaminergic neurons of the tuberomammillary nucleus (TMN). As mentioned in Chapter 33, the TMN projects widely to the cerebral cortex and maintains the awake state by activating H1 receptors on cortical neurons. Narcolepsy is a sporadic disorder and believed to have (not yet proven) an autoimmune basis.

Drugs that promote wakefulness are the first-line medications. Because of its low potential for abuse and minimal side effects, *modafinil* (or *armodafinil*) is now the first-line therapy and assumed to act as a dopamine reuptake inhibitor. Amphetamine and methylphenidate are other stimulants used more frequently in the past that have a mode of action that prevents reuptake or increases the release of monoamines, dopamine in particular.

Treatment of cataplexy begins with a serotonin/norepinephrine reuptake inhibitor (typically prescribed for depression), but the most potent medication is *sodium oxybate*, a metabolite of GABA. Its effect is mediated by GABA-B receptors, but its potential for drug abuse necessitates prescription monitoring.

CLINICAL PANEL 29.2 Seizures

- **Epileptic seizure**: transient occurrence of signs and/or symptoms secondary to abnormal excessive or synchronous neuronal activity in the brain.
- **Epilepsy**: disorder of the brain characterised by an enduring predisposition to generate epileptic seizures, and by the neurobiological, cognitive, psychological, and social consequences of this condition. (This requires at least two unprovoked seizures, one unprovoked seizure and a high probability of another seizure, or diagnosis of an epilepsy syndrome.) Epilepsy can resolve if it is an age-dependent disorder or when a patient remains seizure free while off medications for a period of time.

The term 'seizure' or 'ictus' refers to the clinical manifestations brought about by an abnormal burst firing of neurons in the cerebral cortex. The 'interictal period' is the time interval between seizures. The overall *incidence* (probability of someone being diagnosed with a disease in a given period) of epilepsy varies, but in the UK it is estimated at 51/100,000 per year and is highest for children under the age of 5 years and the elderly; the *prevalence* (total number of cases divided by the population) is 9.7/1000.

The clinical manifestation and mode of onset of epileptic seizures allow them to be placed into two broad groups. **Generalised onset seizures** originate at some point, but rapidly become bilateral through networks of cortical and subcortical structures. The most frequent types are tonic–clonic and absence, together accounting for approximately 80%.

Tonic–clonic seizures (formerly known as grand mal seizures) are characterised by sudden onset of unconsciousness. The body stiffens for up to a minute (tonic stage), and then exhibits jerky movements of all four limbs, and chewing movements of the mouth for about another minute (clonic stage) and is followed by a period of unconsciousness and amnesia of the event. EEG recordings taken at the onset of this kind of seizure show simultaneous bilateral burst firing all over the cortex (Fig. 29.10).

In those at risk, hyperventilation, or photic stimulation by strobe lighting (Fig. 29.7), can precipitate tonic–clonic attacks and these 'activation' techniques are carefully used in the performance of a diagnostic EEG in the evaluation of a patient suspected of having a seizure and perhaps epilepsy.

Absence seizures (formerly, petit mal) are characterised by a generalised 3-Hz spike-and-wave activity on EEG (Fig. 29.11). These seizures usually occur between the ages of 4 and 14 years.

The typical case is a child who, upon relaxing after some physical or mental activity, passes through 'blank' periods (absences) of 10 to 30 seconds, usually with detectable twitching of muscles of the face or fingers. Dozens of such episodes may occur over a period of several hours, often so mild that low-level activities such as walking are not interrupted. The child is unaware of individual episodes, which may occur a hundred or

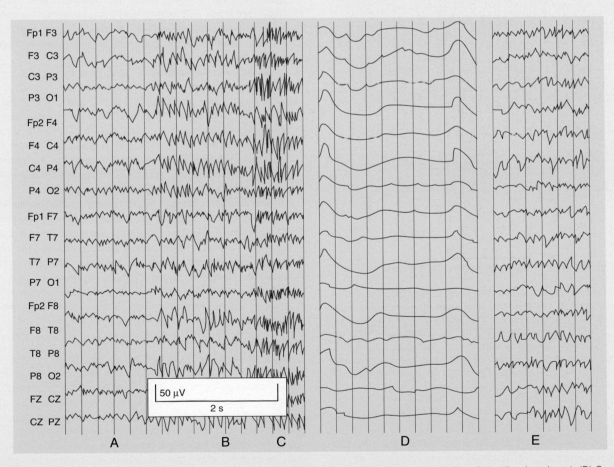

Fig. 29.10 Characteristic 'frenzied' pattern of a tonic–clonic seizure. (A) End of interictal period (preceding the epileptic seizure). (B) Generalised seizure pattern (no clear focal area of origin) involving all electrode positions. (C) In less than 1 second the electroencephalogram (EEG) seizure pattern is obscured by superimposed artefact caused by muscle contraction during the generalised tonic muscle spasm. (D) Immediate postictal period, with slow waveform pattern throughout. (E) Resumption of normal waveforms.

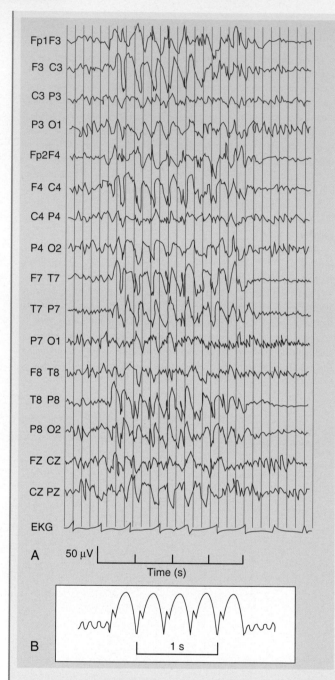

Fp1F3
F3 C3
C3 P3
P3 O1
Fp2F4
F4 C4
C4 P4
P4 O2
F7 T7
T7 P7
P7 O1
F8 T8
T8 P8
P8 O2
FZ CZ
CZ PZ
EKG

A   50 µV

Time (s)

B   1 s

Fig. 29.11 Absence seizure. (A) This episode was recorded over a period of 4 seconds. The spike-and-slow wave pattern is bilateral and generalised. It is important to note that before and immediately after there is no clear abnormality noted in the electroencephalogram (EEG) and no clinical symptoms evident in the individual. (B) The EEG appearance of a typical 3/second spike-and-slow-wave pattern characteristic of the EEG seen during an ictal episode of an individual with absence epilepsy.

more times in one day, and there is no postictal confusion. The 'blank' periods are brought about by prolonged inhibitory postsynaptic potentials on sensory thalamic relay neurons that are generated by thalamic reticular neurons made hyperactive by corticothalamic excitatory discharges.

Focal onset seizures originate within one hemisphere, may be discretely localised, and onset is consistent from one seizure to another.

TABLE 29.1 Loci of Origin of Focal Simple Seizures.

Motor	Movement of any part of the motor homunculus, sometimes with aphasia
Somatosensory	Contralateral numbness/tingling of face, fingers, or toes
Primary visual cortex	Flashes of light or patches of darkness in contralateral visual field
Basal occipitotemporal junction	Formed visual images of people or places, sometimes accompanied by sounds
Superior temporal gyrus (unusual)	Tinnitus, sometimes garbled word sounds

The episode may be associated with awareness and either a motor or nonmotor onset or impaired awareness (previously referred to as 'complex partial' or 'temporal lobe' seizures because of the assumed or frequent site of cerebral origin). Loci of origin of focal seizures and clinical manifestations are shown in Table 29.1.

Jacksonian seizure (named after neurologist John Hughlings Jackson) involves sequential activation of adjacent areas of the motor cortex, for example, ankle, knee, hip; shoulder, elbow, hand; lips, tongue, and larynx. A Jacksonian seizure may be followed by weakness/paralysis of the affected limb(s) for a period of hours or days; this is known as ***Todd paralysis***, which can be encountered in other focal onset seizures.

Benign rolandic epilepsy is a relatively common focal epilepsy disorder in childhood with focal spikes and slow waves over the centrotemporal area on EEG. The seizures result in unilateral facial sensorimotor and oropharyngogutteral symptoms, hypersalivation, and speech arrest. Somatosensory attacks (Fig. 29.12) originate behind the fissure and are described in Table 29.1. A diagnosis of benign rolandic epilepsy requires EEG confirmation, but the seizure type is the hallmark of the disease. The frequency of attacks dwindles and typically completely resolves by the age of 16 years. The EEG often normalises.

Two conditions deserve further comment. ***Status epilepticus*** consists of continuous seizures and incomplete recovery between them; it represents a neurologic emergency that can lead to death or permanent neurologic injury unless promptly treated. The other is ***sudden unexpected death in epilepsy (SUDEP)***, which is unexpected death not caused by injury, drowning, or other known causes. It is the leading cause of death in those with chronic refractory epilepsy and is assumed to represent seizure-induced respiratory dysfunction or a cardiac arrhythmia.

Drug therapy

Antiepileptic drugs (AED), administered in appropriate amounts, control approximately 70% of seizures in those with epilepsy. The drugs are of a broadly predictable nature and newer antiepileptic drugs demonstrate better tolerability. Most of them reduce abnormal neuronal firing by reducing sodium channel activity, reduce calcium conduction, reduce glutamatergic excitatory activity, or enhance γ-aminobutyric acid (GABA)-mediated inhibitory processes. Treatment begins with monotherapy and selection considers efficacy for a specific seizure type, side effects, and modes of use (e.g. dosing schedule, etc.); see Table 29.2.

Mechanism of action of some current drugs include:

- Sodium channel inhibitors: phenytoin, carbamazepine, and lamotrigine reduce high-frequency repetitive firing (Chapter 8) by making those ion

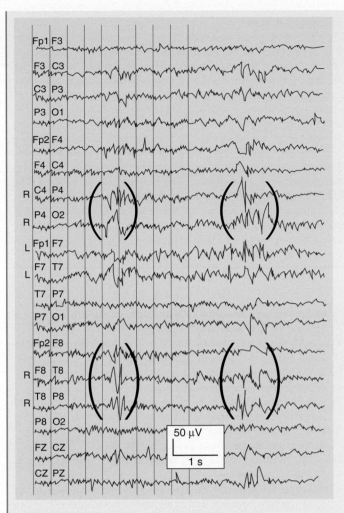

Fig. 29.12 Focal seizure. Seizure originating in the right somatic sensory cortex *(R)* and expressed by 'pins and needles' along the left arm (called a focal seizure with sensory manifestation). There is some spread to the left sensory cortex *(L)*. (Refer to Fig. 29.2 for R and L electrode positions.) The brackets on the figure indicate the abnormality.

TABLE 29.2 Efficacy of Some Anticonvulsant Medications.

Antiepileptic Drug	Focal Onset Seizure	Generalised Onset (Tonic–Clonic Seizure)	Generalised Onset (Absence Seizure)
Carbamazepine	X	Probably	
Ethosuximide			X
Lacosamide	X		
Lamotrigine	X	X	Probably
Levetiracetam	X	X	Probably
Phenytoin	X	Probably	
Topiramate	X	X	
Valproate	X	Probably	X
Zonisamide	X	Probably	Probably

channels less permeable to sodium and/or calcium. Lacosamide blocks sodium channels that enhance their inactivation.

- GABA agonists: benzodiazepines and barbiturates enhance the hyperpolarising effect of GABA on glutamate neurons, as illustrated in Fig. 8.9. Sodium valproate has multiple actions that include blocking the transaminase enzyme that converts GABA to glutamate within adjacent astrocytes (Chapter 8), thereby extending GABA's time in the synaptic cleft. It also blocks sodium channels and T-type calcium channels. Topiramate also has multiple modes of action that include augmenting GABA activity and blocking sodium channels.
- The most widely used and most effective drug for absence seizures is ethosuximide. Ethosuximide is a specific T-type calcium channel blocker (which also inhibits slow sodium channels and inhibits glutamate release). At appropriate dosage, excitability of thalamic relay neurons is sufficiently reduced to prevent them entering burst-firing. Zonisamide also blocks T-type calcium channels and blocks sodium channels.
- Levetiracetam is unique as it binds to a synaptic vesicle protein (SV2A) and has a nonspecific effect by decreasing neurotransmitter release in neuronal hyperactivity.

⬥ Core Information

The oscillations recorded in the *electroencephalogram (EEG)* arise from the collective extracellular currents generated by the summation of excitatory and inhibitory postsynaptic potentials of pyramidal cells within cortical cell columns. The grid-like standard arrangement of the recording electrodes in an EEG permits overall sampling of electrical activity in a manner that is applicable to both children and adults.

Sleep

The awake state EEG displays a desynchronised (irregular) background frequency, sometimes with a *beta frequency* (14 to 40 Hz) in recordings from the frontal area. During quiet rest with eyes closed, *alpha rhythm* (8 to 14 Hz) appears, most prominent over the parietooccipital area. Sleep is an active process and defined as having two components or stages: *nonrapid eye*

movement (NREM) sleep and *REM sleep.* NREM sleep is further characterised into three different stages, based on EEG patterns and physiological changes. Stage 1 NREM sleep shows a transition of the EEG to slower frequencies (*theta rhythm* at 5 to 8 Hz) and slowing of physiological rhythms, i.e. heart rate. During stage 2, the background rhythm of theta waves is interrupted by brief bursts of activity referred to as *sleep spindles* and *K complexes.* Stage 3 is often referred to as 'slow wave sleep' as the EEG slows further (delta range of 3 to 5 Hz) and heart rate and breathing are at their lowest levels. This stage of sleep is necessary for you to feel refreshed upon awakening and it may be difficult to awaken during this stage. The final stage of sleep is REM and your EEG appears similar to awake recordings as breathing, heart rate, and blood pressure increase and become irregular. Most dreaming occurs during REM sleep and while eye movements can be seen, arm and leg muscles become temporarily paralysed. Each of these cycles, from NREM through REM last approximately 90 minutes and cycle throughout the night, and the amount of REM per cycle increases, whereas NREM decreases as sleep progresses.

Narcolepsy is a chronic sleep disorder of hypersomnia that includes daytime sleepiness, sleep attacks, *hypnopompic hallucinations* (vivid visual hallucinations) upon awakening, *cataplexy* (momentary muscle paralysis), and *sleep paralysis* usually upon awakening.

Abnormal EEG Rhythms

Focal abnormalities are usually indicative of underlying cortical dysfunction or injury. Generalised abnormalities without seizures are often caused by metabolic abnormalities, hypoglycaemia, hypoxia, and dementias, any of which may replace normal background activity by diffuse slowing expressed in a theta frequency. Disorders involving cerebral white matter may produce more prominent slowing of the EEG and generalised delta frequencies (4 Hz or slower) that appear either symmetric or polymorphic.

Epileptic Seizures

The clinical manifestation and mode of onset of an epileptic seizure allows them to be placed into two broad groups. *Generalised onset seizures* originate at some point, but rapidly become bilateral through networks of cortical and subcortical structures; they include those with motor features (tonic–clonic) or not (absence seizures). *Focal onset seizures* originate within one hemisphere, may be discretely localised, and further classified according to the patient's awareness. Focal seizure onsets with maintenance of awareness are either associated with a motor or nonmotor onset, whereas the second group are *focal seizures with impaired awareness* (replaces the term 'complex partial seizure'). *Epilepsy* is diagnosed when an individual has at least two unprovoked seizures more than 24 hours apart or one seizure and a 60% probability of having another within the next 10 years.

Antiepileptic drugs have one or more effects. Most enhance GABA-mediated inhibitory activity; some inhibit glutamate activity by either inhibiting glutamate synthesis or by blocking voltage-gated sodium channels at glutamatergic nerve terminals.

SUGGESTED REFERENCES

Abou-Khalil BW. Update on antiepileptic drugs 2019. *Continuum.* 2019;25:508–536.

Baud MO, Rao VR. Gauging seizure risk. *Neurology.* 2018;91:967–973.

Chen H. Electroencephalography in epilepsy evaluation. *Continuum.* 2019;25:431–453.

Golden EC, Lipford MC. Narcolepsy: diagnosis and management. *Cleve Clin J Med.* 2018;85:959–969.

Joiner WJ. The neurobiological basis of sleep and sleep disorders. *Physiology.* 2018;33:317–327.

Jones LA, Thomas RH. Sudden death in epilepsy: insights from the last 25 years. *Seizure.* 2017;44:232–236.

Kanner AM, Ashman E, Gloss D, et al. Practice guideline update summary: efficacy and tolerability of the new antiepileptic drugs I: treatment of new-onset epilepsy: report of the Guideline Development, Dissemination, and Implementation Subcommittee of the American Academy of Neurology and the American Epilepsy Society. *Neurology.* 2018;91:74–81.

Krause AJ, Simon EB, Mander BA, et al. The sleep-deprived human brain. *Nat Rev Neurosci.* 2017;18:404–418.

Pack AM. Epilepsy overview and revised classification of seizures and epilepsies. *Continuum.* 2019;25:306–321.

Pennell PB. Antiepileptic drugs in pregnancy – quick decisions with long-term consequences. *JAMA Neurol.* 2018;75:652–665.

Raible F, Takekata H, Tessmar-Raible K. An overview of monthly rhythms and clocks. *Front Neurol.* 2017;8:189.

Saper CB, Fuller PM. Wake-sleep circuitry: an overview. *Curr Opin Neurobiol.* 2017;44:186–192.

VanHaerents S, Gerard EF. Epilepsy emergencies: status epilepticus, acute repetitive seizures, and autoimmune encephalitis. *Continuum.* 2019;25:454–476.

Veasey SC, Rosen IM. Obstructive sleep apnea in adults. *N Engl J Med.* 2019;380:1442–1449.

Evoked Potentials

STUDY GUIDELINES

1. Describe the general methodology performed to record sensory evoked potentials, the sensory modalities assessed, and an example of clinical disorders and expected abnormality.
2. Contrast the performance of a motor evoked potential versus a motor nerve conduction study.
3. Provide an example of how motor evoked potentials can be used to detect physiologic changes in the motor cortex.
4. Provide an example of how acupuncture may have its clinical effect.

SENSORY EVOKED POTENTIALS

The term *sensory evoked potentials* is used to define the response of the central nervous system (CNS) to specific sensory stimulation. In clinical neurophysiology, the specific stimuli relate to vision, hearing, and cutaneous sensations.

A difficulty with these evoked potentials is that their low amplitudes, of 20 μV or even less, render them undetectable in routine electroencephalogram (EEG) recordings because of the interference from the normal and higher amplitude background EEG.

However, advantage is taken of the regularity of the evoked response to repeated stimuli of the same type. With repetitive stimulation followed by computer averaging, irregular background rhythms cancel each other out and the evoked potentials can be clearly seen.

The three basic kinds of sensory evoked potentials are described as *visual*, *auditory*, and *somatosensory*.

Visual Evoked Potentials

The speed and amplitude of impulse conduction in the visual pathway are tested by a technique known as *pattern reversal* or *pattern shift visual evoked potential (VEP)*. With one eye covered at a time, the patient stares at a spot in the centre of a screen illuminated in a black-and-white checkerboard pattern (small optic nerve lesions can be detected by the technique of *multifocal VEP* where separate responses can be obtained from up to 60 different regions of the central visual field). Once or twice per second, the pattern is reversed (to white and black), for a total of 100 repetitions. Averaging is performed on the first 500 ms of data from a bipolar recording at the occipital and parietal midline EEG sites (OZ and PZ).

The wave peak of interest is called P1 (or P100). In healthy subjects it is a positive deflection 100 ms post stimulus (Fig. 30.1). In the clinical example shown, taken from a patient with a presumptive diagnosis of multiple sclerosis (MS), the normal P1 wave from the right-eye test indicated that both optic tracts and both optic radiations were clear. The P1 wave from the left eye was both delayed and of reduced amplitude, suggesting the presence of a defect in optic nerve conduction, anterior to the optic chiasm. This type of abnormality is encountered in demyelinative optic neuropathies such as one caused by myelin degeneration from multiple sclerosis and in this example, involving the left optic nerve. (*Note:* On screen and in printouts, it is now customary for these waveforms to be 'flipped', with positive responses registering as upward deflections.) Conduction defects caused by demyelination are more often expressed in the form of *latency delays* of the kind shown than in the form of amplitude abnormalities.

In the absence of any evidence for MS elsewhere, an abnormal P1 amplitude from one eye may be caused by an ocular disease such as glaucoma or by compression or ischemia of the optic nerve; visual evoked potential abnormalities do not specify aetiology. Bilateral abnormal P1 recordings can indicate pathology in one or both optic radiations.

Brainstem Auditory Evoked Potentials

Remarkably, it is possible to follow the sequence of electrical events in the auditory pathway, step by step, from cochlea to primary auditory cortex. Following placement of temporal scalp recording electrodes, 0.1 ms click sounds are presented at approximately 10 Hz to each ear in turn through conventional audiometric earphones. Click intensity is adjusted to 60 to 65 decibels (60 to 65 dB nHL; decibels relative to the threshold of a control population) above the click hearing threshold for the ear being tested. The contralateral ear is 'masked' by white noise. (The number of stimuli necessary to elicit clear waveforms is in the order of several thousand, in part because of their small relative amplitude.)

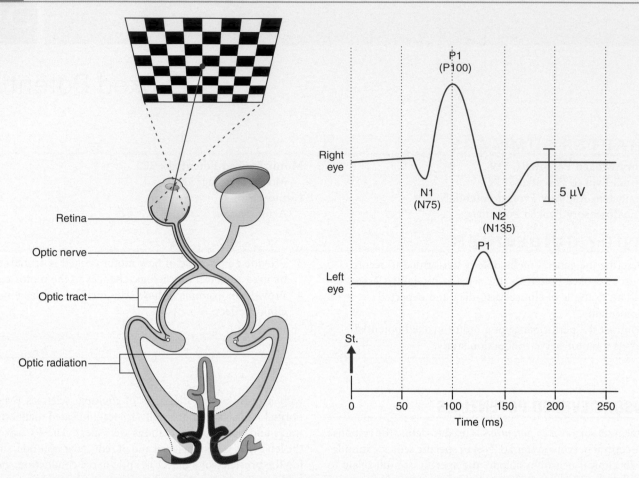

Fig. 30.1 Visual evoked potentials. The patient's right eye has been tested and is now shielded. The left eye is fixated on the spot in the centre of the checkerboard during pattern reversal episodes. The pattern from the right eye is normal, showing a positive deflection at 100 ms post stimulus. In the recording from the left eye, the P1 is both delayed and reduced in amplitude. The combined results indicate the presence of a lesion in the left eye or left optic nerve. The waveforms are identified with their typical nomenclature (*N1* indicates the first negative waveform, a negative polarity is indicated by a downward trace; *P1* the first positive, *N2* the second negative) as well as an alternative nomenclature which combines the surface recorded polarity as well as the average time for the signal to appear in a normal control population (*P100* is the waveform of positive polarity that appears on average at 100 ms). Both forms of nomenclature are used clinically.

A sequence of seven averaged-out waves (I to VII) constitutes the brainstem auditory evoked response (BAER). They are accounted for in the caption to Fig. 30.2.

Pathology anywhere along the auditory pathway results in reduction or abolition of the wave above that level. The technique is a sensitive screening test for *acoustic neuroma*. A diagnostic feature here is *I to III interpeak latency separation*. (*Interpeak latency* refers to the time interval between the recorded waveforms; *separation* refers to extension of the interval, in this case between waves I and III, which is caused by a conduction delay along the affected cochlear nerve that also causes a characteristically reduced amplitude wave II. While the absolute latency of subsequent waves is delayed, the interpeak latency between wave III and V is normal.)

In about 30% of patients who have MS with no clinical evidence of brainstem lesions, BAER is abnormal. The most frequent abnormalities are reduced amplitude of wave V and overall slowing of conduction indicated by increased inter-wave intervals.

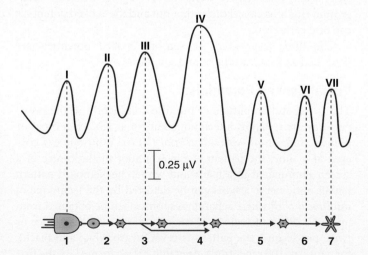

Fig. 30.2 Brainstem auditory evoked potentials. Sources of evoked potentials: *1,* distal auditory nerve (cochlear hair cells); *2,* cochlear nucleus and distal auditory nerve; *3,* cochlear nucleus and superior olivary complex; *4,* lateral lemniscus; *5,* inferior colliculus (inferior brachium); *6,* medial geniculate nucleus (auditory radiation); *7,* primary auditory cortex.

Another clinical application of the BAER technique is the assessment of cochlear function in infants under suspicion of congenital deafness. Assessment of brainstem auditory evoked potentials is also important in the medicolegal domain, to assess deafness induced by environmental noise in industry.

Evidence for a 'Where?' Auditory Pathway. When recording electrodes are specifically deployed over the temporoparietal region and brief sounds are emitted from loudspeakers placed in the left and right visual fields, a cortical response can be detected over the posterior part of the temporal plane, close to the temporoparietal junction. The right posterior temporal plane gives a stronger response, suggesting a right-sided dominance for auditory and visual space analysis.

Somatosensory Evoked Potentials

Somatosensory evoked potentials are the waveforms recorded at surface landmarks in route from the point of stimulation of a peripheral nerve to the CNS where they represent the electrical activity of summated postsynaptic potentials. The rate and amplitude of impulse conduction provide valuable information about the status of myelinated nerve fibres in both peripheral nerves and central pathways.

The nerve of choice for stimulation in the upper limb is the median at the wrist, and in the lower limb, the common peroneal at the knee. Repetitive electrical pulses are delivered to the nerve through a surface or needle electrode. The larger myelinated fibres are stimulated. Computer averaging is required to distinguish the stimulated responses from background noise, notably within the CNS. In the example shown in Fig. 30.3, impulse traffic along the median nerve is detected by a sequence of active electrodes attached to the skin for the purpose of recording speed and amplitude of nerve conduction in sequential segments as follows:

- Over the brachial plexus, to assess the median nerve segment extending from the wrist to the posterior triangle of the neck;

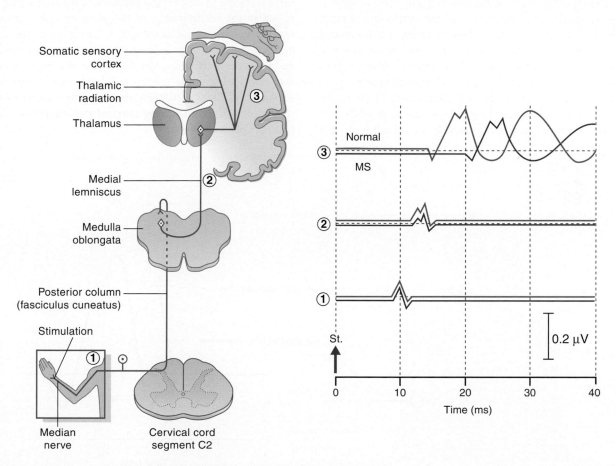

Fig. 30.3 Short latency somatosensory evoked potentials derived from stimulation of the median nerve at the wrist. The pathway has three segments. *1* is purely peripheral nervous system (PNS) recorded over Erb point (over the brachial plexus). *2* is PNS from the brachial plexus to the spinal cord and central nervous system (CNS) within the cord, recorded over the cervical spine. *3* is purely CNS. In the recordings from a patient with multiple sclerosis *(MS)*, the trace in *blue* is normal and *red* is abnormal. Trace 1 is normal; trace 2 shows reduced amplitude of the negative (upward) peak; trace 3 shows a latency delay as well as reduced amplitude. The abnormal red trace suggests that there is a 'conduction delay' of the response that appears to be between the recording site for 2 and 3.

- Over the spine of the C2 vertebra, to record the waveform when it arrives at the dorsal nerve roots and ipsilateral dorsal column (fasciculus cuneatus);
- The ipsilateral scalp over the sensory cortex, to 'pick up' stimulus traffic ascending the medial lemniscus; and
- Over the contralateral sensory cortex, to detect activity in the thalamocortical projection.

In the various peripheral neuropathies mentioned in Chapter 9, the first segment (wrist to brachial plexus) reveals slowing, usually with a reduction of amplitude. The second segment (brachial plexus to nucleus gracilis) may be affected in the first few milliseconds of its time course as a result of dorsal nerve root compression by osteophytes in patients with cervical spondylosis or by involvement of the spinal cord or medulla (Chapter 14). Responses recorded over cortical sites are delayed or affected by CNS lesions and are a common finding in patients suffering from MS.

MOTOR EVOKED POTENTIALS

Motor evoked potentials are compound motor action potentials (CMAPs) detected in surface electromyogram (EMG) recordings following controlled excitation of the corticospinal tract. The technique was mentioned in Chapter 18 because it revealed that the pyramidal tract pathway to sternocleidomastoid spinal motor neurons is essentially crossed, rather than being ipsilateral as previously thought. The most frequent objective is to determine *central motor conduction time (CMCT)* along the corticospinal tract. The procedure is both safe and painless. It uses a subtraction approach comparable in principle to that

used to determine peripheral nerve conduction times (see Fig. 30.3).

The procedure is known as *transcranial magnetic stimulation (TMS)* and Fig. 30.4 illustrates the concept in action. Stimulation is by means of a magnet in the form of a circular coil about 10 cm in diameter. To stimulate the pyramidal cells of the corticospinal tract supplying left ventral horn motor neurons, the magnet is handheld a little to the right side of the vertex and the patient maintains the selected limb muscle (biceps brachii in this example) in a state of slight contraction. A few very brief (200 ms) currents are pulsed at an intensity comfortably above the threshold required to elicit a twitch. The patient feels only a small 'tap' sensation on the scalp. The procedure is then repeated with the magnet touching the skin of the neck overlying the spine of the C5 vertebra, again eliciting a 'tap' sensation. It is generally agreed that the second pulse depolarises the axons of ventral nerve roots exiting the vertebral canal.

The latencies and amplitudes of the CMAPs are measured. The same procedure can be performed for the lower limb, the spinal stimulus being delivered in the lumbar region.

In neurophysiology units, CMCT can be measured when there is reason to suspect the presence of demyelinating plaques of MS in the white matter of the brain or spinal cord; where muscle wasting in the arms and/or legs leads to the suspicion that both upper and lower motor neurons may be degenerating; and in patients where moderate muscle weakness on one side, associated with brisk tendon reflexes, raises suspicion of a stroke. CMCT has also been used intraoperatively to monitor spinal cord function during surgical procedures on the spine that may place it at risk.

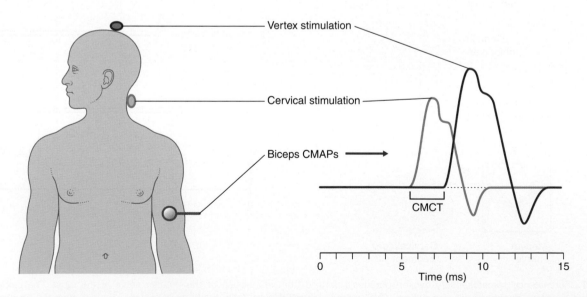

Fig. 30.4 Laboratory estimation of central motor conduction time *(CMCT)*. The *(red)* coil over the vertex has delivered a 200 ms current to pyramidal tract neurons serving upper limb spinal motor neurons. A large compound motor action potential (CMAP) is elicited in the biceps. The *(green)* coil over the cervical spine has delivered a weaker pulse to cervical ventral nerve roots eliciting a smaller CMAP. The difference between the two latencies (stimulus–response intervals) represents CMCT.

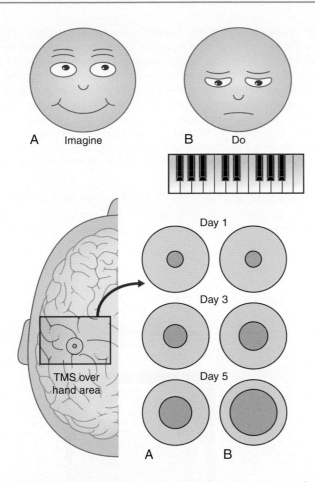

Fig. 30.5 Five-Finger Exercise. As explained in the main text, Group A volunteers imagined performing a daily five-finger piano exercise for the right hand, whereas Group B performed it. TMS showed remarkable enlargement of the area of motor cortex activating the finger flexors and extensors in both groups. (Based on data in Pascul-Leone A, Dang N, Cohen LG. Modulation of muscle responses evoked by transcranial magnetic stimulation during the acquisition of new motor skills. *J Neurophysiol.* 1995;74:1037–1045.)

Motor Training

A remarkable degree of plasticity in the healthy motor cortex has been demonstrated by TMS studies. Fig. 30.5 represents the outcomes of five-finger piano-playing exercises. A small magnetic coil was used over the scalp to locate the modules primarily involved in flexion and extension of the fingers of the right hand. This small scalp area was marked in three sets of volunteers, and the baseline size was measured for each subject. Group A *imagined* doing the five-finger exercise for 2 hours per day for 5 days; Group B *did* the exercises for the same periods; and Group C did not participate in any way prior to attempting the task once on day 5. As indicated in the figure, merely thinking about performance led to a major increase in the number of modules that activated the fingers when stimulated on days 3 and 5. Group B—the actual performers—showed the greatest increase of participating motor modules. The performance skills on day 5 were substantially better in Group B than in Group A, and Group A's performance was better than that of Group C.

There is general agreement that dramatic alterations such as those shown in this group experiment are best explained in terms of *unmasking preexisting connections* or *neuroplasticity*, as in the case of rapid expansion of the cortical sensory territory of one thalamocortical projection following experimental inactivation of a neighbouring projection. The most likely mechanism of additional pyramidal cell recruitment appears to be one of *disinhibition*, probably by the premotor cortex, involving activation of sequential pairs of γ-aminobutyric acid (GABA) ergic neurons in the manner illustrated in Fig. 6.10.

In this general context, it has also been shown that performance improvement in weightlifting is optimal when subjects *mentally rehearse* weightlifting during the days between performing the exercises.

Finally, Clinical Panel 30.1 includes an experiment in which TMS has been used to assess the supposed usefulness of acupuncture in improving motor performance.

CLINICAL PANEL 30.1 Acupuncture

Sensation

For relief of pain, fine (0.25 mm) needles are inserted bilaterally through appropriate acupoints, coming to rest among superficial muscle fibres underlying the subcutaneous fat (Fig. 30.6). The needle is then briefly spun to excite Type II and III sensory nerve fibres in its immediate neighbourhood. A subjective sense of numbness or heaviness in the acupoint area is usually reported.

The accepted explanation of the rapid pain relief produced by this form of stimulation is release of enkephalin by (a) spinal antinociception via the segmental reflex mentioned in 'rubbing the sore spot' combined with (b) supraspinal antinociception via spinoreticular activation of the antinociceptive pathway shown in Fig. 24.9. Pain relief is not achieved if the subject has received a prior injection of the opiate antagonist naloxone.

The term *acupuncture analgesia* refers to low-frequency (1 Hz) electrical stimulation of needles inserted at appropriate acupoints (*electroacupuncture*). The remarkable result is analgesia reported to be so complete as to permit open surgery in alert, awake patients. Clearly the ascending reticular activating system is not paralysed, unlike the case with general anaesthesia. Animal experiments indicate that electroacupuncture, in addition to the above-mentioned effects, produces corelease of β-endorphin from the arcuate nucleus of the hypothalamus and adrenocorticotropic hormone (ACTH) from the adenohypophysis.

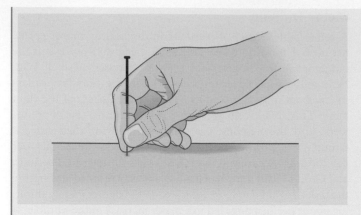

With availability of *functional magnetic resonance imaging* (*fMRI*) as a research tool, attention is being focused on the effects of acupuncture on higher-level sensory functions. Fig. 30.7 is composite, reproducing the remarkable results of two quite separate experiments. In each volunteer, needling was performed bilaterally, one acupoint being traditional for relief of disorders of vision and the other for disorders of hearing. Areas of increased cortical blood flow closely resemble those associated with retinal/cochlear activation. Surprisingly, the volunteers did not report visual/auditory hallucinations. An obvious question persists concerning the mysteriously specific anatomic pathways from the acupoints to the appropriate areas of cortex.

Movement

Movement disorders also have traditional therapeutic acupoints. One of these acupoints, on the lateral side of the proximal forearm, has been selected for low frequency (1 Hz) electroacupuncture in the experiment illustrated in Fig. 30.8.

Fig. 30.6 Standard positioning of an acupuncture needle.

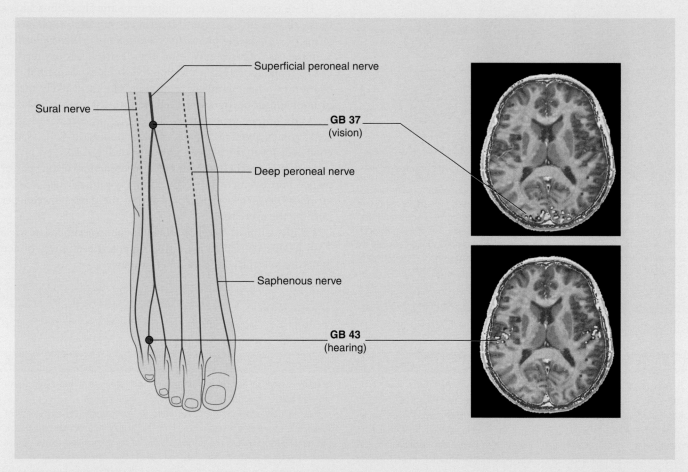

Fig. 30.7 Bilateral needling of acupoint GB 37 generates increased blood flow in the visual cortex. Bilateral needling of acupoint GB 43 generates increased blood flow in the auditory cortex. (Modified from Cho ZH, Na CS, Eng WK, et al. Functional magnetic resonance imaging of the brain in the investigation of acupuncture. In: Litscher G, Cho ZH, eds. Computer-controlled acupuncture. Lengerich: Pabst; 2000:45—64, with permission of Pabst.)

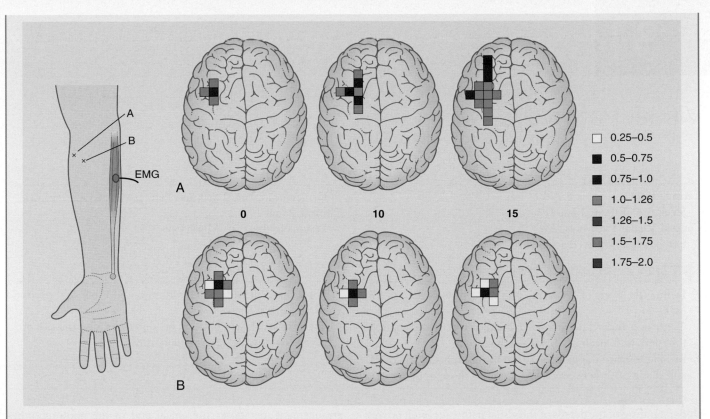

Fig. 30.8 Surface EMG activity recorded over flexor carpi ulnaris muscle in response to tms over and beyond the arm area of the left motor cortex. *A* marks an acupoint traditionally used to improve motor function; *B* marks the sham needling point (needling in the same manner 2 cm medial to A). Both points are well clear of ulnar nerve motor and sensory territories. Numbers *0, 10,* and *15* refer to baseline (no needling), 10 minutes with needle in place, and 15 minutes after needle removal, respectively. The table records voltage of compound motor action potentials in response to TMS over equal areas of the frontal lobe at each time interval. The upper three figures show expansion of the cortical area eliciting a twitch response in the EMG records related to acupoint needling; the lower three, related to sham needling, show no significant expansion. (Based on Lo YL, Cui SL, Fook-Ching S. The effect of acupuncture on motor cortex excitability and plasticity. *Neurosci Lett.* 2005;384:385–389.)

✦ Core Information

Sensory Evoked Potentials

Recordings of sensory evoked potentials are used to assess conduction rates and amplitudes in central neural pathways when they may be involved, based on clinical grounds.

Potentials in the visual cortex are evoked by means of checkerboard pattern reversal, one eye being tested at a time. Conduction deficits caused by demyelination are usually expressed in the form of latency delays.

Potentials in the auditory cortex are evoked by click sounds. The montage normally shows seven successive waveforms generated by the seven cell groups involved in the pathway from the cochlea to the auditory cortex. The auditory evoked potential technique is a sensitive test for detection of an acoustic neuroma.

Potentials in the somatosensory cortex are elicited by electrical pulses delivered to a peripheral nerve, for example, the median at the wrist and common peroneal at the knee, with recording electrodes in place to detect waveforms in the brachial/lumbar plexus, dorsal columns of the spinal cord, brainstem, and thalamocortical projection. Different disorders impair conduction in different segments of the pathway from skin to cortex.

Motor Evoked Potentials

Transcranial magnetic stimulation (TMS) is used clinically to estimate conduction time in the pyramidal tract, in patients with motor weakness originating in the CNS. Surface EMG recordings of compound action potentials are taken from selected muscles while a magnetic coil delivers very brief currents over the scalp to excite the motor cortex. These brief currents are repeated over the cervical and/or lumbar spine to excite ventral nerve roots innervating the selected muscle(s). Central motor conduction time is obtained by subtraction of the peripheral nerve time segment from the total cortex-to-muscle time. TMS is also used in neurophysiology laboratories to study activity changes in the motor cortex occurring in the course of training for motor skill or strength tasks, clinically in evaluation of motor deficits of unclear origin, and intraoperatively to monitor spinal cord function.

SUGGESTED READINGS

Cho Z, Na C, Wong E, et al. Investigation of acupuncture using fMRI. In: Litscher G, Cho Z, eds. *Computer-Controlled Acupuncture*. Berlin: Pabst; 2000:45–64.

Legatt AD. Electrophysiology of cranial nerve testing: auditory nerve. *J Clin Neurophysiol.* 2018;35:25–38.

Macerolo A, Brown MJN, Kilner JM, Chen R. Neurophysiological changes measured using somatosensory evoked potentials. *Trends Neurosci.* 2018;41:294–310.

Misulis KE, Fakhoury T. *Spehlman's Evoked Potential Primer.* 3rd ed. Boston: Butterworth-Heinemann; 2001.

Phil-Jensen G, Schmidt MF, Frederiksen JL. Multifocal visual evoked potentials in optic neuritis and multiple sclerosis: a review. *Clin Neurophysiol.* 2017;128:1234–1245.

Takeda M, Yamaguchi S, Mitsuhaa T, et al. Intraoperative neurophysiologic monitoring for degenerative cervical myelopathy. *Neurosurg Clin N Am.* 2018;29:159–167.

Wilson MT, Fulcher BD, Fung PK, et al. Biophysical modeling of neural plasticity induced by transcranial magnetic stimulation. *Clin Neurophysiol.* 2018;129:1230–1241.

Visual Pathways

STUDY GUIDELINES

1. Define the layers of the retina and the cell types located in each.
2. Contrast a rod versus a cone cell with respect to structure, function, and localisation within the retina.
3. Be able to trace the pathway from retina to occipital cortex and distinguish between the function of those optic nerve fibres that will end in the midbrain and those that project to the cortex.
4. Given a visual field pattern, be able to localise the site of involvement within the visual pathway.

Understanding of the details of the visual pathways often proves helpful in the diagnosis of diseases of the forebrain. The visual pathway extends from the retinas of the eyes to the occipital lobes of the brain. Their great length makes them especially vulnerable to demyelinating diseases such as multiple sclerosis, to tumours of the brain or pituitary gland, to vascular lesions in the territory of the middle or posterior cerebral artery, and to head injuries.

The visual system comprises the retinas, the visual pathways from the retinas to the brainstem and visual cortex, and the cortical areas devoted to higher visual functions. The retinas and visual pathways are described in this chapter. Higher visual functions are described in Chapter 28.

RETINA

The retina and the optic nerves are part of the central nervous system. In the embryo, the retina is formed by an outgrowth from the diencephalon called the optic vesicle (Chapter 1). The optic vesicle is invaginated by the lens and becomes the two-layered optic cup.

The outer layer of the optic cup becomes the pigment layer of the mature retina. The inner, nervous layer of the cup gives rise to the retinal neurons.

Fig. 31.1 shows the general relationships in the developing retina. The nervous layer contains three principal layers of neurons: *photoreceptors*, which become applied to the pigment layer when the *intraretinal space* is resorbed; *bipolar neurons*; and *ganglion cells*, which give rise to the optic nerve and project to the thalamus and midbrain.

Note that the retina is *inverted*: light must pass through the layers of optic nerve fibres, ganglion cells, and bipolar neurons to reach the photoreceptors. The 'rationale' for an arrangement where the photoreceptors are 'farthest away' from their source of stimulation, light, or photons, is multifold. First, this arrangement juxtaposes the apical end of the photoreceptors (which houses their light sensitive photopigment) against the retinal pigment layer that can absorb any scattered light or light that does not react with these photoreceptor cells. Second, the retinal pigmented epithelial cells also fulfil a phagocytic role. The light sensitive photopigment within the rod photoreceptor cells has a short half-life and needs to be continually replaced. New photopigment is generated at the base of the rod cells and migrates towards the cell apex, while the aged apical components are shed, phagocytised by the retinal pigmented epithelial cells, and the proteins recycled (cones do not shed). Finally, the photoreceptor cells have a high metabolic rate, and at this inner-most retinal position, they are closest to capillaries within the

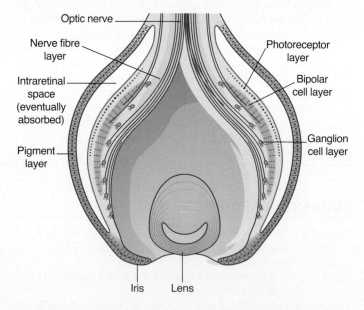

Fig. 31.1 Embryonic retina. *Green* and *red* represent rods and cones, respectively.

choroid (which underlies this pigment epithelium) that supply their nourishment.

At the point of central vision, the *foveola*, the bipolar and ganglion cell layers lean away from a central pit (fovea), and light strikes the photoreceptors directly with minimal distortion (see Foveal Specialisation, later). In the mature eye, the fovea is about 1.5 mm in diameter and occupies the centre of the 5 mm wide *macula lutea* ('yellow spot') where many of the photoreceptor cells contain yellow pigment. The fovea is the point of highest visual acuity and lies in the *visual axis*—a line passing from the centre of the visual field of the eye, through the centre of the lens, to the fovea (Fig. 31.2). To *fixate* or *foveate* an object is to gaze directly at it so that light reflected from its centre registers on the fovea.

The axons of the ganglion cells enter the optic nerve at the *optic nerve head (optic papilla)*, which is devoid of retinal neurons and constitutes the physiologic **blind spot**.

The visual fields of the two eyes overlap across two-thirds of the total visual field. Outside this *binocular field* is a *monocular (temporal) crescent* on each side (Fig. 31.3). During passage through the lens, the image of the visual field is reversed, with the result that objects in the left part of the binocular visual field register on the right half of each retina and objects in the upper part of the visual field register on the lower half. This arrangement is preserved all the way to the visual cortex in the occipital lobe.

From a clinical standpoint, it is essential to appreciate that *vision is a crossed sensation*. The visual field on one side of the visual axis registers on the visual cortex of the opposite side. In effect the right visual cortex 'sees the left visual field' or space and vice versa. Only half of the visual information from each retina crosses in the *optic chiasm*, as the other half has already crossed the midline before it impinges on the retina of the eye opposite to its origin.

Visual defects caused by *interruption of the visual pathway are always described from the patient's point of view*, that is, in terms of the visual fields, and not in terms of retinal topography.

Structure of the Retina

In addition to the serially arranged photoreceptors, bipolar cells, and ganglion cells shown in Fig. 31.1, the retina contains two sets of neurons arranged transversely: **horizontal cells** and **amacrine cells** (Fig. 31.4). A total of eight layers are described for the retina.

The ganglion cells generate action potentials providing the 'requisite speed for conduction' to the thalamus and midbrain. For the other cell types, distances are very short and passive electrical charge (*electrotonus*) or graded changes within their cell membrane potential are sufficient for intercellular communication, whether by gap-junctional contact or transmitter release.

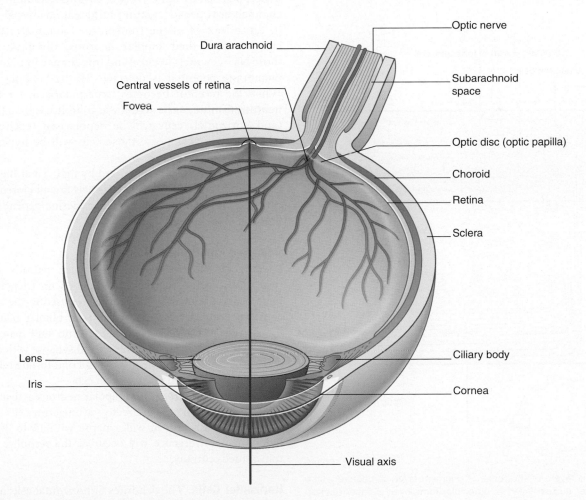

Fig. 31.2 Horizontal section of the right eye, showing the visual axis.

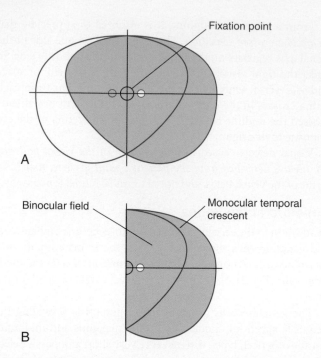

Fig. 31.3 (A) Visual fields of both eyes when targeted on the fixation point. The visual field of the right eye is shaded *blue*. (B) The right visual field. The *white spot* represents the blind spot of the right eye.

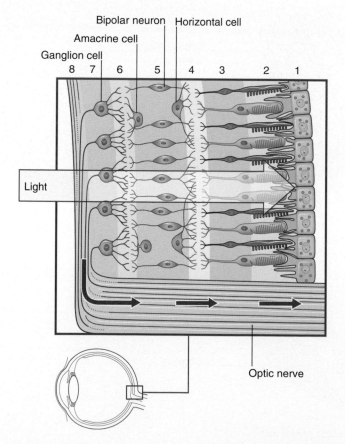

Fig. 31.4 The layers of the retina. *1,* Pigment layer; *2,* photoreceptor layer; *3,* outer nuclear layer; *4,* outer plexiform layer; *5,* inner nuclear layer; *6,* inner plexiform layer; *7,* ganglion cell layer; *8,* nerve fibre layer.

Photoreceptors. The photoreceptor neurons comprise *rods* and *cones*.

Rods function only in dim light and are not sensitive to colour (electromagnetic wavelength energy). They are scarce in the outer part of the fovea and absent from its centre. Cones respond to bright light, are sensitive to colour and to shape, and are most numerous in the fovea. (In the human eye it is estimated that there are 130 million photoreceptor cells; rods outnumber cone cells by 20 to 1 and with the exception of the fovea, are distributed throughout the retina.)

Each photoreceptor cell has an outer and an inner segment and a synaptic end-foot. In the *outer segment* (light sensing 'organelle') there are hundreds of stacked membranous discs (rods) or membrane infoldings (cones) that incorporate a visual pigment (***rhodopsin*** is the photopigment that absorbs light or photons and initiates a molecular cascade that results in a change in the photoreceptor membrane potential and alters the release of neurotransmitter at its synaptic end-foot; this process is called ***phototransduction***); new discs are formed in the *inner segment of rods* and transported to the outer segment; old discs are shed from the apical portion of the outer segment. The *synaptic end-foot* makes contact with bipolar neurons and horizontal cell processes in the *outer plexiform layer*.

A surprising feature of the photoreceptors is that they are hyperpolarised by light. During darkness, sodium ion (Na^+) channels are opened, creating sufficient positive electrotonus to cause leakage of the transmitter (glutamate) from their end-feet onto their bipolar neurons. Illumination causes those Na^+ channels to close and this change in photoreceptor membrane potential is detected by their bipolar neurons. When the receptor becomes hyperpolarised it releases less neurotransmitter as its action was inhibitory; then the bipolar (and horizontal) cells will be depolarised (excited), but if its action was excitatory, those cells will be hyperpolarised (inhibited).

Rod cells are all hyperpolarised by light, so at high levels of illumination their membrane channels are all closed and their contribution to vision is minimal, and vision depends upon the function of the cones.

Cone and Rod Bipolar Neurons

Cone bipolar neurons. Cone bipolar neurons are of two types. **ON** bipolar neurons are switched on (depolarised) by light, being inhibited by transmitter released in the dark. They converge onto ON ganglion cells. **OFF** bipolar neurons have the reverse response and converge onto OFF ganglion cells (Fig. 31.5). Typically, one cone cell will synapse with a few cone bipolar neurons, but at the fovea it is a one-to-one relationship; each will synapse with one ganglion cell.

Rod bipolar neurons. Rod bipolar neurons activate ON and OFF cone ganglion cells indirectly via amacrine cells (Fig. 31.5). One rod bipolar neuron will synapse with 15 to 30 rod cells (additional convergence will occur as the response is further transmitted centrally).

Horizontal Cells. The dendrites of horizontal cells are in contact with photoreceptors. The peripheral dendritic branches

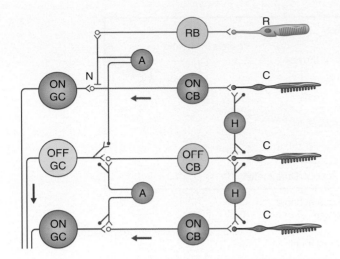

Fig. 31.5 Retinal circuit diagram. *A,* Amacrine cell; *C,* cone; *CB,* cone bipolar neuron; *GC,* ganglion cell; *H,* horizontal cell; *N,* nexus (gap junction); *R,* rod; *RB,* rod bipolar. (Modified from Massey SC and Redburn DA. Transmitter circuits in the vertebrate retina. *Prog. In Neurobiol.* 1987;28:55–96.)

give rise to axon-like processes, which make inhibitory contacts with bipolar neurons.

The function of horizontal cells is to inhibit bipolar neurons outside the immediate zone of excitation. The excited bipolar cells and ganglion cells are said to be 'on-line' and the inhibited ones 'off-line'.

Amacrine Cells. Amacrine cells have no axons. Their appearance is octopus-like; the dendrites all emerge from one side of the cell. Dendritic branches come into contact with bipolar neurons and ganglion cells.

More than a dozen different morphologic types of amacrine cells have been identified, as well as several different transmitters, including acetylcholine, dopamine, and serotonin. Possible functions include contrast enhancement and movement detection. For the rods, they convert large numbers from OFF to ON with respect to their ganglion cells.

Ganglion Cells. The ganglion cells receive synaptic contacts from their bipolar neurons in the inner plexiform layer. The typical response of ganglion cells to bipolar activity is 'centre-surround'. The *centre* of the receptive field represents the direct connections the ganglion cell receives from its photoreceptors; the *surround* of the receptive field are the connections it receives from adjacent photoreceptors via horizontal cells. An ON ganglion cell is excited by a spot of light and inhibited by a surrounding annulus (ring) of light. Horizontal cells cause the inhibition. OFF ganglion cells give the reverse response.

Coding for colour. There are three types of cone photoreceptor cells with respect to spectral sensitivity. One type is sensitive to red (also called L cones based on the 'longer' frequency of light they detect), one to green (M cone), and one to blue (also called S cones, but making up perhaps only 5% to 10% of the cones). The sensitivity is determined by the particular visual pigment of each cone cell type. While the light

frequency that results in maximal stimulation identifies the particular cone type, the cones actually respond to a broader spectrum of light frequency, and the three cone types overlap one another. Colour is perceived not by one cone cell, but by comparing the activity of different cone cells to a particular frequency or colour of light. Groups of each type are connected to ON or OFF ganglion cells. (Processing of colour begins at the retina but continues at the lateral geniculate nucleus and cortex.)

The characteristic response of ganglion cells is one of *colour opponency* (one colour will activate a group of cone cells and their particular ganglion cell while its 'opponent' will inhibit it, or they can be considered as mutually exclusive):

- Ganglion cells that are on-line for green are off-line for red and ganglion cells that are on-line for red are off-line for green.
- Ganglion cells that are on-line for blue are off-line for yellow and ganglion cells that are on-line for yellow are off-line for blue.
- Finally, there is a similar process for white and black or luminance.

Coding for black and white. White light is a mixture of green, red, and blue. In bright conditions, it is encoded by the three corresponding cones, all of them converging onto common ganglion cells. Both ON and OFF ganglion cells are involved in black-and-white vision, just as in colour vision.

In very dim conditions, such as starlight, only rod photoreceptors are active, and objects appear in varying shades of grey. The rods are subject to the same rules as cones, showing centre-surround antagonism between white and black, and being connected to ON or OFF ganglion cells.

Most rod and cone ganglion cells are small (*parvocellular* or 'P'), having small receptive fields and being responsive to colour and shape. A minority are large (*magnocellular* or 'M'), having large receptive fields and being especially responsive to movements within the visual field.

Foveal Specialisation. The relative density of cones increases progressively, and their size diminishes progressively, from the edge of the fovea inwards (Fig. 31.6). The central one-third of the fovea, little more than 100 μm wide and known as the *foveola*, contains only *midget* cones. Two special anatomic features assist the foveal cones in general, and the midget cones in particular, in transducing the maximum amount of information concerning the form and colour values of an object under direct scrutiny. First, the more superficial layers of the retina lean outward from the centre, and their neurites are exceptionally long, with the result that the outer two-thirds of the foveola are little overlapped by bipolar cell bodies and the inner third is not overlapped at all; light reflected from the object strikes the cones of the foveola without any diffraction. Second, one-to-one synaptic contact between the midget cones and midget bipolar neurons, and between these and midget ganglion cells, enhances fidelity of central transmission. Outside the foveola, the amount of cone-to-bipolar-to-ganglion cell convergence increases progressively.

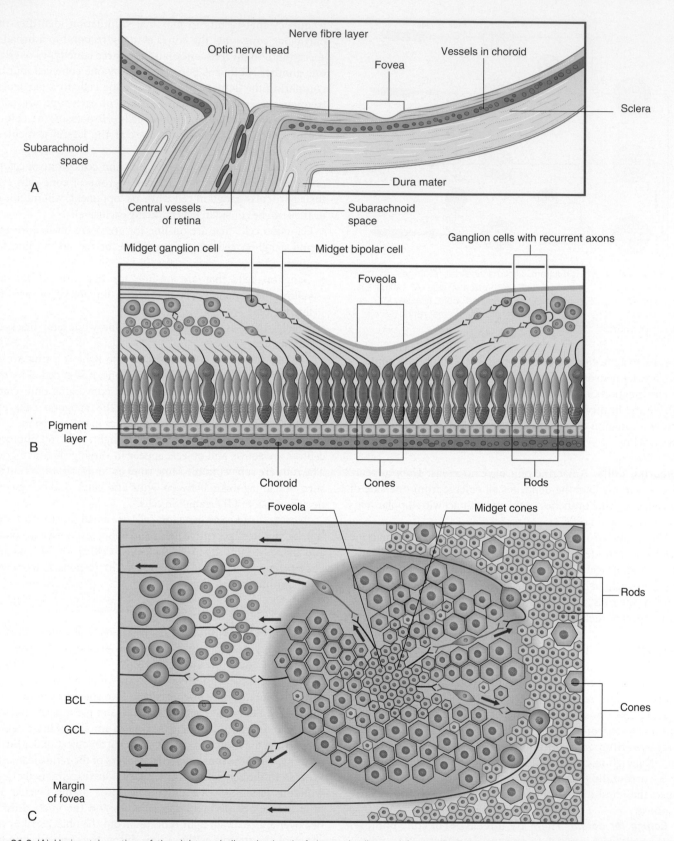

Fig. 31.6 (A) Horizontal section of the right eyeball at the level of the optic disc and fovea. (B) Enlargement from (A). Recurrent axons sweep around the fovea as shown in (C). (C) Surface view of the fovea and neighbouring retina. Cones have been omitted at intervals to show the 'chain' sequence of neurons. *BCL,* bipolar cell layer; *GCL,* ganglionic cell layer.

CENTRAL VISUAL PATHWAYS

Optic Nerve, Optic Tract

The optic nerve is formed by the axons of the retinal ganglion cells. The axons acquire myelin sheaths as they leave the optic disc.

The number of ganglion cells varies remarkably between individuals but is about 1 million. Since every ganglion cell contributes to the optic nerve, the number of axons in the optic nerve is correspondingly variable.

The retinal ganglion cells are homologous to the sensory projection neurons of the spinal cord. The optic nerve is homologous to spinal cord white matter and is *not* a peripheral nerve. As explained in Chapter 9, true peripheral nerves, whether cranial or spinal, contain Schwann cells and collagenous sheaths and are capable of regeneration. The optic nerve contains neuroglial cells of central type (astrocytes and oligodendrocytes) and is not capable of regeneration in mammals. In addition, the nerve is invested with meninges containing an extension of the subarachnoid space—a feature largely responsible for the changed appearance of the fundus oculi when the intracranial pressure increases (*papilloedema*, Chapter 5).

At the optic chiasm, fibres from the nasal hemiretina (medial half of the retina) enter the contralateral optic tract, whereas those from the temporal (lateral) hemiretina remain uncrossed and enter the ipsilateral tract. Information from the retina is transmitted to the midbrain (contributes to eye movement control, pupillary size, and circadian rhythms) and lateral geniculate nucleus of the thalamus (transmitted on to the visual cortex to subserve the various components of vision) by different groups of ganglion cells.

As already noted in Chapter 34, some optic nerve fibres enter the suprachiasmatic nucleus of the hypothalamus, which is the 'central clock' and responsible for helping to maintain circadian rhythms. This connection has been invoked to account for the beneficial effect of bright artificial light, for several hours per day, in the treatment of wintertime depression.

Each optic tract winds around the midbrain and divides into a medial and a lateral root.

Medial Root of the Optic Tract.
The medial root contains 10% of the optic nerve fibres. It enters the side of the midbrain. It contains four distinct sets of fibres:

1. Some fibres, mainly from retinal M cells, enter the superior colliculus and provide for automatic scanning, such as reading this page.
2. Some fibres are relayed from the superior colliculus to the pulvinar of the thalamus; they belong to the extra-geniculate pathway to the visual association cortex (Chapter 28).
3. Some fibres enter the pretectal nucleus and serve the pupillary light reflex (Chapter 23).
4. Some fibres enter the parvocellular reticular formation, where they have an arousal function (Chapter 24).

Lateral Root of the Optic Tract and Lateral Geniculate Body.
The lateral root of the optic tract terminates in the lateral geniculate body (LGB) of the thalamus. The LGB shows six cellular laminae, three of which are devoted to crossed fibres and three to uncrossed fibres (layers 2, 3, and 5; 'U-235'). The two deepest laminae (one for crossed and one for uncrossed fibres) are magnocellular and receive axons from retinal M ganglion cells concerned with detection of *movement* (location, speed, and direction). The other four are parvocellular and receive the axons of P cells concerned with *particulars*, namely visual detail and colour.

The circuitry of the LGB resembles that of other thalamic relay nuclei and includes inhibitory (γ-aminobutyric acid; GABA) terminals derived from interneurons and from the thalamic reticular nucleus. (The portion of the reticular nucleus serving the LGB is called the *perigeniculate nucleus*.) Corticogeniculate axons arise in the primary visual cortex and synapse upon distal dendrites of relay cells as well as upon inhibitory interneurons. Cortical synapses on relay cells are twice as numerous as those derived from retinal ganglion cells. Cortical stimulation usually enhances the response of relay cells to a given retinal input. A likely, but unproven, function could be that of selective enhancement of particular features of the visual scene, such as when searching for an object of known shape or colour. Functional magnetic resonance imaging (fMRI, Chapter 28) is capable of detecting areas of increased neuronal activity in the brain. fMRI has shown that when volunteers expect to see an object of interest onscreen, metabolic activity in the LGB increases *before* the stimulus is presented.

Geniculocalcarine Tract and Primary Visual Cortex

The **optic radiation** (*geniculocalcarine tract*) is of major clinical importance because it is frequently compromised by vascular occlusion or tumours in the posterior part of the cerebral hemisphere. The tract travels from the LGB to the primary visual cortex.

The anatomy of the optic radiation is shown in Figs. 31.7 to 31.10. Fibres destined for the lower half of the primary visual cortex sweep forward into the temporal lobe, as the **Meyer loop**, before turning back to accompany those traveling to the upper half. The tract enters the retrolenticular part of the internal capsule and continues in the white matter underlying the lateral temporal cortex. It runs alongside the posterior horn of the lateral ventricle before turning medially to enter the occipital cortex.

The **primary visual cortex** occupies the superior and inferior banks of the calcarine sulcus along its entire length (the sulcus is 10 mm deep). It emerges onto the medial surface of the hemisphere for 5 mm both above and below the sulcus, and onto the occipital pole of the brain for 10 mm. Its total area is about 28 cm^2. In the freshly cut brain, it is easily identified by a thin band of white matter (the *visual stria of Gennari*) within the grey matter—hence an alternative term, **striate cortex**. The left and right eyes are represented in the cortex in alternating stripes called *ocular dominance columns* (Fig. 31.10).

Retinotopic Map.
The contralateral visual field is represented upside down. The plane of the calcarine sulcus represents the

horizontal meridian. Retinal representation is posteroanterior, with a greatly magnified foveal representation in the posterior half of the calcarine cortex (Fig. 31.10).

The clinical effects of various lesions of the visual pathway are described in Clinical Panel 31.1.

In the left retina and optic nerve, the neural representation of the image is reversed side to side. It is also inverted top to bottom. The right retina and optic nerve are inactive because this eye is shielded.

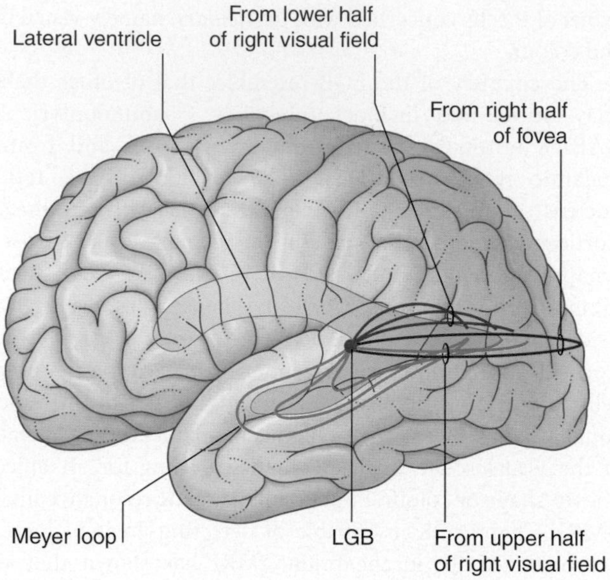

Fig. 31.7 Left optic radiation. *LGB,* Lateral geniculate body.

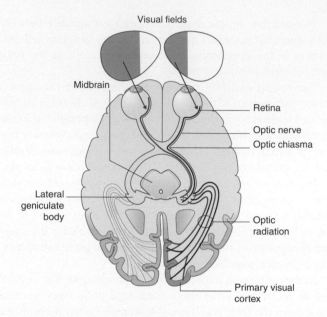
Fig. 31.9 Diagram of the visual pathways. The two visual fields (left and right eye) are represented separately, without the normal overlap.

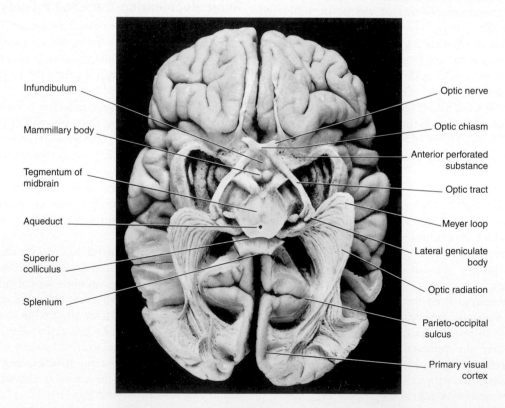
Fig. 31.8 A dissection of the visual pathways viewed from below. (Photograph reproduced from Gluhbegovic N, Williams TW. *The Human Brain. A Photographic Guide,* 1980; Hagerstown: Harper and Row, by kind permission of the authors and of J.B. Lippincott, Inc.)

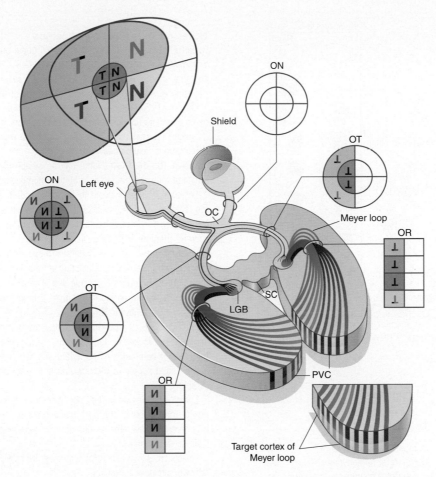

Fig. 31.10 Pathway from the visual field of the left eye to the primary visual cortex. *T* denotes the temporal (outer) half of the left visual field; *N* denotes the nasal (inner) half of the left visual field. *LGB,* Lateral geniculate body; *OC,* optic chiasm; *ON,* optic nerve; *OR,* optic radiations; *OT,* optic tract; *PVC,* primary visual cortex; *SC,* superior colliculus.

At the optic chiasm the axons forming the nasal half of the left optic nerve cross the midline and form the medial half of the right optic tract. Those forming the lateral half of the nerve form the lateral half of the left optic tract. Each set synapses in the corresponding LGB.

The optic radiations are fan-like (compare with Fig. 31.7), with the axons carrying the foveal input initially in the middle of the fan.

As they approach the occipital pole, the foveal axons (red in Fig. 31.10) in both hemispheres move to the back and enter the posterior part of the primary visual cortex. Note the striped pattern of delivery to the cortex on both sides. The blank intervals between are the same width and contain the axons and cortex responsible for the visual field of the *right* eye.

CLINICAL PANEL 31.1 Lesions of the Visual Pathways

The following points arise in testing the visual pathways:

The patient may be unaware of quite extensive blindness—sometimes even of a hemianopia.

Large visual defects can often be detected by simple confrontation, as follows. The patient covers one eye at a time and focuses on the examiner's nose. The examiner, seated opposite, looks the patient in the eye while bringing one or other hand into view from various directions, with the index finger wiggling.

In a blind area the patient does not see blackness; the patient does not see anything.

Visual defects are described from the patient's viewpoint, in terms of the visual fields. *(To foster the concept of visual field representations, numbered 1 through 9, a dark colour is used to signify the area where vision is lost. In actuality, visual field diagrams signify where vision is retained, the opposite of what is shown diagrammatically; the blind spot is also not indicated but would be located temporal (lateral) to the central spot of visual fixation.)*

Possible sites of injury to the visual pathways are shown in Fig. 31.11. The effects produced correspond to the numbers in the following list:

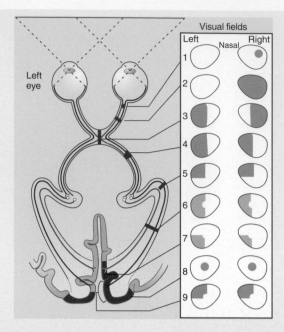

Fig. 31.11 Visual field defects following various lesions of the visual pathways.

LESION #	Visual Field Defects
1. Partial optic nerve	Ipsilateral scotoma[a]
2. Complete optic nerve	Blindness in that eye
3. Optic chiasm	Bitemporal hemianopia
4. Optic tract	Contralateral homonymous[b] hemianopia
5. Meyer's loop	Contralateral homonymous superior quadrantanopia
6. Optic radiation	Contralateral homonymous hemianopia (with macular sparing)
7. Primary visual cortex (upper bank)	Contralateral homonymous inferior hemianopia (with macular sparing)
8. Bilateral macular cortex	Bilateral central scotomas
9. Posterior visual cortex (lower bank)	Contralateral homonymous superior quadrantanopia (with macular sparing)

[a]Patch of blindness.
[b]Matching.

Notes on the Numbered Lesions

Lesion #1: Eccentric lesions of the optic nerve produce scotomas in the nasal or temporal field of the affected eye. *When a young adult presents with a scotoma, multiple sclerosis must always be suspected.*

Lesion #2: Results from a complete lesion of the optic nerve.

Lesion #3: Compression of the middle of the chiasm is most often caused by an adenoma (benign tumour) of the pituitary gland.

Lesion #4: Lesions of the optic tract are rare and result in contralateral homonymous hemianopia.

Lesion #5: The Meyer loop may be selectively caught by a tumour in the temporal lobe resulting in contralateral homonymous superior quadrantanopia.

Lesion #6: Lesions involving the optic radiation include tumours arising in the temporal, parietal, or occipital lobe. The visual fields of both eyes tend to be affected to an equal extent (*congruously*) and in this case the macula is spared. Tumours impinging on the radiation from below produce an upper quadrantic defect at first, whereas those impinging from above produce a lower quadrantic defect. The stem of the radiation occupies the retrolentiform part of the internal capsule and is often compromised for some days by oedema, following haemorrhage from a branch of the middle cerebral artery (classic stroke, Chapter 35).

Thrombosis of the posterior cerebral artery produces a homonymous hemianopia. The notches in field chart no. 7 represent macular sparing. Sparing of the macular hemifields is inconstant and, when present, is often attributed to a dual blood supply of the occipital pole from both the middle and posterior cerebral artery.

Lesion #7: A lesion in the upper bank of the primary visual cortex is usually due to thrombosis of the posterior cerebral artery. The field defect produced is a contralateral homonymous inferior quadrantanopia with macular sparing ("pie on the floor").

Lesion #8: Bilateral central scotomas are most often caused by a backward fall with occipital contusion.

Lesion #9: A lesion in the lower bank of the primary visual cortex is also likely due to a thrombus in the posterior cerebral artery. The field defect produced is a contralateral homonymous superior quadrantanopia with macular sparing ("pie in the sky"). Sparing of the macula is inconstant and, when present, is often attributed to a dual blood supply of the occipital pole from the branches of the middle and posterior cerebral arteries.

✳ Core Information

The embryonic retina is an outgrowth of the diencephalon. The embryonal optic cup is composed of an outer pigment layer and an inner nervous layer, with an intraretinal space between. The nervous layer contains three sets of radially disposed neurons, photoreceptors, bipolar cells, and ganglion cells, and two tangential sets, horizontal cells and amacrine cells. Except at the fovea centralis, light must pass through the other layers to reach the photoreceptors. The visual image is inverted and reversed by the lens. Two-thirds of the visual field are binocular; the outer one-sixth on each side is monocular. Visual defects are described in terms of visual fields.

Rod photoreceptors function in dim light and are absent from the fovea. Cones are most numerous in the fovea; they are responsive to shape and have three kinds of sensitivity to colour. Ganglion cell responses are concentric, showing centre-surround colour opponency. M ganglion cells are relatively large, are movement detectors, and project their axons to the two magnocellular layers of the LGB. P ganglion cells signal particular features of the image as well as colour and project to the four parvocellular layers of the LGB. The LGB is binocular, receiving signals from the contralateral nasal hemiretina (via the optic chiasm) and from the ipsilateral temporal hemiretina. Both sets of axons arrive by the optic tract, which also gives offsets to the midbrain for lower-level visual reflexes.

The optic radiation (geniculocalcarine tract) arises from M and P cells of the LGB and swings around the side of the lateral ventricle to reach the primary visual cortex, in the walls of the calcarine sulcus.

Distinctive visual field defects occur following damage at any of the five major components of the visual pathway (optic nerve, optic chiasm, optic tract, optic radiation, and visual cortex).

SUGGESTED READINGS

Burr DC, Morrone MC. Constructing stable spatial maps of the world. *Perception.* 2012;41:1355—1372.

Dhande OS, Huberman AD. Retinal ganglion cell maps in the brain: implications for visual processing. *Curr Opin Neurobiol.* 2014;24: 133—142.

Hout MC, Goldinger SD. To see or not to see. *Sci Amer Mind.* 2013;24:60—67.

Krauzlis RJ, Lovejoy LP, Zénon A. Superior colliculus and visual spatial attention. *Annu Rev Neurosci.* 2012;36:165—182.

Maya-Vetencourt JF, Origlia N. Visual cortex plasticity: a complex interplay of genetic and environmental influences. *Neural Plast.* 2012;2012:631965.

Pietrasanta M, Restani L, Caleo M. The corpus callosum and the visual cortex: plasticity is a game for two. *Neural Plast.* 2012;2012:838672.

Qin W, Yu C. Neural pathways conveying novisual information to the visual cortex. *Neural Plast.* 2013;2013:864920.

Schmidt KE. The visual callosal connection: a connection like any other? *Neural Plast.* 2013;2013:397176.

Sung CH, Chuang JZ. The cell biology of vision. *J Cell Biol.* 2010;190: 953—963.

Hemispheric Asymmetries

STUDY GUIDELINES

1. List the different cognitive domains and their individual roles.
2. Describe and contrast the clinical outcome of injuries to the Broca and Wernicke areas.
3. Describe the 'steps' performed when reading in relation to areas of the brain involved.
4. Discuss the different clinical manifestations of frontal lobe injuries.
5. Discuss the different clinical manifestations of right parietal lobe injuries.

The two cerebral hemispheres are *asymmetrical* in several respects. Some of the asymmetries have to do with handedness, language, and complex motor activities, but other more subtle differences exist. (Limbic asymmetries are described in Chapter 33.)

HANDEDNESS

Handedness often determines the hemisphere that is dominant for motor control. Left hemisphere/right-hand dominance is the rule. Advances in ultrasound technology have made it possible for the observation of motor behaviour in the fetus, and handedness (and brain asymmetries) established before birth based on the preferred hand used for thumb sucking during fetal life.

In 96% of right-handed subjects, the left hemisphere is dominant for language, and while this asymmetry of language dominance is true for most left-handed subjects, it varies with respect to the 'strength' of their left-handedness. Those who are strongly left-handed have a higher incidence of right hemisphere language dominance (27%), while in those who are ambidextrous the right hemisphere is dominant in 15%. Handedness, hemispheric language dominance, and other left versus right body asymmetries may represent a polygenic trait, but are not limited to humans and functional brain asymmetries exist in the great apes and other vertebrates.

Modular Organisation of Language and Higher Cognitive Functions

Clarifying the function of and interrelationships between brain structures has transitioned beyond the insights gathered by studying those who have suffered focal brain lesions. New techniques such as neuroimaging with functional magnetic resonance imaging (fMRI) and neurophysiologic techniques (e.g. transcranial magnetic stimulation) allow investigation of those with and without cerebral dysfunction and have substantiated some prior interpretations, but just as often have led us to question or revise them.

As exemplified by speech and language, different cognitive functions or domains consist of a network ('connectome') of interconnecting anatomical areas, and within each are 'hubs' that support integrative processing and adaptive behaviour. Critical for the broad display of normal function, hub dysfunction results in disorders that are more expansive and remote than predicted by only the 'size' of the cortical area involved. (*Diaschisis* was a term originally suggested to signify neurophysiologic changes in an area remote from the area of injury. Now with connectomics, it signifies changes at a structural and connectivity level that may be distant from a focal brain lesion.)

Involvement of hubs and dysfunction of their network(s) are associated with or proposed to explain the clinical manifestations of disorders such as Alzheimer disease and schizophrenia. In some cases a hub may demonstrate observable morphologic differences, but in other cases such a clear relationship is absent, as the difficulty had instead disrupted its connections to another area. In addition, one anatomical area may contribute or play a role in more than one cognitive domain.

These cognitive functions or domains include the following that are the most anatomically and functionally distinct:
- A *language network* involves cortical areas around the Sylvian fissure including Broca and Wernicke's area.
- A *behavioural/emotion network* includes prefrontal and cingulate cortical areas and the amygdala.

- *Spatial awareness* is based on centres in the posterior parietal cortex, premotor cortex, supplementary cortex, and the frontal eye fields.
- *Face-object recognition* centres are in the midtemporal and temporopolar cerebral cortex.
- The *executive function network* includes the lateral prefrontal and orbitofrontal cerebral cortex (through its connections with other cortical areas, the prefrontal cortex contributes to and influences other cortical domains).
- *Working memory and learning* include the hippocampus, medial temporal lobe, and prefrontal cortex.
- The *attention network* includes the frontal, parietal, and cingulate cortex.

Language Areas

Our classical way of understanding language was to assign function to discrete areas of the cortex, separating language production from comprehension. At the bedside, this remains a useful conceptualisation for initial localisation and is referred to as the *Wernicke-Lichtheim-(Geschwind) model (WLG)*, after those individuals who pioneered clinical studies of language. While this model remains useful, language depends on multiple cortical and subcortical areas. Currently a *dual stream model*, a concept not limited to language, more accurately describes speech and language organisation. Speech production occurs through a *dorsal stream* that extends from parietal to frontal cortex of the left hemisphere and ends with acoustic speech signals 'mapped' onto cortical areas specific for articulation, resulting in fluent speech. The *ventral stream* involves the lateral temporal lobes, extending anteriorly into the inferior frontal lobe and posteriorly into the inferior parietal lobe, providing meaning to auditory information. Production and comprehension of language through these two systems are dynamically linked and both necessary for successful comprehension and communication.

Broca Area (Fig. 32.1). The French pathologist Pierre Broca assigned a 'motor' or speech production function to the inferior

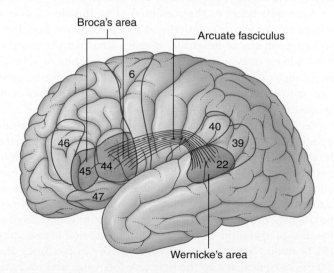

Broca's area

Arcuate fasciculus

6

40

46

39

45 44

22

47

Wernicke's area

Fig. 32.1 The broca and wernicke language areas and the arcuate fasciculus.

frontal gyrus of the left side in 1861. The principal area concerned occupies the pars opercularis and pars triangularis parts of the inferior frontal gyrus corresponding to Brodmann areas 44 and 45. Broca's area represents a node within the anterior portion of the dorsal language stream that includes adjacent Brodmann area 47, premotor cortex (the ventral part of area 6) and the dorsal stream extends posteriorly to the supramarginal gyrus.

A language disorder described as a **Broca** or **expressive aphasia** is attributed to lesions involving the Broca area, where fluency (speech production) is disrupted to a greater extent than comprehension (see Clinical Panel 32.1), but all language disorders can be considered expressive. However, the functional role and manifestations of dysfunction attributed to Broca area lesions have extended beyond the original WLG model. Cytoarchitectonic and connectivity differences are more extensive and dynamic with functional separation into areas that serve a role in *phonology* (how sounds are organised and used in natural languages), *syntax* (arrangement of words and phrases to create well-formed sentences), and *semantics* (meaning of words, phrases, sentences, or even larger units).

We now consider the Broca area (and its connectivity) as not 'language specific', but a role it does fulfil through its connectivity with language-relevant areas. It participates in other cognitive domains such as music and a role in other actions (increasing a listener's attention when specific utterances occur, while decreasing attention to utterances when engaged in 'cocktail speech', or modifying a speaker's utterances in ways that will enhance the meaning of his or her communication to a specific listener). Similarly, its connectivity to Wernicke's area via the arcuate fasciculus (see Fig. 32.1) is more extensive and includes other relevant language areas within the frontal, temporal, and parietal cortex.

Output from the Broca area does facilitate speech articulation through sequences of oral motor and respiratory activity of the adjacent premotor and motor cortex. It also serves to direct and focus attention, and to ensure appropriate behavioural interactivity (e.g. waiting your turn to speak, speaking in the appropriate tone or manner) through interaction with the dorsolateral prefrontal cortex (DLPFC), anterior cingulate gyrus, and parietal cortex. Connectivity with the temporal cortex as well as inferior parietal areas is necessary when accessing memories with respect to knowledge type and the associated phonological, syntax, and semantic forms. In view of these multiple roles, the Broca area is referred to as the *Broca region*, as different functional roles reflect its subparcellation.

As an 'entrenched' bedside clinical localisation, Broca aphasia will likely remain, but eventually replaced by a more appropriate clinical phenomenology.

Wernicke Area (see Fig. 32.1). The German neurologist Karl Wernicke made extensive contributions to the understanding of language processing in the late 19th century. He designated the posterior part of Brodmann area 22 in the superior temporal gyrus of the left hemisphere as a 'sensory area' concerned with understanding the spoken word. Lesions involving this Wernicke area in adults are associated with a **Wernicke** or **receptive aphasia** (Clinical Panel 32.1), where comprehension is impaired to a greater extent than fluency of speech.

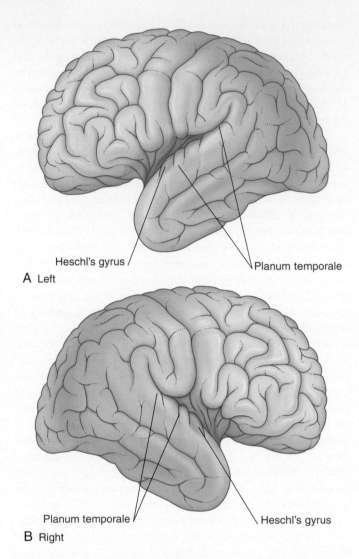

Heschl's gyrus
A Left
Planum temporale

Planum temporale
B Right
Heschl's gyrus

Fig. 32.2 Views of the opened lateral sulcus, showing the upper surface of the temporal lobes.

The upper surface of the Wernicke area includes the ***planum temporale*** *(temporal plane)* (Fig. 32.2) that comprises the superior temporal gyrus (posterior portion of Brodmann area 22) just posterior to the primary auditory cortex (Heschl gyrus) and the supramarginal gyrus, area 40. The planum temporale facilitates spatiotemporal discrimination and identification of auditory stimuli that are crucial for speech (*phonemes*; the smallest unit of speech in a language that is capable of conveying a distinction in meaning), as well as being involved in or modulated by auditory attention when selecting stimuli from the left versus right ear. (The volume of cerebral cortex in the planum temporale is larger on the left side in 65% of right-handed subjects but does not match the more than 90% left-hemisphere dominance for speech.)

The Wernicke area is linked to the Broca area through association fibres of the *arcuate fasciculus* that curve around the posterior end of the lateral fissure within the underlying white matter (see Fig. 32.1). Additional pathways of connectivity for language areas are delineated by magnetic resonance imaging

(MRI) in humans (and suggested by tract-tracing studies in monkeys) between the frontal, temporal, parietal, and occipital cortex. These occur through the uncinate, superior, and inferior longitudinal fasciculi and extreme capsule (see Fig. 2.20).

These multiple pathways further support the concept of a ventral stream (analogous to visual processing) for language. The *ventral stream* relates auditory information to meaning as well as to proper syntax phrase construction.

Like the clinical use of the term Broca aphasia, Wernicke aphasia will likely remain in the clinical realm for some time. However, lesions restricted to the Wernicke area are associated with difficulty in speech production, word retrieval, and speech that is associated with paraphasic (substitution of the correct word by a similar speech sound, incorrect word, or nonsensical word) errors, but word comprehension remains intact. The syndrome of Wernicke aphasia (paraphasic speech production and comprehension impairment) results from injury to the Wernicke area and additional areas within the lateral temporal lobe and parietal cortex.

Angular Gyrus. The angular gyrus (area 39) belongs descriptively to the inferior parietal lobule. The *left* angular gyrus receives a projection from the inferior part of area 19 (the lingual gyrus, shown in Fig. 2.5), and itself projects to the planum temporale. It is commonly included as a part of the Wernicke area.

Right Hemisphere Contribution. During normal conversation there is an increase in blood flow in both left and right superior temporal cortical regions that mediate speech perception and comprehension at a *lexical* (words or vocabulary of a language) level. In addition, it is believed that the right hemisphere may be concerned with melodic aspects of speech—cadences, emphases, and nuances—collectively called *prosody*, that convey both affective and nonaffective information. *Affective prosody* refers to the emotional meaning of the utterance (e.g. happy, angry). *Nonaffective prosody* plays a linguistic role or conveys the intention of what is said (e.g. a question or a statement).

Aprosodia refers to the condition of an individual who is unable to express or comprehend affective and/or nonaffective components of language. Usually seen in right cerebral hemispheric lesions, it can occur with left cerebral or subcortical injury (Clinical Panel 32.1), and a classification scheme that is in parallel to the left hemispheric aphasias has been proposed.

Recovery of speech function—when it occurs—depends upon the age of the subject and in adults, upon the extent of the lesion. Occasional cases have been reported of recovery of near-normal speech in right-handed patients 7 years of age or younger following complete removal of the left hemisphere as a treatment for intractable epilepsy. This can only be explained by language processing, including speech, not fully lateralised at the time of operation. In adults, positron emission tomography (PET) studies have shown increased activity in the Broca and Wernicke equivalents on the right side following cerebrovascular accidents on the left. However, significant improvement is possible only if the left planum temporale is sufficiently viable to be able to process signals passed to it from the right side through the corpus callosum.

Listening to Spoken Words

The auditory system, from cochlea to cortex, is uniquely 'tuned' to natural sounds and their associated frequencies, and especially those related to spoken words. Fig. 32.3 contrasts regional increases in blood flow during PET scanning when a volunteer listens to words ('active listening') versus random tone sequences ('passive listening'). As expected, tone sequences activate the primary auditory cortex (bilaterally). The Wernicke area (left side) also becomes active, probably in screening out this nonverbal material from further processing. Area 9 in the frontal lobe is thought to be part of a supervisory and vigilance system.

The process of actively listening to words is believed to occur through pathways between the temporal and inferior frontal cortex and from the inferior frontal lobe to the temporal cortex. Listening 'begins' in the primary auditory cortex when words (versus pseudowords) are first recognised by their acoustic pattern. The Wernicke area and the adjacent cortex provide interpretation of syntax and semantics, then the anterior portion of the superior temporal gyrus provides further information regarding the word class or category as the syntactic phrase is constructed. This information is now 'submitted' to the inferior frontal cortex (Broca region) where grammatical relationships between phrases are developed.

The Broca region projects back to the anterior portion of the superior temporal lobe as well as to the posterior portion of the superior temporal gyrus. These connections are assumed to exert a level of 'top-down' control with regards to semantics as well as grammatical relationships. Knowledge type may result in other areas of the parietal or temporal cortex becoming involved. Activity in the *dorsolateral prefrontal cortex (DLPFC)* and anterior cingulate gyrus may be recruited to ensure attention is directed to relevant information. When listening to one's own voice, the areas of the temporal lobe identified above become active. An important function served is meta-analysis (*post hoc* analysis) of speech, whereby 'slips of the tongue' are identified. Speech meta-analysis is singularly lacking in cases of so-called Wernicke aphasia (Clinical Panel 32.1).

Neuroanatomy of Reading (Fig. 32.4)
Glossary

- *Graphemes.* A letter or a combination of letters that represents a sound (phoneme) within a language.
- *Orthography* (*Gr.* 'correct writing'). Representation of the sounds of a language by written or printed symbols.
- *Phonemes* (*Gr.* 'sounds'). The sounds of syllables. 'Cat' is a single syllable containing three phonemes: [k], [a], and [t].
- *Phonology.* The rules governing the sounds of words. Testing could include: 'How many of these words have two syllables?' or 'How many of these words rhyme with one another?'
- *Retrieval.* Matching words, phrases, and sentences with those previously entered into memory.
- *Semantics* (*Gr.* 'meaning'). Meaning of words and sentences.

Reading Sequence (a Suggested Sequence and Process)

A. *Perform visual processing*
Visual processing is performed bilaterally in areas 17, 18, and 19. It includes analysis of letter shapes for their identification, distinguishing between letters in upper versus lower case, and between real letters and meaningless shapes ('false fonts'). Processed information in the right extrastriate cortex (areas 18 and 19) is transferred to the left side through the forceps major traversing the splenium of the corpus callosum—a point of clinical significance (see later).

B. *Perform orthographic processing*
Orthographic processing means discerning whether each letter string in a sentence represents a real or a pseudoword, for example, 'word' versus 'wurd'. Medial area 19 (V4) is especially involved.

C. *Perform phonological assembly*
Phonological processing means the conversion of graphemes to phonemes. The angular gyrus (area 390) and middle temporal gyrus (area 21) participate.

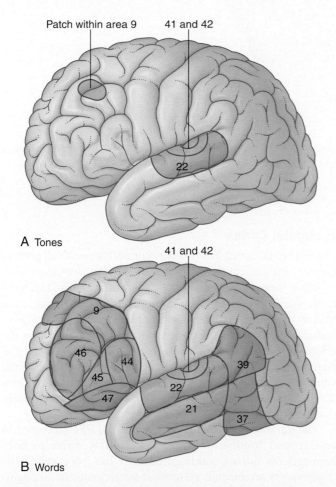

Patch within area 9   41 and 42

A Tones

41 and 42

B Words

Fig. 32.3 Regions of increased blood flow during listening (A) to tones and (B) to words.

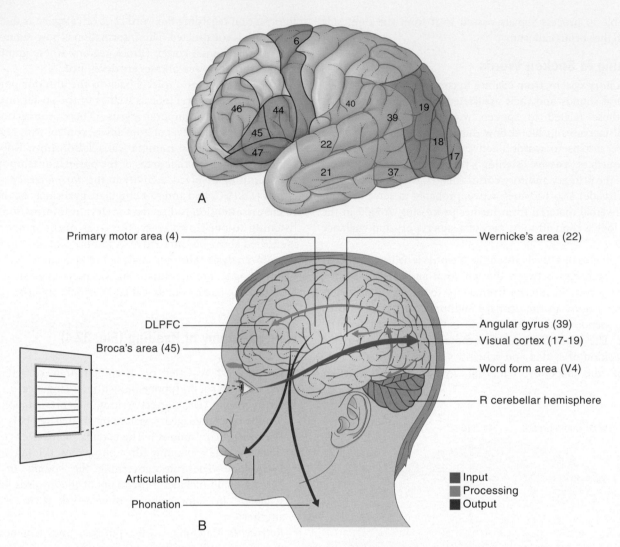

Fig. 32.4 (A) Areas of increased cortical blood flow in the left hemisphere observed in PET scans during reading aloud. (B) Diagram representing input *(blue)*, processing *(green)*, and output *(red)* pathways active during reading aloud. *DLPFC*, Dorsolateral prefrontal cortex.

D. *Perform semantic retrieval*

Semantic retrieval means performance of a memory search using both orthographic and phonological cues from the text to extract the meaning of words and sentences. The anterior part of the Broca area (area 45) becomes active at this advanced stage, together with area 37 in the posterior temporal lobe and area 40 (supramarginal gyrus) in the inferior parietal lobule.

E. Execution of motor plans (phonological execution) is the performance of 'inner speech' (subvocal articulation). The Broca area becomes active, as do the adjacent parts of the premotor and motor cortex, the supplementary motor area (medial area 6), and the contralateral cerebellar hemisphere. The same four areas become much more active during reading aloud.

The left lateral prefrontal cortex in and around area 46 is 'switched on' throughout steps A to E. Also active is part of area 32 in the left anterior cingulate cortex, which is involved in all cognitive activities requiring attention.

Prefrontal Cortex

The prefrontal cortex has two-way connections with all parts of the neocortex except the primary motor and sensory areas, with its fellow through the genu of the corpus callosum, and with the mediodorsal nucleus of the thalamus. It is uniquely large in the human brain and is concerned with the highest brain functions, including abstract thinking, decision making, anticipating the effects of courses of action, and social behaviour. It can also be demonstrated that structural changes occur in the grey and white matter of the brain when practicing motor or cognitive skills. These changes are referred to as *experience-dependent structural plasticity*.

The ***dorsolateral prefrontal cortex*** (**DLPFC**), centred in and around Brodmann area 9, is strongly active in both hemispheres during waking hours. It has been called the 'supervisory attentional system'. It participates in all cognitive activities and is essential for conscious learning of all kinds. During conscious learning it operates *working* *memory*, whereby memories appropriate to the task (work) in hand are retrieved and 'held in the mind' for ongoing processing.

The *medial prefrontal cortex* has auditory and verbal associations. The *orbitofrontal cortex* is described as the 'neocortical representative of the limbic system', being richly connected to the amygdala, septal area, and the cortex of the temporal pole — the three limbic structures described in Chapter 33.

In general terms the left prefrontal cortex has an 'approach' bias, being engaged in all language-related activities, including the 'inner speech' that accompanies investigative activities. The right prefrontal cortex has a 'withdraw' bias, being particularly activated by fearful contexts, whether real or imagined.

Aspects of frontal lobe dysfunction are described in Clinical Panel 32.2.

Parietal Lobe (Fig. 32.5)

The parietal lobe—especially the *right* one—is of prime importance for appreciation of spatial relationships. There is also evidence that the parietal lobe—especially the *left* one—is concerned with initiation of movement. (Most of the following is based on observations made on individuals who have suffered cerebral injuries, usually vascular stroke in origin.) The parietal lobe dynamically integrates motor, visual, and cognitive

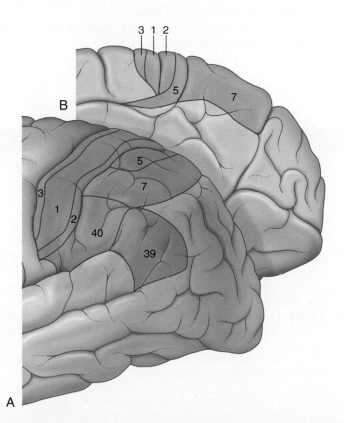

Fig. 32.5 Brodmann areas in the parietal lobe. (A) Lateral view. (B) Medial view. 3/1/2, Somaesthetic cortex; 5, somaesthetic association area; 7, posterior parietal cortex; 39, angular gyrus; 40, supramarginal gyrus.

information that facilitate a range of behavioural and task-related motor activities.

Superior Parietal Lobule and the Body Schema. The term *body schema* refers to an awareness of the existence and spatial relationships of body parts, based on previous (stored) and current sensory experience. The reality of the body schema has been established by the condition known as **contralateral neglect**, in which a patient with a lesion involving the superior parietal lobule ignores the contralateral side of the body.

The syndrome of neglect is much more common following a right than a left parietal lobe lesion. Under normal conditions, however, each parietal lobe exchanges information freely with its partner through the corpus callosum, and the left and right hand are equally adept at distinguishing a key from a coin in a coat pocket without the aid of vision (*stereognosis*, see Chapter 28).

Patients with a right hemisphere lesion involving the superior parietal lobule have difficulty in distinguishing between unseen objects of different shapes with the left hand. They have **astereognosis** *(tactile agnosia)*. Patients with a comparable lesion in the left hemisphere can make this distinction using the right hand but they have difficulty in announcing the *function* of a selected object. The left supramarginal gyrus participates in phonological retrieval, as already noted, and the deficit, although a semantic one, may be related to interference with the 'inner speech' that usually accompanies problem solving.

Parietal Lobe and Movement Initiation. There are several sites for movement initiation in different behavioural contexts. The present context is the performance of learned movements of some complexity: examples would include turning a doorknob, combing one's hair, blowing out a match, and clapping. It is logical to anticipate a starting point within the dominant hemisphere because they can all be performed in response to a verbal command (oral or written). This notion receives support from the observation that if the corpus callosum has been severed surgically, the patient can perform a learned movement on command using the right hand but not on attempting it with the left hand.

Apraxias reflect a disorder of sensory-motor integration in the setting of intact strength, sensation, cerebellar function, basal ganglia function, and an understanding of the task requested. They signify a disturbance within this network of cortical areas and their subcortical pathways that connect the frontal cortex, parietal cortex and other subcortical areas that are responsible for learning and producing these complex motor activities. In addition to planning and initiating movement, concurrent feedback systems from the visual and somatosensory system provide the necessary feedback to make any corrections and ensure the original prediction and intention of the movement be achieved.

Failure to perform a learned movement on request is called **ideomotor apraxia**, or *limb apraxia*, and can occur when there is a disconnection between where the motor act is planned and the centre where it will eventually be executed. The individual may be observed to 'automatically' perform the entire motor act or portions of it, which signifies that there is no underlying

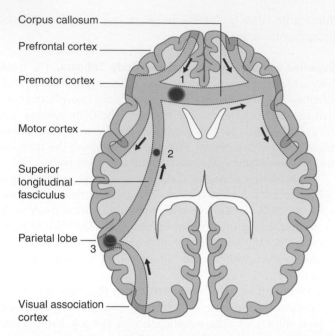

Corpus callosum

Prefrontal cortex

Premotor cortex

Motor cortex

Superior
longitudinal
fasciculus

Parietal lobe

Visual association
cortex

Fig. 32.6 Association and commissural pathways serving motor responses to sensory cues and resulting in a *disconnection syndrome*; damage to the association fibres or commissural fibres in the cerebral cortex that are independent of any lesions to the cortex. The premotor cortex is under higher control by the prefrontal cortex. Lesions at site 1 effectively sever the anterior part of the corpus callosum and produce ipsilateral limb apraxia (left lesion, left limb). Lesions at either site 2 (superior longitudinal fasciculus) or site 3 (angular gyrus) may produce *bilateral* limb apraxia. In practice, a large lesion may render right-limb apraxia impossible to assess because of associated right hemiplegia or receptive aphasia. (Modified from Kertesz A, Ferro JM, Shewan CM. Apraxia and aphasia: the functional-anatomical basis for their dissociation. *Neurology.* 1984;34:40–47.)

primary motor or sensory deficit, and they may be able to describe what is requested of them but cannot execute or pantomime it on command.

Ideomotor apraxia can be accounted for if the dominant parietal lobe is considered to contain a repertoire of learned movement programs, which, on retrieval, elicit appropriate responses by the premotor cortex on one or both sides under directives from the prefrontal cortex. (The basal ganglia would also be involved, as described in Chapter 26.) Ideomotor apraxia has been repeatedly observed immediately following vascular lesions at the sites listed and described in Fig. 32.6; involvement of the supramarginal gyrus is a more frequent 'cause' of apraxia and a left-sided lesion results in bilateral limb involvement, while right-sided lesions result in apraxia limited to the left side. In Fig. 32.6 a vascular stroke at site 2 injuring corticospinal fibres descending from the hand area of the motor cortex may cause clumsiness of movement of both hands, whereas a similar lesion on the right side may only compromise movements of the left hand.

Ideational apraxia is an inability to formulate a complex motor plan that requires the execution of several different components (properly identify a tool but cannot properly complete the set of actions associated with its use). It is most often evident bilaterally and is usually the result of diffuse cerebral involvement, but it can be seen with focal lesions, such as within the left posterior parietal cortex. The actual movements that occur will appear disorganised or performed in the wrong order or sequence (as may be demonstrated when trying to put on a garment, referred to as a *dressing apraxia*).

Clinical Panel 32.3 provides a brief account of clinically observed syndromes of parietal lobe dysfunction.

CLINICAL PANEL 32.1   Bedside Evaluation of Aphasia

Aphasia is a disturbance of language function caused by a lesion of the brain. The usual cause is a stroke produced by vascular occlusion in the cortical territory of the left middle cerebral artery.

General Neurologic Evaluation

Particular attention is paid to the presence of a hemiparesis (frontal lobe involvement), visual field deficit (occipital lobe or optic radiation), and apraxia (parietal lobe involvement); these findings further support localisation of the lesion producing the aphasia.

Language Evaluation

- **Spontaneous speech.** Particular attention is paid as to whether speech production is *fluent* (rate, quantity, and effort related to speech production) versus nonfluent (effortful), and to any evidence of *paraphasias* (incorrect words for the intended word). Word-finding difficulty in general is called *anomia*. (A condition that can be seen in aphasia, but more commonly results from poor muscle control leading to impaired articulation, is **dysarthria**; language testing is otherwise normal in individuals so afflicted.)
- **Repetition.** Requires an individual to demonstrate that they can repeat a phrase without errors; one preferred phrase is 'No ifs, ands, or buts'.

- **Comprehension.** Auditory comprehension can often be judged when the history is elicited. However, observing the response to simple commands, yes/no questions, and asking the individual to point to objects within the room should be employed.
- **Naming.** Usually assessed by having the person name objects within the room, body parts, or colours.
- **Reading.** Reading is evaluated by having the individual read a sentence out loud or by determining if they can silently read and follow a written command (e.g. 'Close your eyes'); when reading is impaired it is referred to as *alexia*.
- **Writing.** Evaluation requires more than having the individual write his or her name; when impaired this is referred to as *agraphia*. For evaluation, ask the patient to write a short sentence that may describe how they are feeling, comment about the weather, or why they like their favourite hobby. They should also write a sentence dictated to them.

Performing the different parts of this bedside evaluation provides clues that allow the clinical classification of the aphasia as well as a suggested site of cerebral involvement, as indicated in Fig. 32.7. Some idealised findings on bedside evaluation are included in this table.

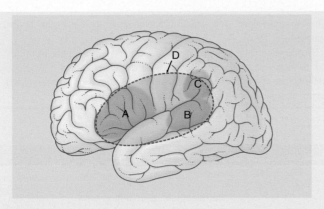

Fig. 32.7 (A) Lesion involving the Broca area. (B) Lesion involving the Wernicke area. (C) Lesion involved in conduction aphasia. (D) Shaded area involved in a global aphasia.

Aprosodia

Lesions of the right hemisphere may affect speech in subtle ways. Lesions that include area 44 on the right (corresponding to the Broca area on the left) tend to change the patient's speech to a dull monotone *(nonaffective prosody)*. On the other hand, lesions that involve area 22 on the right (corresponding to the Wernicke area) may lead to listening errors, such as being unable to detect inflections of speech; the patient may not know whether a particular remark is intended as a statement or as a question *(affective prosody)*.

Type	Fluency	Comprehension	Repetition	Naming	Site (Fig. 32.7)
Broca (e.g. anterior or motor aphasia)	Poor and effortful	Good	Poor	Poor	A
Lesion site — posterior portion of the inferior frontal gyrus (Broca area), and surrounding premotor, motor, and subcortical white matter.					
Wernicke (e.g. posterior or sensory aphasia)	Good, but with paraphasic errors	Poor	Poor	Poor	B
Lesion site — posterior third of the superior temporal gyrus (Wernicke area).					
Conduction aphasia	Good	Good	Poor	Good	C
Lesion site — supramarginal gyrus or primary auditory cortex and insular cortex.					
Global aphasia	None	Very poor	Very poor	Very poor	D
Lesion site — involves the perisylvian area that includes the Broca area, the Wernicke area, and the cortex that is interposed between them.					

Developmental Dyslexia

It is generally agreed that reading is a more skilled activity than speech, because it requires an exquisite level of integration of visual scanning and auditory (inner speech) comprehension.

Developmental dyslexia are hereditary neurologic disorders of severe and persistent reading and/or spelling difficulties, despite normal intelligence; it represents a language problem with decoding or processing of sounds as a major contributor while comprehension is more intact. *Phonological awareness* (awareness of the sound structure of words) is a predictor of reading skills in languages with inconsistent *orthographies* (the representation of the sounds of a language by written or printed symbols) and serial naming in consistent orthographies.

Two commonly used classroom tests to detect *phonological impairment* (slow and inaccurate processing of the sound structure of language) are *rhyming*, for example, to identify the eight letters in the alphabet that rhyme with the letter B, and to pronounce *nonwords (pseudowords)* within a word string; for example, 'door', '*melse*', 'farm', '*duve*', 'miss'.

Dyslexia is widespread across cultures, affecting an estimated 7% of children (comorbidities such as attention-deficit hyperactivity disorder and other language disorders may coexist and further impact school performance). There is a 30% incidence in siblings of affected children and a similar incidence in one or the other parent. There is a slightly higher incidence in boys, and in left-handed children of either gender.

A consistent finding in PET and fMRI studies during reading is diminished activity (compared with peers) in the left temporoparietal region (areas 22, 39, and 40) associated with structural abnormalities. The causes of dyslexia are likely multifactorial, but candidate genes have been identified, some related to neuronal migration and axonal guidance, and there is the suggestion of gene–environment interactions *(bioecological genes)* because heritability declines with declining parental education.

CLINICAL PANEL 32.2 Frontal Lobe Dysfunction

Symptoms of *early* frontal lobe disease typically involve subtle changes in personality and social function rather than diminution of cognitive performance on objective tests. (*Theory of mind (ToM)* refers to the ability of an individual to reason about the feelings of others and predict their behavioural responses. It appears that areas in the right inferior and orbital frontal cortex have a role in sharing another individual's emotional state, while the right prefrontal cortex has a role in recognising the emotional state of another person. The right anterior temporal lobe, cingulate, insula cortex, and amygdala appear to integrate these two areas.)

Lack of foresight (failure to anticipate the consequences of a course of action), distractibility (poor concentration), loss of the ability to perform voluntary actions or to make decisions *(abulia)*, and difficulty in 'switching cognitive sets' (e.g. inability to switch easily from one subject of conversation to another) are characteristic. These general symptoms are more often associated with bilateral cerebral disease with impending dementia than with a brain tumour. With increasing disease, especially if bilateral, the *gait* is affected. *Marche à petits pas* ('walk with small steps') refers to a characteristic short, shuffling gait often associated with disequilibrium (tendency to fall), and 'freezing' (e.g. when the patient is turned suddenly, for a brief period of time he/she is unable to step or takes short steps). This syndrome may give rise to a mistaken suspicion of Parkinson disease.

Large *dorsolateral lesions* are associated with slowing of mental processes of all kinds, leading to hypokinesia, apathy, and indifference to surrounding events. In those cases, cortical blood flow may not show the anticipated increase in the dorsolateral region in response to appropriate psychological tests.

Large *orbitofrontal* lesions are associated with hyperkinesia, and with increased instinctual drives in relation to food and sexual behaviour. With disease more pronounced (or only) in the right orbitofrontal cortex, the 'fearful' side of the patient's nature may be lost, leading to puerile jocularity and compulsive laughter. Compulsive crying may be a clue to left-sided disease. A well-known stereotypic cause of orbitofrontal disturbance is a meningioma arising in the groove occupied by the olfactory nerve; *anosmia* (loss of the sense of smell) may be discovered on testing, and optic atrophy may follow pressure on the optic nerve where it emerges from the optic canal on that same side.

Hyperkinetic frontal lobe and psychiatric disorders in the past 'were treated' by means of *prefrontal leucotomy* — a surgical procedure in which the white matter above the orbital cortex was severed through a temporal incision or through an orbital route as a form of 'psychosurgery'.

CLINICAL PANEL 32.3 Parietal Lobe Dysfunction

Anterior Parietal Cortex

Lesions of the somatic sensory cortex and somaesthetic association area tend to occur together, causing cortical-type sensory loss and inaccurate reaching movements into the contralateral visual hemispace (e.g. at mealtimes the patient may tend to knock things over). (Directing attention is not limited to the parietal lobe but reflects a dynamic relationship and network that exists with the frontal lobe.)

Supramarginal Gyrus

Lesions affecting the supramarginal gyrus (area 40) are usually vascular (middle cerebral artery) and usually concomitant with contralateral hemiplegia with or without hemianopia. However, the blood supply to the gyrus is sometimes selectively occluded, giving rise to a state known as *personal hemineglect*. The patient ignores the opposite side of the body unless attention is specifically drawn to it. A male patient will shave only the ipsilateral (with respect to the side of the injury) side of the face; a female patient will comb her hair only on the ipsilateral side. Patients who demonstrate neglect may also lack awareness of their neurological deficit (e.g. hemiplegia) or demonstrate behaviour that does not consider it; this is referred to as *anosognosia*.

Not consistently seen in such cases is when a patient may be able to acknowledge a tactile stimulus to the contralateral side when tested alone; simultaneous testing of both sides will only be acknowledged ipsilaterally *(sensory extinction)*.

Angular Gyrus

Lesions of the anteroventral part of the angular gyrus (area 39, see Fig. 32.8) are notably associated with *spatial (extrapersonal) hemineglect*. The patient fails to perceive or orient to the contralateral visual hemispace, even if the visual pathways remain intact, and *visual extinction* (contralaterally) to simultaneous bilateral stimuli can be demonstrated, such as when the clinician wiggles index fingers in both visual fields simultaneously. Hemineglect

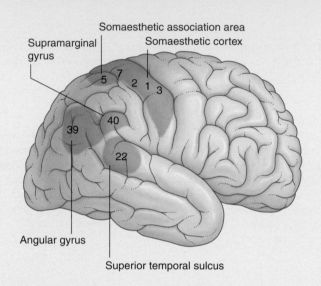

Fig. 32.8 Angular gyrus (brodmann area 39), supramarginal gyrus (brodmann area 40).

is at least five times more frequent following lesions on the *right* side, especially at the temporoparietal junction, irrespective of handedness.

An isolated vascular lesion of the posterior part of the left angular gyrus (very rare) produces *alexia* (complete inability to read) and *agraphia* (inability to write); letters on the page are suddenly without any meaning. If the planum temporale is uninjured, patients can still name words spelt aloud to them.

For *ideomotor apraxia*, see main text.

✳ Core Information

Hemispheric asymmetries are 'exemplified' by handedness and language, which show left cerebral localisation predominance. People who are left-handed show a similar left cerebral localisation, but less so if they are strongly left-handed (right hemisphere dominant in 27%) versus those who are ambidextrous.

Language and speech function surround the Sylvian fissure with the *Broca* speech area occupying the inferior frontal gyrus and lesions give rise to what is still commonly referred to as 'motor or expressive aphasia' because speech production and writing appear more affected than comprehension. The *Wernicke area* is in the posterior portion of the superior temporal gyrus, and when affected gives rise to a 'sensory or receptive aphasia' in which speech production is fluent but often nonsensical and understanding of language is affected. These conceptualisations are useful for bedside localisation of aphasia, but now informed by a more nuanced understanding that language is an integrated process that involves the left frontal, temporal, and parietal cortex, as well as the right cerebral hemisphere.

The prefrontal cortex is involved in multiple cognitive roles. The *dorsolateral prefrontal cortex (DLPFC)* contains a supervisory attentional system especially involved in conscious learning, where it operates working memory appropriate to the task. The orbitofrontal cortex is a neocortical representative of the limbic system. General signs of frontal lobe disease include lack of foresight, distractibility, and difficulty in switching cognitive sets. The gait may take the form of short shuffling steps with instability and 'freezing' or sudden occurrences of immobility. DLPFC lesions lead to slowing of mental processes, apathy, and indifference. Orbitofrontal lesions tend to produce a hyperkinetic state with increased instinctual drives and puerile behaviour.

The inferior parietal lobule is concerned with the body schema; lesions here may result in neglect of personal and (sometimes) extrapersonal space on the opposite side. The left parietal lobe may be responsible for integrating and properly sequencing complex motor programs that otherwise cannot be explained by weakness, sensory loss, or understanding *(apraxia)*.

SUGGESTED READINGS

Basilakos A, Smith KG, Fillmore P, et al. Functional characterization of the human speech articulation network. *Cerebral Cortex.* 2018;28:1816–1830.

Binder JR. The Wernicke area: modern evidence and a reinterpretation. *Neurology.* 2015;85:2170–2175.

Brandler WM, Morris AP, Evans DM, et al. Common variants in left/right asymmetry genes and pathways are associated with relative hand skill. *PLoS Genet.* 2013;9:e1003751.

Carrera E, Tononi G. Diaschisis: past, present, future. *Brain.* 2014;137:2408–2422.

Coslett HB. Apraxia, neglect, and agnosia. *Continuum.* 2018;24:768–782.

Crossley NA, Mechelli A, Scott J, et al. The hubs of the human connectome are generally implicated in the anatomy of brain disorders. *Brain.* 2014;137:2382–2395.

Dale ML, Curtze C, Nutt JG. Apraxia of gait- or apraxia of postural transitions? *Parkinsonism Relat Disord.* 2018;50:19–22.

Dick AS, Tremblay P. Beyond the arcuate fasciculus: consensus and controversy in the connectional anatomy of language. *Brain.* 2012;135:3529–3550.

Dronkers NF, Plaisant O, Iba-Zizen MT, et al. Paul Broca's historic cases: high resolution MR imaging of the brains of Leborgne and Lelong. *Brain.* 2007;130:1432–1441.

Freedman DJ, Ibos G. An integrative framework for sensory, motor, and cognitive functions of the posterior parietal cortex. *Neuron.* 2018;97:1219–1234.

Fridriksson J, Yourganov G, Bonilha L, et al. Revealing the dual streams of speech processing. *Proc Natl Acad Sci USA.* 2016;113:15108–15113.

Fridriksson J, den Ouden DB, Hillis AE, et al. Anatomy of aphasia revisited. *Brain.* 2018;141(3):848–862.

Gajardo-Vidal A, Lorca-Puls DL, Hope TMH, et al. How right hemisphere damage after stroke can impair speech comprehension. *Brain.* 2018;141:3389–3404.

Gervain J, Geffen MN. Efficient neural coding in auditory and speech perception. *Trends Neurosci.* 2019;42:56–65.

Hagoort P. Nodes and networks in the neural architecture for language: Broca's region and beyond. *Curr Opin Neurobiol.* 2014;28:136–141.

Knecht S, Dräger B, Deppe M, et al. Handedness and hemispheric language dominance in healthy humans. *Brain.* 2000;123:2512–2518.

Lupyan G, Winter B. Language is more abstract than you think, or, why aren't languages more iconic? *Philos Trans R Soc Lond B Biol Sci.* 2018;373(1752).

Mesulam MM. Fifty years of disconnexion syndromes and the Geschwind legacy. *Brain.* 2015;138:2791–2799.

Patel GH, Kaplan DM, Snyder LH. Topographic organization in the brain: searching for general principles. *Trends Cogn Sci.* 2014;18:351–363.

Poeppel D. The neuroanatomic and neurophysiological infrastructure for speech and language. *Curr Opin Neurobiol.* 2014;28:142–149.

Rogers LJ, Vallortigoia G, Andrew RJ. *Divided brains: the biology and behavior of brain asymmetries.* New York: Cambridge University Press; 2013.

Tate MC, Herbet G, Moritz-Gasser S, et al. Probabilistic map of critical functional regions of the human cerebral cortex: Broca's area revisited. *Brain.* 2014;137:2773–2782.

Wandell BA, Rauschecker AM, Yeatman JD. Learning to see words. *Annu Rev Psychol.* 2014;63:31–53.

Zarate JM. The neural control of singing. *Front Hum Neurosci.* 2013;7:237.

Olfactory and Limbic Systems

STUDY GUIDELINES

Olfactory System

In most vertebrates, the olfactory system is altogether more important than it is in humans. Although damage to the olfactory pathway on one side is associated with anosmia on that side, olfactory deficits are often found in neurodegenerative disorders.

Limbic System

Cortical and subcortical limbic areas are prominent features of the brain in primitive mammals where they are intimately concerned with mechanisms of attack and defence, procreation, and feeding. The principal effector elements of the limbic system are the hypothalamus and the reticular formation.

The elements, pathways, and transmitters of the human limbic system provide the bedrock on which most of psychiatry and clinical psychology are built.

THE OLFACTORY SYSTEM

The olfactory system is remarkable in four respects:

1. The somas of the primary afferent neurons occupy a surface epithelium.
2. The axons of the primary afferents enter the cerebral cortex directly; second-order afferents are not interposed.
3. The primary afferent neurons undergo continuous turnover, being replaced from basal stem cells.
4. The pathway to the cortical centres in the frontal lobe is entirely ipsilateral.

The olfactory system consists of the olfactory epithelium and olfactory nerves, the olfactory bulb and tract, and several areas of the olfactory cortex.

Olfactory Epithelium

The olfactory system possesses a dynamic neuroepithelium from which olfactory neurons project to the brain. Due to their location, the olfactory sensory neurons are vulnerable to damage. The olfactory epithelium retains neural stem and progenitor cells in the basal layers, providing the tissue an ability to effect self-repair.

The olfactory epithelium occupies the upper one-fifth of the lateral and septal walls of the nasal cavity. The epithelium contains three cell types (Fig. 33.1):

1. *Olfactory neurons* are bipolar neurons, each with a dendrite extending to the epithelial surface and an unmyelinated axon contributing to the olfactory nerve. The dendrites are capped by immotile cilia containing molecular receptor sites. The axons run upward through the cribriform ('sieve-like') plate of the ethmoid bone and enter the olfactory bulb. The axons (some 3 million on each side) are grouped into fila (bundles) by investing Schwann cells. The collective fila constitute the *olfactory nerve*.

2. *Sustentacular cells* are interspersed among the bipolar neurons.

3. *Basal stem cells* lie between the other two cell types. Olfactory bipolar neurons are unique in that they undergo a continuous cycle of growth, degeneration, and replacement. The basal cells transform into fresh bipolar olfactory neurons, which survive for about a month. Replacement declines over time accounting for the general reduction in olfactory sensitivity with age.

Olfactory Bulb (Fig. 33.1)

The olfactory bulb is small in comparison to the neocortex, but it is a functionally complex structure that is central to the processing and transmission of olfactory information. Research findings strongly suggest that the human adult olfactory bulb is a highly plastic structure. The exact mechanisms of the plasticity are as yet unclear.

Anatomically, the olfactory bulb consists of a three-layered allocortex surrounding the commencement of the olfactory tract. The chief cortical neurons are some 50,000 **mitral (or tufted) cells**, which receive the olfactory nerve fibres and give rise to the olfactory tract.

Contact between olfactory fibres and mitral cell dendrites takes place in some 2000 **glomeruli**, which are sites of innumerable synapses and have a glial investment, but each receives its input from sensory neurons that respond to the same stimulus (*odorant*). Glomeruli that are 'on-line' (active) inhibit neighbouring, 'off-line' glomeruli through the mediation of γ-aminobutyric acid (GABA)ergic **periglomerular cells** (cf. the horizontal cells of the retina), representing an initial stage of signal (specific odour) processing. Mitral cell activity is also sharpened at a deeper level by **granule cells** that are devoid of axons (cf. the amacrine cells of the retina), representing the next stage of signal processing and contrast enhancement between mitral cells. The granule cells receive excitatory dendrodendritic contacts from active mitral cells, and they suppress neighbouring mitral cells through inhibitory (GABA) dendrodendritic contacts.

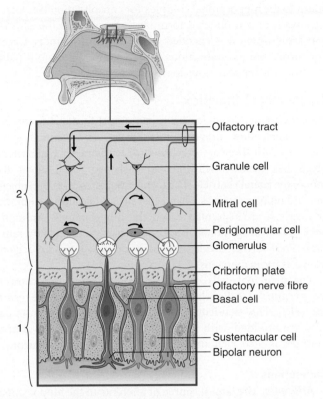

Fig. 33.1 Connections of the olfactory epithelium *(1)* and the olfactory bulb *(2)*. The second glomerulus from the left is 'on-line' (see text).

Labels: Olfactory tract; Granule cell; Mitral cell; Periglomerular cell; Glomerulus; Cribriform plate; Olfactory nerve fibre; Basal cell; Sustentacular cell; Bipolar neuron

Central Connections. Mitral cell axons run centrally in the **olfactory tract** (Fig. 33.2). The tract divides in front of the anterior perforated substance into **medial** and **lateral olfactory striae**.

The medial stria contains axons from the **anterior olfactory nucleus**, which consists of multipolar neurons scattered within the olfactory tract. Some of these axons travel to the septal area via the *diagonal band* (see later, under Limbic System). Others cross the midline in the anterior commissure and inhibit mitral cell activity in the contralateral bulb (by exciting granule cells there). The result is a relative enhancement of the more active bulb, providing a directional cue to the source of olfactory stimulation.

The lateral olfactory stria terminates in the **piriform lobe** of the anterior temporal cortex. The human piriform lobe includes

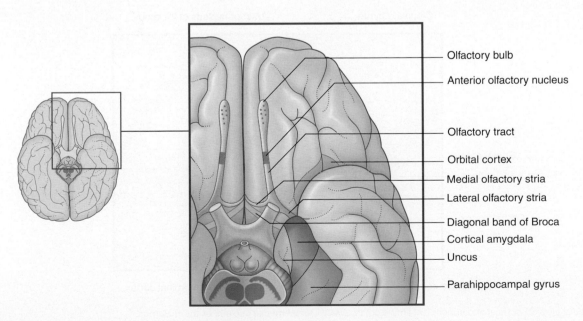

Labels: Olfactory bulb; Anterior olfactory nucleus; Olfactory tract; Orbital cortex; Medial olfactory stria; Lateral olfactory stria; Diagonal band of Broca; Cortical amygdala; Uncus; Parahippocampal gyrus

Fig. 33.2 Brain viewed from below, showing cortical olfactory areas.

the cortical part of the amygdala, the uncus, and the anterior end of the parahippocampal gyrus. The highest centre for olfactory discrimination is the posterior part of the orbitofrontal cortex, which receives connections from the piriform lobe via the dorsomedial nucleus of the thalamus.

The *medial forebrain bundle* links the olfactory cortical areas with the hypothalamus and brainstem. These linkages trigger autonomic responses such as salivation and gastric contraction and arousal responses through the reticular formation.

Points of clinical interest are mentioned in Clinical Panel 33.1.

LIMBIC SYSTEM

The term 'limbic system' is most useful when defined as the limbic cortex (further defined below) and related subcortical nuclei. The term 'limbic' (Broca, 1878) originally referred to a *limbus* or rim of cortex immediately adjacent to the corpus callosum and diencephalon. The limbic cortex is now taken to include the three-layered *allocortex* of the hippocampal complex and septal area, together with transitional *mesocortex* in the parahippocampal gyrus, cingulate gyrus, and insula. The principal subcortical component of the limbic system is the amygdala, which merges with the cortex on the medial side of the temporal pole. Closely related subcortical areas are the hypothalamus, the reticular formation, and the nucleus accumbens. Cortical areas closely related to the limbic system are the orbitofrontal cortex and the temporal pole (Fig. 33.3).

Fig. 33.4 is a graphic reconstruction of mainly subcortical limbic areas.

Parahippocampal Gyrus

The parahippocampal gyrus is a major junctional region between the cerebral neocortex and the allocortex of the hippocampal complex. Its anterior part is the **entorhinal cortex (area**

28 *of Brodmann)*, which is six layered but has certain peculiar features. The entorhinal cortex can be said to face in two directions. Its *neocortical face* exchanges massive numbers of afferent and efferent connections with all four association areas of the neocortex. Its *allocortical face* exchanges abundant connections with the hippocampal complex. In the broadest terms, the entorhinal cortex receives a constant stream of cognitive and sensory information from the association areas of the neocortex, transmits it to the hippocampal complex for consolidation (see later), retrieves it in consolidated form, and returns it to the association areas where it is encoded in the form of memory traces. The fornix and its connections form a second, circuitous pathway from the hippocampus to neocortex.

Hippocampal Complex

The hippocampal complex (or hippocampal formation) consists of the **subiculum**, **hippocampus proper**, and **dentate gyrus** (Fig. 33.5). All three are composed of temporal lobe allocortex, which has tucked itself into an S-shaped scroll along the floor of the lateral ventricle. The fornix originates from the subiculum and hippocampus as a band-like structure called the fimbria. The early neuroanatomists called the hippocampus 'Ammon's horn' (or cornu ammonis), because it looked to them like a ram's horn. They further divided the hippocampus into four regions known as *cornu ammonis (CA)* 1 to 4 (Fig. 33.6A).

The principal cells of the subiculum and hippocampus are **pyramidal cells**; those of the dentate gyrus are **granule cells**. The dendrites of both granule and pyramidal cells are studded with dendritic spines. The hippocampal complex is also rich in inhibitory (GABA) interneurons.

Connections

Afferents. The largest source of afferents to the hippocampal complex is the **perforant path**, which projects from the

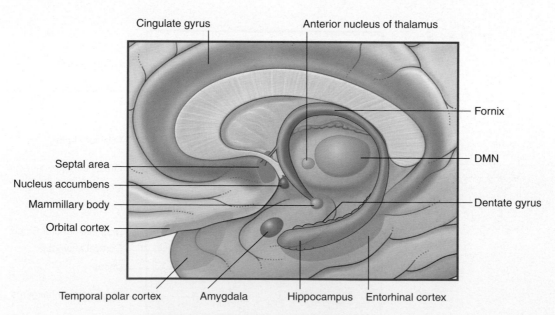

Fig. 33.3 Medial view of cortical and subcortical limbic areas. *DMN,* Dorsal medial nucleus of the thalamus.

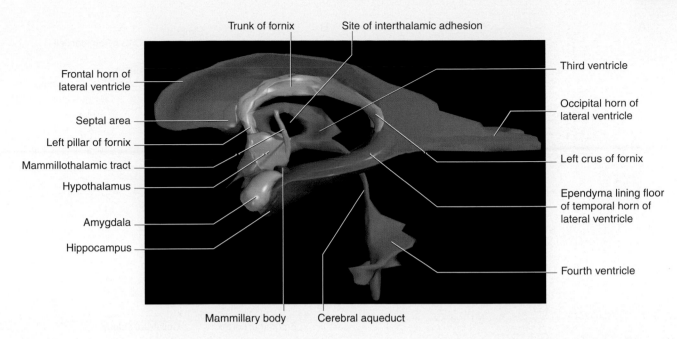

Fig. 33.4 Three-dimensional computerised reconstruction of postmortem brain showing components of the limbic system in relation to the ventricular system. (Excerpt of figure from Kretschmann and Weinrich, 1998, with kind permission of the authors and the publisher.)

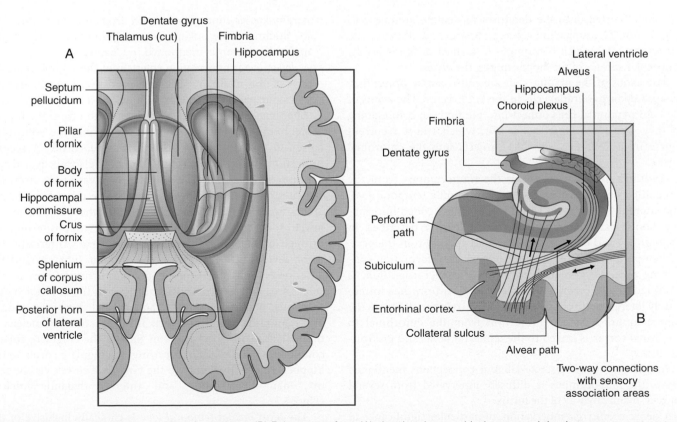

Fig. 33.5 Hippocampal complex. (A) View from above. (B) Enlargement from (A) showing the entorhinal cortex and the three component parts of the hippocampal complex. *Arrows* indicate direction of transmission.

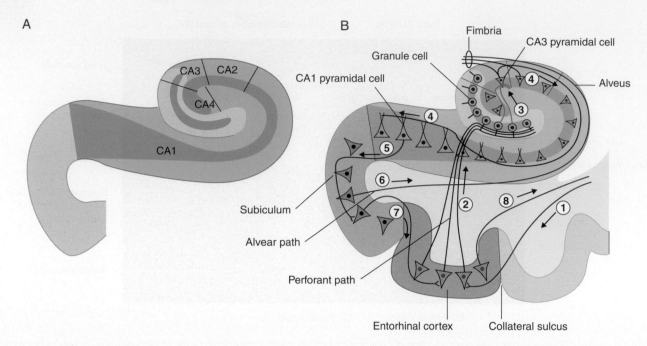

Fig. 33.6 (A) The four sectors of Ammon's horn. (B) Input—output connections of the hippocampal complex. *1,* Afferent from the sensory association cortex; *2,* Entorhinal cortex projecting perforant path fibres to the dentate gyrus; *3,* Dentate granule cell projecting to CA3; *4,* CA3 principal neuron projecting into the fimbria and CA1; *5,* CA1 principal cell projecting to the subiculum; *6,* Subicular principal cell projecting into the fimbria; *7,* Subicular principal cell projecting into the entorhinal cortex; *8,* Entorhinal pyramidal cell projecting to the sensory association cortex. *CA,* Cornu ammonis.

entorhinal cortex onto the dendrites of dentate granule cells (Fig. 33.6B). The subiculum gives rise to a second afferent path, the *alvear path*, which contributes to a sheet of fibres on the ventricular surface of the hippocampus, the ***alveus***.

The axons of the granule cells are called ***mossy fibres***; they synapse upon pyramidal cells in the CA3 sector. The axons of the CA3 pyramidal cells project into the fimbria; before doing so they give off *Schaffer collaterals*, which run a recurrent course from CA3 to CA1. CA1 projects into the entorhinal cortex.

Auditory information enters the hippocampus from the association cortex of the superior and middle temporal gyri. The supramarginal gyrus (area 40) transmits coded information about personal space (the *body schema* described in Chapter 32) and extrapersonal (visual) space. From the occipitotemporal region on the inferior surface, information concerning object shape and colour, and facial recognition, is projected to the cortex called *perirhinal* or *transrhinal*, immediately lateral to the entorhinal cortex. From here it enters the hippocampus. A return projection from the entorhinal to perirhinal cortex is linked to the temporal polar and prefrontal cortex.

In addition to the discrete afferent connections mentioned above, the hippocampus is diffusely innervated from several sources, mainly by way of the fornix:

• A dense *cholinergic* innervation, of particular significance in relation to memory, is received from the septal nucleus.
• A *noradrenergic* innervation is received from the locus coeruleus.

• A *serotonergic* innervation enters from the raphe nuclei of the midbrain. The linkage between serotonin depletion and major depression is mentioned in Chapter 34.
• A *dopaminergic* innervation enters from the ventral tegmental area of the midbrain. The linkage between dopamine and schizophrenia is discussed in Clinical Panel 33.2.

Efferents. The largest efferent connection from the hippocampal complex is a massive projection via the entorhinal cortex to the association areas of the neocortex. A second projection is the ***fornix*** (Fig. 33.5A). The fornix is a direct continuation of the ***fimbria***, which receives axons from the subiculum and hippocampus proper. The ***crus*** of the fornix arches up beneath the corpus callosum, where it joins its fellow to form the ***trunk*** and links with its opposite number through a small ***hippocampal commissure***. Anteriorly, the trunk divides into two ***pillars***. Each pillar splits around the anterior commissure sending *precommissural* fibres to the septal area and *postcommissural* fibres to the anterior hypothalamus, mammillary body, and medial forebrain bundle. The mammillary body projects into the anterior nucleus of the thalamus, which projects in turn to the cingulate cortex, completing the ***Papez circuit*** from the cingulate cortex to the hippocampus with return to the cingulate cortex via the fornix, mammillary body, and anterior thalamic nucleus (Fig. 33.7).

The term *medial temporal lobe* is clinically inclusive of the hippocampal complex, parahippocampal gyrus, and amygdala. The term is most often used in relation to seizures (Clinical Panel 33.3).

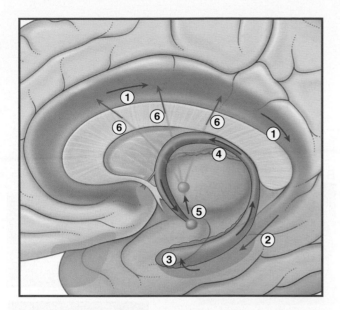

Fig. 33.7 The papez circuit. *1*, Backward-projecting neurons in the cingulate gyrus; *2*, Projection into the entorhinal cortex; *3*, Projection into the hippocampus; *4*, Fornix; *5*, Mammillothalamic tract; *6*, Projections from the anterior nucleus of the thalamus to the cingulate cortex. *Arrows* indicate direction of transmission.

Memory function of the hippocampal complex. The evidence for a *mnemonic* (memory-related) function in the hippocampal complex is discussed at considerable length in psychology texts. Some insights are given below.

Glossary

- **Short-term memory**: Holding one or more items of new information briefly in mind (e.g. a new telephone number while pressing the buttons).
- **Long-term (remote) memory**: Stored information capable of retrieval at appropriate moments. Two kinds of long-term memory are recognised: explicit and implicit.
  - *Explicit memory* has to do with recollections of facts and events of all kinds that can be explicitly stated or declared, hence the term *declarative memory*. The term *episodic memory* is also used, in the autobiographical sense of recollection of episodes involving personal experience. Yet another term, *semantic memory*, was devised in the context of memory for the meaning of written and spoken words, but is now also used to include knowledge of facts and concepts.
  - *Implicit memory* has to do with performance of learned motor procedures, such as riding a bicycle or assembling a jigsaw puzzle. The term *procedural memory* is commonly used.
- **Working memory**: Effortless brief simultaneous retrieval of several items from long-term memory stores for a task in hand, such as driving a car along a familiar route while making appropriate decisions based on previous experience.
- **Consolidation**: The process of storing new information in long-term memory. Novel factual information is relayed from the relevant sensory association areas to the hippocampal complex for encoding. Following a prolonged period of processing, the encoded information is relayed back to the same association areas and (with the exception of strongly autobiographical episodes) no longer depends on the hippocampal complex for retrieval.

Clinical and Experimental Observations.

Bilateral damage or removal of the anterior part of the hippocampal complex is followed by *anterograde amnesia*, a term used to denote absence of conscious recall of newly acquired information for more than a few minutes. When asked to name a commonplace object, the patient will have no difficulty because access to long-term memories does not require the anterior hippocampus. However, when the same object is shown a few minutes later, the patient will not remember having seen it. There is loss of explicit/ declarative memory.

Procedural (how-to-do) memory is preserved. If asked to assemble a jigsaw puzzle, the patient will do it in the normal way. When asked to repeat the exercise the next day, the patient will do it faster, although there will be no recollection of having seen the puzzle previously. *The hippocampus is not required for procedural memory.* We have previously noted that the basal ganglia are the storehouse of routine motor programs and that the cerebellum is the storehouse of motor adaptations to novel conditions.

Long-term potentiation (LTP) is uniquely powerful in the dentate gyrus and hippocampus. It is regarded as vital for preservation (consolidation) of memory traces. Under experimental conditions, LTP is most easily demonstrated in the perforant path—dentate granule cell connections and in the Schaffer collateral—CA1 connections. A strong, brief (milliseconds) stimulus to the perforant path or Schaffer collaterals induces the target cells to show long-lasting (hours) sensitivity to a fresh stimulus. LTP is associated with a cascade of biochemical events in the target neurons, following activation of appropriate glutamate receptors, as described in Chapter 8 in the context of pain sensitisation. Repetitive stimuli may cause cyclic adenosine 3′,5′-monophosphate (cAMP) to increase its normal rate of activation of protein kinases involved in phosphorylation of proteins that regulate gene transcription. The outcome is increased production of proteins (including enzymes) required for transmitter synthesis and of other proteins for construction of additional channels and synaptic cytoskeletons (Fig. 33.8).

LTP is described as an *associative* phenomenon because the required expulsion of the magnesium plug from the *N*-methyl-D-aspartate (NMDA) receptor (Fig. 33.8) is facilitated when the powerful depolarising stimulus is coupled with a weaker stimulus to the depolarised neuron from another source. *Norepinephrine* and *dopamine* are suitable associative candidates, one or both being released during elevation of the attentional or motivational state at the appropriate time.

Cholinergic activity in the hippocampus is also significant for learning. In human volunteers, administration of scopolamine, which inhibits acetylcholine (ACh) transmission, severely impaired memory for lists of names or numbers, whereas a

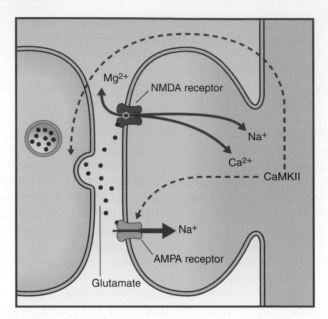

Fig. 33.8 Long-term potentiation. *AMPA*, -amino-3-hydroxy-5-methyl-4-isoxazolepropionic acid; *CaMKII*, calcium-dependent protein kinase II; *NMDA*, N-methyl-D-aspartate.

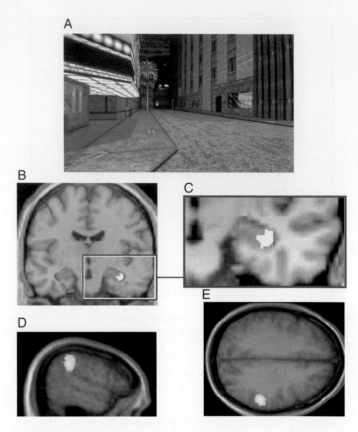

Fig. 33.9 Navigation in a Virtual Environment. (A) Scene from a virtual town. Subjects navigated through the town using a keypad to stay clear of obstacles. PET scans taken during the virtual journey showed increased activation, (B) and (C), within the right hippocampus, and (D) and (E), within the right supramarginal gyrus. Orientation (L, R) of the MRIs is for a more general readership. (Kindly provided by Dr Eleanor Maguire, Wellcome Department of Cognitive Neurology, Institute of Neurology, University College, London, UK, and with permission from the Editor of *Current Opinion in Neurobiology*.)

cholinesterase inhibitor (physostigmine) actually enhanced recall of the same lists. Clinically, hippocampal cholinergic activity is severely reduced in patients suffering from Alzheimer disease (AD), a condition that is particularly associated with impaired memory function (see Clinical Panel 33.4).

Kindling ('lighting a fire') is a property unique to the hippocampal complex and amygdala although its relationship to learning is not obvious. Kindling is the progressively increasing group response of neurons to a repetitive stimulus of uniform strength. In both humans and experimental animals, it can spread from the mesocortex to neocortex and cause generalised convulsive seizures.

The contribution of the fornix projection to memory is uncertain. Indirect evidence has been inferred from *diencephalic amnesia*, a state of anterograde amnesia that may follow bilateral damage to the diencephalon. Such damage may interrupt the *Papez circuit* linking the fornix to the cingulate gyrus by way of the mammillary body and the anterior nucleus of the thalamus. Particularly impaired is relational memory (e.g. recollection of the sight and sound of a particular event in which accompanying sensations are a significant part of the memory, such as the sound of a waterfall when close or the sight or feel of the blowing spray).

Left versus right hippocampal functions. In keeping with known hemispheric asymmetries, the left anterior hippocampus and dorsolateral prefrontal cortex (DLPFC) are engaged in encoding novel material involving language function. Also consistent is the finding that the right hippocampus and right inferior parietal lobe are engaged in spatial tasks such as driving a car (Fig. 33.9). Blood flow in the DLPFC increases more on the left side during driving presumably because of the 'inner speech' that occurs when exploring novel territory.

Anterior versus posterior hippocampal functions. The hippocampus is about 8 cm in length, and there is evidence for anteroposterior functional specialisation with respect to novelty versus familiarity, for example, when novel material is being read on a screen the left anterior hippocampus is especially active; but with development of familiarity with repeated exposure, activity shifts to the posterior part, suggesting that this region is involved in encoding material into long-term memory.

Long-term medial temporal lobe dependency. Autobiographical recollections typically are visual whereby we revisit scenes from the past, sometimes from childhood. Clinical studies indicate that medial temporal lobe damage may severely impair recall of ego-centred (personal) memories, while leaving intact allocentric (nonpersonal) memories such as for a place or object. On the other hand, damage to the visual association cortex has the opposite effect.

Prefrontal cortex and working memory. Volunteers have been examined under functional magnetic resonance imaging (fMRI) while preparing to give a motor response to one or more sensory cues. The midregion of the prefrontal cortex (area 46) tends to be especially active at these times. Its possible role is to tap into memory stores in relevant sensory association areas and to organise motor responses, including speech.

Insula

The anterior insula is a cortical centre for pain (Box 33.1). The central region is continuous with the frontoparietal and temporal opercular cortex, and it seems to have a *language* rather than a limbic function. During language tasks, PET scans show activity there as well as in the opercular speech receptive and motor areas, but not in people with congenital dyslexia, where it remains silent (see Chapter 32). The posterior insula is interconnected with the entorhinal cortex, and the amygdala and is therefore presumed to participate in emotional responses; perhaps in the context of pain evaluation.

Cingulate Cortex and Posterior Parahippocampal Gyrus

The cingulate cortex is part of the Papez circuit receiving a projection from the anterior nucleus of the thalamus and becoming continuous with the parahippocampal gyrus behind the splenium of the corpus callosum.

The *anterior* cingulate cortex belongs to the *rostral limbic system*, which includes the amygdala, ventral striatum, orbitofrontal cortex, and anterior insular cortex.

Six functional areas can be discerned in the anterior cingulate cortex (Fig. 33.12):

1. An *executive area* is connected directly with the DLPFC and with the supplementary motor area (SMA). The executive area becomes active prior to execution of willed movements, including voluntary saccades (see Chapter 28),

---

BOX 33.1 Pain and the Brain

The international association for the study of pain has given the following definition: *Pain is an unpleasant sensory and emotional experience associated with actual or potential tissue damage or described in terms of such damage.* See Table 33.1 for glossary of pain terminology.

TABLE 33.1 Glossary of Pain Terminology.

Term	Meaning
Allodynia	Pain produced by normally innocuous stimuli. Examples: stroking sunburned skin; moving an inflamed joint.
Central pain-projecting neurons (CPPNs)	An inclusive conventional term denoting all dorsal horn neurons projecting pain-encoded information to contralateral brainstem and thalamic nuclei. Pathways included are *spinothalamic*, the lateral pain pathway to the posterior nucleus of the thalamus; *spinoreticulothalamic*, the medial pain pathway to the medial and intralaminar nuclei of the thalamus via the brainstem reticular formation; *spinoamygdaloid*, to the amygdala via the reticular formation; and *spinotectal*, to the superior colliculus.
Central pain state	A state of chronic pain, resistant to therapy, sustained by hypersensitivity of peripheral and/or central neural pathways.
Wind-up phenomenon	Sustained state of excitation of CPPNs induced by glutamate activation of NMDA receptors.
Fast pain	Stabbing pain perceived following activation of Aδ nociceptors.
Hyperalgesia	Hypersensitivity to stimulation of injured tissue, and of surrounding uninjured tissue. Causes include mechanical or thermal damage, bacterial/viral inflammation, small-fibre peripheral axonal neuropathy, and radiculopathy (dorsal nerve root injury).
Neurogenic inflammation	Inflammation caused by liberation of substance P (in particular) following antidromic depolarisation of fine peripheral nerve fibres.
Neuropathic pain	Chronic stabbing or burning pain resulting from injury to peripheral nerves. Examples: postherpetic neuralgia; amputation neuroma.
Nociceptors	Peripheral receptors whose activation generates a sense of pain. These receptors occupy the plasma membrane of fine nerve endings and contain transduction channels that convert the requisite physical or chemical stimulus into trains of impulses decoded by the brain as a sense of pain.
Polymodal nociceptors	Peripheral nociceptors (notably in skin) responsive to noxious thermal, mechanical, or chemical stimulation.
Sensitisation	Lowering the threshold of peripheral nociceptors by histamine (in particular) following peripheral release of peptides via the axon reflex.
Slow pain	Aching pain perceived following activation of C-fibre nociceptors.

This definition emphasises the *affective* (emotional) component of pain. Its other component is *sensory-discriminative* ('where and how much?').

Peripheral Pain Pathways

As already noted in Chapter 9, pain is served by finely myelinated (Aδ) and unmyelinated (C) fibres belonging to unipolar spinal ganglion cells. These fibres are loosely known as 'pain fibres' although others of similar diameters are purely mechanoreceptors and others again elicit pain only when discharging at high frequency, notably mechanical nociceptors and thermoreceptors. The latter are referred to as *polymodal nociceptors* in the general context of pain.

From somatic tissues including skin, parietal pleura and parietal peritoneum, muscle, joint capsules, and bone, the distal processes of the ganglion cells travel in all of the spinal nerves. The proximal processes branch within the dorsal root entry zone and span five or more segments of the spinal cord within the dorsolateral tract of Lissauer before terminating in laminae I, II, and IV of the dorsal grey horn. The corresponding fibres of the trigeminal nerve terminate in the spinal nucleus of that nerve.

From the viscera, the distal processes share perineural sheaths with postganglionic fibres of the sympathetic system. The proximal processes mingle with the somatic fibres within the Lissauer tract and terminate in the same region. As noted in Chapter 13, overlap of somatic and visceral afferent terminals on the dendrites of central pain-projecting neurons is thought to account for *referred pain* in visceral disorders such as myocardial infarction and acute appendicitis.

Sensitisation of Nociceptors

Injured tissue liberates molecules such as bradykinin, prostaglandin, and leukotrienes, which lower the activation threshold of nociceptors. Injured C fibres also initiate axon reflexes (see Chapter 11), whereby substance P ± calcitonin gene-related peptide (CGRP) is liberated into the adjacent tissue, causing histamine release from mast cells. Histamine receptors may develop on the nerve terminals and (as already noted in Chapter 8) produce arachidonic acid by hydrolysis of membrane phospholipids. The enzyme *cyclooxidase* converts arachidonic acid into a prostaglandin. (The main action of aspirin and other nonsteroidal antiinflammatory analgesics is to inactivate that enzyme, thereby reducing synthesis of prostaglandins.)

The net result is sustained activation of large numbers of C-fibre neurons and sensitisation of mechanical nociceptors, manifested by *allodynia*, where even gentle stroking of the area may elicit pain; and by *hyperalgesia*, where moderately noxious stimuli are perceived as very painful.

As already noted in Chapter 13, *irritable bowel syndrome* is characterised by sensitisation of nociceptive *interoceptors* in the bowel wall. That event also underlies the painful urinary bladder condition known as *interstitial cystitis*.

Sensitisation of C-fibre neurons may include *gene transcription* (see Chapter 8) whereby abnormal sodium channels are inserted into the cell membrane of the parent neurons in the dorsal root ganglion. Spontaneous trains of impulses generated here are thought to account for occasional failure of quite high-level nerve blocks to abolish the pain.

Neuropathic Pain

When a peripheral nerve is severed, and the proximal and distal stumps are separated by developing scar tissue, trapped regenerating axons form thread-like balls, called *neuromas*, which are exquisitely sensitive to pressure. Repetitive activation may prolong the victim's suffering by engendering a central pain state (see below). *Postherpetic neuralgia* is a neuropathic pain that may be a sequel to *herpes zoster* ('creeping girdle') manifested by clusters of watery blisters, usually along the cutaneous territory of an intercostal nerve. The virus concerned may perpetuate the pain by precipitating the gene transcription mentioned above.

Central Pain Pathways

Central pain-projecting neurons are of two kinds as described in Chapter 15: nociceptive-specific, with small peripheral sensory fields (about 1 cm^2), and wide dynamic range, with fields of 2 cm^2 or more; these are mechanical nociceptors encoding tactile stimuli by low-frequency impulses and noxious stimuli by high-frequency impulses.

The current consensus is that the *spinothalamic* (or *anterolateral* based on its position within the spinal cord) *pathway* is a composite of tracts that contribute to both the discriminative features of pain, temperature, and touch (*neospinothalamic tract* or *direct pathway*), and the arousal, affective, motor, and autonomic attributes (*paleospinothalamic tract* or *indirect pathway*) in relation to pain (Figs. 33.10 and 33.11).

Direct Pain Pathway

For the trunk and limbs, the direct pathway arises in the dorsal grey horn of the spinal cord and projects into the spinothalamic tract to the posterior part of the contralateral ventral posterolateral nucleus of the thalamus. For the head and neck, it commences in the spinal nucleus of the trigeminal nerve and occupies the trigeminothalamic projection to the contralateral posterior medial thalamic nucleus. The onward projection is mainly to the primary somatic sensory cortex (SI) and partly to the upper bank of the lateral sulcus (SII). The arrangement is somatotopic, as can be seen on PET scanning when a noxious heat stimulus is applied to different parts of the body. Animal investigations demonstrate intensity responsive, nociceptive-specific neurons in SI, having appropriately small peripheral receptive fields, ideal candidates for encoding the 'Where and how much?' aspects of pain.

Onward projections to the posterior parietal cortex and SII are indicated in Figs. 33.10 and 33.11.

Not surprisingly the spinothalamic early warning system stimulates orientation of head and eyes towards the source of pain. As mentioned in Chapter 15 the *spinotectal tract* ascends alongside the *spinothalamic tract* and terminates in the superior colliculus. Its imprint is somatotopic, and it elicits a *spinovisual reflex* to orient the eyes/head/trunk towards the area stimulated. In addition to activation of this phylogenetically ancient (reptilian) reflex, the 'Where?' visual channel (see Chapter 28) is engaged by association fibres passing to the posterior parietal cortex from SI.

Nociceptive neurons in SII are less numerous, and many also receive visual inputs. They are linked to the insula, which also receives direct inputs from the thalamus. Insular stimulation may elicit autonomic responses such as a rapid pulse rate, vasoconstriction, and sweating. Surprisingly, preexisting lesions of the insula may abolish the aversive quality of painful stimuli while preserving the location and intensity aspects. The condition is known as *asymbolia for pain*.

Indirect Pain Pathway

The indirect pathway is polysynaptic, via the spinoreticular and trigeminoreticular tracts to the contralateral dorsomedial thalamic nucleus (among others), with onward projection to the anterior cingulate cortex. That this area is concerned with the affective component of pain experience is strongly supported by the effect of surgical undercutting (cingulotomy) or removal (cingulectomy) as a treatment for chronic pain. Patients report that the intensity of their pain is unchanged but that it has lost its aggressive nature. Precisely the same result follows morphine injection—presumably because the anterior cingulate has the greatest number of opiate receptors in the cerebral cortex.

Following cingulotomy, oedema of the bladder control area frequently causes temporary urinary incontinence. More importantly, more than half of all patients show permanent 'flatness of affect', that is, low experience of either elation or depression.

An unexpected stab of pain from any source is likely to generate an immediate sense of fear. This is attributable to activation of *spinomesencephalic* fibres projecting to the midbrain reticular formation, with onward projection to the amygdala, a nucleus particularly associated with the sense of fear (see main text). Some of the fibres are believed to ascend in or alongside the dorsolateral tract of Lissauer; they may account for the persistence of pain perception in some patients following the cordotomy procedure.

Central Pain States

Central pain states are almost always generated by wind-up of the central pain-projecting neurons (CPPNs) of the spinothalamic and spinoreticular pathways. One or more of three mechanisms may be responsible:

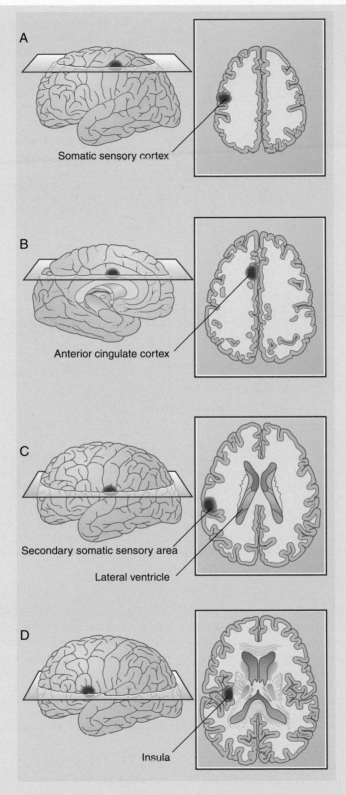

Fig. 33.10 Areas showing increased metabolic activity following application of noxious heat to the right forearm. Shown in horizontal sections: (A) somatic sensory cortex; (B) anterior cingulate cortex; (C) secondary somatic sensory area; (D) insula.

- Repetitive activation of NMDA glutamate receptors by dorsal nerve root inputs, over a period of weeks or months, tends to induce a state of long-term potentiation of CPPNs.
- The threshold of CPPNs may be lowered further by gene transcription whereby additional glutamate receptors are inserted into their dendrites.

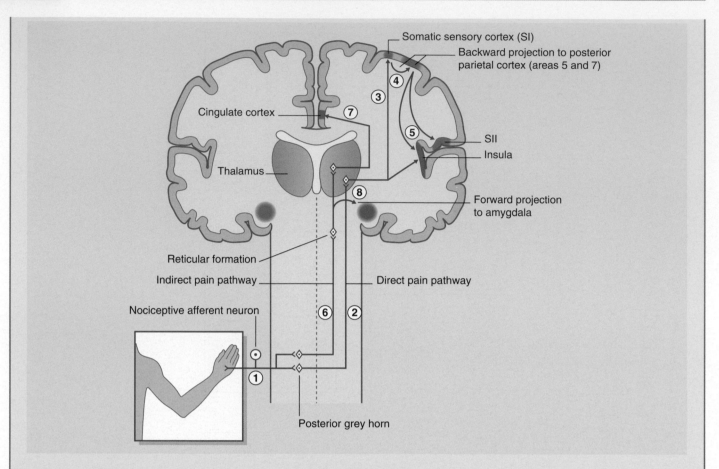

Fig. 33.11 Pain pathways. *Violet* signifies areas having emotional significance. The amygdala is in fact anterior to the plane of section in the diagram, and areas 5 and 7 are posterior to it. *1,* Peripheral nociceptive neurons project to dorsal grey horn; *2,* 'Fast' central pain projecting neurons project direct to the contralateral posterolateral thalamus and *3,* relay to the somatic sensory cortex *(SII); 4,* Association fibres connect SI to the posterior parietal cortex both for 'Where?' and 'How much?' tactile analysis, and to provide a 'Where?' visual alert; *5,* The posterior parietal cortex projects to lateral sulcus *(SIII)* for tactile–visual integration. Onward relay to the insular cortex, supplemented by some direct thalamic inputs there, may elicit autonomic and emotional responses; *6,* 'Slow' CPPNs relay via the reticular formation to the medial thalamus, with forward projection to the prefrontal cortex (not shown here) for overall evaluation; *7,* Upward projection to the cingulate cortex normally generates an aversive (*L.* 'turn away') emotional evaluation; *8,* Some CPPNs excite reticular neurons projecting to the amygdala, where they are likely to generate a sense of fear.

- The term 'paradoxical' seems appropriate for the third mechanism. Reference was made in Chapter 24 to *supraspinal antinociception*, whereby serotonergic neurons projecting from the medullary magnus raphe nucleus (MRN) to the dorsal grey horn may *inhibit CPPNs* by activating encephalinergic interneurons. Evidence from animal experiments now indicates that while either of the first two mechanisms may initiate a central pain state, its maintenance requires that nonserotonergic neurons in or near the MRN *facilitate CPPNs* by a direct excitatory transmitter of uncertain nature. Following limb amputation, an ultimate expression of wind-up is *phantom limb pain,* where severe pain may be experienced in the distal part of the missing limb.

  As mentioned in Chapter 25, the central pain state known as *thalamic syndrome* may develop following a vascular lesion in the white matter close to the ventroposterior nucleus of the thalamus. Explanation of the bouts of severe contralateral pain sensation may lie in elimination of the normal inhibitory feedback to the posterior thalamus from the surrounding thalamic reticular nucleus.

and even prior to the SMA itself. The executive area is thought to have special significance, together with the DLPFC, in generating *appropriate motor plan selection* by the SMA.

2. A *pain perception area* receives afferents from the dorsomedial nucleus of the thalamus (Box 33.1).

3. An *emotional area* lies close to the pain perception area. When volunteers 'think happy' while undergoing PET scans, the anterior cingulate cortex 'lights up' and the amygdala 'switches off'. A reverse result occurs when volunteers 'think sad'. Although rarely performed today, anterior cingulectomy was once used to reduce aggressive behaviour in patients with psychiatric disorders.

4. A *bladder control area* becomes increasingly active during bladder filling (see Chapter 24).

5. A *vocalisation area* becomes active, together with the DLPFC, during *decision making* about appropriate sentence construction during speech activity. Electrical

stimulation of this area causes jumbling of speech. *Stammering* in children is associated with *reduced* blood flow in the left anterior cingulate gyrus during speech. Blood flow there is also reduced in people suffering from *Tourette syndrome* which is characterised by brief, loud utterances of a single syllable or phrase at times offensive to the ear.

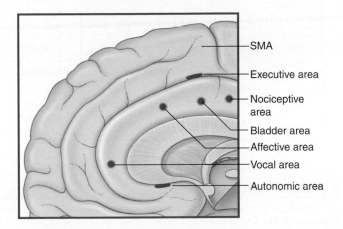

Fig. 33.12 Functional areas in the anterior cingulate cortex. *SMA,* Supplementary motor area.

6. An *autonomic area*, below the rostrum of the corpus callosum, elicits autonomic and respiratory responses when stimulated electrically. This area is thought to participate in eliciting the visceral responses typical of emotional states.

The posterior cingulate gyrus (area 23) merges with the posterior parahippocampal gyrus (area 36). This cortical complex is richly interconnected with visual, auditory, and tactile/spatial association and evidently contains memory stores related to these functions because PET studies reveal increased activity there when scenes or experiences are conjured up in the mind. The complex is also engaged during reading (see Chapter 32).

Amygdala

The **amygdala** (*Gr.* 'almond'; also called the *amygdaloid body* or *amygdaloid complex*) is a large group of nuclei above and in front of the temporal horn of the lateral ventricle and anterior to the tail of the caudate nucleus. *The amygdala is primarily associated with the emotion of fear,* as identified by the fMRI response when looking at an angry or fearful face (Fig. 33.13). Clinical and experimental studies are currently under way in an effort to gain diagnostic and therapeutic insights into the role of the amygdala with regard to various *phobias* and *anxiety states* prevalent in both the young and the adult populations. The

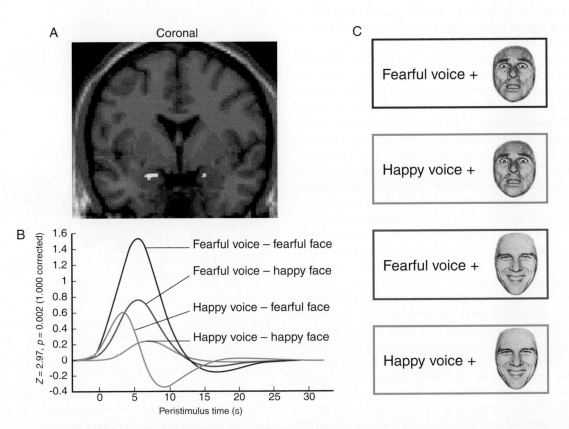

Fig. 33.13 Cross-modal emotional responses. (A) Coronal structural MRI image showing a superimposed fMRI map of bilateral activation of the amygdala in a volunteer observing a fearful face accompanied by a fearful voice (see C). At the opposite end of the spectrum, amygdala activity was below normal level in the presence of a happy face and voice. (B) The associated graph shows experimental condition-specific fMRI responses in the amygdala. (Kindly provided by Professor R.J. Dolan, Wellcome Department of Cognitive Neurology, Institute of Neurology, University College, London, UK.)

TABLE 33.2 Afferents to the Lateral Nucleus of the Amygdala.

Nature	Subcortical Source	Cortical Source
Tactile	Ventral posterior nucleus of the thalamus	Parietal lobe
Auditory	Medial geniculate body	Superior temporal gyrus
Visual	Lateral geniculate body[a]	Occipital cortex
Olfactory	—	Piriform lobe
Mnemonic	—	Hippocampus/entorhinal cortex
Cardiac	Hypothalamus	Insula
Nociceptive	Midbrain reticular formation	—
Cognitive	—	Orbital cortex
Attention-related	Locus coeruleus	Basal nucleus of Meynert

[a]Afferents from the lateral geniculate body to the amygdala have yet to be clearly identified.

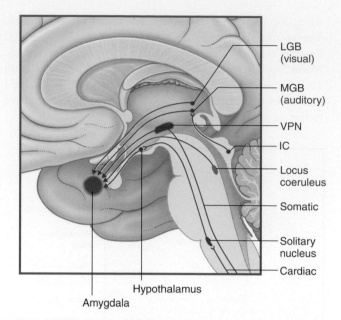

Fig. 33.14 Subcortical afferents to the lateral nucleus of the amygdala. *IC*, Inferior colliculus; *LGB*, lateral geniculate body; *MGB*, medial geniculate body; *VPN*, ventral posterior nucleus of the thalamus.

connections of the amygdala (inasmuch as these are understood) are consistent with the present perception of its pivotal position in the perception and expression of fear.

Afferent pathways. Within the amygdala, nuclear groups receiving afferents are predominantly laterally placed and are usually referred to collectively as the *lateral nucleus*. In Table 33.2 and related figures, the afferents are segregated into subcortical and cortical.

Subcortical access, depicted in Fig. 33.14, is thought to be especially important in infancy and childhood, at a time when the amygdala, which is developing faster than the hippocampus, is capable of acquiring fearful memory traces without hippocampal participation. Such memories cannot be *consciously* recalled at any later time despite generating physical responses of an 'escape' nature. The general-sense and special-sense pathways listed and depicted are sufficiently comprehensive to account for the acquisition of almost any specific 'unexplained' phobia (e.g. enclosed spaces, smoke, heights, dogs, faces).

As indicated in Fig. 33.15, all sensory association areas of the cortex have direct access to the lateral nucleus of the amygdala. These areas are also linked to the prefrontal cortex through long association fibre bundles, rendering all conscious sensations subject to cognitive evaluation.

Activity of the visual association cortex is especially important in connection with phobias and anxiety states. Area V4 on the inferior surface of anterior area 19 is a link in the object/face recognition pathway. V5, on the lateral surface of anterior area 19, is a link in the movement detection pathway. Both are connected to the amygdala via the hippocampus, where fearful visual memories may be recalled by the current visual scene. The visual association cortex is also important in that fearful visual images conjured in the mind independently of current sensation may activate the amygdala. This capability may be related to *posttraumatic stress disorder*, in which a seemingly innocent scene may cause the afflicted individual to 'relive' a horrific visual experience up to 20 years or more after the event. In the multimodal anterior region of the superior temporal

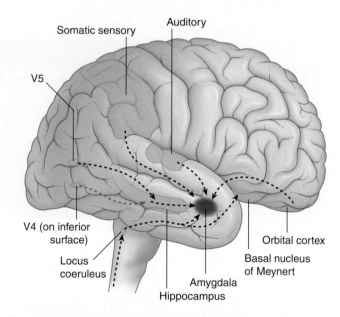

Fig. 33.15 Cortical afferents to the lateral nucleus of the amygdala. *V4*, object/face recognition area; *V5*, motion detection area.

gyrus, where sound and vision coalesce, a door banged shut may induce a 'virtual reality' reenactment of a horrific encounter, such as of a haunting war experience.

The orbital prefrontal cortex of the right side, with its bias towards 'withdrawal' rather than 'approach' (see Chapter 32), is commonly active (in PET scans) along with the right amygdala in fearful situations, such as when a specific phobia is presented to a susceptible subject. On the one hand, this offers the 'downside' potential to 'feed on one's fear'. On the other hand, expert social/psychological conditioning may eventually suffice to reduce the 'negative drive' of the orbital cortex. When conditioning is combined with use of anxiolytic drugs, specific phobias may be abolished completely.

The insula is omitted from Fig. 33.15 but, as noted earlier, its posterior part also has direct access to the amygdala and has a function probably related to the emotional evaluation of pain.

Finally, the *basal nucleus of Meynert* is listed. The cholinergic projection from this nucleus is thought to be significant in facilitating activity in cortical cell columns in the context of situations having negative emotional valence. Meynert activity appears to be heightened in association with anxiety that generates a raised level of autonomic activity involving the amygdala (and/or the adjacent bed nucleus of the stria terminalis, mentioned below).

Efferent Pathways (Table 33.3).

Easily identified in the postmortem brain is the **stria terminalis** (Fig. 33.16), which upon emerging from the central nucleus of the amygdala, follows the curve of the caudate nucleus and accompanies the thalamostriate vein along the *sulcus terminalis* between the thalamus and caudate nucleus. The stria sends fibres to the septal area and hypothalamus before entering the *medial forebrain bundle* and (downstream) the *central tegmental tract*. Some fibres of the stria terminate in a *bed nucleus* above the anterior commissure. The bed nucleus is regarded by some workers as part of the 'extended amygdala'; it may be more active than the amygdala proper, on PET scans, in anxiety states.

A second efferent projection, the **ventral amygdalofugal pathway**, passes medially to synapse within the nucleus accumbens (Fig. 33.17). This connection is considered in the context of schizophrenia (Clinical Panel 33.2).

Notes on the efferent target connections. *Periaqueductal grey matter.* A source of *supraspinal antinociception* was described in Chapter 24, namely the opioid-containing axons from the hypothalamus that disinhibit the excitatory projection from the periaqueductal grey matter to the serotonergic cells of origin of the raphespinal tract. The excitatory cells of the *dorsal periaqueductal grey matter* are directly stimulated by axon terminals entering from the amygdala via the medial forebrain bundle.

In laboratory animals, stimulation of the ventral periaqueductal grey matter causes *freezing*, where a fixed, flexed posture is adopted. The ventral periaqueductal grey matter contains neurons projecting to the cells of origin of the medullary reticulospinal tract. This tract activates flexor motor neurons during the walking cycle, and intense activation may cause a frightened person to 'go weak at the knees' and perhaps fall down.

Locus coeruleus. Facilitation of excitatory cortical neurons by the noradrenergic projection from this pontine nucleus is to be expected.

Medullary adrenergic neurons. As noted in Chapter 24, these neurons are a component of the baroreflex pathway sustaining the blood pressure against gravitational force. Sudden stimulation by the direct projection from the amygdala may send the heart pounding and cause a major elevation of systemic blood pressure.

Hypothalamus. Fibres of the stria terminalis synapse upon two sets of hypothalamic neurons. The first, located in the anterolateral region, sends axons into the dorsal longitudinal fasciculus to synapse in cells of origin of the vagal supply to the heart. The well-known condition, referred to as a **vasovagal episode** or *neurocardiogenic syncope* (fainting at the sight of

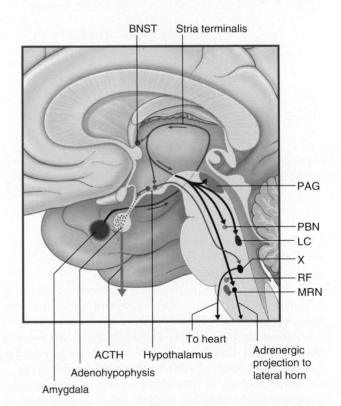

Fig. 33.16 Efferents from the central nucleus of the amygdala via the stria terminalis. The only postsynaptic pathways shown are autonomic. The periaqueductal grey matter *(PAG)* projects to magnus raphe neurons *(MRN)*, giving rise to the raphespinal tract. *ACTH,* Adrenocorticotropic hormone; *BNST,* bed nucleus of the stria terminalis; *LC,* locus coeruleus; *PBN,* parabrachial nucleus; *RF,* reticular formation; *X,* dorsal nucleus of the vagus.

TABLE 33.3 Efferents From the Central Nucleus of the Amygdala.	
Target Nucleus/Pathway	**Function/Effect**
Periaqueductal grey matter (to medulla/ raphespinal tract)	Antinociception
Periaqueductal grey matter (to medullary reticulospinal tract)	Freezing
Locus coeruleus	Arousal
Norepinephrine medullary neurons (projection to lateral grey horn)	Tachycardia/hypertension
Hypothalamus/dorsal nucleus of vagus (to heart)	Bradycardia/fainting
Hypothalamus (liberation of corticotropin-releasing hormone)	Stress hormone secretion
Parabrachial nucleus (to medullary respiratory nuclei)	Hyperventilation

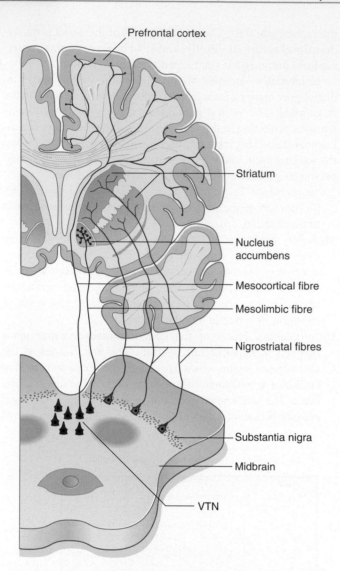

Fig. 33.17 Coronal section at the level of the nucleus accumbens highlighting distribution of dopaminergic fibres arising in the ventral tegmental nuclei *(VTN)* of the midbrain.

blood at the scene of an accident), is characterised by initial sympathetic excitation followed by vagus-induced bradycardia, causing the individual to collapse (faint).

The second set of neurons secrete corticotropin-releasing hormone (CRH) into the adenohypophysis via the hypophyseal portal system, with consequent release of adrenocorticotropin (ACTH). Curiously, these CRH neurons send collateral branches into the central nucleus of the amygdala with positive feedback enhancement of its activity.

Parabrachial nucleus. In individuals subject to *panic attacks*, hyperventilation, together with a sense of fear, may be triggered by what may appear to be relatively trivial environmental challenges. Normally, the respiratory alkalosis produced by washout of carbon dioxide reduces the respiratory rate causing the blood pH to return to normal, whereas susceptible individuals continue to hyperventilate. Because selective serotonin reuptake

inhibitors (SSRIs) are highly successful in treatment, the prevailing view is that the normal inhibitory role of serotonergic terminals within the nucleus accumbens (see later) becomes deficient. However, overactivity of the locus coeruleus has also been implicated because yohimbine (a drug that once found favour as a weight-loss agent and as a treatment for sexual dysfunction in men) can induce a panic attack, apparently through norepinephrine release.

Limbic striatal loop. This circuit is depicted in Chapter 26, passing from the prefrontal cortex through the nucleus accumbens and dorsomedial nucleus of the thalamus with return to the prefrontal cortex. However, the central nucleus of the amygdala participates in this circuit through an excitatory projection to the nucleus accumbens. In the right hemisphere this projection is likely to facilitate a withdrawal response; in the left, it may facilitate an approach response.

Bilateral ablation of the amygdala was once carried out in humans for treatment of *rage attacks*, characterised by irritability building up over several hours or days to a state of dangerous aggressiveness. This controversial operation was 'successful' in eliminating such attacks. In monkeys, bilateral ablation leads to placidity together with a tendency to explore objects orally and to exhibit hypersexuality (*Klüver–Bucy syndrome*). A comparable syndrome has occasionally been observed in humans.

At the other end of the spectrum, PET studies of incarcerated murderers have revealed that the amygdala of the majority remains 'silent' even when gruesome scenes are presented on screen.

Nucleus Accumbens

The full name is *nucleus accumbens septi pellucidi*, 'the nucleus leaning against the septum pellucidum'. More accurately, the nucleus abuts septal nuclei located in the base of the septum. Figs. 33.17 and 33.18C show this relationship. The accumbens is one of many deep-seated brain areas where electrodes have been inserted on a therapeutic trial basis notably in the hope of providing pain relief. Stimulation of the accumbens induces an intense sense of well-being *(hedonia)*, comparable to that experienced by intake of drugs of addiction such as heroin (see Clinical Panel 33.5). This 'high' feeling is attributed to flooding of the nucleus, and of the medial prefrontal cortex, by synaptic and volume release of dopamine from the neurons projecting from the ventral tegmental area. Normally, dopamine is released in small amounts and quickly retrieved from the extracellular space by a specific dopamine reuptake transporter.

Septal Area

The septal area consists of the **septal nuclei**, merging with the cortex directly in front of the anterior commissure, together with a small extension into the septum pellucidum (Fig. 33.19).

Afferents to the septal nuclei are received from the following:
- The amygdala, via the *diagonal band (of Broca)*, a slender connection passing alongside the anterior perforated substance;
- The olfactory tract, via the medial olfactory stria;
- The hippocampus, via the fornix; and
- Brainstem monoaminergic neurons, via the medial forebrain bundle.

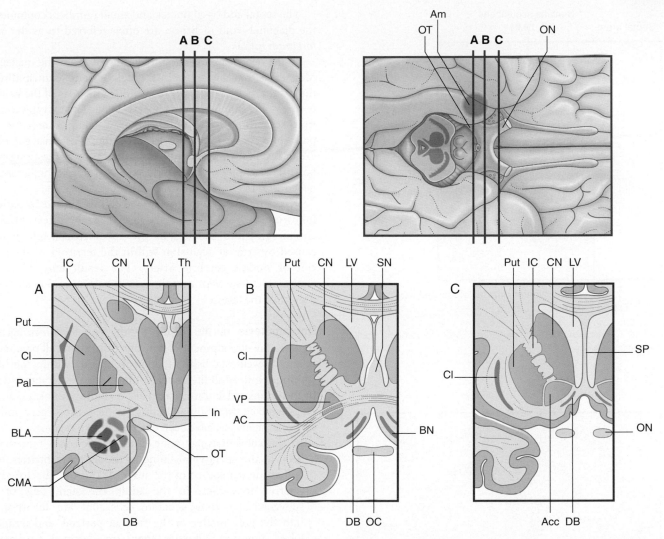

Fig. 33.18 (A–C) Coronal Sections of the Basal Forebrain in the Planes Indicated. *AC*, Anterior commissure; *Acc*, nucleus accumbens; *Am*, amygdala; *BLA*, basolateral amygdala; *BN*, basal nucleus of Meynert; *Cl*, claustrum; *CMA*, corticomedial amygdala; *CN*, caudate nucleus; *DB*, diagonal band of Broca; *IC*, internal capsule; *In*, infundibulum; *LV*, lateral ventricle; *OC*, optic chiasm; *ON*, optic nerve; *OT*, optic tract; *Pal*, pallidum; *Put*, putamen; *SN*, septal nucleus; *SP*, septum pellucidum; *Th*, thalamus; *VP*, ventral pallidum.

The two chief *efferent* projections are as follows:
- **Stria medullaris**, a glutamatergic strand running along the junction of side wall and roof of the third ventricle to synapse upon cholinergic neurons in the **habenular nucleus**, in Fig. 33.19. The habenular nuclei of the two sides are connected through the **habenular commissure** located close to the root of the pineal gland, as shown earlier, in Fig. 17.19. The habenular nucleus sends the cholinergic **habenulo-interpeduncular tract** *(fasciculus retroflexus)* to synapse in the **interpeduncular nucleus** of the reticular formation in the midbrain (Fig. 17.19). The interpeduncular nucleus is believed to participate in the sleep—wake cycle together with the cholinergic neurons beside the locus coeruleus, identified earlier (Fig. 24.1B).
- **Septohippocampal pathway**, running to the hippocampus by way of the fornix (Fig. 33.20). It is responsible for generating the slow-wave *hippocampal θ rhythm* detectable in electroencephalogram (EEG) recordings from the temporal lobe. Glutamatergic neurons in this pathway are pacemakers that

determine the *rate* of θ rhythm; cholinergic neurons determine the *size* of the θ waves. θ rhythm is produced by synchronous discharge of groups of hippocampal pyramidal cells and is significant in the development of biochemical alterations within pyramidal glutamate receptors during the long-term potentiation involved in laying down episodic memory traces. The strength of θ rhythm is greatly reduced in Alzheimer disease, reflecting the substantial loss of both cholinergic neurons and episodic memory formation and retrieval in this disease.

Electrical stimulation of the human septal area produces sexual sensations akin to orgasm. In animals, an electrolytic lesion may evince signs of extreme displeasure (so-called 'septal rage'). This surprising response may be due to destruction of a possible inhibitory projection from the septal area to the amygdala.

Basal Forebrain

The basal forebrain extends from the bifurcation of the olfactory tract as far back as the infundibulum and from the midline to

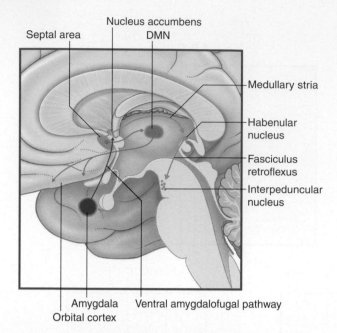

Fig. 33.19 Connections of the septal area. *DMN*, Dorsomedial nucleus of the thalamus.

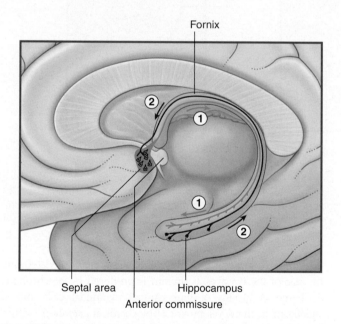

Fig. 33.20 Septohippocampal pathway *(1)* with return projection from hippocampus *(2)*.

the amygdala (Fig. 33.18). In the floor of the basal forebrain is the **anterior perforated substance**, named for its appearance that results from being pierced by anteromedial central branches arising from the arterial circle of Willis (Chapter 4). Here the cerebral cortex is replaced by scattered nuclear groups of which the largest is the **magnocellular basal nucleus of Meynert**.

The *cholinergic neurons of the basal forebrain* have their somas mainly in the septal nuclei and basal nucleus of Meynert (Fig. 33.21). The basal nucleus projects to all parts of the cerebral neocortex, which also contains scattered intrinsic cholinergic neurons.

The septal and basal nuclei, and small numbers contained in the diagonal band of Broca, are often referred to as the *basal forebrain nuclei*.

In the neocortex the cholinergic supply from the nucleus of Meynert is tonically active in the waking state, contributing to the 'awake' pattern on EEG recordings. All areas of the neocortex are richly supplied. Tonic liberation of ACh activates muscarinic receptors on cortical neurons, causing a reduction of potassium conductance, making them more responsive to other excitatory inputs. The cholinergic supply promotes long-term potentiation and training-induced synaptic strengthening of neocortical pyramidal cells.

The general psychic slowdown often observed in patients following a stroke may be accounted for by interruption of cholinergic fibre bundles in the subcortical white matter, caused by arterial occlusion within the territory of the anterior or middle cerebral artery. The result may be virtual cholinergic denervation of the cortex both at and posterior to the site of the lesion.

Neurogenesis in the Adult Brain. The term *neurogenesis* signifies the development of neurons from stem cell precursors. It is now well-established that neurogenesis within the brain continues into adult life and, at a much lower rate, into old age. In the brains of laboratory animals, including monkeys, and in biopsies taken from human brains during neurosurgery, mitotic neuronal stem cells have been detected in two regions:

- In the subventricular zone, that is the zone immediately deep to the ependymal lining of the lateral ventricles. This is the original source of the stem cells of the olfactory bulb referred to earlier. In the adult, the stem cells of the subventricular zone generate cells that are incorporated into the grey matter of the frontal, parietal, and temporal lobes; however, whether they are destined to become neurons or neuroglia is uncertain.
- Within the hippocampal complex in the zone immediately deep to the granule cell layer of the dentate gyrus. In all species examined, including humans, these stem cells, when followed in cell cultures, exhibit branching and acquire electrical activity. Serial histologic studies in rats prove that they become mature, integrated granule cells.

In adult rats, the numbers of mitotic stem cells may increase dramatically in response to appropriate sensory stimulation. For example, the numbers in the olfactory bulb increase fivefold in the presence of an odour-rich environment; in the dentate subgranular zone, a sharp increase is observed in the presence of learning opportunities provided by tread-wheels and mazes. These observations lend credence to the belief that continuing to exercise body and mind is beneficial to humans entering their retirement years.

There is evidence from animal experiments that existing pharmacologic therapies for neurodegenerative and neuropsychiatric disorders exert beneficial neurotrophic effects. A high level of serotonin in the extracellular fluid of the dentate gyrus stimulates the proliferation of neurons there, notably following administration of serotonin reuptake or monoamine oxidase inhibitors.

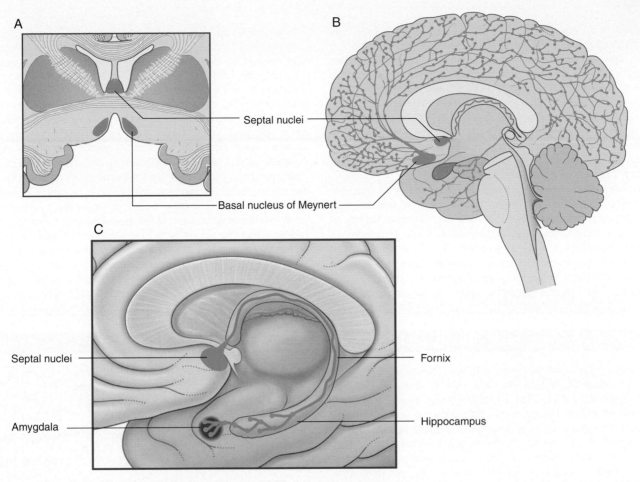

Fig. 33.21 Cholinergic Innervation of the Cerebral Cortex From the Basal Forebrain Nuclei. (A) Section at level indicated in (B). (B) Cortical innervation. (C) Septohippocampal pathway via the fornix. The amygdala is also supplied via this route.

CLINICAL PANEL 33.1 Olfactory Disturbance

A routine test of olfactory function is to ask the patient to identify strong-smelling substances such as coffee and chocolate through each nostril in turn. If it is unilateral, loss of smell, or **anosmia**, may not be detected by the patient without testing. If it is bilateral, the complaint may be one of loss of taste because the flavour of foodstuffs depends on the olfactory qualities of volatile elements. In such cases, the four primary taste sensations (sweet, sour, salty, bitter) are preserved.

Unilateral anosmia may be caused by a *meningioma* compressing the olfactory bulb/tract or by a head injury with fracture of the anterior cranial fossa. Anosmia may be a clue to a fracture and should prompt tests for leakage of cerebrospinal fluid into the nasal cavity.

Olfactory auras are a typical prodromal feature of *uncinate epilepsy* (see Clinical Panel 33.3).

CLINICAL PANEL 33.2 Schizophrenia

Schizophrenia occurs in about 1% of the population in all countries where the prevalence has been studied. It is a heritable illness with about a 10% risk of occurrence if a person's first-degree relative is affected and as much as a 50% risk of occurrence if both parents or an identical co-twin is affected. Although the onset of illness is typically in early adulthood, there is substantial evidence for neurodevelopmental disturbance in the illness with increased rates of birth complications, early developmental insults, and childhood social, motor, and academic underperformance in those who later develop schizophrenia. Cognitive dysfunction is present in the illness, but relatively stable throughout life, unlike the progressive dementias.

Magnetic resonance imaging (MRI) studies reveal enlargement of lateral ventricles and regionally specific atrophy predominantly affecting frontal and temporal parts of the cortex, the medial temporal lobe, and thalamus. There is a reduction or even a reversal of the usual left—right difference in the size of the temporal plane on the upper surface of the superior temporal gyrus. There

is some progression of these neuroimaging abnormalities in the early years of the illness, which then plateau. Postmortem studies indicate that the atrophy identified by imaging studies is related to loss of neuropil and reduced neuronal size rather than neuronal loss. No evidence of astrogliosis or of neurodegenerative disease pathology has been identified. Consistent with neurodevelopmental disturbance, underlying the illness are findings of aberrantly located neurons, for example, in the entorhinal cortex and in white matter.

The clinical presentation is quite variable but the symptoms and behavioural changes can be categorised into two broad spectra: positive symptoms and negative symptoms.

- *Positive psychotic symptoms* include hallucinations, delusions, and disorganised thoughts and behaviour. Hallucinations are typically auditory (the patient hears voices that are commonly derogatory in nature and refer to the patient in the third person). Delusions often take a paranoid form with a belief that the patient is being monitored or the subject of a conspiracy. Other typical delusions include a belief that one's thoughts and actions are being controlled by an outside agency and that thoughts are not private but are somehow accessible by other people. Thought processes frequently become disorganised with the normal flow and logic of speech breaking down and in severe cases becoming incoherent. Disorganised behaviour includes disinhibited, socially inappropriate behaviour or in some cases physical aggression in response to hallucinations or delusions. Although positive symptoms cause great distress to patients and their families, they are much more responsive to antipsychotic medication treatment than the negative ones, which in the long-term are more disabling.

- *Negative (deficit) psychotic symptoms* refer to an inability to engage in normal emotional and social interactions with people and frequently lead to impaired capacity to self-care. The patient lacks motivation, has little to say, and rambles from one inconsequential theme to another in conversation. There is a loss of emotional responsiveness *(flattening of affect)*, including inability to experience pleasure *(anhedonia)*. Personal hygiene and ability to live independently and manage affairs are often impaired. The negative symptoms appear to be associated with

'hypofrontality,' that is, diminished prefrontal function. Functional imaging studies using functional MRI (fMRI) and positron emission tomography (PET) support this idea by demonstrating failure of the normal response of the dorsolateral prefrontal cortex to standard tests of cognitive function.

Medications used to treat psychotic disorders such as schizophrenia are called *antipsychotics, neuroleptics,* or *major tranquillisers.* All such antipsychotic medications block dopamine D_2 receptors to some extent (e.g. haloperidol or olanzapine). In the normal brain, the D_2 receptors are on spiny (excitatory) stellate cells in the mesocortical projection territory of the ventral tegmental nucleus. D_2 receptors are inhibitory for one or more of three possible reasons noted in Chapter 8. Interestingly, symptoms closely resembling the positive psychotic ones of schizophrenia may be induced by consuming excessive amounts of dopamine-stimulating drugs such as cocaine or amphetamine ('speed'). Amphetamine is known to increase the amount of dopamine in the forebrain extracellular space (Clinical Panel 33.5). In schizophrenia, dopaminergic overactivity seems not to be a matter of overproduction but of greater effectiveness through an increased number of postsynaptic dopamine receptors on the spiny stellate neurons. (The assistance of Professor Colm McDonald, Department of Psychiatry, NUI, Galway, Ireland, is gratefully appreciated.)

CLINICAL PANEL 33.3 'Temporal Lobe' Epilepsy

Focal onset with impaired awareness seizures are synonymous with the older term of temporal lobe epilepsy. The initial event, or *aura*, may be a focal onset seizure whose electrical activity escapes into the temporal lobe. Many originate in a focus of runaway neural activity within the temporal lobe and spread over the general cortex within seconds to trigger a *secondarily generalised* tonic–clonic seizure (Fig. 33.22) as mentioned in Chapter 29. Types of temporal lobe auras include well-formed visual or auditory hallucinations (scenes, sound sequences), a sense of familiarity with the surrounding scene ('déjà vu'), a sense of strangeness ('*jamais vu*'), or a sense of fear. Attacks originating in the uncus are ushered in by unpleasant olfactory or gustatory auras. Bizarre *psychic* auras can occur where the patient has an 'out of body experience' in the form of a sensation of floating in the air and looking down at themselves and any others present.

Following accurate localisation of the ictal (seizure) focus by means of recording electrodes inserted into the exposed temporal lobe, a tissue block including the focus may be removed with abolition of seizures in four out of five cases. Histologic examination of the surgical biopsy typically reveals *hippocampal sclerosis*: the picture is one of glial scarring with extensive neuronal loss in CA2 and CA3 sectors. The granule cells of the dentate gyrus are relatively well-preserved. Loss of inhibitory, GABA interneurons has been blamed in the past, but these cells have recently been shown to persist. Instead the granule cells appear to be *disinhibited* because of loss of minute, inhibitory basket cells from among their dendrites.

Because 30% of sufferers from temporal lobe epilepsy have first-degree relatives similarly afflicted, often from childhood, a genetic influence must be significant. One possibility could be 'faulty wiring' of the hippocampus during midfetal life. Histologic preparations show areas of congenital misplacement of hippocampal pyramidal cells, some lying on their sides or even in the subjacent white matter. The sclerosis is regarded as a typical central nervous system healing process following extensive loss of neurons. The neuronal loss in turn seems to be inflicted by *glutamate toxicity*, a known effect of excessively high rates of discharge of pyramidal cells in any part of the cerebral cortex. Dentate granule cells are the main source of burst-firing which is no surprise in view of their natural role in long-term potentiation and kindling (see main text).

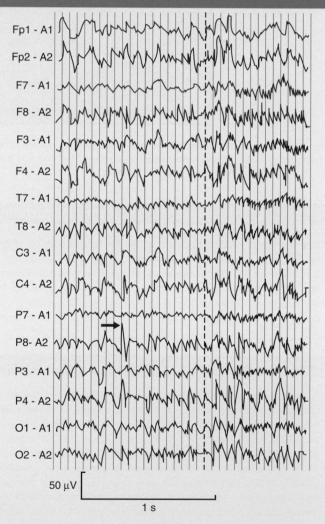

Fp1 - A1
Fp2 - A2
F7 - A1
F8 - A2
F3 - A1
F4 - A2
T7 - A1
T8 - A2
C3 - A1
C4 - A2
P7 - A1
P8- A2
P3 - A1
P4 - A2
O1 - A1
O2 - A2

50 μV

1 s

Fig. 33.22 Focal onset with impaired awareness ("temporal lobe") seizure. The ictal focus *(arrow)* occupies the middle–posterior junctional zone of the right temporal lobe (cf. electrode positions in Fig. 29.2). Within a second, the entire cortex exhibits a secondarily generalised seizure (to the right of the dashed line).

CLINICAL PANEL 33.4 Alzheimer Disease

Dementia is defined as a severe loss of cognitive function without impairment of consciousness. Alzheimer disease (AD) is the commonest cause of dementia afflicting 5% of people in their seventh decade and 20% of people in their ninth. AD patients fill 20% of all beds in psychiatric institutions.

MRI brain scans usually reveal severe atrophy of the cerebral cortex with widening of the sulci and enlargement of the ventricular system. As seen in Fig. 33.23, the medial temporal lobe (hippocampal complex and entorhinal cortex) areas are most severely affected. The primary sensory and motor areas and the upper regions of the prefrontal cortex are relatively well-preserved.

Postmortem histologic studies of the cerebral cortex reveal:
* Extensive loss of pyramidal neurons throughout the brain.
* **Amyloid plaques** and **neurofibrillary tangles** notably in the hippocampus and amygdala. The plaques begin in the walls of small blood vessels and have been explained in terms of an enzyme defect resulting in abnormal β-*amyloid* protein production. The tangles are made up of clumps of microtubules associated with an abnormal variant of a microtubule-associated θ protein. The tangles are progressively replaced by amyloid.
* Loss of up to 50% of the cholinergic neurons from the basal nucleus of Meynert and from the septal area, together with their extensive projections through the cerebral isocortex and mesocortex. Indeed, degenerating ACh terminals seem to contribute to the neurofibrillary tangles in the temporal lobe.

Hypometabolism can be shown on PET scans arranged to detect glucose utilisation. This is attributable in part to loss of pyramidal cells and in part to loss of cholinergic innervation of the pyramidal cells remaining. Healthy pyramidal neurons have excitatory ACh receptors in their cell membranes.

Although the pattern of degeneration varies from case to case, its general trend is to commence in the medial temporal lobe and to travel upwards and forwards. The following clinical features are explained in that sequence:
* *Dwindling hippocampal function.* Anterograde amnesia leads to *forgetfulness*, such as recounting a personal event within minutes of telling it (loss of present-time episodic memory); difficulty in finding one's way around familiar streets, or alarming misjudgements while driving an automobile (hippocampal activity is required to sustain parietal lobe *spatial sense*); and *attentional deficit*, whose earliest manifestation is an inability to switch attention from one thing to another.
* *Dwindling occipitotemporal function.* Damage to area 37 leads to an inability to read and write. Damage to the temporal polar region leads to a distressing failure to recognise the faces of family and friends. Involvement of the supramarginal and angular gyri leads to an inability to write.
* *Dwindling frontal lobe function.* Usually within 3 years of onset, the patient is 'spaced out', staring at walls and seemingly unaware of what is going on in the room. This 'vacant' state lasts for up to 5 or 6 years antemortem.

An unusual variant, known as *early-onset AD*, shows clear evidence of an autosomal dominant trait. The illness appears during the fourth or fifth decade. Chromosomal analyses have revealed a specific mutation in the gene coding for amyloid precursor protein on the long arm of chromosome 21. This mutation is also found in Down syndrome, in which sufferers surviving into middle age usually develop AD.

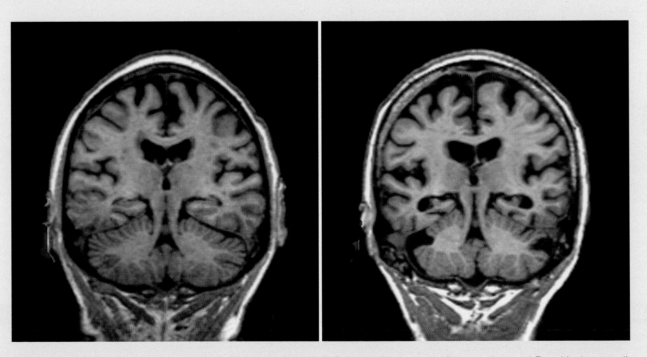

Fig. 33.23 Coronal MRI slices. (A) Normal control. (B) Alzheimer patient. Colours added: *green,* Hippocampus; *red,* Entorhinal cortex. (Images supplied by Professor Clifford R. Jack, Jr., and the Alzheimer's Disease Research Center at the Mayo Clinic.)

CLINICAL PANEL 33.5   **Drugs of Dependency**

Experimental evidence from the injection of drugs of abuse has yielded the following results (Figs. 33.24 and 33.25):

- Cocaine binds with the dopamine reuptake transporter blocking reuptake of the normal secretion with consequent dopamine accumulation in the extracellular space.

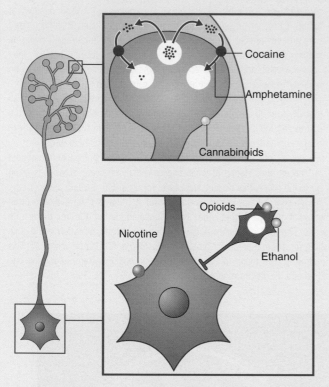

Fig. 33.24 Mesolimbic neuron supplying the nucleus accumbens, showing sites of action of some drugs of dependency.

- Amphetamine and methamphetamine are potent dopamine-releasing agents and also tend to block the reincorporation of dopamine into synaptic vesicles. These two drugs are also significantly active within the terminal dopaminergic network in the prefrontal cortex.
- Cannabinoids activate specific, excitatory, cannabinoid receptors on dopamine nerve endings.

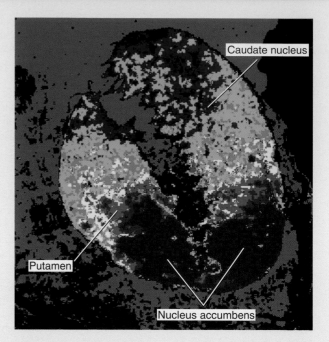

Fig. 33.25 Intense Activation (red) of D3 Receptors (D2 variants) in the Nucleus Accumbens of a Cocaine Addict. (From Staley and Mash, 1996, with permission.)

- Nicotine attaches to specific excitatory receptors in the plasma membrane of parent somas in the midbrain.
- Opioids such as morphine and dihydromorphine (heroin) activate specific *inhibitory* receptors located in the plasma membrane of GABAergic interneurons within the nucleus. These neurons normally exert a tonic braking action on the projection cells of the ventral tegmental nuclei. Opioid-induced hyperpolarisation of the interneurons leads to functional disinhibition of the projection cells with consequent increased activity of both mesolimbic and mesocortical neurons.
- Ethanol also interferes with normal GABAergic activity. It binds to postsynaptic GABA membrane receptors throughout the brain without activating them; again, the target neurons become more excitable.

Serotonergic and noradrenergic neurons projecting to the limbic system and hypothalamus have also been implicated in connection with drug dependency, notably in expressing some of the effects of abrupt drug withdrawal.

✳ Core Information

Olfactory system

The olfactory system consists of the olfactory epithelium in the nose, the olfactory nerves, olfactory bulb, and olfactory tract, and several patches of olfactory cortex. The epithelium consists of bipolar olfactory neurons, supporting cells, and basal cells, which renew the bipolar neurons at a diminishing rate throughout life. Central processes of the bipolar neurons form the olfactory nerves, which penetrate the cribriform plate of the ethmoid bone and synapse upon mitral cells in the bulb. Mitral cell axons form the olfactory tract, which has several low-level terminations in the anterior temporal lobe. Olfactory discrimination is a function of the orbitofrontal cortex, which is reached by way of the dorsal medial nucleus of the thalamus.

Limbic system

The limbic system consists of the limbic cortex and related subcortical nuclei. The limbic cortex includes the hippocampal complex, septal area, parahippocampal gyrus, and cingulate gyrus. The principal subcortical nucleus is the amygdala. Closely related are the orbitofrontal cortex, temporal pole, hypothalamus and reticular formation, and the nucleus accumbens.

The anterior part of the parahippocampal gyrus is the entorhinal cortex, which receives cognitive and sensory information from the cortical association areas, transmits it to the hippocampal complex for consolidation, and returns it to the association areas where it is encoded in the form of memory traces.

The hippocampal complex consists of the subiculum, hippocampus proper, and dentate gyrus. Sectors of the hippocampus are called CA1, CA2, CA3, and CA4.

The perforant path projects from the entorhinal cortex on to the dendrites of dentate granule cells. Granule cell axons synapse on CA3 pyramidal cells, which give Schaffer collaterals to CA1. CA1 projects back to the entorhinal cortex, which is heavily linked to the association areas.

The fornix is a direct continuation of the fimbria, which receives axons from the subiculum and hippocampus. The crus of the fornix joins its fellow to form the trunk. Anteriorly the pillar of the fornix divides into precommissural fibres entering the septal area and postcommissural fibres entering the anterior hypothalamus, mammillary bodies, and medial forebrain bundle.

Bilateral damage to or removal of the hippocampal formation is followed by anterograde amnesia with loss of declarative memory. Procedural memory is preserved. Long-term potentiation of granule and pyramidal cells is regarded as a key factor in the consolidation of memories.

The insula has functions in relation to pain and to language. The anterior cingulate cortex has functions in relation to motor response selection, emotional tone, bladder control, vocalisation, and autonomic control. The posterior cingulate responds to the emotional tone of what is seen or felt.

The amygdala, above and in front of the temporal horn of the lateral ventricle, is the principal brain nucleus associated with the perception of fear. Its afferent, lateral nucleus receives inputs from olfactory, visual, auditory, tactile, visceral, cognitive, and mnemonic sources. The central, efferent nucleus sends fibres via the stria terminalis to the hypothalamus, activating corticotropin release and vagus-mediated bradycardia, and to the brainstem, activating dorsal and ventral periaqueductal grey matter and influencing respiratory rate and autonomic activity. The amygdalofugal pathway from the central nucleus facilitates defensive/evasive activity via the limbic striatal loop.

The nucleus accumbens is a clinically important component of the mesolimbic system in the context of drug dependency based upon its abundance of dopaminergic nerve terminals derived from ventral tegmental nuclei. Dopamine levels in the extracellular space in the nucleus accumbens and medial prefrontal cortex are raised by cocaine and amphetamines, which interfere with local dopamine recycling, and by cannabinoids, which activate specific terminal receptors. Nicotine activates specific receptors in the parent tegmental neurons. Opioids and ethanol interfere with the normal braking action of GABA tegmental interneurons.

The septal area consists of two main nuclear groups. One sends a set of glutamatergic fibres in the stria medullaris thalami to the habenular nucleus, which in turn sends the cholinergic fasciculus retroflexus to the interpeduncular nucleus, which participates in the sleep—wake cycle. The other forms the septohippocampal pathway to synapse upon hippocampal pyramidal cells. Glutamatergic and cholinergic elements govern the rate and strength, respectively, of hippocampal θ rhythm, which facilitates formation of episodic memories.

The basal forebrain is the grey matter in and around the anterior perforated substance. It includes the cholinergic, nucleus basalis of Meynert which projects to all parts of the neocortex, and the cholinergic, septal nucleus projecting to the hippocampus. Both lose about half of their neurons in Alzheimer disease, and the neocortical distribution is vulnerable to stroke.

SUGGESTED READINGS

Bekkers JM, Suzuki N. Neurons and circuits for odor processing in the piriform cortex. *Trends Neurosci.* 2013;36:429—438.

Catani M, Dell'Acqua F, de Schotten MT. A revised limbic system model for memory, emotion and behavior. *Neurosci Biobehav Rev.* 2013;37:1724—1737.

Chen NK, Chou YH, Sundman M, et al. Alteration of diffusion-tensor magnetic resonance imaging measures in brain regions involved in early stages of Parkinson's disease. *Brain Connect.* 2018;8(6):333—339.

Choi R, Goldstein BJ. Olfactory epithelium: cells, clinical disorders, and insights from an adult stem cell niche. *Laryngoscope Investig Otolaryngol.* 2018;3(1):35—42.

DeMaria S, Ngai J. The cell biology of smell. *J Cell Biol.* 2010;191:443—452.

Frankland PW, Kohler S, Josselyn SA. Hippocampal neurogenesis and forgetting. *Trends Neurosci.* 2013;36:497—503.

Grady C. The cognitive neuroscience of ageing. *Nat Rev Neurosci.* 2012;13:491—505.

Hillis AE. Inability to empathize: brain lesions that disrupt sharing and understanding another's emotions. *Brain.* 2014;137:981—997.

Kandel ER, Dudai Y, Mayford MR. The molecular and systems biology of memory. *Cell.* 2014;157:163—186.

Kretschmann H-J, Weinrich W. *Neurofunctional Systems: 3D Reconstructions with Correlated Neuroimaging: Text and CD-ROM.* New York: Thieme; 1998.

Lacy JW, Stark CEL. The neuroscience of memory: implications for the courtroom. *Nat Rev Neurosci.* 2013;14:649—658.

Leech R, Sharp DJ. The role of the posterior cingulate cortex in cognition and disease. *Brain.* 2014;137:12—32.

Lepousez G, Valley MT, Lledo PM. The impact of adult neurogenesis on olfactory bulb circuits and computations. *Annu Rev Physiol.* 2013;75:339—363.

Kumar A, Pareek V, Faiq MA, Ghosh SK, Kumari C. Adult neurogenesis in humans: a review of basic concepts, history, current research, and clinical implications. *Innov Clin Neurosci.* 2019;16(5-6):30—37.

Maren S, Phan KL, Liberzon I. The contextual brain: implications for fear conditioning, extinction and psychopathology. *Nat Rev Neurosci.* 2013;14:417—428.

Nieuwenhuys R. The insular cortex: a review. *Prog Brain Res.* 2012;195:123—163.

Pessoa L. Emotion and cognition and the amygdala: from "what is it?" to "what's to be done?". *Neuropsychology.* 2010;48:3316—3329.

Ranganath C, Ritchey M. Two cortical systems for memory-guided behavior. *Nat Rev Neurosci.* 2012;13:713—726.

Sadeh T, Ozubko JD, Winocur G, et al. How we forget may depend on how we remember. *Trends Cogn Sci.* 2014;18:26—36.

34

Pituitary and Hypothalamus

STUDY GUIDELINES

1. The pituitary gland (hypophysis cerebri) is in the hypophyseal fossa of the sphenoid bone and is intimately linked to the hypothalamus. It is composed of two parts: the adenohypophysis and the neurohypophysis.
2. Hypothalamic neuroendocrine cells fulfil the basic criteria both for neurons and for endocrine cells. Small neuroendocrine cells control release of hormones by the purely endocrine cells of the anterior pituitary gland. Large neuroendocrine cells have their terminals in the posterior pituitary, where they release hormones directly.
3. Some neurons confined to the hypothalamus are involved in control of body temperature, food and fluid intake, and sleep. Others, involved in attack and defence responses, and memory, are controlled by the limbic system.

The hypothalamus develops as part of the limbic system, which is concerned with preservation of the individual and of the species. Therefore, it is logical that the hypothalamus should have significant controls over basic survival strategies, including reproduction, growth and metabolism, food and fluid intake, attack and defence, temperature control, the sleep—wake cycle, and aspects of memory.

Most of its functions are expressed through its control of the pituitary gland and of both divisions of the autonomic nervous system.

GROSS ANATOMY

The hypothalamus occupies the side walls and floor of the third ventricle. It is a bilateral, paired structure. Despite its small size (it weighs only 4 g), it has major functions in homeostasis and survival. Its homeostatic functions include control of body temperature and circulation of blood. Its survival functions include regulation of food and water intake, the sleep—wake cycle, sexual behaviour patterns, and defence mechanisms against attack.

Boundaries

The boundaries of the hypothalamus are as follows (Figs. 34.1 and 34.2):
- *Superior*: the **hypothalamic sulcus** separating it from the thalamus
- *Inferior*: the **optic chiasm**, **tuber cinereum**, and **mammillary bodies**. The tuber cinereum shows a small swelling, the **median eminence**, immediately behind the **infundibulum** ('funnel') atop the pituitary stalk

- *Anterior*: the lamina terminalis
- *Posterior*: the tegmentum of the midbrain
- *Medial*: the third ventricle
- *Lateral*: the internal capsule

Subdivisions and Nuclei

In the sagittal plane, it is customary to divide the hypothalamus into three regions: *anterior* (supraoptic), *middle* (tuberal), and *posterior* (mammillary). These areas are small, even in large mammals, and the descriptive use of 'regions' has been convenient for animal experiments involving placement of lesions and often serves us well in the clinical setting with humans. Named nuclei in the three regions are listed in Table 34.1.

In the coronal plane, the hypothalamus can be divided into *lateral*, *medial*, and *periventricular* regions. The full length of the lateral region is occupied by the **lateral hypothalamic nucleus**. Merging with the lateral nucleus is the **medial forebrain bundle**, carrying aminergic fibres to the hypothalamus and to the cerebral cortex.

The Pituitary Gland

The pituitary gland (hypophysis cerebri) is in the hypophyseal fossa of the sphenoid bone and is intimately linked to the hypothalamus.

All endocrine glands have a rich vascular supply, to satisfy the high energy needs of the endocrine cells, but the veins and capillaries are the ductal system for hormone secretion.

The pituitary consists of two distinct parts:

The anterior adenohypophysis, which arose embryonically from the roof of the primitive pharynx, is composed of glandular cells. There are two regions, the tuberal or infundibular part

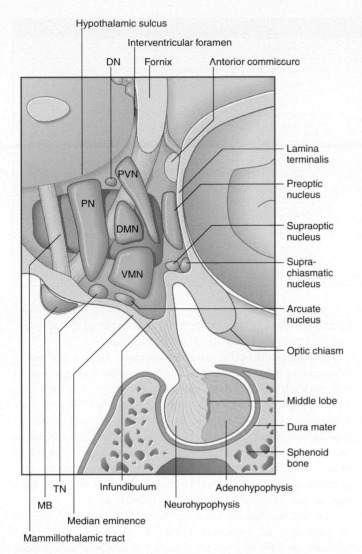

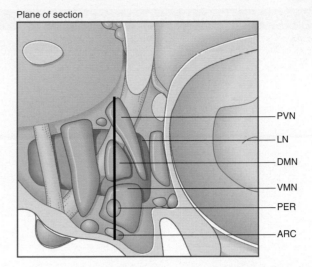

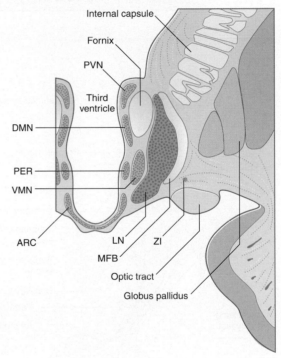

Fig. 34.1 Hypothalamic nuclei and hypophysis viewed from the lateral side. *DMN,* Dorsomedial nucleus; *DN,* dorsal nucleus; *MB,* mammillary body; *PN,* posterior nucleus; *PVN,* paraventricular nucleus; *TN,* tuberomammillary nucleus; *VMN,* ventromedial nucleus. The lateral hypothalamic nucleus is shown in *pink.*

Fig. 34.2 Hypothalamic nuclei, and related neural pathways, in a coronal section. *ARC,* Arcuate nucleus; *DMN,* dorsomedial nucleus; *LN,* lateral nucleus; *MFB,* medial forebrain bundle; *PER,* periventricular nucleus; *PVN,* paraventricular nucleus; *VMN,* ventromedial nucleus; *ZI,* zona incerta.

which is a narrow extension of cells from the main region the anterior pars distalis. Trophic hormone secreting gland cells can be classified into chromophobes and chromophils depending on staining affinity. Further classification of cell type is dependent upon staining characteristics, often using immunocytochemistry.

The key glandular cell types (and hormonal products) found within the adenohypophysis include: somatotrophs (growth hormone), mammotrophs (prolactin), gonadotrophs (follicle stimulating hormone (FSH) and luteinizing hormone (LH)), thyrotrophs (thyrotrophin), and corticotrophs (adrenocorticotrophic hormone (ACTH)).

The second part of the pituitary gland is the posterior neurohypophysis, which is formed from a downgrowth from the floor of the third ventricle and is composed of nerve fibres and nerve endings. The neurohypophysis continues superiorly as the pituitary stalk (infundibulum) above the

subarachnoid space at the base of the brain. The nerves contained are neurosecretory fibres originating in the supraoptic and paraventricular nuclei of the hypothalamus, releasing the hormones oxytocin and vasopressin (antidiuretic hormone (ADH)).

FUNCTIONS

Hypothalamic Control of the Pituitary Gland

The arterial supply of the pituitary gland comes from hypophyseal branches of the internal carotid artery (Fig. 34.3). One set of

TABLE 34.1 Main Hypothalamic Nuclei.

Location	Nucleus	Function
Posterior	Posterior	Blood pressure, pupillary dilation, shivering
		Vasopressin
	Mammillary	Memory
Middle	Tuberomammillary	Arousal/sleep, memory/learning, energy, balance
	Paraventricular	Releasing hormones for thyrotropin and corticotropin
		Oxytocin, vasopressin and somatostatin release
	Dorsomedial	Heart rate, blood pressure, GI stimulation
	Lateral	Orexin. Wakefulness, energy expenditure modulates visceral function
		Regulating nociception
	Ventromedial	Satiety, thermoregulation, and sexual activity
	Arcuate	Growth hormone releasing hormone
		Feeding, prolactin inhibition
Anterior	Preoptic	Gonadotrophin releasing hormones, thermoregulation
	Supraoptic	Vasopressin and oxytocin
	Suprachiasmatic	Circadian rhythms

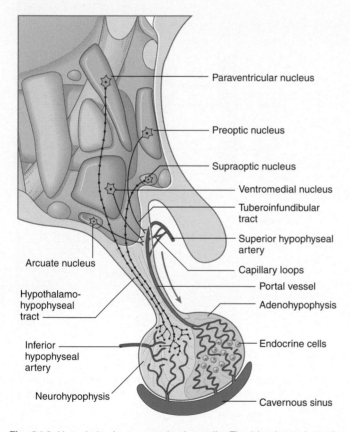

Labels (top to bottom, right side): Paraventricular nucleus; Preoptic nucleus; Supraoptic nucleus; Ventromedial nucleus; Tuberoinfundibular tract; Superior hypophyseal artery; Capillary loops; Portal vessel; Adenohypophysis; Endocrine cells; Cavernous sinus.

Labels (left side): Arcuate nucleus; Hypothalamo-hypophyseal tract; Inferior hypophyseal artery; Neurohypophysis.

Fig. 34.3 Hypothalamic neuroendocrine cells. The blood supply to the hypophysis, including the endocrine cells of the adenohypophysis, is also shown (*arrow* indicates direction of blood flow in the portal system).

branches supplies a capillary bed in the wall of the infundibulum. These capillaries drain into **portal vessels**, which pass into the adenohypophysis (anterior lobe). There they break up to form a second capillary bed, which bathes the endocrine cells and drains into the cavernous sinus.

The neurohypophysis receives a direct supply from the inferior hypophyseal arteries. The capillaries drain into the cavernous sinus, which delivers the secretions of the anterior and posterior lobes into the general circulation.

Secretions of the pituitary gland are controlled by two sets of **neuroendocrine cells**. Neuroendocrine cells are true neurons in having dendrites and axons and in conducting nerve impulses. They are also true endocrine cells because they liberate their secretions into capillary beds (Fig. 34.4). With one exception (mentioned below), the secretions are peptides, synthesised in clumps of granular endoplasmic reticulum and packaged in Golgi complexes. The peptides are attached to long-chain polypeptides called *neurophysins*. The capillaries concerned are outside the blood—brain barrier and are fenestrated.

The somas of the neuroendocrine cells occupy the *hypophysiotropic area* in the lower half of the preoptic and tuberal regions. Contributory nuclei include the **preoptic, supraoptic, paraventricular, ventromedial**, and **arcuate** (infundibular). Two classes of neurons can be identified: *parvocellular* (small) **neurons** reaching the median eminence and **magnocellular** (large) **neurons** reaching the posterior lobe of the pituitary gland.

The Parvocellular Neuroendocrine System. Parvocellular neurons of the hypophysiotropic area give rise to the **tuberoinfundibular tract**, which reaches the infundibular capillary bed. Action potentials travelling along these neurons result in calcium-dependent exocytosis of *releasing hormones* from some and *inhibiting hormones* from others, for transport to the adenohypophysis via the portal vessels. The cell types of the adenohypophysis are stimulated/inhibited in accordance with Table 34.2. In the left-hand column, the only nonpeptide parvocellular hormone is the prolactin-inhibiting hormone, which is *dopamine*, secreted from the arcuate (infundibular) nucleus.

The releasing/inhibiting hormones are not wholly specific: they typically have major effects on a single cell type and minor effects on one or two others.

Multiple controls exist for parvocellular neurons of the hypophysiotropic area. The controls include the following: depolarisation by afferents entering from the limbic system and

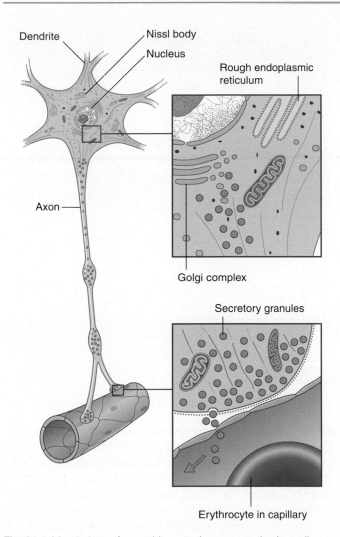

Dendrite · Nissl body · Nucleus · Rough endoplasmic reticulum · Golgi complex · Axon · Secretory granules · Erythrocyte in capillary

Fig. 34.4 Morphology of a peptide-secreting neuroendocrine cell.

TABLE 34.2 Hypothalamic Parvocellular Releasing/Inhibiting Hormones (RH/IH).

RH/IH	Anterior Lobe Hormone
Corticotropin RH	Adrenocorticotrophic hormone
Thyrotropin RH	Thyrotropin
Growth hormone RH	Growth hormone
Growth hormone IH (Somatostatin)	Growth hormone
Prolactin RH	Prolactin
Prolactin IH (Dopamine)	Prolactin
Gonadotropic hormone RH	Follicle stimulating hormone/luteinizing hormone

from the reticular formation; hyperpolarisation by local-circuit γ-amino butyric acid (GABA) neurons, some of which are sensitive to circulating hormones; and inhibition of transmitter release by opiate-releasing interneurons, which are numerous in the intermediate region of the hypothalamus. The picture is further complicated by the fact that opiates and other modulatory peptides may be released into the portal vessels and activate receptors on the endocrine cells of the adenohypophysis. *Stress* causes increased secretion of ACTH, which in turn stimulates the adrenal cortex to raise the plasma concentration of glucocorticoids, including cortisol. Normally, cortisol exerts a negative feedback effect by exciting inhibitory hypothalamic neurons having glucocorticoid receptors. In patients suffering from major depression, this feedback system fails (Clinical Panel 34.1).

The Magnocellular Neuroendocrine System. Magnocellular neurons in the supraoptic and paraventricular nuclei give rise to the *hypothalamohypophyseal tract* (or *supraopticohypophyseal tract*), which descends to the neurohypophysis (posterior lobe) (Fig. 34.3). Minor contributions to the tract are received from opiatergic and other peptidergic neurons in the periventricular region of the hypothalamus, and from aminergic neurons of the brainstem.

Two hormones are secreted by separate neurons located in both the supraoptic and paraventricular nuclei: *antidiuretic hormone (ADH; vasopressin)* and *oxytocin*. Axonal swellings containing the secretory granules for these hormones make up nearly half the volume of the neurohypophysis. The largest swellings, called *Herring bodies*, may be as large as erythrocytes. The Herring bodies provide a local depot of granules for release by smaller, terminal swellings into the capillary bed.

Antidiuretic hormone. ADH continuously stimulates water uptake by the distal convoluted tubules and collecting ducts of the kidneys. The chief regulator of electrical activity in the ADH-secreting neurons is the osmotic pressure of the blood. A rise of as little as 1% in the osmotic pressure causes the plasma to be diluted to normal levels by means of increased water uptake. The neurons are themselves sensitive to osmolar changes, but they are facilitated by inputs from osmolar and volume detectors elsewhere, notably from the *vascular* and *subfornical circumventricular organs* (Basic Science Panel 34.1).

Some ADH neurons also synthesise *corticotropin-releasing hormone* (CRH); the two hormones are released together from collateral branches into the capillary pool of the infundibulum. It is of interest that ADH neuronal activity is increased when the body is stressed and that the output of ACTH is boosted by the presence of ADH in the adenohypophysis.

Withdrawal of ADH secretion results in *diabetes insipidus* (Clinical Panel 34.2).

Oxytocin. The principal function of oxytocin is to participate in a *neurohumoral reflex* when an infant is suckling at the breast. The afferent limb of this reflex is provided by impulses travelling from the nipple to the hypothalamus via the spinoreticular tract. Oxytocin is liberated by magnocellular neurons in response to suckling. Having entered the general circulation, it causes the expression of milk by stimulating myoepithelial cells surrounding the lactiferous ducts of the breast.

Oxytocin also has a mild stimulating action on uterine muscle during labour. The afferent stimulus in this case originates in the genital tract once labour gets underway. Oxytocin and vasopressin have been found to have broader roles including learning, anxiety, sexual and maternal behaviour, and aggression.

See also under *stress*, later.

Other Hypothalamic Connections and Functions

The hypothalamus either directly or indirectly coordinates a group of diverse functions that help to maintain homeostasis. These functions include autonomic control, thermoregulation, osmoregulation, sexual function, responses to stress, and sleep—wake cycles. In some circumstances discrete lesions can produce specific deficits, but often the observed deficits are more complex. As a generalisation, the nuclei near the third ventricle (periventricular) are concerned with neuroendocrine function; the medial nuclei are concerned with thermoregulation, osmoregulation, and responses to stress; and the lateral nuclei play a role in the sleep—wake cycle, arousal, and behaviours related to feeding and drinking.

Autonomic Centres. In animals, stimulation of the anterior hypothalamic area produces *parasympathetic effects*: slowing of the heart, constriction of the pupil, salivary secretion, and intestinal peristalsis. In contrast, stimulation of the posterior hypothalamic area produces *sympathetic effects*: increase in heart rate and blood pressure, pupillary dilation, and intestinal stasis. Axons from both areas project to autonomic nuclei in the brainstem and spinal cord. In the midbrain and pons this projection occupies the dorsal longitudinal fasciculus as seen in Chapter 17.

Temperature Regulation. The preoptic nucleus in the anterior hypothalamus contains *thermosensitive neurons*, which initiate appropriate responses to changes in the core temperature of the body. Activity of these neurons is reinforced by information received (via the spinoreticular tract) from thermosensitive neurons supplying the skin (see Chapter 11).

Core temperatures are maintained through mechanisms coordinated by the anterior hypothalamus. Elevation of the core temperature can be corrected by the hypothalamic nucleus, which sends axons to synapse on the preganglionic thoracolumbar lateral horn neurons of the spinal cord, directing blood flow into the skin and activating sweat glands. Heat-generating mechanisms in the posterior hypothalamus are also inhibited.

Hypothalamic control of the sympathetic system diminishes with age. For this reason, the elderly are particularly prone to develop hypothermia in cold weather.

Hyperthermia is characteristic of fevers. Infectious agents (bacteria, viruses, parasites) cause tissue macrophages to liberate *endogenous pyrogen*, a protein that causes the hypothalamic 'thermostat' to be reset to a higher value. (Pyrogens accomplish this by inducing the local production of prostaglandins within the hypothalamus.) The chief mechanisms used to raise the body temperature to the new set point are cutaneous vasoconstriction and shivering.

Drinking. The chief centre controlling the intake of water appears to be the medial preoptic nucleus that integrates information from peripheral receptors that detect blood volume and pressure, decreased blood flow, and elevated levels of angiotensin hormone (*subfornical organ*; Fig. 34.5), and changes in osmolality (*vascular organ of the lamina terminalis*; Fig. 34.5). This information is transmitted to the cerebral cortex, which then initiates the necessary behaviour to correct a deficit (e.g. sensation of thirst).

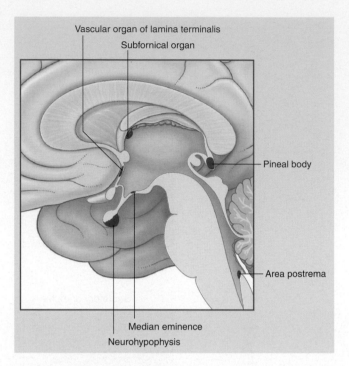

Fig. 34.5 Circumventricular organs.

Eating. Eating habits have obvious social and cultural components, causing dietary practice to vary widely among individuals and among communities. The arcuate nucleus of the hypothalamus integrates input that is related to feeding in the form of interplay between the lateral and ventromedial nuclei, which together provide a baseline for caloric and nutrient intake that constitutes the *appestat* (appetite set point). The arcuate nucleus is sensitive to glucose levels and to various secreted peptides that stimulate feeding behaviour (*ghrelin* is secreted by the stomach and stimulates feeding; *leptin* is secreted by adipocytes and suppresses feeding). Destruction of the lateral hypothalamus or '*feeding centre*' causes a cat or rat to refuse to eat. Conversely, lesions of the ventromedial portion of the hypothalamus or '*satiety centre*' cause animals to persistently overeat and become grossly obese. Of interest here is that serotonin can alter the appestat, by inhibiting the lateral nucleus. People with anorexia nervosa tend to have a raised level of serotonin production, and those with bulimia nervosa have a reduced level.

Hypothalamic Response to Psychological Stress. A stressful event (psychological, physical, or physiologic) disrupts normal homeostasis, and physiologic systems attempt to restore the imbalance. The hypothalamus, specifically the *hypothalamus—pituitary—adrenal (HPA) axis,* is an integral part of this restorative mechanism.

The paraventricular nucleus receives inputs from brainstem structures that respond to various physiologic stressors as well as from the limbic system, which is involved in emotion (see Chapter 33). CRH released by the paraventricular nucleus (and fortified by vasopressin corelease) leads to ACTH release by the adenohypophysis. ACTH activates release of cortisol from the adrenal cortex. Cortisol in turn activates energy stores throughout the body.

There does appear to be a gender difference in how men and women respond to stress, both psychologically and biologically. Functional magnetic resonance imaging (fMRI) studies have shown that in males there is activation of the lateral prefrontal cortex (a significant *decision* centre in the context of approach or withdrawal; see Chapter 28), while the predominant activation in females is in the cingulate gyrus, the predominant cortical *emotional* control centre (see Chapter 33). Whether complex behaviours can be attributed to changes identified on fMRI remains unclear.

There are no specific neuropathological structural anomalies in the brain of patients with mood disorders. There is an intricate network of stress-related circuits which includes nuclei in the brainstem, amygdala, habenula, prefrontal cortex, and hypothalamus. The hypothalamic nuclei are at the centre of these networks. They play a key role in the symptoms of depression, such as disordered circadian rhythm, eating, sex, and disturbed cognitive functions. A better understanding of these brain regions may allow a better understanding of the neurobiological system in the depressed patient, and that will allow customised antidepressive therapy.

Rage and Fear. The lateral and ventromedial nuclei are concerned with *mood* as well as food. Cats that are overweight in consequence of ventromedial lesions tend to also be highly aggressive. Conversely, animals rendered underweight by ventromedial stimulation tend to be unduly docile (see also the section on the amygdala in Chapter 33).

Sleeping and Waking. The hypothalamus plays a critical role in both arousal and sleep—wake cycles. The tiny (0.34 mm^3) *suprachiasmatic nucleus* embedded in the upper surface of the optic chiasm receives a direct input from the retina and is the circadian pacemaker for the brain. It participates in setting the normal sleep—wake cycle through its effects on endocrine, autonomic, and behavioural functions (e.g. its connections with the pineal gland and its secretion of melatonin).

Lesions of the posterior hypothalamic area may cause hypersomnolence or even coma. This area contains the *tuberomammillary nucleus* (Fig. 34.1), housing hundreds of *histaminergic neurons*, which project widely to the grey matter of the brain and spinal cord. Some of the fibres run rostrally within the medial forebrain bundle, in company with aminergic fibres of brainstem origin. Histaminergic fibres destined for the cerebral cortex fan out below the genu of the corpus callosum. They branch within the superficial layers of the frontal cortex and run back to supply the cortex of the parietal, occipital, and temporal lobes.

In animals, there is abundant physiologic evidence in support of an *arousal function* for the histaminergic system. The tuberomammillary nucleus is normally activated during the awake state by the peptide **orexin** liberated by a small group of neurons in the lateral hypothalamus. Failure of orexin production appears to underlie the disabling sleep attacks characteristic of narcolepsy (see Chapter 29).

Sexual Arousal. A subset of neurons (*third interstitial nucleus of the anterior hypothalamus, INAH$_3$*) within the medial part of the preoptic nucleus is more than twice as large in males as in females. It is also rich in androgen receptors and activated by circulating testosterone. In females, oestrogen-rich neurons are contained within the ventromedial nucleus. In laboratory animals, electrical stimulation of these nuclei elicits appropriate sexual responses, and it has been proposed that similar roles exist in humans.

Memory. The mammillary bodies belong to a *limbic (or Papez) circuit* involving the fornix, which sends fibres to it, and the *mammillothalamic tract* which projects to the anterior nucleus of the thalamus. This circuit has a function in relation to memory (see Chapter 33).

CLINICAL PANEL 34.1 Major Depression

Major depression is a state of depressed mood occurring without an adequate explanation in terms of external events. The condition affects about 4% of the adult population, and there is a genetic predisposition: about 20% of first-degree relatives have it too. Phases of depression may begin in childhood or adolescence.

Major depression is characterised by at least several of the following features:
- Depressed general mood, with loss of interest in normal activities and outside events.
- Diminished energy, easy fatigue, loss of appetite and sex drive, constipation.
- Impairment of self-image, with a feeling of personal inadequacy.
- Disturbance of the sleep—wake cycle, typically shown by early morning wakefulness.
- Aches and pains; recurrent abdominal pains may simulate organ disease.
- Periods of agitation, with restlessness and perhaps suicidal tendency.

Involvement of *monoamines* was first indicated by the chance observation that the use of reserpine in treatment of hypertension produced depression as a side effect. Reserpine depletes monoamine stores (serotonin, norepinephrine, and dopamine).

The symptoms listed above are also characteristic of *chronic stress*. It is therefore not surprising to find that the suprarenal cortex is hyperactive in depressed patients. Serum cortisol levels are elevated. As already mentioned, a rising serum cortisol level normally inhibits production of CRH by the hypothalamus. In depressed patients, the central glucocorticoid receptors are relatively insensitive. This change forms the basis of the *dexamethasone suppression test*. Dexamethasone is a potent synthetic glucocorticoid that reduces ACTH secretion in healthy individuals.

Some of the CRH neurons send branches into the brain itself. In the midbrain, CRH inhibits mesocortical dopaminergic neurons, which are normally associated with positive motivational drive. In the midbrain they also inhibit raphe serotonergic neurons critically involved with diurnal rhythms, mainly through intense innervation of the suprachiasmatic nucleus.

The front line of therapy is dominated by drugs that enhance serotonergic transmission. The range of antidepressants is large, and their sites of action vary. For example, some inhibit reuptake from the synaptic cleft, others inhibit degradation by monoamine oxidase (see Chapter 13). They take several weeks to take effect; the latent interval is taken up with desensitising (inhibitory) autoreceptors on serotonergic cell membranes.

Electroconvulsive therapy (ECT) is at least as effective as the antidepressants. It seems to desensitise autoreceptors, to sensitise (excitatory) serotonin receptors on target neurons, and to depress noradrenergic transmission.

CLINICAL PANEL 34.2 Hypothalamic Disorders and Pituitary Dysfunction

The most dramatic disorder of hypothalamic function is **diabetes insipidus**, which is brought about by interruption of the hypothalamohypophyseal pathway; sometimes by tumours in the region, sometimes by head injury. The patient drinks upwards of 10 litres of water per day and excretes a similar amount of urine. Historically, the term insipidus refers to the absence of taste sensation from the urine, in contrast to *diabetes mellitus*, in which the urine is sweet-tasting (mellitus) owing to its sugar content.

Hypophysectomy (surgical removal of the pituitary gland) can be performed in the treatment of other diseases, without causing more than temporary diabetes insipidus, provided the pituitary stalk is sectioned at a low level. Within a short period, enough ADH is secreted into the capillary bed of the median eminence to ensure adequate water conservation.

Hypothalamic nuclei are key regulators that maintain homeostasis and a wide variety of hypothalamic dysfunctions have been reported in the clinical literature. Causes are also varied and include tumours, congenital malformations, and head injury. Inflammation in the hypothalamus can result in disruption to these control regions; this has been linked to somatic diseases such as obesity, diabetes, hypertension, and cachexia. Hypothalamic inflammation also may also affect aging and lifespan. A better understanding of the links between somatic diseases and hypothalamic function may lead to the development of novel therapeutic approaches for their treatment.

Pituitary dysfunction occurs in up to 40% of patients who have moderate or severe traumatic brain injury with resultant hormonal disturbances. These disturbances have been implicated in morbidity and increased mortality in traumatic brain injury patients. The exact mechanisms behind posttraumatic pituitary damage have yet to be understood. The development of appropriate preventive medical measures to limit possible damage to the pituitary gland and hypothalamic pituitary axis in order to maintain or re-establish near-normal physiologic functions is vital in order to reduce the effects of traumatic brain injury.

BASIC SCIENCE PANEL 34.1 Circumventricular Organs

Six patches of brain tissue close to the ventricular system contain neurons and specialised glial cells abutting fenestrated capillaries. These are the **circumventricular organs (CVOs)** (Fig. 34.5). The **median eminence** and **neurohypophysis** are described in the main text. The **vascular organ of the lamina terminalis** and the **subfornical organ** close to the interventricular foramen send axons into the supraoptic and paraventricular nuclei of the hypothalamus and facilitate depolarisation of neurons secreting ADH. In conditions of lowered blood volume, the kidney secretes renin, which, on conversion to angiotensin II, stimulates these two CVOs to complete a positive feedback loop.

The **pineal gland** synthesises *melatonin*, an amine hormone implicated in the sleep–wake cycle. Melatonin is synthesised from serotonin, the requisite enzymes being unique to this gland. Melatonin is liberated into the pineal capillary bed at night and has a sleep-inducing effect; it may have other benefits, including clearance of harmful free radicals liberated from tissues during the aging process. Daytime secretion is suppressed by activity in sympathetic fibres reaching it from the superior cervical ganglia by way of the walls of the straight venous sinus. The relevant central pathway is from the paired suprachiasmatic nuclei via the dorsal longitudinal fasciculus.

From the third decade onward, calcareous deposits ('pineal sand') may accumulate within astrocytes in the pineal gland. Calcification is often detectable in plain radiographs of the head. A shift of the gland may denote a space-occupying lesion within the skull. However, a normal pineal gland may lie slightly to the left, because the right cerebral hemisphere is usually a little wider than the left at this level.

The **area postrema** is embedded in the roof of the fourth ventricle at the level of the obex. It is the *chemoreceptor trigger zone*, or *emetic* (vomiting) *centre*. The emetic centre contains neurons sensitive to a wide range of toxic substances, and it serves a protective function by reflexly eliciting emesis via connections with the hypothalamus and reticular formation.

✳ Core Information

The **hypothalamus** is a bilateral structure beside the third ventricle. In the sagittal plane, it can be divided into an anterior (supraoptic) region containing three nuclei, an intermediate (tuberal) region with five nuclei, and a posterior (mammillary) region with three nuclei. In the coronal plane lateral, medial, and periventricular regions are described.

The **pituitary gland** (hypophysis cerebri) is in the hypophyseal fossa of the sphenoid bone and is intimately linked to the hypothalamus. It is composed of two parts:

The *anterior adenohypophysis* produces the hormonal products growth hormone (GH), prolactin (luteotropic hormone, PRL), follicle stimulating hormone (FSH), luteinizing hormone (LH), thyrotropin (thyroid stimulating hormone, TSH) and adrenocorticotrophic hormone (ACTH).

The second part is the *posterior neurohypophysis*. The nerves contained within are neurosecretory fibres originating in the supraoptic and paraventricular nuclei of the hypothalamus. These nerves release the hormones oxytocin and vasopressin (antidiuretic hormone, ADH).

The pituitary gland is controlled by hypothalamic neuroendocrine cells, which are characterised by impulse transmission and hormonal secretion into capillary beds. Parvocellular neuroendocrine cells project to the median eminence. They secrete releasing/inhibiting hormones into the capillary bed. These hormones are transported to the adenohypophysis in a portal system of vessels. Large (magnocellular) neuroendocrine cells form the hypothalamohypophyseal tract, which liberates ADH and oxytocin into the capillary bed of the neurohypophysis.

Circumventricular organs, which lack a blood–brain barrier, comprise the median eminence and neurohypophysis; the vascular organ of lamina terminalis and subfornical organ (both of these involved in a feedback loop regulating plasma volume); the pineal gland, which secretes melatonin; the emetic centre or area postrema; and the subfornical organ.

Anterior and posterior regions of the hypothalamus contain neurons that activate the parasympathetic and sympathetic system, respectively. Thermoregulatory neurons maintain the body temperature set point, mainly by manipulating the sympathetic system.

Stimulation of the lateral hypothalamic area provokes an increase in food and water consumption. Destruction of this area, or stimulation of a ventromedial satiety centre, results in refusal to eat.

The **suprachiasmatic nucleus** participates in control of the sleep–wake cycle. The medial preoptic area contains androgen-sensitive neurons, and the ventromedial nucleus contains oestrogen-sensitive neurons. The mammillary bodies receive inputs from the limbic system via the fornix, and have a function in relation to memory.

SUGGESTED READINGS

Albrecht U. Timing to perfection: the biology of central and peripheral circadian clocks. *Neuron.* 2012;74:246–340.

Alvarez EO. The role of histamine in cognition. *Behav Brain Res.* 2008;199:183–189.

Andrews J, Ali N, Pruessner JC. Reflections on the interaction of psychogenic stress systems in humans: the stress coherence/ compensation model. *Psychoneuroendocrino.* 2014;38:947–961.

Bao AM, Swaab DF. The human hypothalamus in mood disorders: the HPA axis in the center. *IBRO Rep.* 2018;6:45–53.

Bechtold DA, Loudon ASI. Hypothalamic clocks and rhythms in feeding behaviour. *Trends Neurosci.* 2013;36:74–82.

Benarroch E. Thermoregulation: recent concepts and remaining questions. *Neurology.* 2007;69:1293–1297.

Benarroch EE. Neural control of feeding behavior. Overview and clinical correlations. *Neurology.* 2010;74:1643–1650.

Dietrich MO, Horvath TL. Hypothalamic control of energy balance: insights into the role of synaptic plasticity. *Trends Neurosci.* 2013;36:65–73.

Kousaku O, Sakurai T. Orexin neuronal circuitry: role in the regulation of sleep and wakefulness. *Front Neuroendocrinol.* 2008;29:70–87.

Motofei IG, Rowland DL. The ventral-hypothalamic input route: a common neural network for abstract cognition and sexuality. *BJU Int.* 2014;113:296–303.

Mravec B, Horvathova L, Cernackova A. Hypothalamic inflammation at a crossroad of somatic diseases. *Cell Mol Neurobiol.* 2019;39 (1):11–29.

Neumann ID, Landgraf R. Balance of brain oxytocin and vasopressin: implications for anxiety, depression, and social behaviors. *Trends Neurosci.* 2012;35:649–659.

Saper CB. The neurobiology of sleep. *Continuum (Minneap Minn).* 2013;19:19–31.

Sav A, Rotondo F, Syro LV, Serna CA, Kovacs K. Pituitary pathology in traumatic brain injury: a review. *Pituitary.* 2019;22:201.

Sawchenko PE. Toward a new neurobiology of energy balance, appetite, and obesity: the anatomists weigh in. *J Comp Neurol.* 1998;402:435–441.

Schneeberger M, Gomis R, Claret M. Hypothalamic and brainstem neuronal circuits controlling homeostatic energy balance. *J Endocrinol.* 2014;220:T25–T46.

Sellayah D, Sikder D. Food for thought: understanding the multifaceted nature of orexins. *Endocrinology.* 2013;154:3990–3999.

Stemson SM. Hypothalamic survival circuits: blueprints for purposive behaviors. *Neuron.* 2013;77:810–824.

Swaab DF, Hofman MA. Age, sex and light: variability in the human suprachiasmatic nucleus in relation to its functions. *Prog Brain Res.* 1994;100:341–345.

Szymusiak R, McGinty D. Hypothalamic regulation of sleep and arousal. *Ann NY Acad Sci.* 2008;1129:275–286.

Taylor SE, Klein LC, Lewis BP, et al. Biobehavioral responses to stress in females: tend-and-befriend, not fight-or-flight. *Psychol Rev.* 2000;107:411–429.

Wang J, Korczykowski M, Rao H, et al. Gender difference in neural response to psychological stress. *Soc Cogn Affect Neurosci.* 2007;2:227–239.

Cerebrovascular Disease

STUDY GUIDELINES

1. Review the blood supply of the central nervous system and the relevance of the circle of Willis (circulus arteriosus) in limiting the deficit from a cerebral artery occlusion (see Chapter 4).
2. Define stroke, transient ischaemic attack, and subarachnoid haemorrhage.
3. Describe the clinical features expected with a stroke within the anterior, middle, and posterior cerebral artery.
4. Describe the clinical features expected with posterior circulation occlusions.
5. Describe the clinical features and stroke location for the following lacunar syndromes: pure motor stroke, pure sensory stroke, dysarthria-clumsy hand syndrome.
6. An objective of this chapter is to demonstrate the value of understanding the regional as well as systems anatomy of the brain, because strokes cause injury to specific regions, with consequent effects on multiple neurological systems.

STROKE DEMOGRAPHICS, DEFINITIONS, AND SYNDROMES

Despite the impact of more intensive management of risk factors (especially hypertension and hypercholesterolemia) and a decrease in stroke incidence, stroke remains a major worldwide cause of morbidity and mortality, with a global lifetime risk of stroke from the age of 25 years onward of 25%. There remains large geographic and ethnic variance; prevalence of stroke increases with age and the impact of associated risk factors that are modifiable (e.g. hypertension, diabetes, smoking, inactivity) and nonmodifiable (e.g. age, gender, genetics).

A *stroke* is defined clinically as a focal neurologic deficit of ischaemic vascular origin involving the central nervous system (CNS) or retina and lasting for more than 24 hours. A *transient ischaemic attack (TIA)* is a focal neurological dysfunction lasting less than 24 hours (90% last less than 10 minutes) and with no evidence of infarction. While the deficit is transient, recognition of TIAs involving the cerebral circulation is important because up to 20% of individuals with stroke will originally present with a TIA. Up to 80% of strokes after TIA can be prevented.

Stroke syndromes or specific combinations of neurological findings can be associated with occlusion of a specific cerebral vessel and this results from the 'predictability' of the vascular supply to the brain. When combined with various imagining

techniques (e.g., magnetic resonance imaging, angiography), not only is anatomic involvement clarified, but so is the probable pathogenesis and mechanism that can guide further diagnostic and therapeutic decisions.

Ischaemic Strokes

While there are multiple potential aetiologies for a stroke, initial classification is ischaemic, comprising 85% of all strokes, and the remainder are haemorrhagic. For ischaemic stroke the underlying mechanism is either vessel pathology that leads to occlusion (e.g., atherothrombosis) or a source (e.g. the heart) generating a 'particle' that results in embolic occlusion of a vessel (e.g. cardiac). A third group of ischaemic stroke involves occlusion of cerebral small vessels that results in small subcortical infarctions within the territory of those perforating arterioles and on neuroimaging (and postmortem) the appearance of fluid-filled cavities called lacunes, hence the name *lacunar strokes*. There is a subgroup of these small-vessel arteriole strokes that, based on their clinical presentation, identify *lacunar syndromes* that reflect injury to specific white matter tracks or subcortical structures (Clinical Panel 35.4). Historically chronic hypertension (a risk factor for cerebrovascular disease) was the assumed primary cause of these occlusions, but now the proposed aetiology is dysfunction in endothelial cells and

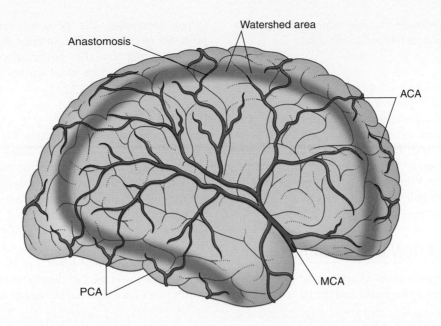

Anastomosis

Watershed area

ACA

PCA

MCA

Fig. 35.1 Watershed area of anastomotic overlap between the middle cerebral artery *(MCA)* and the anterior and posterior cerebral arteries *(ACA, PCA)*.

disruption of the blood–brain barrier that eventually leads to arteriole injury, degeneration, and occlusion.

Atherosclerosis signifies 'fatty deposits' in the intimal lining of the internal carotid and vertebrobasilar system—most notably in the internal carotid trunk or in one of the vertebral arteries. The deposits pose a dual threat: in situ enlargement may cause progressive occlusion of a main artery; and breakaway deposits may form emboli ('plugs') blocking distal branches within the brain. Embolic strokes can also arise from blood clots in the left side of the heart, in association with coronary or valvular disease.

The expected deficit from the gradual occlusion of a vessel may be minimised by routing of blood through alternative, collateral, blood vessels. For example, an internal carotid artery may be progressively occluded over a period of 10 years or more without apparent brain damage; the contralateral internal carotid artery utilises the circle of Willis to perfuse both pairs of the anterior and middle cerebral arteries. Or the external carotid can bypass the occlusion through collateral vessels that originate from branches of the facial artery and anastomose with the ophthalmic artery on the affected side. Similarly, occlusion of the stem of one of the three cerebral arteries may be compensated by small (less than 0.5 mm) anastomotic arteries in the depths of cortical sulci, perfused by the other two cerebral arteries. The number of such small arteries varies greatly between individuals and this 'crescent-shaped' anastomotic region is known as the *watershed area* (Fig. 35.1). On the other hand, all arteries penetrating the brain substance are end arteries and their communications with neighbouring penetrating arteries are too fine to prevent ischaemic injury for most cerebral arterial occlusions.

Haemorrhagic Strokes

The remaining 15% of acute strokes are haemorrhagic, either intracerebral (10%) or from subarachnoid haemorrhage (5%).

Most haemorrhagic strokes represent spontaneous rupture of a small cerebral vessel and hypertension is the most common aetiological factor. The remainder reflect bleeding from various vascular malformations or abnormalities of blood coagulation that predispose to bleeding.

Nontraumatic *subarachnoid haemorrhage (SAH)* is most frequently (80%) the result of rupture of an intracranial aneurysm ('berry aneurysm'). A typical sequence of clinical events is the sudden onset of headache ('worst headache of my life') followed by altered mental status and signs of meningeal irritation (neck stiffness with pain on motion secondary to the irritative effects of blood). Morbidity is significant and mortality is up to 50%.

Intracranial aneurysms originate near the circle of Willis, but some arise at arterial bifurcation points within the brain. This location explains the fact that when these aneurysms rupture, blood directly enters the subarachnoid space and bleeding continues until the intracranial pressure increases and stops bleeding at the aneurysmal rupture site and thrombus forms. In up to 40% of cases there is an earlier rupture, less catastrophic, but serving as a warning or *'sentinel leak'* weeks before the more serious event. This serves as the rationale for a high suspicion of SAH if an individual presents with a sudden, severe, and unusual headache.

The cranial cavity is a rigid structure and any increase in volume is associated with an increase in intracranial pressure. Cerebral infarcts (or haemorrhage) result in *cytotoxic oedema* that consists of an increase in intracellular water in the area of ischaemic injury. This causes an increase in intracranial pressure and displacement of cerebral structures that can result in effects at a distance by causing subfalcine or tentorial herniation of the brain in the manner of a tumour (see Chapter 5), and cerebral blood flow in initially unaffected vessels can also be affected. Cerebral oedema typically reaches its maximum in 72 to 120 hours and cytotoxic oedema does not respond to steroid administration (the oedema frequently encountered with brain tumours is extracellular, *vasogenic oedema*, and does respond to steroids).

Stroke Mimics

There are other clinical conditions that can mimic a stroke as they present with neurological impairment, but symptoms are often vague and lack the localising features seen in stroke syndromes. These include seizure, brain tumour, migraine with aura, metabolic derangements that result in dysfunction of the brain, and *encephalopathy* (e.g. hypoglycaemia, electrolyte disturbance, drugs) as the most frequent. When history, exam, and neuroimaging are inconclusive, such individuals may initially be evaluated and treated as a stroke until time allows further clarification.

ANTERIOR CIRCULATION OF THE BRAIN

Clinicians refer to the internal carotid artery and its branches as the ***anterior circulation of the brain*** and the vertebrobasilar

system (including the posterior cerebral arteries) as the ***posterior circulation***. The anterior and posterior circulations are connected by the posterior communicating arteries (Fig. 35.2). About 75% of all strokes originate in the anterior circulation.

Internal Capsule

The following details supplement the account of the arterial supply of the internal capsule in Chapter 4.

The blood supply of the internal capsule is shown in Fig. 35.3. The three sources of supply are the ***anterior choroidal***, a direct branch of the internal carotid; the ***medial striate***, a branch of the anterior cerebral; and ***lateral striate (lenticulostriate)*** branches of the middle cerebral artery.

The contents of the internal capsule are shown in Fig. 35.4. The anterior choroidal branch of the internal carotid artery supplies the lower part of the posterior limb and the retrolentiform part of the internal capsule and the inferolateral part of

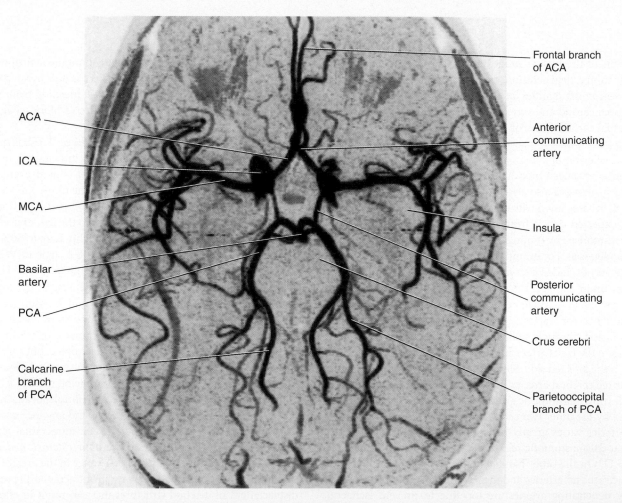

Fig. 35.2 Circle of willis and its branches. This is a magnetic resonance (MR) angiogram based on the principle that flowing blood generates a different signal to that of stationary tissue, without injection of a contrast agent. Conventional angiograms, for example those in Chapter 4, require arterial perfusion with a contrast agent. The vessels shown here are contained within a single thick MR 'slice'. Some, for example the calcarine branch of the posterior cerebral artery, could be followed further in adjacent slices. *ACA*, Anterior cerebral artery; *ICA*, internal carotid artery; *MCA*, middle cerebral artery; *PCA*, posterior cerebral artery. (From a series kindly provided by Professor J. Paul Finn, Director, Magnetic Resonance Research, Department of Radiology, David Geffen School of Medicine at UCLA, CA, USA.)

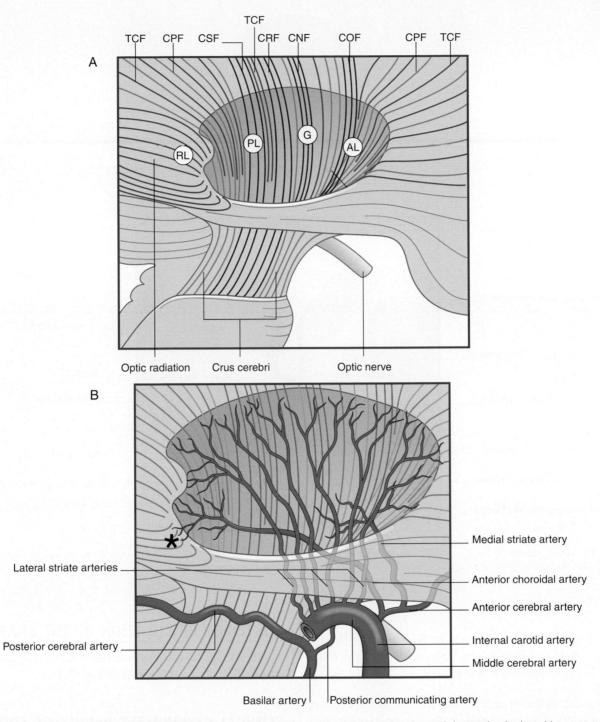

Fig. 35.3 Internal capsule. (A) Pathways. Lateral view of the right cerebral hemisphere showing the oval depression in the white matter following removal of the lentiform nucleus. The internal capsule occupies the floor of the depression. (B) Blood supply. The medial striate branch of the anterior cerebral artery is the *recurrent artery of Heubner*. Only three of the six lateral striate branches of the middle cerebral artery shown are labelled. *Arterial supply from the anterior choroidal artery to the inferolateral part of the lateral geniculate body. *AL*, Anterior limb; *CNF*, corticonuclear fibres; *COF*, corticooculomotor fibres; *CPF*, corticopontine fibres; *CRF*, corticoreticular fibres; *CSF*, corticospinal fibres; *G*, genu; *IC*, internal capsule; *LGB*, lateral geniculate body; *PL*, posterior limb; *RL*, retrolenticular; *SC*, superior colliculus; *TCF*, thalamocortical fibres.

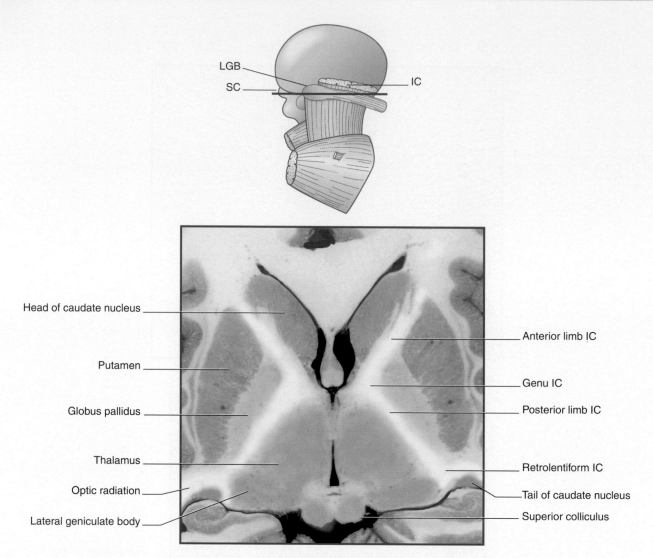

Fig. 35.4 Horizontal section of the internal capsule at the level indicated (based on Fig. 2.12), depicting its boundaries and parts (left) and stroke-relevant motor contents (right). *IC*, Internal capsule; *LGB*, lateral geniculate body; *SC*, superior colliculus.

the lateral geniculate body. Some of its branches (not shown) supply a variable amount of the temporal lobe of the brain and the choroid plexus of the inferior horn of the lateral ventricle.

The medial striate branch of the anterior cerebral artery (*recurrent artery of Heubner*) supplies the lower part of the anterior limb of the internal capsule, genu of the internal capsule, and the head of the caudate.

The lateral striate arteries penetrate the lentiform nucleus and give multiple branches to the anterior limb, genu, and posterior limb of the internal capsule.

POSTERIOR CIRCULATION OF THE BRAIN

Additional information is confined to the stem branches of the posterior cerebral artery shown in Fig. 35.5.

CLINICAL SYNDROMES RESULTING FROM VASCULAR OCCLUSION

In the Clinical Panels, clinical aspects or findings with occlusion of arteries within the anterior and posterior circulation are summarised.

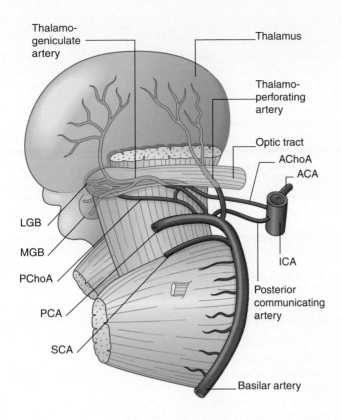

Fig. 35.5 Central branches of the posterior cerebral artery (PCA). Although only two arteries are shown, each in fact comprises several branches from the PCA. The thalamoperforating artery shown pierces the posterior perforated substance and supplies the anterior one-third of the thalamus. The thalamogeniculate artery shown supplies the geniculate bodies and the posterior two-thirds of the thalamus. *ACA*, Anterior cerebral artery; *AChoA*, anterior choroidal artery; *ICA*, internal carotid artery; *LGB*, lateral geniculate body; *MGB*, medial geniculate body; *PChoA*, posterior choroidal artery; *SCA*, superior cerebellar artery.

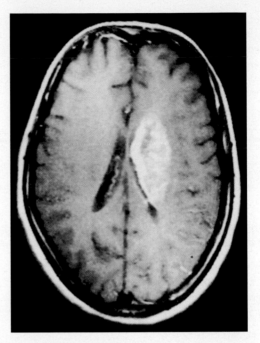

Fig. 35.6 Contrast-enhanced magnetic resonance image taken from a patient 11 days after an embolic stroke (This patient suffered a right hemiplegia and right hemisensory loss. Their MRI shows extensive infarction of the white matter of the left side at the junctional region between the corona radiata and external capsule, with compression of the lateral ventricle). (From Sato A, Takahashi S, Soma Y, et al. Cerebral infarction: early detection by means of contrast-enhanced cerebral arteries at MR imaging. *Radiology*. 1991;178:433–439, with kind permission from Dr S. Takahashi, Department of Radiology, Tohoku University School of Medicine, Sendai, Japan, and the editors of *Radiology*.)

CLINICAL PANEL 35.1 Anterior Choroidal Artery Occlusion (see Fig. 35.3)

- Contralateral hemiparesis (face = arm = leg) — lower part of the posterior limb and retrolentiform part of the internal capsule.
- Contralateral hemianaesthesia — posterior ventral lateral thalamus.
- Contralateral incongruent quadrantanopia or hemianopia — lateral geniculate body. Similarity between the visual field deficit in both eyes is referred to as *congruency* and is most marked the closer the lesion is to the visual cortex where visual pathway fibres that originate from corresponding retinal areas lie close together. The lateral geniculate receives its blood supply through the

anterior (branch of the internal carotid artery) and lateral (posterior) choroidal artery (branch of the posterior cerebral artery; referred to as a 'single artery', it usually consists of up to 10 or 11 arteries divided into medial posterior choroidal artery and lateral posterior choroidal artery groups). Occlusion of the anterior choroidal artery can result in an incongruent upper quadrantanopia or both upper and lower quadrants can be involved, with vision spared along that horizontal meridian of the visual field supplied by the lateral choroidal artery.

CLINICAL PANEL 35.2 Anterior Cerebral Artery Occlusion

Complete interruption of flow in the proximal anterior cerebral artery (ACA) is rare because the opposite artery has direct access to its distal territory through the anterior communicating artery. However, branch occlusions are well recognised, with corresponding variations in the clinical picture:

Left ACA
- Right leg numbness (cortical sensory loss) and weakness
- Transcortical motor aphasia
- Ipsilateral or contralateral ideomotor apraxia

Right ACA
- Left leg numbness (cortical sensory loss) and weakness
- Motor neglect
- Ipsilateral or contralateral ideomotor apraxia

ACA branch occlusion — orbital or frontopolar branch
- The usual result is an apathetic state with some memory loss.

ACA branch occlusion – medial striate artery (recurrent artery of Heubner)

- Dysarthria — compromise of the motor supply to the contralateral nuclei supplying the muscles of the mandible (V), lips (VII), and tongue (XII).
- Hoarseness and dysphagia — when the supranuclear supply to the nucleus ambiguus is interrupted.

ACA branch occlusion – callosomarginal

- Contralateral motor weakness and cortical-type sensory loss — this branch supplies the dorsomedial prefrontal cortex, the supplementary motor area (SMA), and the lower limb and perineal areas of the sensorimotor cortex and the supplementary sensory area (SSA).

- Urinary incontinence — may occur for some days owing to contralateral weakness of the pelvic floor.
- Abulia (lack of initiative) — damage to the prefrontal cortex.
- Mutism (left-sided stroke) — involvement of the SMA (collaborates with the Broca area in the initiation of speech).
- Ideomotor apraxia — damage to the SMA.

ACA branch occlusion – pericallosal

- Ideomotor apraxia — the anterior part of the corpus callosum may result in ideomotor apraxia. (The lesion would be comparable to lesion 1 in Fig. 32.6.)
- Tactile anomia — midregion of the corpus callosum (interference with the transfer of tactile information from right to left parietal lobe).

CLINICAL PANEL 35.3 Middle Cerebral Artery Occlusion (see Fig. 35.6)

Left middle cerebral artery (MCA)

- Right face/arm > leg numbness (cortical sensory)/weakness
- Aphasia
- Gaze preference to left side

Right MCA

- Left face/arm > leg numbness (cortical sensory)/weakness
- Left hemispatial neglect
- Graphaesthesia and astereognosis
- Gaze preference to right

MCA branch occlusion – anterosuperior division

- Contralateral face/arm > leg weakness

- Dysarthria — damage to supranuclear pathways involved in speech articulation
- Broca aphasia (left-sided stroke)
- Gaze preference to side of stroke

MCA branch occlusion – posteroinferior division

- Contralateral incongruent hemianopia
- Confused and agitated state — involvement of limbic pathways to the temporal lobe
- Wernicke aphasia (left-sided stroke)
- Neglect and ideomotor apraxia (right-sided stroke)

CLINICAL PANEL 35.4 Lacunar Syndromes

- **Pure motor** — contralateral hemiparesis; localisation to the posterior limb of the internal capsule, corona radiata, or basis pontis. Occlusion of the lenticulostriate artery (middle cerebral artery) or perforating arteries from the basilar artery. Fig. 35.7 shows the typical posture during walking: the

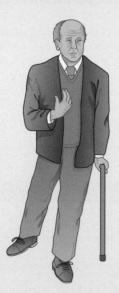

elbow and fingers are flexed, and the leg must be circumducted during the swing phase (unless an ankle brace is worn) because of the antigravity tone of the musculature. During the early rehabilitation period an arm sling is required in order to protect the shoulder joint from downward subluxation (partial dislocation). This is because the supraspinatus muscle is normally in continuous contraction when the body is upright, preventing slippage of the humeral head.

- **Pure sensory** — contralateral hemisensory loss; localisation to the ventral posterolateral and ventral posteromedial nuclei of the thalamus (VPL and VPM). Occlusion of the lenticulostriate artery (middle cerebral artery) or thalamoperforator arteries from the posterior cerebral artery.
- **Sensorimotor** — contralateral weakness and numbness; localisation to the thalamus and adjacent internal capsule. Occlusion of the lenticulostriate artery (middle cerebral artery).
- **Ataxic hemiparesis** — contralateral hemiparesis and limb ataxia out of proportion to severity of weakness; localisation to the posterior limb of the internal capsule of basis pontis. Occlusion of the lenticulostriate artery (middle cerebral artery) or perforating arteries from the basilar artery.
- **Dysarthria-clumsy hand syndrome** — dysarthric speech and fine motor weakness of the contralateral hand; localisation to the rostral portion of the basis pontis. Occlusion of perforating arteries from the basilar artery.

Fig. 35.7 Hemiplegic gait. The patient's right side is affected.

The lumen of the internal carotid artery may become progressively obstructed by atheromatous deposits. Common sites of obstruction are the point of commencement in the neck, and the cavernous sinus. A slowly progressive obstruction may be compensated for by the opposite internal carotid artery, through the circle of Willis. Additional blood may also be provided through various external—internal collateral anastomoses (e.g., the orbit from the facial artery). At the other extreme, sudden occlusion may cause death from infarction of the entire anterior and middle cerebral territories, and sometimes the posterior cerebral artery territory as well.

Warning signs of carotid occlusion can take the form of transient ischaemic attacks (TIAs). As with TIAs elsewhere, the physician is unlikely to be present during an attack and must interpret the account given by the patient or relative. The territory of the middle cerebral artery is most often affected, and symptoms tend to occur in isolation and include any of the following: a feeling of heaviness/weakness/numbness/tingling in one arm or leg, halting or slurring of speech. A TIA can also involve the ophthalmic artery and cause transient monocular blindness (one eye may be perceived as filled with fog or white steam) or *amaurosis fugax*.

In all cases where a TIA or stroke is experienced, evaluation includes imaging of the cerebral circulation, intracranial and extracranial, to determine the aetiology for the event. In all cases medical management is used to address risk factors for cerebrovascular disease and accompanied by the judicious use of antiplatelet/antithrombotic, antihypertensive, and lipid-lowering therapy. When narrowing of the lumen of the internal carotid artery is detected, further interventions are considered that include angioplasty (accomplished by carotid endarterectomy) or vessel stenting to directly address and 'resolve' the assumed aetiology (occlusive lesion or embolic source) of the person's TIA or stroke.

The clinical phrase **long tract signs** is most often used in the context of brainstem lesions. It refers to evidence of a lesion in one or more of the three long tracts: the pyramidal tract, the dorsal column—medial lemniscal pathway, and the spinothalamic pathway. All the long tract signs occur in the limbs on the side opposite to the lesion.

Superior Cerebellar Artery
- Ipsilateral limb and gait ataxia

Anterior Inferior Cerebellar Artery
- Vertigo and ipsilateral deafness
- Ipsilateral facial weakness and ataxia

Posterior Inferior Cerebellar Artery
- Ipsilateral limb and gait ataxia
- Wallenberg syndrome (lateral medullary syndrome, Clinical Panel 19.2)

Basilar Artery
- 'Locked in syndrome' — impairment of horizontal eye movements, quadriplegia, and intact wakefulness
- 'Top of the basilar syndrome' — decreased consciousness or coma, bilateral visual field deficits, vertical gaze palsies, hemiparesis (unilateral or bilateral)

Brainstem syndromes carry various eponyms and result from occlusion of perforating arteries that arise from the posterior cerebral or basilar artery and involve midbrain, pons, or medulla. They localise to the side of the cranial nerve deficit and long tract findings are on the contralateral side:

Midbrain — Paramedian (Benedict Syndrome); Ventral Mesencephalic Tegmentum
- CN III palsy (ipsilateral); involvement of the fascicular portion of CN III
- Ataxia (contralateral); involvement of the red nucleus

Midbrain — Paramedian (Weber Syndrome); Cerebral Peduncle
- CN III palsy (ipsilateral); involvement of the fascicular portion of CN III

- Hemiplegia (contralateral); corticospinal tract involvement within the cerebral peduncle

Pons — paramedian (Raymond syndrome); dorsomedial pons
- CN VI palsy (ipsilateral); fascicular portion of CN VI
- Hemiplegia (contralateral); corticospinal tract within the basis pontis

Pons — Paramedian (Foville Syndrome): Caudal Pontine Tegmentum Involving Facial Colliculus
- Gaze palsy (ipsilateral); PPRF/CN VI
- CN VII palsy (ipsilateral); VII nucleus/fascicular portion of CN VII
- Hemiplegia (contralateral); corticospinal tract within the basis pontis

Pons — Lateral (Millard—Gubler Syndrome); Dorsolateral Pons
- CN VII palsy (ipsilateral); fascicular portion of CN VII
- Hemiplegia (contralateral); corticospinal tract within the basis pontis

Medulla — Paramedian (Dejerine Syndrome); Medial Medulla
- CN XII palsy (ipsilateral); CN XII nucleus
- Hemisensory loss (contralateral); medial lemniscus
- Hemiparesis (contralateral); pyramidal tract

Medulla — Lateral (Wallenberg Syndrome); Lateral Medulla (Clinical Panel 19.2)
- Facial sensory loss and pain (ipsilateral); CN V nucleus
- Ataxia limb and gait (ipsilateral); posterior and rostral anterior spinocerebellar fibres
- Nystagmus, vertigo, and nausea/vomiting (ipsilateral); vestibular nucleus
- Hoarseness and dysphagia (ipsilateral); nucleus ambiguus
- Impaired taste (ipsilateral): nucleus of the solitary tract
- Horner syndrome (ipsilateral); descending sympathetic fibres
- Hemisensory loss of the body (contralateral); spinothalamic tract

A variety of effects may follow occlusion of branches of the posterior cerebral artery. Usually the occlusion is limited to a branch to the brainstem or to the cerebral cortex.

Thalamus (See Clinical Panel 25.1)
- Anterior territory — *tuberothalamic arteries* that arise from the posterior communicating artery supply the anterior nucleus, ventral anterior, and

part of the ventral lateral (12% of thalamic strokes). Infarction results in cognitive (anterograde amnesia, perhaps in part secondary to disruption of the mammillothalamic tract and superimposition of unrelated information when speaking) and behavioural changes (apathy and perseveration or repeating the same comment or action), and impaired visuospatial processing.

- Paramedian territory — *thalamoperforating arteries* that arise from the posterior cerebral artery (P1 segment or the portion between the top of the basilar artery and the origin of the posterior communicating artery) supply the intralaminar group and most of the dorsomedial nucleus (35% of thalamic strokes). After infarction there can be a period of loss of consciousness or somnolence that with resolution is followed by behavioural (disinhibited behaviour or speech, apathy, or motivation) and cognitive impairment (amnesia, confusion, aphasia) accompanied by vertical gaze impairment.
- Inferolateral territory — *thalamogeniculate arteries* whose origin is the posterior cerebral artery (P2 segment or the portion after the posterior communicating artery) provide circulation to the ventral lateral nuclear groups (45% of thalamic strokes). Infarction results in some degree of *hypoaesthesia* (diminished sensory loss, but possible sparing of proprioception) and ataxia accompanied by difficulties with planning, initiating, and regulating goals and behaviour (*executive functions*).
- Posterior territory — *posterior choroidal artery* that originates from the P2 segment supplies the lateral geniculate and the pulvinar (8% of thalamic strokes). After infarction there can be hypoesthesia, visual field deficit (because of involvement of the lateral geniculate and producing a contralateral *homonymous horizontal sectoranopia*), and deficits in attentional processes related to visual stimuli.
- Occlusion of a thalamoperforating branch may destroy the small subthalamic nucleus. After this injury, *hemiballism* (abrupt onset of wild, flailing movements) can be seen on the contralateral side, usually affecting the arm (Clinical Panel 26.2).

Occlusion of a thalamogeniculate branch can result in infarction of the posterior lateral nucleus of the thalamus (which receives the spinothalamic tract and medial lemniscus), and sometimes of the lateral geniculate nucleus also. The usual result is a contralateral sense of numbness, perhaps with hemianopia. A rare and unpleasant *thalamic pain syndrome* (or *central poststroke pain, CPSP*) may result after a period of complete sensory loss on the contralateral side of the body, and bouts of severe pain occurring either spontaneously or in response to tactile stimuli develop. While unexplained, it is associated with the combination of spinothalamic dysfunction and anterior pulvinar nucleus involvement.

Midbrain
Paramedian (Benedict syndrome); ventral mesencephalic tegmentum
- CN III palsy (ipsilateral); involvement of the fascicular portion of CN III
- Ataxia (contralateral); involvement of the red nucleus
Paramedian (Weber syndrome); cerebral peduncle
- CN III palsy (ipsilateral); involvement of the fascicular portion of CN III
- Hemiplegia (contralateral); corticospinal tract involvement within the cerebral peduncle

Left Posterior Cerebral Artery
- Alexia without agraphia, as a result of a disconnection between visual input from the intact right occipital cortex and language areas within the left brain; infarction of the left occipital lobe and selenium of the corpus callosum

Posterior Cerebral Artery
- Homonymous hemianopia, with sparing of macular vision assumed to be secondary to dual supply from the middle cerebral artery or bilateral representation of the fovea in the primary visual cortex (contralateral); involvement of occipital

Bilateral Posterior Cerebral Artery Occlusion
- *Cortical blindness (Anton's syndrome)* — complete visual loss on confrontation testing and lack of awareness *(anosognosia)* for the deficit; bilateral lesions of the primary visual cortex
- *Prosopagnosia* — inability to recognise people or their faces; bilateral lesions of the *fusiform gyrus* (inferior occipitotemporal cortex)
- *Achromatopsia* — inability to match or name colours presented visually, but able to name the colour associated with specific objects; bilateral lesions of the inferior occipitotemporal cortex

---

CLINICAL PANEL 35.8   Subarachnoid Haemorrhage

Blister-like 'berry' aneurysms 5 to 10 mm in diameter are a routine autopsy finding in about 1% to 2% of people. Most are in the anterior half of the circle of Willis. Spontaneous rupture of an aneurysm into the interpeduncular cistern usually occurs in early or late middle age. The characteristic presentation is a sudden blinding headache, with collapse into unconsciousness or coma within a few seconds. On physical examination, a diagnostic feature (absent in one-third of cases) is nuchal (neck) rigidity. This is caused by movement of blood into the posterior cranial fossa, where the dura mater is supplied by cervical nerves 2 and 3 (see Chapter 5). The term *meningismus* is sometimes used for this sign.

The massive rise in intracranial pressure may be fatal within a few hours or days. Recovery may be impeded by a secondary elevation of intracranial pressure caused by blood clot obstruction of cerebrospinal fluid circulation through the tentorial notch or even within the arachnoid granulations.

About a quarter of all cases develop a neurologic deficit 4 to 12 days after the initial attack. The deficit is fatal in a quarter of those who get it. The immediate cause is spasm of the main, conducting segments of the cerebral arteries. The amount of spasm is proportionate to the size of the surrounding blood clot in the interpeduncular cistern.

It is usual practice to define the aneurysm by means of angiography, and to ligate it surgically or via endovascular repair, and pack the aneurysm with platinum coils which leads to thrombosis within the aneurysm. Without operation, most aneurysms will rupture again at some future date.

CLINICAL PANEL 35.9   Motor Recovery after Stroke (See Fig. 35.8)

Very Early Recovery — Up To 24 Hours
- Within hours of a stroke associated with severe hemiplegia caused by embolic occlusion of a major artery of supply to the corona radiata or internal capsule, some patients show remarkable recovery of motor function, to a level where only a moderate weakness of an arm or leg may persist. One or both of two explanations are possible:
  - The embolus has undergone fragmentation, freeing up some or all of the primary branches of the artery.
  - Collapse of the blood pressure within the territory of the blocked artery has permitted retrograde filling of the peripheral branches through the small-artery anastomoses along the border zone illustrated in Fig. 35.1.

Early Recovery — The First Few Days
- A more limited improvement, during a period of a week or more, is attributable to resolution of the surrounding oedema, permitting resumption of oxygen and glucose supply to viable neurons.

Later Recovery

- During the ensuing months, slow but progressive recovery of motor function is the rule, especially with the assistance of remedial exercises supervised by a physical therapist.
- A consistent feature on functional magnetic resonance imaging scans is a widespread hyperexcitability of cortical areas connected to the lesion site. The hyperexcitability, associated with reduced local activity of inhibitory, smooth stellate (γ-aminobutyric acid, GABA) neurons, appears within days and gradually diminishes over a period of up to a year or even more.

Reorganisation Within the Affected M1

- Cell columns adjacent to those inactivated by the infarct, now liberated from lateral (surround) inhibition, become especially active. Previously

silent hand-specific columns within the arm and shoulder representations are likely to become active. Existence of outlying hand-specific columns would be analogous to the cortical representation of the tongue, which in the homunculus is shown entirely below that for the face, although outlying tongue-specific columns extend halfway up the motor cortex.

- *Change of allegiance.* In monkeys, a significant contribution to recovery from paralysis (e.g., of the hand) produced by excising a patch of motor cortex arises from neighbouring (e.g., arm-related) cortical cell columns activating hand rather than arm motor neurons in the cord. This phenomenon is easily explained by the extensive overlap of cortical motor territories in the spinal cord, the focusing factor normally being the recurrent (Renshaw cell) inhibitory shield surrounding the zone of maximal

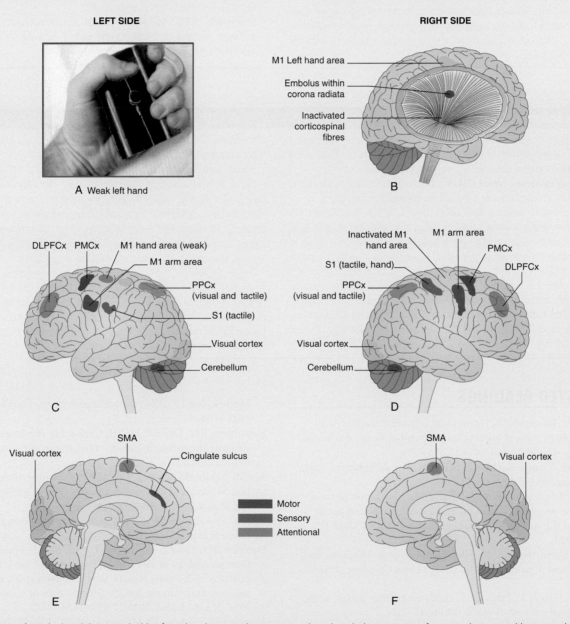

Fig. 35.8 Areas of cortical activity revealed by functional magnetic resonance imaging during recovery from stroke caused by an embolus within the white matter containing the right corticospinal tract. (A) The 'manipulandum' used by Ward et al. to register the squeezing power of the affected hand. (B) Depiction of embolic compromise of the right corticospinal tract. (C) Lateral view of areas of increased cortical activity in the left (contralateral) cortex of the cerebrum and cerebellum. (D) Corresponding view of the right (lesional) side. (E) Medial view of the left side. (F) Medial view of the right side. *DLPFCx*, Dorsolateral prefrontal cortex; *M1*, primary motor cortex; *PMCx*, premotor cortex; *PPCx*, posterior parietal cortex; *S1*, somatic sensory cortex; *SMA*, supplementary motor area. (Assistance of Dr. Nick Ward, Honorary Consultant Neurologist, National Hospital for Neurology and Neurosurgery, Queen Square, London, is gratefully acknowledged.)

activation. Suspended activation of spinal cell columns includes loss of surround inhibition, thereby rendering the silent motor neurons accessible to excitation by collateral branches of nearby corticospinal fibres.

Contributions Originating Outside the Affected M1

- Active secondary motor areas contributing to the contralateral (left) corticospinal tract include the premotor cortex, SMA, and anterior cingulate cortex, and the arm/shoulder area of the left M1 (Fig. 35.8). All three are active during the recovery period. Functional magnetic resonance image (fMRI) monitoring indicates that, in those patients with greatest damage to the corticospinal tract, there is greatest reliance on secondary motor areas to generate some motor output. Their recruitment is often bilateral, presumably because of bilateral hand representations. Opinions differ concerning the contribution of the *hand* area of the left M1 to motor recovery, although some contribution would be expected in view of its 10% contribution to the left lateral corticospinal tract.

- The cerebellum and motor thalamus (ventrolateral nucleus) are also active bilaterally throughout and share the progressive reduction of activity during later stages. Cerebellar activity during *motor learning* was touched upon in Chapter 27, whereby a 'reference copy' of pyramidal tract activity is sent to the cerebellar cortex via the red nucleus and inferior olivary nucleus, representing intended movements. Sensory feedback during movement enables the cerebellum to detect any discrepancy between intention and execution, leading to adjustment of the cerebellar discharge via the thalamus to the motor cortex. As accuracy improves, cerebellar corrective activity declines.

Sensory System Contributions

- Visual and tactile areas of the cortex show above-normal activation during the recovery period; so too does the dorsolateral prefrontal cortex. These activities suggest a heightened level of sensory attention, with the objective of optimising task performance.
- Collectively, fMRI observations reveal the recruitment of alternative pathways capable of activating the ventral horn cells that have been functionally deprived by the stroke.

✳ Core Information

A ***stroke*** ('brain attack') is neurological dysfunction from a focal infarction in the central nervous system or retina, within a cerebrovascular territory and based on clinical and/or objective (e.g., radiological) evidence.

A ***transient ischaemic attack (TIA)*** is a focal neurological dysfunction lasting less than 24 hours (usually minutes) and with no evidence of infarction.

Ischaemic strokes comprise 85% of all strokes, and in the majority the underlying mechanism is either vessel pathology that leads to occlusion (e.g., atherothrombosis) or a source (e.g., heart) generating a 'particle' that results in embolic occlusion of a vessel (e.g., cardiac). A third group of ischaemic stroke involves occlusion of cerebral small vessels that results in small subcortical infarctions within the territory of those perforating arterioles and on neuroimaging (and postmortem) the appearance of fluid-filled cavities called lacunes, hence the name ***lacunar strokes***. Historically, chronic hypertension (a risk factor for cerebrovascular disease) was the assumed primary aetiology of these occlusions, but now the proposed aetiology is dysfunction in endothelial cells

and disruption of the blood—brain barrier that eventually leads to arteriole injury, degeneration, and occlusion.

Fifteen percent of acute strokes are haemorrhagic, either intracerebral (10%) or from subarachnoid haemorrhage (5%). Nontraumatic subarachnoid haemorrhage is most frequently (80%) the result of rupture of an intracranial aneurysm ('berry aneurysm'). A typical sequence of clinical effects is the sudden onset of headache ('worst headache of my life'), followed by altered mental status and signs of meningeal irritation (neck stiffness with pain on motion). Morbidity is significant and mortality is up to 50%.

The predictability of the vascular supply to the brain allows specific stroke syndromes (neurological findings associated with involvement of different cerebral vessels) to be identified, and when supported by various imagining techniques, facilitates further diagnostic and therapeutic decisions. The Clinical Panels describe the expected clinical findings associated with strokes resulting from specific cerebral vessel involvement.

SUGGESTED READINGS

Brown RD Jr, Broderick JP. Unruptured intracranial aneurysms: epidemiology, natural history, management options, and familial screening. *Lancet Neurol.* 2014;13:393—404.

Coupland AP, Thapar A, Qureshi MI, et al. The definition of stroke. *J Royal Soc Med.* 2017;110:9—12.

de Boer IH, Bakris G, Cannon CP. Individualizing blood pressure targets for people with diabetes and hypertension: comparing the ADA and the ACC/AHA recommendations. *JAMA.* 2018;319: 1319—1320.

Hassan TF, Rabinstein AA, Middlebrooks EH, et al. Diagnosis and management of acute ischemic stroke. *Mayo Clin Proc.* 2018;93: 523—538.

Hope TMH, Friston K, Price CJ, et al. Recovery after stroke: not so proportional after all. *Brain.* 2019;142:15—22.

Kim DE, Park JD, Schellingerhout D, et al. Mapping the supratentorial cerebral arterial territories using 1160 large artery infarcts. *JAMA Neurol.* 2019;76:72—80.

Meschia JF, Klass JP, Brown RD Jr, Brott TG. Evaluation and management of atherosclerotic carotid stenosis. *Mayo Clinic Proc.* 2017;92:1144—1157.

Muehlschlegel S. Subarachnoid hemorrhage. *Continuum.* 2018;24: 1623—1657.

Regenhardt RW, Das AS, Lo EH, Caplan LR. Advances in understanding the pathophysiology of lacunar stroke: a review. *JAMA Neurol.* 2018;75:1273—1281.

Sato A, Takahashi S, Soma Y, et al. Cerebral infarction: early detection by means of contrast-enhanced cerebral arteries at MR imaging. *Radiology.* 1991;178:433—439.

Solomon RA, Connolly ES Jr. Arteriovenous malformations of the brain. *N Engl J Med.* 2017;376:1859—1866.

Sweeney MD, Zhao Z, Montagne A, et al. Blood—brain barrier: from physiology to disease and back. *Physiol Rev.* 2019;99:21—78.

The GBD 2016 Lifetime Risk of Stroke Collaborators, et al. Global, regional, and country-specific lifetime risks of stroke, 1990 and 2016. *N Engl J Med.* 2018;379(25):2429—2437.

Vartiainen N, Perchet C, Magnin M, et al. Thalamic pain: anatomical and physiological indices of prediction. *Brain.* 2016;139:708—722.

GLOSSARY

ABBREVIATIONS: Ch. or Chs, Chapter(s) containing main reference. Fr. signifies French origin; Gr. signifies Greek origin; L. signifies Latin origin; CNS, central nervous system.

A

Abducens L. 'leading away'. Abducens nerve innervates the lateral rectus muscle that abducts the eyeball (Ch. 23).

Absence seizures A generalised seizure disorder with an onset in childhood and manifested as frequent brief spells of unresponsiveness ('absence') (Ch. 29).

Absolute refractory period Time interval following generation of an action potential, during which the membrane is refractory to a second stimulus because of the inactivation of voltage-gated Na+ channels (Ch. 7).

Abulia Gr. 'lack of will'. Loss of willpower associated with prefrontal cortical disorders (Ch. 32).

Accommodation Process where the eye changes its focus from a distant to a near image by changing the shape of the lens to a more convex shape (Ch. 23).

Action potential A brief fluctuation in membrane potential caused by rapid opening and closure of voltage-gated ion channels that actively propagates along an axon (Ch. 7).

Action tremor See *Intention tremor*.

Active zone Site of release of neurotransmitter through the presynaptic membrane (Ch. 10).

Adaptation Attenuation of response to a sustained sensory stimulus (Ch. 11).

Adrenaline Synonym for epinephrine (Ch. 13).

Adrenoceptor Sympathetic junctional receptor (Ch. 13).

Affective disorder A disorder of mood, e.g. major depression (Ch. 34).

Afferent L. 'carrying toward'. Strictly, applies to nerve impulses traveling toward CNS along sensory fibres; is loosely applied within CNS, e.g. afferent connections of the cerebellum (Ch. 2). See also *Centripetal*.

Agnosia Gr. 'without knowledge'. Inability to interpret sensory information (Ch. 28).

Agraphia Gr. 'without writing'. Inability to express oneself in writing, owing to a central lesion (Ch. 32).

Akinesia Gr. 'without movement'. Refers to immobility often seen in Parkinson disease (Ch. 26).

Alexia Gr. 'without reading'. Inability to read (Ch. 32).

Allocortex Gr. 'other cortex'. Phylogenetically old, three- layered cortex in the temporal lobe (Ch. 28).

Allodynia Pain produced by normally innocuous stimulation (Ch. 33).

Alpha (α) motor neuron The motor neuron that innervates extrafusal skeleton muscle fibres (Ch. 10).

Alveus Gr. 'trough'. Refers to the thin layer of white matter on the surface of the hippocampus (Ch. 28).

Alzheimer disease Most common form of neurodegenerative dementia (Ch. 33).

Amino acid transmitters Glutamate, γ-aminobutyric acid (GABA), glycine (Ch. 8).

Amnesia Loss of memory (Ch. 33).

Amygdala Gr. 'almond'. Nucleus at the tip of the inferior horn of the lateral ventricle, part of the limbic system (Ch. 2).

Amyotrophic lateral sclerosis See *Motor neuron disease* (Ch. 16).

Analgesia Gr. 'without pain'. Absence of perception of a noxious stimulus (Ch. 15).

Aneurysm Gr. 'widening'. Localised dilation of an artery (Ch. 35).

Angiogram Image of blood vessels obtained by intraarterial injection of radiopaque fluid (Ch. 4).

Anomia Gr. 'without names'. Inability to name common objects (Ch. 32).

Anopsia Gr. 'without vision'. A defect in the visual field (Ch. 31).

Anterior circulation The territory of the internal carotid artery and its branches (contributes to the Circle of Willis) (Chs 4, 35).

Anterograde amnesia Inability to lay down new memories (Ch. 34).

Anterograde transport Axonal transport from soma to nerve terminals (Ch. 6).

Anterolateral system (ALS) Conjoint anterior and lateral spinothalamic tracts (Ch. 15).

Antidromic Gr. 'running against'. Conduction along an axon that is opposite to its normal direction of propagation (e.g. towards the soma in a motor axon) (Ch. 11).

Aphasia Gr. 'without speech'. An acquired language disorder of the brain usually as a result of an injury in the perisylvian area of the left cerebral hemisphere (e.g. motor aphasia, sensory aphasia) (Ch. 32).

Apperceptive tactile agnosia A form of tactile agnosia usually from a right parietal lobe injury (Ch. 32).

Apraxia Gr. 'without movement'. Inability to carry out voluntary movements despite normal strength and comprehension (Ch. 32).

Aprosodia Absence of normal variations of pitch, rhythm, and stress in the speech (Ch. 32).

Arachnoid Gr. 'spider-like'. Refers to the fine delicate web-like nature of the arachnoid mater (Ch. 5).

Archi- (arche-) Gr. 'beginning'. Refers to oldest areas, e.g. archicerebellum (Ch. 27).

Area postrema L. 'back end area'. It is a circumventricular organ in the medulla oblongata and is located in the inferior posterior part on the floor of the fourth ventricle (Ch. 17).

Arnold–Chiari malformation A condition in which the inferior poles of the cerebellar hemispheres and the medulla protrude through the foramen magnum into the spinal canal due to a maldevelopment of the posterior cranial fossa. It is one of the causes of hydrocephalus and is usually accompanied by spina bifida cystica and meningomyelocele (Ch. 14).

Ascending reticular activating system (ARAS) A group of nuclei within the brain stem (neuromodulatory system) that regulate alertness and sleep—wake states (Ch. 24).

Assistance reflex During voluntary movement, positive feedback from actively stretched neuromuscular spindles assists the movement (Ch. 16). Cf. *Resistance reflex*.

Association cortex Area of cortex receiving afferents from one or more primary sensory areas (Ch. 28).

Associative agnosia Left parietal lobe style of tactile agnosia (Ch. 32).

Astereognosis Gr. 'without knowledge of solid'. Refers to the inability to identify common objects by touch alone (Ch. 28).

Astrocyte The 'star-like' glial (nonneuronal) cell that plays a prominent role in maintaining the neuronal microenvironment (Ch. 6).

Asymbolia for pain Abolition of the aversive quality of painful stimuli while preserving the location and intensity aspects (Ch. 33).

Ataxia Gr. 'without order'. Impaired coordination and control of voluntary movements and balance; often associated with posterior column (Ch. 15) or cerebellar (Ch. 27) disease.

Atherosclerosis Arterial degenerative disorder associated with fatty subintimal plaques capable of detachment with consequent embolism within the arterial territory (Ch. 35).

Athetosis Gr. 'without stability'. Describes the continuous writhing movements sometimes associated with damage to the basal ganglia (Ch. 26).

Autogenetic inhibition Negative feedback from Golgi tendon organs causing a muscle to relax (Ch. 10).

Autonomic Self-regulating (Ch. 13).

Autoreceptor A presynaptic receptor acted on by the transmitter released at the same nerve ending (Chs 8, 13).

Autoregulation The capacity of a tissue to regulate its own blood supply (Ch. 4).

Axolemma Gr. 'husk'. Cell membrane of an axon (Ch. 6).

Axon reflex Activation of the reflex arc producing the triple response in the skin (Ch. 11).

Axoplasm Gr. 'substance'. The cytoplasm of the axon (Ch. 6).

Axoplasmic transport Orthograde or retrograde transport of materials within an axon (Ch. 6).

B

Babinski sign Reflex fanning of the toes with dorsiflexion of the great toe, following stroking stimulus to the lateral part of the sole of the foot; sign of corticospinal tract disorder (Ch. 16).

Ballism/Ballismus Gr. 'throwing'. A type of involuntary movement affecting the proximal limb musculature, manifested in jerking, flinging movements of the extremity; caused by a lesion of the contralateral subthalamic nucleus. Usually only one side of the body is involved, resulting in hemiballismus (Ch. 26).

Baroreceptor Gr. 'weight' receptor. Refers to the blood pressure receptors of the carotid sinus and aortic arch (Ch. 24).

Baroreceptor reflex (Baroreflex) Reflex increase of sympathetic vascular tone in response to a fall in intracranial blood pressure, e.g. on assuming the upright position (Ch. 24).

Barosympathetic reflex Reflex reduction of sympathetic tone in response to a rise of arterial blood pressure (Ch. 24).

Barovagal reflex Reflex reduction of heart rate in response to a rise of arterial blood pressure (Ch. 24).

Bell palsy Subacute onset of peripheral facial nerve paralysis assumed to result from a viral infection and associated with swelling of the nerve resulting in its compression against the wall of the bony facial canal (Ch. 22).

Benign essential tremor A rhythmic, involuntary oscillation of part of the body (usually the upper extremity or head), usually symmetric and most evident with posture (Ch. 26).

Benign rolandic epilepsy of childhood An age related, idiopathic, localisation related epilepsy syndrome (e.g. disorder having an ictal focus of origin in front of or behind the fissure of Rolando or the central sulcus) (Ch. 29).

Berry aneurysm A small saccular aneurysm within the circle of Willis or nearby cerebral artery (Ch. 35).

Binocular visual field Vision that involves focusing on an object with both eyes simultaneously. It is important in judging distance (Ch. 31).

Bipolar recording A particular pattern of variable pairs of electrode connections used in recoding an EEG (Ch. 29). Cf. *Referential recording*.

Bitemporal hemianopia Blindness in the temporal half of the visual field in each eye resulting from involvement of the optic chiasm and which can result from compression from a pituitary adenoma (Ch. 31).

Blind sight Patients with cortical blindness may perceive or respond to movement in that peripheral visual field where they do not consciously see (Ch. 31).

Blinking-to-light reflex Reflex blinking in response to a flash of bright light (Ch. 22).

Blinking-to-noise reflex Acousticofacial reflex causing the orbicularis oculi to twitch in response to a loud sound (Ch. 22).

Blood trauma phobia Fainting at the sight of blood (Ch. 33).

Body schema Consciousness of the relative position of body parts and the space around them (Ch. 32).

Border zone or Watershed area Border zone area between the territories of major arteries of the brain (Ch. 35).

Bradykinesia Gr. 'slow movement'. Slowness of initiation and performance of voluntary movements; characteristic of Parkinson disease (Ch. 26).

Brain attack or Stroke Neurological deficit secondary to a vascular aetiology (Ch. 35).

Brain-derived neurotrophic factor (BDNF) A 'nourishing' factor that promotes survival and normal functioning of cortical neurons (Ch. 6).

Brainstem Comprises midbrain, pons, and medulla oblongata (Ch. 3). In the embryo, also includes the diencephalon (Ch. 1).

Brainstem auditory evoked potentials Electrical potentials recorded from the surface of the skull, evoked by click (sound) stimulation of the ear and generated by action potentials as they traverse the auditory pathway (Ch. 30).

Broca aphasia (Expressive aphasia) A nonfluent aphasia caused by damage to the posterior portion of the inferior frontal gyrus in the dominant cerebral hemisphere (Broca area) (Ch. 32).

Broca area Pars triangularis (area 44) and pars opercularis (area 45) of the frontal operculum, involved in generating speech (Ch. 32).

Brown–Sequard syndrome The constellation of signs that follows hemisection or injury to one side of the spinal cord; ipsilateral weakness and position sense loss and contralateral impairment of pain and temperature (Ch. 16).

Bulbar L. 'bulb' of the brain. A discredited term usually meaning medulla oblongata.

C

Calcar avis L. 'spur of a bird'. Refers to the elevation produced by the calcarine sulcus in the medial wall of the atrium of the lateral ventricle (Ch. 2).

Cataplexy Gr. 'struck down'. Term used to signify sudden, brief episodes of loss of muscle tone triggered by emotion, notably by surprise of any kind and representing a disorder of regulation of sleep and wake cycles (Ch. 29).

Catecholamines The neurotransmitters dopamine, norepinephrine, and epinephrine, comprising amines attached to catechol rings (Ch. 8).

Cauda equina L. 'horse's tail'. Collection of dorsal and ventral nerve roots below the caudal end of the spinal cord and traversing the lumbar cistern to their respective intervertebral foramina (Ch. 14).

Caudal anaesthesia Pelvic–perineal anaesthesia produced by injection of local anaesthetic through the sacral hiatus into the epidural space (Ch. 14).

Caudate L. 'having a tail', e.g. caudate nucleus (Ch. 26).

Centre-surround receptive field A visual receptive field having a centre surrounded by a ring of opposite sign (Ch. 31).

Central motor conduction time Measurement of corticospinal tract conduction time using a combination of transcranial magnetic stimulation and surface electromyography.

Central pain state A state of chronic pain, resistant to therapy, sustained by hypersensitivity of peripheral and/or central neural pathways (Ch. 33).

Central pattern generator A neural circuit giving rise to rhythmic motor activity.

Centrifugal L. 'fleeing the centre'. See *Efferent*.

Centripetal L. 'seeking the centre'. See *Afferent*.

Cerebellar ataxia Ataxia of cerebellar origin. See *Ataxia* (Ch. 27).

Cerebellar cognitive affective syndrome Cerebral functional deficits that can include cognitive, speech, affective, and emotional behaviour following injury to the cerebellum (Ch. 27).

Cerebellar signs Ataxia or intention tremor (in particular) associated with cerebellar pathology (Ch. 27).

Cerebellum L. 'little brain'. The convoluted region of the brain located at the back of the cerebrum and located dorsal to the pons that is primarily concerned with coordination of motor activity by helping to ensure that intention matches outcome (Ch. 27).

Cerebrum L. 'brain'. It is the upper expanded part of the forebrain derived from the telencephalon. The two cerebral hemispheres are separated by median longitudinal fissure. It is the highest level of control in the hierarchy of the nervous system. It is involved in sensory integration, control of voluntary movements, and all higher intellectual functions (Ch. 28).

Cervical spondylosis A form of vertebral arthritis accompanied by bony outgrowths around the margins of cervical facet joints, resulting in compression of cervical nerve roots and spinal cord (Chs 12, 14).

Cervicogenic headache A secondary type of headache disorder attributed to head or neck injury and resulting in neck pain associated with headache (Ch. 14).

'Change of allegiance' Plastic response to motor cortical injury, whereby neighbouring neurons are recruited to serve a lost motor function (Ch. 35).

Chemical synapse Distinguished from electrical synapses by release of a neurotransmitter (Ch. 8).

Chemoreceptor A sensory receptor (e.g. carotid body) selective for a chemical substance (Ch. 24).

Chiasm Gr. 'crossing'. Refers mainly to the optic chiasm (Ch. 31).

Chorea Gr. 'dance'. Irregular, involuntary movements that seem to extend from one area of the body to the next and interfere with voluntary motor activities (Ch. 26).

Choroid plexus Gr. a 'membranous network' of capillaries invested with choroidal epithelium and located within the ventricles of the brain; responsible for the production of cerebrospinal fluid (Ch. 5).

Chromatolysis Gr. 'dissolution of colour'. Loss of Nissl substance (granular endoplasmic reticulum and ribosomes) within a neuron following injury to the cell body or axon (Ch. 9).

Cingulotomy Sectioning or resection of the anterior cingulate cortex, once done for relief of intractable pain (Ch. 33).

Cingulum L. the 'girdle' of white matter within the cingulate gyrus (Chs 2, 33).

Clasp knife rigidity Initial resistance to passive movement followed by collapse of resistance; a sign of upper motor neuron disease (Ch. 16).

Claustrum L. the 'barrier'. Thin band of grey matter (technically part of the basal ganglia) between the external and extreme capsules (Ch. 2).

Clonus L. 'turmoil'. Involuntary rhythmic, alternating contraction of agonist and antagonist muscles that occur in rapid succession that results in a rapid beating movement at ankle or wrist produced by sudden passive extension; associated with upper motor neuron disease (Ch. 16).

Coactivation Simultaneous activation of α and γ motor neurons (Ch. 10).

Cocontraction Simultaneous contraction of agonist and antagonist muscles (Ch. 16).

Cognition Refers to the conscious and unconscious mental processes that include variable aspects of memory, language, visuospatial, and executive functions dysfunction (Ch. 32).

Cognitive style A term from cognitive psychology that describes the different processes used to think, perceive, and remember information (Ch. 32).

Cogwheel rigidity A ratchet-like interruption in muscle tone that can be felt as the limb is passively moved. It is thought of as rigidity with a superimposed tremor and is classically seen in Parkinson disease (Ch. 26).

Colliculus L. 'little hill'. Four colliculi (corpora quadrigemina) comprise the tectum of the midbrain (Chs 3, 20).

Column A term used interchangeably for the posterior/dorsal funiculus of the spinal cord (Ch. 15).

Combined processing Simultaneous engagement of more than one sensory modality in a particular sensory task (Ch. 25).

Commissure L. 'link'. Axons connecting similar areas of the two sides of the nervous system, e.g. white commissure of the spinal cord (Ch. 3), anterior commissure of the brain, corpus callosum (Ch. 2).

Compensation reflex Vestibuloocular reflex compensating for movement of the head; associated with fixation (foveation) (Ch. 23).

Complex focal (partial) seizure An epileptic seizure involving one cerebral hemisphere (usually frontal or temporal lobe) and associated with impairment of awareness (Ch. 29).

Complex spikes Multiple action potentials generated from Purkinje cells to stimulation of their dendritic tress by olivocerebellar fibres and believed to play a role in motor learning (Ch. 27).

CMAP Compound motor action potential represents the surface recording of the underlying membrane depolarisation of muscle fibres elicited by stimulation of their respective motor nerve (Ch. 12).

Concussion A type of traumatic brain injury (TBI) usually caused by a blow to the head (Ch. 5).

Conduction aphasia Aphasia caused by damage to the arcuate fasciculus that manifests as impaired repetition with relatively intact comprehension and fluency of speech (Ch. 32).

Conductive deafness Deafness caused by disease in the outer ear canal or middle ear (Ch. 20).

Conjugate eye movement Movement of both eyes in the same direction that allows bilateral visual fixation, e.g. ocular saccades (Ch. 23).

Conscious proprioception Perceived sensations arising within the body, notably from muscle spindles (Ch. 15).

Consolidation The process of storing information in long-term memory (Ch. 33).

Continuous conduction Mode of impulse conduction along unmyelinated nerve fibres (Ch. 7).

Contralateral L. Refers to opposite side of the body (cf. *Ipsilateral*, 'same side').

Convolution L. A gyrus (Ch. 2).

Cordotomy Involves the sectioning of the anterolateral pathways in the spinal cord, done to relieve intractable pain (Ch. 15).

Corneal reflex Blinking in response to corneal contact (Ch. 22).

Corona radiata L. 'radiating crown'. White matter of ascending and descending projections from cerebral cortex to internal capsule and vice versa (Ch. 2).

Corpus callosum L. 'hard body'. Refers to the great transverse commissure of white matter interconnecting homotopic areas of the cerebral hemispheres (Ch. 2).

Corpus striatum L. 'striated body'. Part of the basal ganglia, comprising the caudate and lentiform nuclei (Chs 2, 26).

Cortex L. the 'bark'. Outer grey matter at the surface of the cerebrum and cerebellum (Ch. 2).

Cortical blindness Blindness owing to damage to the primary visual cortex (Ch. 31).

Cortical mosaic Mosaic arrangement created by interdigitating of cortical modules of different kinds (Ch. 28).

Cortical-type sensory loss Diminution of tactile perception associated with damage to the primary sensory cortex (Ch. 28).

Crossed hemiplegia Follows unilateral brainstem lesion affecting one or more motor cranial nerve nuclei (resulting in ipsilateral paralysis) together with corticospinal fibres (resulting in contralateral hemiplegia or hemiparesis) (Ch. 35).

Crus L. 'leg', e.g. crus of fornix (Ch. 2), crus of midbrain (Ch. 2).

Cuneate L. 'wedge-like', e.g. cuneate fasciculus (Chs 3, 15).

Cuneus L. 'wedge', e.g. the gyrus of that shape in the occipital lobe (Ch. 2).

D

Declarative memory Memory for facts and events that can be consciously recalled (Ch. 33).

Decussation L. From Roman numeral X. Refers to X-shaped crossing of nerve bundles at junctional regions, e.g. pyramidal decussation (spinomedullary junction, Chs 3 and 16), decussation of superior cerebellar peduncles (pons—midbrain, Ch. 3).

Déjà vu Fr. Epileptic aura where an event currently being experienced is associated with the sensation of it having occurred in the past (Ch. 29).

Delta waves EEG waveforms characteristic of slow-wave sleep and a frequency of less than 4 Hz (Ch. 29).

Dementia Loss of cognitive abilities in the presence of intact motor and sensory systems (Ch. 33).

Dendrite(s) Gr. 'tree(s)'. Refers to the neuronal processes receiving synaptic input (usually) from axons of other neurons (Ch. 6).

Dendritic sheaves Within the thalamic reticular nucleus, bundles of dendrites belonging to different neurons, linked to one another by dendrodendritic synapses.

Dentate L. 'toothed', e.g. dentate nucleus of the cerebellum (Ch. 27), dentate gyrus in the temporal lobe anchoring the spinal cord to the dura mater (Ch. 33).

Denticulate L. 'little-toothed', e.g. denticulate ligament of pia mater anchoring the spinal cord (Ch. 5).

Depolarisation block Conduction block along an axon that is produced by high-frequency stimulation (Ch. 7).

Depolarise Make the membrane potential of the neuron less negative (Ch. 7).

Dermatome The strip of skin supplied by a single sensory nerve (Ch. 11).

Detrusor instability 'Unstable bladder' characterised by spontaneous expulsion of urine despite conscious attempts at restraint (Ch. 13).

Developmental dyslexia A hereditary neurologic disorder involving language that manifests as severe and persistent reading and/or spelling difficulties, despite normal intelligence (Ch. 32).

Diabetes insipidus Hypothalamic disorder characterised by polyuria and polydipsia (Ch. 34).

Diencephalic amnesia Amnesia attributed to injury to the diencephalon (Ch. 33).

Diencephalon Gr. 'between-brain', comprising epithalamus, thalamus, and hypothalamus (Ch. 34).

Diffuse noxious inhibitory controls Appropriate neural connections whereby painful stimulation of one part of the body may produce pain relief in all other parts (Ch. 24).

Diffusion tension imaging (DTI) An MRI technique designed to measure diffusion of water molecules along nerve fibres (Ch. 2).

Diplopia Gr. 'double vision' (Ch. 23).

Discriminative touch Fine touch sensibility (Chs 15, 28).

Disinhibition Release of excitatory neurons by inhibition of inhibitory neurons (Chs 6, 26).

Dissociated sensory loss Loss of one sensory modality with preservation of others (Ch. 15).

Dopa Dihydroxyphenylalanine, a precursor of dopamine, norepinephrine, and epinephrine (Ch. 8).

Dopamine Catecholamine neurotransmitter synthesised from dopa (Ch. 8).

Dura mater L. 'hard cover'. Outermost meninx (Ch. 5).

Dynamic (kinetic) labyrinth The semicircular canals (Ch. 19).

Dynamic posturography An instrumental recording that tests postural reflex responses to sudden tilting (Ch. 27).

Dys- Gr. 'difficult'.

Dysarthria Gr. 'difficult articulation'. A group of motor speech disorders caused by a disturbance in the neuromuscular control of speech (Ch. 32).

Dysarthria—clumsy hand syndrome A lacunar stroke syndrome associated with a vascular lesion of the genu of the internal capsule (or pons) and manifested as dysarthria and limb ataxia (Ch. 35).

Dysdiadochokinesia Gr. 'difficult successive movements'. An impairment in making smooth and rapid alternating movements, e.g. difficulty in performing rapid pronation—supination sequences of the forearm (Ch. 27).

Dyskinetic (or extrapyramidal) cerebral palsy Movement disorder seen with cerebral palsy as a result of damage to the basal ganglia (Ch. 26).

Dyslexia Gr. 'difficult reading'. Difficulty reading and interpreting written forms of communication by a person whose vision and general intelligence are otherwise unimpaired (Ch. 32).

Dysmetria Gr. 'difficult measurement'. An inability to control the range of movement of a body part, e.g. trying to touch an object with an index finger (Ch. 27).

Dysphagia Gr. 'difficult in swallowing', e.g. following paralysis of pharyngeal constrictors (Ch. 18).

Dysphasia See *Aphasia* (Ch. 32).

Dysphonia Any impairment of the voice; alteration in the sound of the voice with hoarseness, restriction of vocal performance, or strained vocalisation (Ch. 18).

E

ECT (electroconvulsive therapy) The administration of an electric current to the brain for treatment of drug-resistant or extremely severe depression (Ch. 34).

Ectoderm Gr. 'outer skin'. Refers to the outer germ layer giving rise to the nervous system and to the epidermis of the skin (Ch. 1).

EEG (electroencephalogram) Surface recording of the extracellular alternating currents generated from cortical neurons (Ch. 29).

Efferent L. 'carrying away'. Strictly, applies to nerve impulses traveling away from the CNS; also used regionally, e.g. cerebellar efferents. See also *Centrifugal.*

Ejaculation L. 'throwing'. The action of ejecting semen from the body (Ch. 13).

Electrical potential Voltage.

Electrical synapse Synapse where current can flow from one neuron to another via gap junctions (Chs 6, 7).

Electrodiagnostic examination The combination of nerve conduction studies and electromyography (Ch. 12).

Electromyogram The graphic record of the depolarisation waveforms of muscle fibres at rest and with voluntary muscle contraction (Ch. 12).

Electromyography (EMG) Recording the waveforms generated by selected muscles during voluntary contraction.

Electrotonic potentials The passive spread of a positive or negative change in membrane potential that becomes smaller (decrement) as it spreads along the plasma membrane (Ch. 7).

Electrotonus The passive spread of charge within a neuron (Ch. 7).

Emboliform nucleus Gr. 'plug-like'. With the globose nucleus, forming the interposed deep cerebellar nucleus (Ch. 27).

Embolus Gr. 'plug'. Typically, a blood clot that is carried within the blood stream and causes a blockage or occlusion of a blood vessel (Ch. 35).

EMG See *Electromyography* (Ch. 12).

Endocytosis Vesicular uptake of material from the extracellular space (Ch. 6).

Endogenous opioids Brain-derived neuropeptides (Ch. 24).

Endoneurium Gr. 'within nerve'. Refers to the connective tissue sheath surrounding individual nerve fibres (Ch. 9).

Engram The chemical intraneuronal representation of a memory.

Enteroception L. 'reception from inside'. The reception of sensory stimuli from hollow internal organs (Ch. 13).

Entorhinal Gr. 'in nose'. Refers to entorhinal cortex of the temporal lobe (Ch. 33).

Entrapment neuropathy Peripheral mononeuropathy usually caused by nerve compression beneath ligamentous bridges by stretching at bony angulations (Ch. 12).

Ependyma Gr. 'upper garment'. Refers to the epithelium lining the ventricular system of the brain (Ch. 2) and the central canal of the spinal cord (Ch. 3).

Epidural anaesthesia Anaesthesia procured by injecting analgesic solution into the epidural space, usually in the lumbar region (Ch. 14).

Epinephrine Catecholamine hormone synthesised in adrenal medulla (Ch. 13); also, a neurotransmitter synthesised in the brainstem (Ch. 24). Also known as adrenaline.

Epineurium Gr. 'on nerve'. Refers to a loose connective tissue sheath investing peripheral nerves (Ch. 9).

Episodic memory Ability to recollect episodes of one's own earlier life (Ch. 33).

Epithalamus Gr. 'above thalamus', includes pineal gland (Ch. 27).

Evoked potentials Surface recorded potentials evoked by motor or sensory stimulation. See *brainstem auditory evoked potential, somatosensory evoked potentials and visual evoked potentials* (Ch. 30).

Excitotoxicity Toxic effects on target neurons, of excessive glutamatergic activity (Chs 8, 33).

Expressive aphasia A nonfluent aphasia caused by damage to the posterior portion of the inferior frontal gyrus in the dominant cerebral hemisphere (e.g. Broca aphasia) (Ch. 32).

Extensor plantar response See *Babinski sign.*

Exteroception L. 'reception from outside'. Refers to stimuli transduced at the body surface, rather than within the body wall or limbs (proprioception) or alimentary tract (enteroception).

Extrapyramidal L. 'nonpyramidal'. Refers to pathways involving the basal ganglia (Ch. 26).

Eye-righting reflex Reflex torsion of the eyeballs to maintain horizontal gaze when the head is tilted to the side (Ch. 19).

F

Facilitation Increasing the likelihood of depolarisation (Ch. 7).

Falx L. 'sickle'. Refers to shape, e.g. falx cerebri, falx cerebelli (Ch. 4).

Familial tremor See *Benign essential tremor* (Ch. 26).

Far response Sympathetic activity causing flattening of the lens for far vision (Ch. 23).

Fascicle L. 'small bundle' of nerve or muscle fibres (Ch. 7).

Fasciculation Visible involuntary twitching of muscle fascicles; when prominent and if associated with weakness, a sign of lower motor neuron disease (Ch. 16).

Fasciculation potentials On the EMG record, MUAPs (motor unit action potentials) that appear infrequently and are not under voluntary control; often associated with lower motor neuron disease (Ch. 12).

Fasciculus L. 'small bundle' of anatomically distinct nerve fibres within the CNS, e.g. fasciculus gracilis, fasciculus cuneatus (Ch. 15).

Fast pain Stabbing pain perceived following activation of Aδ nociceptors (Ch. 34).

Fast receptor See *Ionotropic receptor* (Ch. 8).

Fastigial nucleus L. 'apex of a roof'. Fastigial nucleus is one of the deep cerebellar nuclei and located within the roof of the fourth ventricle (Ch. 27).

Feature extraction Separate simultaneous analysis of individual features of the scene by the visual association cortex (Ch. 31).

Fibrillation Denervation supersensitivity of individual muscle fibres that causes them to spontaneously depolarise and contract (Ch. 16).

Fibrillation potentials Spontaneous muscle fibre depolarisation that is neither clinically visible (detected on EMG) or detectable by the patient and signifies muscle fibre denervation (Ch. 12).

Filopodia Antenna-like growth cone processes anchoring growth cones to cell surface adhesion molecules on Schwann cells (Ch. 9).

Fimbria L. 'fringe'. Refers to the fringe of white fibres along the edge of the hippocampus (Ch. 33).

Finger-to-nose-test It is a test of appendicular coordination as well as cerebellar function, in which the patient is asked to alternately touch their nose and the examiner's finger as quickly as possible (Ch. 27).

Fixation Visual targeting of an object so it is projected onto the fovea; cf. *Foveation* (Ch. 23).

Flatness of affect Dearth of emotional expression (Ch. 32).

Focal seizure Seizure originating in a particular lobe (focus) of the brain (Ch. 29).

Foramen L. 'opening'.

Forceps L. 'pair of tongs', e.g. the forceps minor and forceps major of the corpus callosum (Ch. 2).

Fornix L. 'arch'. Refers to the efferent projection of the hippocampal formation (Chs 2, 33).

Fovea L. 'pit', e.g. fovea centralis of the retina (Ch. 23).

Foveation Visual targeting so that the centre of the scene is aligned with the fovea (Ch. 23).

Functional electrical stimulation Muscle rehabilitation by electrical stimulation at the motor point (Ch. 10).

Functional MRI Functional magnetic resonance imaging (Ch. 28).

Functional sympathectomy Preganglionic sympathetic nerve ablation (chemical or surgical) (Ch. 13).

Funiculus One of the three subdivisions of white matter in the spinal cord (Ch. 3).

Fusimotor Pertaining to motor nerve fibres that innervate intrafusal fibres of the muscle spindle (Ch. 10). See *Gamma motor neuron.*

Fusion pore Pore through which transmitter substance passes from terminal bouton into synaptic cleft (Ch. 8).

G

G protein Cell membrane protein subunits that bind with guanine nucleotides (Ch. 8).

GABA Gamma aminobutyric acid; the main inhibitory neurotransmitter (Ch. 8).

Gag reflex Reflex contraction of the pharyngeal constrictors in response to touching the oropharynx (Ch. 18).

Gait ataxia Staggering unsteady gait associated with posterior column (Ch. 15) and cerebellar disease (Ch. 27).

Gamma (γ) motor neuron Neuron with an A diameter axon supplying the intrafusal muscle fibres of a muscle spindle (Ch. 10).

Ganglion Gr. 'knot'. Refers (a) to spinal and peripheral autonomic ganglia (Chs 9, 13); (b) to the basal ganglia (Ch. 26).

Gasserian ganglion The trigeminal ganglion (Ch. 21).

Gating Controlling ease of passage of impulses from one set of neurons to another, e.g. from primary to secondary sensory neurons (Ch. 24).

Gene transcription The process of copying sequences from DNA to form messenger RNA (Ch. 8).

Generator potential Temporal and/or spatial summation of excitatory stimuli that spread to and result in depolarisation of the initial segment of the axon and the production of an action potential (Ch. 7).

Geniculate L. 'knee-form', meaning bent.

Genu L. 'knee', meaning a bend.

Giant motor unit potential Abnormally large motor unit potential identified on EMG and a sequelae of viable motor neurons reinnervating adjacent denervated muscle fibres; usually seen in motor axonal or motor neuron disease (Ch. 12).

Glia Gr. 'glue'. Refers to the supporting neuroglial cells of the CNS (Ch. 6).

Gliosis The proliferation of glial cells in the central nervous system after an injury to the brain or spinal cord (Ch. 6).

Globose nucleus L. 'ball-like'. With the emboliform forms the interposed deep cerebellar nucleus (Ch. 27).

Globus pallidus A nucleus medial to the putamen and source of efferent fibres from basal ganglia (Ch. 26).

Glomerulus L. 'little ball of yarn', e.g. synaptic glomeruli in the cerebellum (Ch. 27) and olfactory bulb (Ch. 33).

Glossopharyngeal Gr. 'lingual-pharyngeal', with reference to the sensory distribution of the glossopharyngeal nerve (and to its motor supply to stylopharyngeus muscle) (Ch. 18).

Glutamate The most common excitatory neurotransmitter in the CNS (Chs 6, 8).

Glutamate toxicity Extensive loss of neurons caused by excessively high rates of discharge of pyramidal cells in any part of the cerebral cortex (Ch. 33).

Gracilis L. 'slender', e.g. gracile fasciculus in the spinal cord (Ch. 15).

Graded potentials See *Electrotonic potentials.*

Grand mal *Fr.* A form of generalised seizure characterised by tonic-clonic motor activity, involving two phases; the tonic phase in which the body becomes rigid, and clonic phase in which there is uncontrolled jerking (Ch. 29).

Grapheme A written syllable (Ch. 32).

Growth cone The conical tip of a growing axon (Ch. 9).

Guillain–Barré syndrome An acute autoimmune inflammatory peripheral neuropathy, usually related to a viral infection and resulting in demyelination of nerves (Ch. 12).

Gustation/gustatory Pertaining to the sense of taste (Ch. 18).

Gyrus L. A convolution of the cerebral cortex (Ch. 2).

H

H response The Hoffman reflex, a test using the tibial nerve to assess conduction of the S1 reflex arc (Ch. 12).

Head-righting reflex A reflex, engaging the static labyrinth and medial vestibulospinal tract, designed to keep the head upright (Ch. 19).

Heel-to-knee-test A test of cerebellar function (Ch. 27).

Hemi- Gr. 'half'.

Hemianopia Gr. 'half-blindness'. Caused by a lesion of the geniculocalcarine pathway or primary visual cortex and resulting in blindness of half of the visual field (Ch. 31).

Hemiballism Gr. 'half-throwing'. Refers to involuntary, 'throwing' movements of arm and/or leg on one side, usually associated with damage to the subthalamic nucleus (Ch. 26).

Hemineglect Lack of awareness of the contralateral side of the body and/or the contralateral visual space (Ch. 32).

Hemiparesis Gr. 'half-weakness'. Weakness of one side of the body associated with upper motor neuron disease (Chs 16, 35).

Hemiplegia Gr. 'half-struck'. Refers to paralysis of one half of the body following a major stroke (Chs 16, 35).

Hering–Breuer reflex Reflex inhibition of the dorsal respiratory centre by pulmonary stretch receptors (Ch. 18).

Hertz (Hz) Cycles per second.

Heteroreceptor A cellular receptor that influences how the cell manufactures and releases neurotransmitters different from the agent that stimulated the receptor (Chs 8, 13).

Hippocampus Gr. 'sea horse'. A cortical area that is part of the limbic system and located in the temporal lobe (Chs 2, 33).

Histaminergic system Widespread histaminergic innervation of the cerebral cortex by the tuberoinfundibular nucleus of the hypothalamus (Ch. 34).

Homonymous Gr. 'matching'. (a) Matching motor neurons (Ch. 10); (b) matching parts of the binocular visual field (Ch. 31).

Horner syndrome Signs of cervical sympathetic paralysis, the complete syndrome comprising miosis, ptosis, and anhidrosis (Chs 13, 23).

Huntington disease A progressive autosomal dominant disorder characterised by dementia, psychiatric symptoms, and typically a hyperkinetic movement disorder (choreoathetosis) (Ch. 26).

Hydrocephalus Gr. 'water head'. An abnormal accumulation of cerebrospinal fluid within the ventricles of the brain (Ch. 5).

Hyper- Gr. 'excessive'.

Hyperacusis An abnormally acute sense of hearing (Ch. 22).

Hyperalgesia An excessive sensitivity to pain due to stimulation of injured tissue and of surrounding uninjured tissue (Ch. 33).

Hypercapnia Excess plasma P_{CO_2} (Ch. 4).

Hyperhidrosis Gr. 'too much watering'. Excessive sweating (Ch. 13).

Hyperkinetic disorder Disorders associated with involuntary movements (Ch. 26).

Hyperpolarization An increase in the resting potential of a cell membrane of a neuron, that causes the inside of the cell to become more negative. This change raises the threshold level for depolarisation, thus making the cell relatively less sensitive to stimuli (Ch. 7).

Hyperreflexia Exaggerated tendon reflexes; associated with upper motor neuron disease (Ch. 16).

Hypnagogic hallucinations Gr. 'accompanying sleep'. In narcolepsy, sleep onset characterised by striking visual imagery (Ch. 29).

Hypo- Gr. 'below'.

I

Ictal focus Locus of origin of seizures (Ch. 29).

Ictus The clinical manifestations brought about by an abnormal burst firing of neurons in the cerebral cortex in a seizure (Ch. 29).

Ideomotor apraxia A disturbance of voluntary movement in which a person cannot translate an idea into movement. People with ideomotor apraxia can still perform automatic movements, such as using scissors. However, they cannot perform such movements upon request. They also cannot copy movements or make gestures (Ch. 32).

Idiopathic Pathology of unknown origin.

Impotence Inability in a man to achieve an erection or orgasm (Ch. 13).

Incontinence Involuntary voiding of urine or faeces (Chs 13, 24).

Infarction L. 'stuffed into'. With respect to the nervous system, it refers to an ischemic stroke resulting from blockage of a blood vessel supplying the brain (Ch. 35).

Infranuclear lesion Lesion of the nucleus and the trunk of a cranial nerve.

Infundibulum L. 'funnel', leading down to the hypophysis (Ch. 34).

Insertional activity Signifies recorded potentials elicited by initial contact of an EMG needle with muscle fibres (Ch. 12).

Insula L. 'island' of cerebral cortex covered by the opercula (Ch. 2).

Intention tremor Tremor (actually an ataxia) appearing during performance of purposive movements; associated with cerebellar disease (Ch. 27).

Internuncial L. 'messenger between'. Refers to small connecting neurons (Ch. 8).

Intra- L. 'within'.

Intrafusal muscle fibres Muscle fibres within the fusiform, spindle-shaped neuromuscular spindle.

Ionotropic receptor Receptor containing transmitter-gated ion channels (Ch. 8).

Ipsilateral L. 'on same side'.

Irritable bowel syndrome A disorder of the brain—gut axis (Ch. 13).

Iso- Gr. 'equal', e.g. isocortex, uniformly containing six layers of neurons (Ch. 28).

Isofrequency stripes Bands of primary auditory cortex responding to particular tonal frequencies (Ch. 28).

J

Jacksonian seizure A focal partial seizure that affects a small area of the brain and then spreads to a larger area of the brain and can result in the sequential activation of adjacent areas of the motor cortex (Ch. 29).

Jamais vu Fr. 'never seen'. Epileptic aura where a familiar scene appears novel (Ch. 33).

Jargon aphasia Jumbled speech associated with a lesion of Wernicke area (Ch. 32).

Jaw jerk Reflex elevation of the mandible in response to a tap on the chin (Ch. 21).

Joint sense The sense of direction of passive movement of a joint; affected in posterior column disease (Ch. 15).

Joint stiffness 'Active' joint stiffness is the element of resistance to movement introduced by autogenetic inhibition and designed to prevent oscillation (Ch. 10). 'Passive' joint stiffness is a progressive resistance to passive movement caused by intramuscular collagen accumulation following an upper motor neuron lesion (Ch. 16).

Jugular foramen syndrome Constellation of symptoms and signs associated with injury to the glossopharyngeal, vagus, and accessory nerves related to the jugular foramen (Ch. 18).

K

Kindling 'Lighting a fire'. Progressively increasing group response of hippocampal neurons to a repetitive stimulus of uniform strength (Ch. 33).

Kinaesthesia Gr. 'perception of movement' (Ch. 15).

Kinetic or dynamic labyrinth The semicircular canals (Ch. 19).

Klüver—Bucy syndrome Constellation of neural and personality changes following bilateral injury to the anterior temporal lobe and amygdaloid nucleus. It is characterised by loss of recognition of people, loss of fear, rage reactions, hypersexuality, uncontrolled appetite, memory deficits, and overreaction to certain stimuli (Ch. 33).

Korsakoff psychosis Permanent state of anterograde amnesia and confabulation (without the intention to deceive, production of distorted memories) resulting from vitamin B1 (thiamine) deficiency (previously related to excessive alcohol use and associated malnutrition) that results in injury to the mammillary bodies, thalamus, and periaqueductal grey (Ch. 33).

L

Lacunar infarct Brain infarct in the form of a lacuna ('little lake') that results from occlusion of one of the small penetrating arteries of the brain; associated with hypertension (Ch. 35).

Latency Stimulus—response interval (Chs 10, 12).

Lateral medullary syndrome (or Wallenberg syndrome) Characteristic symptoms and signs (dysphagia, hoarseness, dizziness, nausea/vomiting, nystagmus, and gait ataxia) following thrombosis of the vertebral or posterior inferior cerebellar artery and infarction of the lateral portion of the medulla oblongata (Ch. 19).

Lead pipe rigidity Uniform resistance to passive joint movement; characteristic of Parkinson disease (Ch. 26).

Lemniscus Gr. 'ribbon'. Used with reference to several afferent pathways (tracts) in the brainstem (Ch. 17).

Lentiform L. Lens-shaped nucleus, part of the corpus striatum (caudate and lentiform nuclei) (Chs 2 and 26).

Leptomeninges Gr. 'thin membranes' comprising the arachnoid and pia mater (Ch. 5).

Limb apraxia See *Ideomotor apraxia*.

Limbic L. 'marginal'. Refers to limbic structures at the inner margin of the cerebral hemisphere (Ch. 33).

Lissauer's tract The posterolateral tract in the spinal cord (Ch. 15).

Locomotor centre Pedunculopontine nucleus (Ch. 24).

Long-tract signs Clinically used to refer to dysfunction of major sensory and motor pathways, especially with spinal cord lesions (e.g. spasticity, hyperreflexia, bladder dysfunction) (Ch. 35).

Lower motor neuron signs Signs of lower motor neuron disease, e.g. atrophy, weakness, and fasciculations (Ch. 16).

LTD Long-term (prolonged) depression of neuronal responsivity following conditioning stimuli (Chs 8, 27).

LTP Long-term potentiation of neuronal responsivity following conditioning stimuli (Chs 8, 33).

Lumbar puncture Spinal tap. Needle puncture of the lumbar cistern to obtain a sample of cerebrospinal fluid (Ch. 5).

M

Macula L. 'spot', e.g. macula of utricle (Ch. 19), macula lutea (yellow) of retina (Ch. 31).

Major depression Prevalent psychiatric disorder associated with depressed mood (Ch. 34).

Mammillary L. 'nipple-like'. Refers to the mammillary bodies.

Marche à petits pas Fr. 'walk with small steps'. Hesitant, short-stepped gait associated with frontal lobe disease (Ch. 32).

Mechanoreceptor Sensory receptor sensitive to mechanical stimuli, e.g. muscle spindles and tendon organs (Ch. 10), some cutaneous receptors (Ch. 11), carotid sinus receptors (Ch. 24), and inner ear hair cells (Chs 19, 20).

Medulla L. 'marrow'. Refers to the marrow-like appearance of the fresh brain and spinal cord within their bony shells.

Medulla oblongata L. 'oblong'. (Elongate) part of the hindbrain (Ch. 3).

Membrane potential The voltage across a cell membrane (Ch. 7).

Meningismus A condition characterised by pain on neck motion with associated neck stiffness, headache, and often photophobia that most often accompanies meningitis (Ch. 5) and subarachnoid haemorrhage (Ch. 35).

Meningomyelocele A form of spina bifida (neural tube defect) with protrusion of the spinal cord and its meninges through a defect in the vertebral arch (Ch. 14).

Meralgia paresthetica Thigh pain with 'pins-and-needles' sensation. Compression of the lateral cutaneous nerve of the thigh where it pierces the inguinal ligament (Ch. 12).

Mesencephalic locomotor centre A complex pattern generator that facilitates locomotion. The pedunculopontine nucleus of the reticular formation is a significant contributor.(Ch. 24).

Mesencephalon The midbrain (Ch. 1).

Mesocortical fibres Dopaminergic fibres projecting to the prefrontal cortex from the ventral tegmental nuclei of the midbrain (Ch. 33).

Mesoderm Gr. 'middle skin'. Refers to the middle germ layer (Ch. 1).

Mesolimbic fibres Dopaminergic fibres projecting to the limbic system from the ventral tegmental nuclei (Ch. 33).

Metabotropic receptor Membrane receptor capable of generating multiple metabolic effects within the cytoplasm of the neuron (Ch. 8).

Metencephalon Gr. 'after the brain'. Comprises embryonic pons and cerebellum (Ch. 1).

Microglia Gr. Small glial cells. A nonneuronal cell that serves an immune function and similar to a peripheral macrophage (Ch. 6).

Microzone The smallest efferent unit of the cerebellar cortex that arises from mossy fibre afferents exciting groups of granule cells whose parallel fibres then facilitate many hundreds of Purkinje cells, arranged in rows beneath those parallel fibres, and those Purkinje cells fire and inhibit neurons in one of the deep nuclei (Ch. 27).

Miosis Gr. 'constriction' of the pupil (Ch. 23).

Mnemonic Gr. 'memory related'. Having to do with memory (Ch. 33).

Modality See *Sensory modality*.

Modulation Effect of neurotransmitters, notably the catecholamines and serotonin, in altering the response of neurons to classic transmitters (Ch. 6).

Module A cell column in the cerebral cortex (Ch. 28).

Monoamines Catecholamines, serotonin, histamine (Ch. 8).

Monocular blindness Blindness in one eye (Ch. 31).

Monocular crescent The visual fields of the two eyes overlap across two-thirds of the total visual field and outside this binocular field is a monocular (temporal) crescent on each side (Ch. 31).

Monoplegia Paralysis of one limb resulting from upper motor neuron disease (Chs 16, 35).

Monosynaptic reflex A simple reflex that involves transmission of information from a sensory neuron to the appropriate motor neuron across a single synapse in the spinal cord. The knee-jerk reflex is an example of a monosynaptic reflex (Ch. 10).

Montage A particular pattern of electrode connections used in performing an EEG recording (Ch. 29).

Motor endplate A specialised synaptic contact between a motor axon and a skeletal muscle cell (Ch. 10).

Motor evoked potentials Single- or repetitive-pulse stimulation of the brain that causes the spinal cord and peripheral muscles to produce neuroelectrical signals known as motor evoked potentials (MEPs). In clinical practice, MEPs are used as a tool for the diagnosis and evaluation of multiple sclerosis and as a prognostic indicator for stroke motor recovery (Ch. 30).

Motor learning The process of improving motor skills through practice, with long-lasting changes in the capability for responding. The cerebellum and basal nuclei play a major role (Ch. 27).

Motor neuron disease Disease of spinal cord or brainstem motor neurons (Ch. 16).

Motor point Motor points are electrophysiologically defined, as the point with the highest excitability of the muscle or the point on the skin where muscle contraction can be elicited by the least electrical stimulation (Ch. 10).

Motor set Posture adopted prior to movement (Ch. 28).

Motor unit action potentials (MUAPs) Individual waveforms representing activation of muscle fibres of an individual motor unit (Ch. 12).

Motor unit An α motor neuron together with all the muscle fibres it supplies (Ch. 10).

Movement synergy Manner of operation of the primary motor cortex (Ch. 28).

MRI Magnetic resonance imaging (Ch. 2).

MUAPs See *Motor unit action potentials*.

Multimodal association cortex See *Polymodal association cortex*.

Multiple sclerosis A primarily demyelinating disease of an autoimmune nature and associated with multifocal areas of demyelination (and axonal injury); pathologically associated with multiple areas of sclerosis (hardening) caused by glial scarring (Ch. 6).

Multiple system atrophy A neurodegenerative disease that affects autonomic, extrapyramidal, cerebellar, and corticospinal systems, classified with respect to the predominant clinical feature; may initially be misdiagnosed as Parkinson disease (Ch. 26).

Muscarinic receptor Acetylcholinergic receptor historically activated by muscarine (Chs 8, 13).

Myasthenia gravis Gr./L. 'serious muscle weakness'. An autoimmune disease that results in dysfunction of motor end plates and a syndrome of variable motor weakness (Ch. 12).

Myelencephalon Gr. 'marrow brain'. Refers to the embryonic medulla oblongata (Ch. 1).

Myelin Gr. 'marrow'. Refers to the myelin sheath of axons (Ch. 6).

Myelocele A form of spina bifida in which the neural tissues of the spinal cord are exposed; open neural tube (Ch. 14).

Myelogram Image of the spinal subarachnoid space produced by injection of a radiopaque substance into the lumbar cistern (Ch. 5).

Myoneural junction Gr. Motor end plate (Ch. 10).

Myotatic reflex Gr. 'muscle touching'. Tendon reflex (Ch. 10).

N

Narcolepsy Gr. 'sleep seizure'. Is a disorder of excessive daytime sleepiness characterised by a distortion of wakefulness and sleep (especially REM sleep) and attributed to a reduction in hypocretin (orexin) secreting neurons in the hypothalamus (Ch. 29).

Near response Passive thickening of the lens, miosis, and convergence, combined for close-up viewing (Ch. 23).

Needle electrode An EMG recording electrode in the lumen of a fine needle (Ch. 12).

Neglect Neglect of contralateral personal or extrapersonal space, associated with inferior parietal lobe disease (Ch. 32).

Neo- Gr. 'new', e.g. neocerebellum (Ch. 27), neocortex (Ch. 28).

Nervi erigentes L. 'erectile nerves'. Parasympathetic nerve fibres responsible for penile erection (Ch. 13).

Neurite Gr. Process of a neuron, whether axon or dendrite (Ch. 6).

Neuroblast Gr. 'nerve germ'. Refers to embryonic neuron (Ch. 1).

Neuroeffector junctions Autonomic nerve endings within target tissues (Ch. 13).

Neurofibril L. Refers to matted neurofilaments seen by light microscopy (Ch. 6).

Neurofibrillary tangles Abnormal accumulations of neurofibrils, most numerous in Alzheimer disease (Ch. 33).

Neurofilament L. The fine filaments seen in neurons by electron microscopy (Ch. 6).

Neurogenic inflammation Inflammation caused by liberation of substance P (in particular) following antidromic depolarisation of fine peripheral nerve fibres (Chs 11, 33).

Neurohumoral reflex Reflex with neural afferent limb and hormonal efferent limb, e.g. the milk ejection reflex (Ch. 34).

Neurolemma Gr. 'nerve sheath'. Comprising chains of Schwann cells that surround axons (Ch. 9).

Neuron Gr. 'nerve'. Refers to the complete nerve cell (Ch. 6).

Neuropathic pain Chronic stabbing or burning pain resulting from injury to peripheral nerves (Ch. 33).

Neuropathy Dysfunction or injury within the peripheral nervous system and presenting as either a generalised dysfunction of nerves (polyneuropathy and clinically may be modality specific) or of one or more peripheral nerves (Ch. 12).

Neurotoxicity Refers to damage inflicted on target neurons by excess glutamate (Ch. 28).

Neurotransmitter A chemical liberated at a nerve terminal that activates postsynaptic and/or presynaptic receptors (Chs 6, 8).

Nicotinic receptor Acetylcholinergic receptor historically activated by nicotine (Chs 8, 13).

Nigrostriatal pathway Dopaminergic projection from substantia nigra to the striatum; especially relevant to Parkinson disease (Ch. 26).

Nociceptive L. 'taking injury'. Responsive to noxious stimulation (Ch. 11).

Nociceptors A somatic or visceral free nerve ending of thinly myelinated and unmyelinated fibres whose activation generates a sense of pain (Ch. 33).

Nonconscious proprioception Sensory signals arising within the body that are not perceived, e.g. spinocerebellar tracts (Ch. 15).

Noradrenergic Neurons using norepinephrine (noradrenaline) as transmitter, e.g. postganglionic sympathetic (Ch. 13), cerulean nucleus (Ch. 17).

Norepinephrine Also called noradrenaline. Hormone released by the adrenal medulla (Ch. 13); also, a brainstem neurotransmitter (Ch. 17).

NREM sleep Nonrapid eye movement sleep (Stages 1–3); also called *slow-wave sleep* (Ch. 29).

Nuclear lesion Lesion of a motor nucleus in the brainstem.

Nucleus L. 'nut'. Refers either to the trophic centre of a cell, or to a group of neurons within the CNS (Chs 6 and 17).

Nystagmus Gr. 'nodding'. Rapid, rhythmic, repetitious, and involuntary eye movements (Ch. 19).

O

Occupational deafness Occupational deafness is a type of sensorineural hearing loss caused by prolonged exposure to high level of noise at the workplace (Ch. 20).

Ocular dominance columns Cell columns in the primary visual cortex activated by geniculostriate neurons (Ch. 28).

Oculomotor hypokinesia Inadequate saccades often associated with Parkinson disease (Ch. 26).

Oculomotor L. 'eye-moving'. Refers to the oculomotor nerve (Ch. 23).

Olfactory aura Epileptic aura accompanied by illusion of an odour (Ch. 33).

Oligodendrocyte Gr. 'few tree cell'. A myelin-forming nonneuronal (neuroglial cell) with few processes within the CNS (Ch. 6).

Operculum L. 'cover'. Adjacent cerebral cortex overlying the lateral sulcus and covering the insula (Ch. 2).

Ophthalmoplegia Gr. 'eye stroke'. Signifies paralysis of extrinsic ocular muscles (Ch. 23).

Organ of Corti The spiral organ of hearing (Ch. 20).

Orthodromic Impulse conduction in a centrifugal direction.

Orthograde transneuronal degeneration Neuronal degeneration in a proximodistal direction (Ch. 9).

Orthograde (also called anterograde) transport Proximodistal axoplasmic transport (Ch. 6).

Orthography Processing of letter shapes by the visual cortex (Ch. 32).

Oscillation Spontaneous burst-firing of large groups of thalamic reticular neurons; thought to be responsible for occurrence of sleep spindles (Ch. 25).

Osteophytes Bony projections that often form where bones meet each other and often where vertebral bones meet to form a joint (Ch. 14).

Otitis media An inflammatory middle ear disease (Ch. 20).

Otosclerosis Ear disease associated with ankylosis of the footplate of stapes (Ch. 20).

Ototoxic Term referring to drugs causing sensorineural deafness (Ch. 20).

P

Pachymeninx Gr. 'thick membrane'. The dura mater (Ch. 5).

Paleo- Gr. 'old', e.g. paleocerebellum (mainly the anterior lobe, Ch. 27), paleocortex (olfactory, Ch. 33), paleostriatum (globus pallidus, Ch. 26).

Pallidotomy Surgical lesion of globus pallidus, a treatment for Parkinson disease (Ch. 26).

Pallidum L. 'pale'. Refers to globus pallidus (Chs 2, 26).

Pallium Gr. 'cloak'. The cerebral cortex.

Papez circuit A circuit of the limbic system involved in consolidation of memories that begins with the hippocampus, then mammillary body, anterior nucleus of the thalamus, cingulate cortex, and then back to the hippocampus; first described by James Papez in 1937 (Ch. 33).

Papilledema Swelling of the optic papilla, usually in association with raised intracranial pressure (Ch. 5).

Para- Gr. 'beside'.

Paradoxical sleep Dreamy light sleep accompanied by EEG voltage patterns resembling those of the awake state (Chs 24, 29). See *REM sleep*.

Paralysis agitans An archaic term. See *Parkinson disease*.

Paralysis Gr. 'disablement'. Loss of voluntary movement.

Paraplegia Gr. 'paralysis'. Refers to paralysis of both lower limbs (Ch. 16).

Paresis Gr. 'weakness'. Incomplete paralysis.

Paraesthesia Gr. 'side feeling'. A sense of numbness or tingling.

Parkinson disease Degenerative CNS disorder, particularly of the dopamine secreting neurons of the substantia pars compacta, that results in a syndrome of rest tremor, rigidity, postural instability, and bradykinesia as its characteristic features (Ch. 26).

Partial seizure See *Focal seizure*.

Passive stiffness Resistance of ankle dorsiflexors to slow passive plantar flexion in patients with long-standing hemiparesis; probably caused by collagen accumulation within these muscles (Ch. 16).

Pattern generators Patterned activities involving cranial or spinal nerves (Chs 16, 24).

Peduncle L. 'little foot'. Refers to stem, e.g. cerebral peduncle (Ch. 2).

Peri- Gr. 'around'.

Peroneal nerve entrapment Compression of the common peroneal nerve usually at the neck of the fibula (Ch. 12).

PET Positron emission tomography (Ch. 28).

PGO pathway Pathway from pontine reticular formation via lateral geniculate body to occipital cortex, responsible for rapid eye movements during light sleep (Ch. 29).

Phase cancellation A recording event (not a physiologic one) that is most evident during compound sensory nerve action potential measurements, where positive and negative phases of adjacent waveforms tend to 'cancel' each other out (Ch. 12).

Phasic motor neurons Motor neurons innervating groups of fast, glycolytic muscle fibres (Ch. 10).

Phoneme A syllable of sound corresponding to a grapheme (Ch. 32).

Phonemic paraphasia In Wernicke aphasia, the use of incorrect but similar-sounding words (Ch. 32).

Phonology The sounds of words (Ch. 32).

Physiological temporal dispersion See *Phase cancellation* (Ch. 12).

Pia mater Gr. 'soft cover'. The innermost layer of the meninges (Ch. 5).

Pineal L. 'pine cone'. The pineal gland is part of the epithalamus (Ch. 25).

Plasticity Ability of the nervous system to change its activity in response to intrinsic or extrinsic stimuli by reorganising its structure, functions, or connections (Ch. 28).

Plexopathy Neuropathy within one or more of the limb plexuses (Ch. 12).

Plexus L. 'interwoven'. Interwoven nerves or blood vessels.

Polymodal afferent Afferent neuron receptive to more than one sensory modality, e.g. touch and pain (Ch. 11).

Polymodal association cortex Association cortex processing signals in more than one sensory modality (Ch. 28).

Polymodal nociceptors Peripheral nociceptors (notably in skin) responsive to noxious thermal, mechanical, or chemical stimulation (Ch. 33).

Polyphasic MUAPs Compound motor unit action potentials having an abnormally large number of positive and negative phases, signifying *reinnervation* of motor end plates vacated by earlier degeneration of their nerve supply, followed by takeover by neighbouring healthy axons (Ch. 12).

Pons L. 'bridge'. Part of brainstem in the interval between midbrain and medulla oblongata (Ch. 2).

Position sense Perception of the position of body parts (Ch. 15).

Positron emission tomography (PET) Imaging technique identifying radioactive atoms that emit positrons (Ch. 28).

Posterior circulation The vertebrobasilar arterial system including the posterior cerebral arteries (Chs 4, 35).

Posterior columns The gracile and cuneate fasciculi (Ch. 3).

Postherpetic neuralgia Neuropathic pain sequel to *herpes zoster* inflammation (Ch. 33).

Postjunctional receptors Receptors in the plasma membranes of autonomic target tissues (Ch. 13).

Postsynaptic inhibition Inhibition of a target neuron (Ch. 6).

Posttraumatic stress disorder (PTSD) A disorder that can occur following a trauma (either observed by or involving the individual) where the individual subsequently relives the trauma through their thoughts, avoids possible situations that may remind them of the trauma, or demonstrates intense inappropriate emotions (Ch. 33).

Postural fixation Fixation of axial musculature prior to voluntary movement of a limb (Ch. 27).

Postural hypotension Fall of arterial blood pressure on assuming the upright posture (Ch. 16).

Posture Attitude or position of the body. The spontaneous body adjustments, requiring vestibular and proprioceptive integration, that maintain the centre of gravity, keep the head and body in alignment, and stabilise body parts, such as the shoulder girdle when the hand reaches for a distant object (Ch. 16).

Prejunctional receptors Receptors in the plasma membrane of postganglionic nerve terminals (Ch. 13).

Pressure coning Displacement of the cerebellar tonsils into the foramen magnum with compression of the medulla oblongata (Ch. 6).

Presynaptic inhibition Mechanisms that suppress release of neurotransmitters from axon terminals. It involves binding of chemical messengers to inhibitory receptors at transmitter release sites on the axon (Ch. 6).

Priapism Persistent involuntary erection of the penis (Ch. 13).

Primary or inherited myopathy Degenerative disorder of a hereditary origin, but possibly unclear pathogenesis, originating in muscle fibres, e.g. muscular dystrophies (Ch. 12).

Primary or inherited neuropathy Degenerative disorder of a hereditary origin, but possibly unclear pathogenesis, originating in peripheral nerve fibres of their soma, e.g. hereditary motor and sensory neuropathies. One specific example is Charcot-Marie-Tooth disease; cf. *Secondary neuropathy* (Ch. 12).

Primary tonic-clonic seizure A generalised seizure type (Ch. 29).

Procedural memory Is a part of the long-term memory that is responsible for knowing how to do things, also known as motor skills (Ch. 33).

Progressive bulbar palsy A form of motor neuron disease characterised by weakness of the laryngeal, pharyngeal, tongue, and facial muscles. The patient experiences progressive dysarthria and dysphagia (Ch. 16).

Projection L. 'forward throw'. Target of a neuronal pathway, e.g. spinothalamic tract projecting to the thalamus (Ch. 15).

Prolapsed intervertebral disk Herniation of the nucleus pulposus into the intervertebral foramen with consequent pressure on spinal nerve roots (Ch. 14).

Proprioception Gr. 'self-perception'. Conscious or unconscious sense by the brain of self-movement and body position, by information from muscles, tendons, and joints (Ch. 15).

Propriospinal tract Fibres of internuncial neurons passing from one segment of the spinal cord to another (Ch. 15).

Prosencephalon The embryonic forebrain (Ch. 1).

Prosody Tonal variations during speech having emotional attributes (Ch. 32).

Prosopagnosia Gr. 'face-no-knowledge'. Inability to recognise faces (Ch. 28).

Pseudobulbar palsy Term given to the clinical picture arising from compromise of the corticonuclear supply to motor cranial nuclei in pons and medulla oblongata, lacking lower motor neuron signs and presenting with dysphagia, dysphonia, and often involuntary emotional lability (Ch. 18).

Psychosis Mental disorder involving a distorted sense of reality, e.g. schizophrenia (Ch. 32).

Ptosis Gr. 'falling'. Drooping of the upper eyelid (Ch. 23).

Pulvinar L. 'cushion'. Refers to posterior bulge of thalamus above the midbrain (Ch. 3).

Pure motor syndrome A lacunar stroke syndrome (most frequent) due to occlusion of one of the small perforating arteries, usually involving the posterior limb of the internal capsule and manifested as hemiparesis not associated with sensory deficits or disturbances of higher cortical function (e.g. aphasia, neglect) (Ch. 35).

Pure sensory syndrome A lacunar stroke syndrome (most frequent) due to occlusion of one of the small perforating arteries, usually involving the thalamus and manifested as hemisensory loss (face, arm, and leg) that is not associated with motor deficits or disturbances of higher cortical function (e.g. aphasia, neglect) (Ch. 35).

Putamen L. 'shell'. Refers to outer part of lentiform nucleus (Ch. 2).

Q

Quadrantic hemianopia Blindness in one quadrant of the visual field (Ch. 31).

Quadriplegia Gr./L. 'four-stroke'. Paralysis of all four limbs (Ch. 16).

R

Radiculopathy L. *Radix*, 'root'. Nerve root pathology (Ch. 12).

Rage attack Associated with a sense of intense violence or anger that may be in response to an external cue, usually in individuals with depression or anxiety, but of uncertain pathophysiology; once attributed to hyperactivity of the amygdala (Ch. 33).

Raphe Gr. 'seam'. Refers to the midline. Greek genitive case is used in nucleus raphe magnus (Ch. 17).

Raynaud phenomenon Intermittent attacks of pallor or cyanosis of the small arteries and arterioles of the fingers as the result of inadequate arterial blood flow; often seen in cold weather and under emotional stress (Ch. 13).

Receptor A term with two distinct meanings: (a) sensory receptors (e.g. photoreceptors, neuromuscular spindles) transduce sensory stimuli;

(b) molecular receptors on or within cells that are protein molecules acted on by messenger molecules, e.g. hormones, neurotransmitters.

Receptor blocker A drug that can occupy a membrane receptor without activating it (Ch. 13).

Receptor potential The membrane potential at a peripheral sensory nerve ending where action potentials are generated (Ch. 7).

Referential recording A particular pattern of electrode connections where electrode pairs have one recording site in common (e.g. auricle or mastoid area) and used in recording an EEG (Ch. 29). Cf. *Bipolar recording.*

Referred pain Perception of pain at a site distant from the locus of nociceptive activity (Ch. 13).

Reflex reversal Term used to signify the 'change of sign' accompanying a switch from reflex resistance to reflex assistance (Ch. 16).

Reflexive impotence Impotence caused by damage to reflex arcs (Ch. 13).

Relative refractory period Time interval after firing one action potential, during which a greater-than-normal negative current is required to generate another (Ch. 7).

REM sleep Rapid eye movement sleep (Chs 24, 29).

Renshaw cells Neurons in the medial part of the anterior horn exerting tonic inhibition on alpha motor neurons (Ch. 16).

Resistance reflex Resistance to passive movement, notably at the knee joint, produced by passive stretching of neuromuscular spindles (Ch. 16). Cf. *Assistance reflex.*

Resting tremor Tremor at rest that is characteristic of Parkinson disease (Ch. 26).

Reticular L. 'net-like', e.g. reticular formation (Ch. 24).

Retrieval Calling up items from memory stores (Chs 32, 33).

Retrograde amnesia Amnesia for past events (Ch. 33).

Retrograde transport Transport of materials from axon terminals to soma (Ch. 6).

Rhinencephalon Gr. 'nose brain'. Parts of the cerebral hemisphere directly related to the sense of smell; forms the paleocortex (Ch. 28).

Rhombencephalon Gr. 'rhomboid-brain' containing the rhomboid fourth ventricle. Embryologically, the hindbrain vesicle (Ch. 1).

Rolandic epilepsy See *Benign rolandic epilepsy.*

Rostral limbic system The anterior cingulate cortex and related areas (Ch. 33).

Rostrum L. 'beak'. Rostrum of corpus callosum extends from genu to lamina terminalis (Ch. 2).

Rubro- L. 'red'. Refers to projections from red nucleus.

S

Saccade A volitional conjugate rapid movement of the eyes that results in an image being placed on the fovea (Ch. 23).

Saltatory conduction Gr. 'jumping'. Impulse transmission that skips from node to node, providing rapid transmission of impulse along myelinated nerve fibres (Ch. 9).

Satellite L. 'attendant', e.g. the satellite cells in spinal ganglia.

Schizophrenia Gr. 'split mind'. Characterised by gross distortion of reality, disturbances of language and cognitive function, withdrawal from social interaction, disorganisation and fragmentation of thought, altered perception, and emotional reaction (Ch. 32).

Scotoma A blind spot in the visual field (Ch. 31).

Second messenger After activation of its receptor, the first messenger (e.g. G-protein-coupled membrane receptor) generates an intracellular second messenger (eg. cyclic AMP) that initiates biochemical events in the cytoplasm and/or nucleus (Ch. 8).

Secondary tonic-clonic convulsion A tonic-clonic seizure whose origin was initially focal, but secondarily generalised (Ch. 33).

Segmental antinociception Relief of pain at segmental level, e.g. by 'rubbing the sore spot' (Ch. 24).

Seizure Uncontrolled electrical activity in the brain, which can produce major or minor physical signs, thought disturbances, or a combination of symptoms (Ch. 29).

Semantic Having to do with meaning of words or other symbols (Ch. 32).

Semantic retrieval Retrieving the meaning of a word from memory stores (Ch. 32).

Sensitisation Lowering the threshold of peripheral nociceptors (by histamine in particular) following peripheral release of peptides via the axon reflex (Ch. 33).

Sensorineural deafness Deafness caused by disease of the cochlea or of the cochlear nerve (Ch. 20).

Sensory competition The capacity of a neuron to process simultaneously multiple stimuli is limited so various mechanisms (e.g. attention) exist to suppress those not immediately relevant to the current situation or task at hand; may be an explanation for cortical sensory plasticity (Ch. 28).

Sensory modality A distinct mode of sensation, e.g. touch versus pain (Ch. 11).

Sensory unit A cutaneous nerve fibre together with all of its sensory terminals (Ch. 11).

Septal rage An archaic term used to apply to a rage attack thought to originate in the septal nuclei (Ch. 33).

Septum pellucidum L. A 'transparent partition' separating the frontal horns of the lateral ventricles (Ch. 2).

Sign An objective indicator of a disorder, e.g. Babinski sign (Ch. 16).

Sleep paralysis A state of awareness that is accompanied by complete paralysis (except breathing and eye movements) at the beginning and/or end of sleep and more frequent in narcolepsy.

Slow pain Aching pain perceived following activation of C-fibre nociceptors (Ch. 33).

Slow receptor See *Metabotropic receptor.*

Slow-wave sleep Stages 1, 2, and 3 of sleep, characterised by slow, delta waves (Ch. 29).

Sodium pump Membrane ion channel capable of simultaneously extruding Na^+ ions while importing K^+ ions (Ch. 7).

Sole plate An accumulation of nuclei, mitochondria, and ribosomes in the sarcoplasm at the myoneural junction (Ch. 10).

Soma Gr. The cell body of a neuron (Ch. 6).

Somatic Gr. 'body-related'. Implies body wall as distinct from viscera.

Somatosensory evoked potentials Electrical potentials recorded from surface landmarks over the spine and surface of the skull, evoked by stimulation of a peripheral nerve (electrical stimulation) and generated by action potentials as they traverse the somatosensory pathway to the somatic sensory cortex (Ch. 30).

Somatotopic Containing a body map.

Somesthetic Somatic sensory, e.g. somesthetic cortex (Ch. 28).

Sound attenuation Dampening of sound by contraction of stapedius or tensor tympani (Ch. 20).

Sound field The peripheral field of sound perception by one ear (Ch. 20).

Spastic State of increased muscle tone induced by an upper motor neuron lesion (Ch. 16).

Spastic diplegia A form of cerebral palsy involving corticospinal fibres destined for lower-limb motor neurons (Ch. 26).

Spatial sense Perception of the position of objects in relation to one another (Ch. 28).

Speech meta-analysis Post hoc analysis of one's own speech (Ch. 32).

Sphincter–detrusor dyssynergia Failure of the urethral sphincter to relax at the onset of micturition; a feature of spinal cord injury (Ch. 16).

Spike Action potential (Ch. 7).

Spina bifida Varying degrees of failure of the embryonic neural arches to unite in the posterior midline (Ch. 14).

Spinal anaesthesia Anaesthesia induced by injection of local anaesthetic into the lumbar cistern (Ch. 5).

Spinal tap Lumbar puncture. Needle puncture of the lumbar cistern to obtain a sample of cerebrospinal fluid (Ch. 5).

Splanchnic Gr. 'visceral'.

Splenium L. 'pad'. Refers to posterior end of corpus callosum (Ch. 2).

Startle response Generalised muscle twitch in response to sudden loud noise (Ch. 20).

Static labyrinth The utricle and saccule (Ch. 19).

Static posturography Study of postural responses on an unstable platform (Ch. 27). Cf. *Dynamic posturography.*

Stellate ganglion The fused inferior cervical and first thoracic sympathetic ganglia whose postganglionic fibres supply the head, neck, and upper limbs, and also the heart (Ch. 13).

Stereoanaesthesia Inability to identify an unseen object held in the hand, as a consequence of cortical-type sensory loss (Ch. 28).

Stereopsis Three-dimensional vision (Ch. 28).

Stimulus-induced analgesia Analgesia induced by electrical stimulation of the periaqueductal grey matter (Ch. 24).

Strabismus Gr. A condition where the eyes are not aligned with one another (colloquially referred to as 'crossed eyes' or 'squinting') (Ch. 23).

Stress incontinence Incontinence brought about by weakness of the pelvic floor (Ch. 13).

Stria terminalis Originating in the amygdala and projecting to the septal area and hypothalamus (Ch. 33).

Striatum L. 'furrowed'. Refers to caudate nucleus and putamen taken together (Ch. 2).

Stroke A persistent neurological deficit the result of inadequate blood flow to a region of the brain (Ch. 35).

Subfalcine herniation Abnormal displacement of brain tissue beneath the falx cerebri (Ch. 6).

Subiculum L. 'little layer'. Refers to transitional zone between six-layered parahippocampal gyrus and three-layered hippocampus (Ch. 33).

Substantia L. 'substance', e.g. substantia gelatinosa of the spinal grey matter (Ch. 15), and substantia nigra of the midbrain (Ch. 17).

Sulcus L. 'groove'.

Supervisory attentional system Attention centre within the dorsolateral prefrontal cortex (Ch. 32).

Supraspinal antinociception Pain suppression by pathways descending to the posterior horn grey matter from the brainstem (Ch. 24).

Symptom Clues about a disorder derived from the patient's account.

Synapse Gr. 'contact'. Refers to sites of contact between neurons (Ch. 6).

Syndrome Gr. 'running together'. A characteristic group of symptoms and signs.

Syringomyelia Gr. 'marrow tube'. Refers to central cavitation of the spinal cord (Ch. 15).

T

T channels Voltage-gated calcium channels causing transient (momentary) bursts of thalamic reticular neuronal activity during slow-wave sleep (Chs 25, 29).

Tactile agnosia Inability to identify common objects by touch alone (Ch. 32).

Tactile meniscus A specialised nerve ending for tactile sensation that is in contact with the base of a Merkel cell.

Tandem gait A test of gait stability when an individual is asked to perform a toe-the-line test and typically used as a test for ataxia (Ch. 15).

Tapetum L. 'carpet'. Fibres from the splenium arch over the atrium of the lateral ventricle and into the temporal lobe (Ch. 2).

Tarsal tunnel syndrome Compression of the tibial nerve within the tarsal tunnel (Ch. 12).

Tectum L. 'roof' of midbrain, comprising the four colliculi.

Tegmentum L. 'covering'. A general term for the area anterior (ventral) to the ventricular system of the midbrain, pons, and medulla (Ch. 17).

Tela choroidea L. 'membranous web', consisting of vascular pia-ependyma, which gives rise to the choroid plexus (Ch. 2).

Telencephalon Gr. 'endbrain', comprising the embryonic cerebral hemispheres (Ch. 1).

Teloglia Gr. 'distant'. Specialised Schwann cells at the end of a motor nerve fibre near the neuromuscular junction. Helps with synaptic transmission and nerve regeneration (Ch. 11).

Temporal lobe epilepsy See *Complex (partial) seizure* (Ch. 32). Now referred to as focal onset epilepsy with impaired awareness.

TENS Transcutaneous electrical nerve stimulation (Ch. 24).

Tentorium cerebelli An extension of dura mater that separates the cerebellum from the inferior portion of the occipital lobe

Tetanus Gr. 'taut'. Spasmodic state of musculature, especially those of the face and lower jaw following infection with *Clostridium tetani* (Ch. 6).

Tetraplegia Gr. 'four-paralysis'. Synonymous with quadriplegia.

Thalamic pain syndrome Syndrome including contralateral sensory loss but associated with intractable pain, following occlusion of the thalamogeniculate artery (Ch. 35).

Thalamus Gr./L. 'meeting place'. The largest component of the diencephalon and composed of multiple separate nuclei and through its diverse connections facilitates sensorimotor integration (Ch. 25).

Thermosensitive neurons Peripheral sensory neurons having sensory receptors activated by heat (Ch. 11).

Theta rhythm Slow-wave temporal lobe rhythm associated with the septohippocampal cholinergic pathway (Ch. 33).

Threshold The membrane voltage level at which action potentials are generated.

Thrombus L. 'clot'. A blood clot within the circulatory system (Ch. 35).

TIA See *Transient ischemic attack.*

Tinnitus A ringing, booming, or buzzing sound heard in one or both ears (Ch. 20).

Todd paralysis A brief episode of weakness or paralysis that usually affects one side of the body (could also be manifested as impairment of speech or vision) following a seizure and resolving completely in less than 48 hours, but of unclear pathophysiology.

Tonic motor neuron Motor neuron innervating a squad of slow, oxidative–glycolytic muscle fibres (Ch. 10).

Tourette syndrome A neurological disorder with onset typically in childhood and affecting males more often than females that is characterised by repetitive, stereotyped, involuntary movements and vocalisations called tics (Ch. 33).

Tracking Slow conjugate eye movements that serve to maintain an image on the fovea and elicited by fixation on a slowly moving object or through the vestibular system; under normal conditions it is not possible to move the eyes smoothly, unless tracking an object, and such attempts usually consist of short saccadic eye movements (Ch. 23).

Tract L. *Tractus*, 'district'. A group of CNS axons having the same origin and destination.

Transcranial electrical stimulation Recording central motor conduction time by means of transcranial magnetic stimulation of the motor cortex (Ch. 30).

Transduction L. 'leading across'. Refers to conversion of sensory stimuli into trains of nerve impulses.

Transient ischemic attack (TIA) Brief (usually minutes) episode of neurologic dysfunction from a focal and temporary episode of cerebral ischemia that is not associated with cerebral infarction (Ch. 35).

Transneuronal atrophy Atrophic neuronal degeneration passing from one neuron to another, in either an orthograde or a retrograde manner (Ch. 9).

Trapezoid L. 'diamond-shaped'. Collection of second-order auditory fibres in the pons (Ch. 20).

Tremor Involuntary trembling of one or more body parts; may accompany cerebellar (Ch. 27) or basal ganglia disease (Ch. 26).

Trigeminal L. 'triplet'. Refers to the ophthalmic, maxillary, and mandibular divisions of the trigeminal nerve (Ch. 21).

Trigger point (or Trigger zone) A point or zone in the initial segment of the axonal membrane where the generator potential arises (Ch. 7).

Triple response The line—flare—wheal response to a sharp stroke to the skin, involving an axon reflex (Ch. 11).

Trochlear L. 'pulley'. Transferred epithet: tendon of superior oblique muscle passes through a fascial pulley, and the name is applied to the nerve of supply (trochlear) (Ch. 23).

Trophic Gr. 'nourishing' (Ch. 9).

Tropic Gr. 'turning'. Chemotropic substances attract ('turn') axonal growth cones (Ch. 9).

Truncal ataxia Inability to maintain the upright position; a feature of midline cerebellar disease (Ch. 27).

Two-point discrimination A test used to assess discriminative touch (Ch. 15).

U

Ulnar nerve entrapment Compression of the ulnar nerve usually at the elbow (Ch. 12).

Uncal herniation Abnormal displacement of the uncus through the tentorial notch (Ch. 6).

Unconscious proprioception See *Nonconscious proprioception.*

Uncus L. 'hook'. A medial protrusion of the anterior temporal lobe from the underlying amygdala (Chs 2, 33).

Unimodal sensory cortex Primary somatic sensory, visual, or auditory cortex (Ch. 28).

Unstable bladder See *Detrusor instability.*

Upper motor neuron Corticonuclear—corticospinal neuron.

Upper motor neuron signs Physical signs indicating presence of upper motor neuron disorder, e.g. spasticity, Babinski sign (Ch. 16).

Up-regulation Increase in the number of membrane receptors (Chs 26, 33).

Urinary retention Inability to void urine (Ch. 13).

Uvula L. 'little grape'. A lobule of the cerebellar vermis (Ch. 27).

V

Vagus L. 'wandering', with reference to the tenth cranial nerve (Ch. 18).

Vallecula L. 'little valley' between the cerebellar hemispheres (Ch. 27).

Ventricle L. 'little belly'.

Verbal paraphasia In Wernicke aphasia, the use of words of allied meaning (Ch. 32).

Vergence Convergence of gaze for close-up viewing (Ch. 23).

Vermis L. 'worm'. The median part of the cerebellum that is positioned between either cerebellar hemisphere (Ch. 27).

Vestibular nystagmus Nystagmus resulting from a vestibular disorder (Ch. 19).

Vestibuloocular reflexes Reflexes that maintain the gaze on a selected target despite movements of the head (Ch. 19).

Vibration sense A test of posterior column function, using a tuning fork placed on a bone, e.g. shaft of tibia (Ch. 15).

Visceral referred pain Visceral pain referred to somatic structures innervated from the same segmental levels of the spinal cord (Ch. 13).

Viscerosomatic pain Pain caused by spread of disease from visceral to somatic structures (Ch. 13).

Visual evoked potentials Electrical potentials recorded from the surface of the skull, evoked by stimulation of the retina (flash of light or watching an alternating checkerboard pattern) and generated by action potentials as they traverse the visual pathway to the visual cortex (Ch. 30).

Volume transmission Nonsynaptic release of neuropeptides into the extracellular space (Ch. 6).

W

Wallerian degeneration Orthograde degeneration of a peripheral nerve distal to the point of injury (Ch. 9).

Warm caloric test A test of kinetic labyrinthine function (Ch. 19).

Wernicke area Area of the temporal lobe where damage results in an aphasia that is characterised as fluent speech, but with impaired comprehension (Ch. 32).

Wind-up phenomenon Sustained state of excitation of central pain-projecting neurons induced by glutamate activation of NMDA receptors (Ch. 33).

Withdrawal reflex Reflex retraction of a limb in response to a noxious stimulus; includes the flexor reflex (Ch. 14).

Working memory Holding relevant memories briefly in mind while performing a task (Ch. 33).

Note: Page numbers followed by *b* indicate boxes, *f* indicate figures, and *t* indicate tables.